Pediatric nursing

Pediatric nursing

HELEN C. LATHAM, R.N., M.L., M.S.

Formerly Associate Professor of Nursing,
Valdosta State College,
Valdosta, Georgia

ROBERT V. HECKEL, B.S., M.S., Ph.D.

Director, Social Problems Research Institute, and
Professor of Psychology,
University of South Carolina,
Columbia, South Carolina

LARRY J. HEBERT, B.S., M.D., F.A.A.P.

Associate Professor of Pediatrics, Louisiana State
University School of Medicine, New Orleans, Louisiana;
Chief of Pediatrics, Louisiana State University
School of Medicine Pediatric Department, Earl K.
Long Memorial Hospital;
Medical Director, Louisiana Child Protection Programs,
Baton Rouge, Louisiana

ELIZABETH BENNETT, R.N., Ed.D.

Associate Professor of Maternal and Child Health,
Tulane University, School of Public Health,
New Orleans, Louisiana

THIRD EDITION

with 253 illustrations and 2 color plates

The C. V. Mosby Company

Saint Louis   1977

THIRD EDITION

Copyright © 1977 by The C. V. Mosby Company

All rights reserved. No part of this book may be reproduced
in any manner without written permission of the publisher.

Previous editions copyrighted 1967, 1972

Printed in the United States of America

Distributed in Great Britain by Henry Kimpton, London

The C. V. Mosby Company
11830 Westline Industrial Drive, St. Louis, Missouri 63141

Library of Congress Cataloging in Publication Data

Main entry under title:

Pediatric nursing.

    First-2d ed. by H. C. Latham and R. V. Heckel.
    Includes bibliographies and index.
    1. Pediatric nursing. I. Latham, Helen C.
Pediatric nursing. [DNLM: 1. Pediatric nursing.
WY159 P373]
RJ245.L3 1977   610.73′62   76-57734
ISBN 0-8016-2877-6

GW/CB/B 9 8 7 6 5 4 3 2 1

CONTRIBUTORS

KAREN K. HARRISON, M.S.

Psychology Department,
Louisiana State University,
Baton Rouge, Louisiana

MARGARET IVES, B.A., M.A., Ph.D.

Formerly Director of Psychological Services,
St. Elizabeth's Hospital,
Washington, D.C.

JOYCE VERMEERSCH, Dr.P.H.

Assistant Professor,
Department of Nutrition,
University of California,
Davis, California

To
ALL CHILDREN
everywhere

PREFACE

Many changes have been made in this third edition: new chapters have been added and other material has been revised and expanded.

Dr. Vermeersch contributed a new chapter, Nutrition During Pregnancy and Lactation. Dr. Bennett has rewritten Chapter 2, Toward Good Health of the Neonate, and Chapter 4, Physical Assessment and Care of the Neonate. She also assisted in the revision of Chapter 1, Home Environment. Dr. Ives has enlarged the chapter on adolescence by adding pertinent new material. Also, there are a number of changes in the chapter on psychological assessment of children.

To emphasize the role of the nurse in promotion of health, the various sections on this subject relative to the infant, the toddler and preschool child, the schoolchild, and the adolescent have been brought together in one chapter. To this chapter are added suggested guides on assessment of the child's health as well as a discussion of differences in growth and health problems at various stages of development.

Although the emphasis in Part II is still on the care of the child with common conditions, Dr. Hebert has added a discussion of several others, including hemophilia, Hodgkin's disease, infectious mononucleosis, hyperthyroidism, omphalocele, and congestive heart failure. Dr. Hebert has greatly expanded the section on the abused child and revised the material on congenital heart disease.

I wish to express my thanks for the cooperation and patience of the co-authors and contributors: Dr. Heckel, Dr. Hebert, Dr. Bennett, Dr. Vermeersch, and Mrs. Harrison. For her many suggestions and contributions, special thanks go to Dr. Margaret Ives. Appreciation goes also to Dr. Mary D. Rastatter, Chief of the Speech Pathology and Audiology Branch, St. Elizabeth's Hospital, Washington, for her contribution to Chapter 10, Psychological Assessment of Children.

For encouragement and general comments, grateful acknowledgement is due Miss Mary Jones, Associate Professor of Nursing, Valdosta State College; Mr. Preston Lee Davidson, Associate Professor, Medical College of Georgia, School of Nursing; and all four of my nieces: Mrs. Ann Berkey, Mrs. Barbara Schwartz, Mrs. Mary Nys, and Mrs. Patricia Cormier.

All of the secretaries who helped typed material for the book were helpful, but the services of Mrs. Laurel McDonald, Miss Vickie Bayham, and Mrs. Andrea Carter deserve special mention.

Helen Cabot Latham

CONTENTS

13 Nursing care of the child with congenital defects, 337

14 Nursing care of the child with a limited hospitalization, 395

15 Nursing care of the child accident victim, 434

16 Nursing care of the child with prolonged medical supervision, 465

PART I

Growth, development, and promotion of health of children

1
HOME ENVIRONMENT

It is particularly important for the nurse to understand how features of the environment can influence the physical and emotional health of children in order to plan effectively for their care. In this respect there is not a more significant environmental circumstance that will determine the success of those efforts than a complete understanding of the child's home.

INFLUENCES ON BEHAVIOR

Certain features of the home environment will influence the behavioral development of the child. Among the most important modifiers of behavior are the culture, the community, the subgroup membership, and the family.

Culture

The development of children occurs within an environment that is influenced by a cultural heritage. No matter where in the world a child is born, he finds himself in an environment that affects who and what he will be and how he will behave.

Cultures have different ways of viewing pregnancy, childbirth and child rearing; however, in no known culture are they ignored or treated with indifference. Each culture has to be studied to develop a deep understanding of the influence of tradition on behavior. Behavior of women and those who assist them in childbirth and child rearing are patterned by customs and are regulated by traditional practice. The mother-child relationship is prescribed by cultural norms. For example, a culture that favors male children creates difficulty for the mother when the child is a girl. Societal acceptance and approval are withheld from both mother and child.

Culture influences the attitude toward illegitimate pregnancies. In the United States and Great Britain there is evidence that increased

mortality and morbidity have occurred with illegitimate pregnancy largely because the prospective mothers have sought and obtained illegal abortions. If the abortion can be performed legally, this problem virtually disappears. Prematurity rates are higher with prenuptial than postnuptial conceptions. In other parts of the world conception prior to marriage is viewed as physical evidence of the ability to bear children. Morbidity, mortality, and prematurity rates are unaffected. These biological events are influenced by culturally imposed attitudes. Where attitudes and reactions are dictated by culture, the large majority of members of that society react virtually the same way.

Since cultural characteristics vary around the world, a home environment desirable for fostering a particular behavior in one country may not be desirable in another. For example, the economic independence of married children from their parents valued in the American culture is facilitated by the custom of maintaining separate living quarters. The child grows up seeing his older brothers and sisters marry and move away. Although parents may continue to support some young couples for a time, the ones who can "make it on their own" are the most admired; thus the child learns to expect and accept responsibility for his own future economic welfare. This value is supported by the American legal system, which does not insist that well-to-do relatives be responsible for their less fortunate kin. The state has established elaborate systems of loans, insurance, and welfare programs to which individuals can turn in times of financial need.

On the other hand, some societies that stress economic interdependence find the extended family system more conducive to maintaining this value. Here the child grows up with grandparents, aunts, uncles, and cousins in the household and learns to feel responsible for their support. Legal codes may enforce this standard by holding relatives responsible for the debts incurred by other family members, thus making organized financial assistance programs largely unnecessary.

It can therefore be seen that culture is the way a society prescribes the behavior of its members. Its institutions, laws, and mores are the means by which the desired behavior is perpetuated and maintained.

A closer examination of the culture of the United States reveals several identifiable attitudes and values. Derived mainly from the Judeo-Christian tradition and the spirit of private enterprise, the American ethos recognizes individual freedom, self-discipline, competition, and productivity. An individual is expected to make continuous attempts to better himself through education, occupational advancement, and spiritual development while maintaining a high level of integrity in his dealings with others. Those who exhibit such qualities are supposedly accorded the highest rewards in terms of socioeconomic status and prestige. However, recent political events have shown that many of those to whom we have looked for leadership have not lived up to these ideals, and the resulting disillusionment of our youth may have serious consequences for the future of the United States.

Community

Within the broad definitions of the culture, certain behaviors of the child will receive impetus from the physical and social circumstances of the community in which he lives. There are established differences between urban and rural life-styles that leave their mark on personality development.

Country and small town living in the United States has traditionally been typified by provincialism; throughout history its most conspicuous feature has been isolation. The agricultural way of life makes for a thinly scattered population where outside contacts on a day-to-day basis are limited. In his developmental years the child may see little of the world beyond the farm. The social contacts he does have are mainly with family and friends with similar backgrounds, similar goals, and similar problems. Such homogeneity has usually meant that the country child tends to develop a conservative outlook and intolerance toward new or unfamiliar persons, places, and ideas.

Limited contacts outside the community foster an intricate network of relationships within the community. The child learns to recognize others in a number of established roles. For example, he sees the local storekeeper not as an anonymous man who merely takes his money in exchange for a new pair of shoes but perhaps as the father of one of his schoolmates, a friend of the family, the husband of his piano teacher, a member of the town council, and so on. In other words, the child's perception of other people is extended to include more of their total personalities as the result of frequent contacts in a variety of situations. This can be contrasted to the urban child who is more likely to relate to individuals by categorizing them in single-faceted functional roles. To most urban children the storekeeper *is* an anonymous man who merely takes their money in exchange for a new pair of shoes.

Another distinction between rural and urban environments that undoubtedly has some effect on personality and behavior is the general pace of living. Sociologists suspect that the noise, the traffic, and the bustling impersonal atmosphere of the city produce more tensions and anxiety than the quiet, less regimented life of the country. The city child must constantly compete with others for recognition in crowded schools, for a seat on a crowded bus, for a place in line at a crowded theater or department store. He needs to develop a set of aggressive and self-assertive behaviors to cope with the social pressures of urban life.

It must be noted that the advance of technological progress into the countryside has blurred the traditional clear-cut differences between American rural and urban life in recent years. Movies, television, freeways, and the "consolidated" school have reduced the isolation of the country child and have brought him into contact with the city. The adoption of scientific farming techniques has forced a change of attitude on the part of many rural parents toward the value of formal and advanced education.

Perhaps today provincialism is a more apt description of the urban slum or the metropolitan suburb than of the modern rural community. Social distance and physical separation have segmented the city so that children growing up in one neighborhood may have little opportunity to meet and experience the life-styles of people of a different race, level of education, or socioeconomic status.

Subgroup membership

A sense of belonging is a universal need. Within the generalized classifications of culture and community, society sees to it that each individual is associated with various subgroups, which serve to establish his identity by anchoring him in time, in space, and in relation to other human beings. For the child, subgroup membership provides a frame of reference through which he can form perceptions of himself and others. It establishes a blueprint for behavior by defining who the child is and what he believes.

Most of the subgroups to which the young child belongs are the result of nonvoluntary associations. For example, the child has no control over the date and place of his birth and hence over his age, sex, race, nationality, ethnicity, and family. In most cases the child's religion and socioeconomic status are prescribed by virtue of his membership in the family. Early socialization to the attitudes and values of these nonvoluntary groups lays the foundations of behavior that will guide the child's choice of voluntary subgroup memberships in later years. They may influence his choice of friends, his choice of occupation, his choice of whether or not he will go to college, and his choice of the college he will attend.

Membership in a subgroup implies that the individual must learn a set of expectations regarding the manner in which he is to behave toward other members of the group and toward people outside the group. He also learns to expect how others will behave toward him. This establishes the individual's role in the subgroup. The child learns his role by observation and imitation of appropriate role models. This is becoming increasingly difficult and causes confusion because of the rapidly changing mores

in this society. For example, the strict role distinction between boys' and girls' activities no longer holds, and even in dress it is sometimes hard to differentiate. The child who is a member of a racial minority group will form perceptions of expected behavior by observing the manner in which other group members respond to their treatment by people outside the group. Minority group membership, however, which formerly often conveyed a feeling of inferior status, is now becoming a source of pride and allows the individual member to acquire status because of his membership, for example, as shown in ''Black is beautiful.''

Another significant pattern of behavior that can be linked to the child's ethnic background is the way he learns to handle emotion. Overt expressions of love, joy, sorrow, and fear are typical of people of Latin descent. The child learns that the pleasures and pains of life are accompanied by an appropriate set of physical gestures and verbal expressions. To the uninitiated the intensity of the reaction may sometimes appear disproportionate to the actual situation. On the other hand, children of Anglo, Germanic, or Oriental backgrounds learn that the emotions are not a matter for public display. Their reactions are likely to be more restrained and internalized. To someone who is unfamiliar with the pattern such behavior might be misconstrued as indifference, but this too is changing in the present generation.

Religion is also a powerful determinant of a child's attitudes, values, and behavior. Membership in a particular church group will provide the child with a rationale for living, a code of morality, and a set of limitations for tolerance and compromise. The church may infuse the child with a sense of responsibility for his own destiny, or it may lead him to believe that his lot in life and ultimate fate are preordained. Most churches also take definite stands on the value of education. Scholarly inquiry may be promoted as a means of revealing truth, or it may be denounced as a threat to faith in God. The child's religious affiliation might determine the kind of school he attends, which in turn might influence his peer group associations and eventually the partner he will choose in marriage.

There is general agreement that the most far-reaching effects on behavioral development are produced by the social class to which an individual belongs. Social class in the United States is often synonymous with socioeconomic status. An individual's placement at a particular socioeconomic level is determined mainly by wealth and occupation (or in the case of the child, by family income, which is greatly influenced by the occupation of his parents). Education is the usual prerequisite for occupational achievement, but certain individuals may acquire their status through inheritance. A person's race, place of residence, or religion can either facilitate or inhibit his chances for education, occupational advancement, and ultimate socioeconomic standing.

Numerous studies have documented differences in child-rearing practices among socioeconomic groups. Lower class parents are found to use more traditional methods that stress obedience, conformity, and discipline. Severe physical punishment is most often the means of quelling undesirable behavior. This is contrasted to a more rational approach employed by the middle class. Middle class parents are inclined to attempt to draw upon the child's sense of guilt by reasoning with him or isolating him as a form of punishment; the child who exhibits undesirable behavior may be scolded and sent to his room in lieu of being spanked. Upper class parents may use even more permissive techniques. They tend to ascribe to a "developmental" approach and condition desirable behavior through positive reinforcement.

In upper and middle class homes more emphasis is placed on school achievement. In addition, parents offer more direction over the child's leisure time and social acquaintances by enrolling him in such activities as music or dance lessons, scouting troops, and the Little League. They are concerned about providing experiences that contribute to the emotional satisfaction of the child.

The typical upper middle class child lives in an enriched environment. He is surrounded by material comforts that can be taken for granted. His parents undoubtedly have at least a high school education, and one or both may hold a college degree. They are engaged in occupations that stress creativity, good judgment, civility, resourcefulness, and reason and therefore automatically tend to employ these faculties in dealing with the child. When the child goes to school, he will encounter a teacher whose mannerisms and speech are not unlike those of his parents, and he will be assigned activities that are not wholly unfamiliar. When the child is encouraged to study hard so he can grow up and get a good job, he will think of his own family history—perhaps how his great-grandparents came to America from the "old country" and made their fortune, how his uncle started his own business, how his older sister went to college and learned to be a nurse. He will take pride in his family tradition and feel a responsibility for continuing it in his own life. The child thus becomes socialized to the behaviors appropriate to the attitudes and values of his culture.

Lower class parents are more concerned about the immediate gratification of the physical needs of the child. The good parent is the good provider—someone who sees to it that the child is well fed, neat, and clean. They are likely to pay less attention to the child's leisure activities so long as he does not "get into trouble." In relation to school, "minding the teacher" may be stressed more than bringing home a report card with good grades.

The typical lower class child comes from a home of material deprivation. His housing may provide shelter but offers little as a source of pride. Although his parents may wish to provide the child with intellectual stimulation, they may be illiterate and thus ill equipped to introduce him to the world of books. There is usually no money to buy the "educational toys" afforded in upper class homes. Job discrimination due to educational level or race leads to a high level of job dissatisfaction among low income males. The United States Bureau of Labor statistics reports that low income women are more readily hired than men. This produces a role reversal in many lower class families in which the mother is the main economic provider. Job insecurity and role reversal threaten the traditional status of the American male in his position of power and authority within the family structure.

Severe physical punishment of the child for misbehavior may be the means of displacing the hostility and aggression stemming from his feeling of impotency. Furthermore, even though the parents may be aware of more "enlightened" child-rearing techniques, isolation is an impractical discipline method when a family of six lives in a two-room apartment.

To provide the disadvantaged child with an opportunity for a good education is a challenging social problem for every community, every state, and the nation as a whole. State and local expenditures for school buildings, teaching equipment, athletic facilities, and teachers' salaries come from taxation of the citizenry. If the child lives in an economically depressed area, the tax base may be inadequate to finance the cost of quality education. The child who has a low educational motivation takes a dim view of his teacher and the school because he has no role models in his family history to support the idea that a promising career through education is a real possibility. In his world those who "make it" do so without the benefit of a high school diploma. For him school is a dead-end street; the most reasonable alternative is to drop out. Such children may have little opportunity to enter occupations that will move them to a higher socioeconomic status. They remain bound in patterns of behavior imposed by their limited education and environment.

Increased concern about the marginal child in our society is evidenced by such programs as Head Start and other bootstrap operations, which seek to minimize the handicaps of the disadvantaged child arising from his deprived environment. These programs are directed toward the provision of suitable social and intellectual experiences that will broaden the child's base of expectancies, strengthen his potential for achievement, and equip him with a set of behaviors that will allow his development to keep pace with that of his more advantaged peers.

Family

From the foregoing discussion it is apparent that most of the influences on behavior from the culture, the community, and subgroup membership will focus on the young child

through the family. The family is the first primary group to which the child belongs, and it is where his psychosocial development begins. The general reaction patterns formed within the family are then extended to external settings, where they mesh or conflict with reaction patterns of other children and adults.

Most of the shaping of the young child's behavior will come from the nuclear or immediate family situation. In families where other key figures such as grandparents, aunts, uncles, or cousins live in the home their influence may also be significant. In the early part of this century families tended to be quite large and included members of the extended family, who helped in a joint effort on family farms or in family businesses. As a result, each of these individuals took part in shaping the child's behavior. The term *baby-sitter* was largely unknown because each family was equipped with built-in baby-sitters. The extended family, which played such an important role in child development in early American culture, is still prevalent in some societies of the world, but in the United States today the major modifiers of the child's behavior in the home are his parents, brothers, and sisters.

The atmosphere in the family and therefore the attitudes of the parents toward each other and toward their children are of primary significance for the adjustment, present and future, of the child in the family. There have been numerous studies of the relationships involved despite the difficulty of obtaining spontaneous interaction with an observer present. Questionnaires, interviews, and home visits have been used intensively. Supposedly spontaneous interactions between parent and child have been observed through a one-way screen in a structured situation. For example, the mother may be instructed to teach her child how to use certain educational toys or other materials, and the behavior of both is carefully observed and rated or coded. One serious difficulty in the interpretation of the results is that usually the subjects used have been middle class; therefore generalization to other social classes may be unwarranted.

The results of several studies (Mussen, Conger, and Kagan, 1974) indicate that neither the authoritarian nor the so-called permissive parent is likely to produce the most mature, autonomous, self-directing child. Authoritarian parents were described as highly controlling and lacking in warmth, nurturance, and affection. They believed in the old saying "Spare the rod and spoil the child." They did not encourage the child to express his views. The children showed some self-reliance and were likely to be quiet and well-behaved but not very happy, outgoing, or trustful.

The children of very permissive parents, who were nondemanding and noncontrolling but warm and nurturant, seemed to be the least mature and the most dependent, lacking in self-reliance but friendly and affectionate. These parents indirectly made few demands for mature behavior and paid little attention to training for independence.

Children of parents who are intermediate between the two extremes seem to be the most mature, friendly, independent, and competent. These parents encourage the child's autonomy, are warm and loving, and communicate well with the children, but they also are firm and decisive, hold to their decisions, and set limits while letting the children know the whys and wherefores of what is expected of them. They encourage understanding and rational thinking on the part of the children, who are treated as worthwhile human beings with ideas that should be listened to and considered. This kind of consideration begins with the infant and toddler. If communication is not established early, it is much more difficult to develop it later.

If the nurse is an observer in a structured situation, she should take note of the spontaneous interactions between parent and child—the mother or father's way of motivating the child, enforcing regulations, reacting to the child's difficulties and frustrations, responding to his questions—generally his or her ability to treat the child as another human being worthy of respect and understanding, whose ideas are of importance. There is no doubt that in a warm, interacting family that encourages learning and intellectual activity, children tend to achieve and function on a more satisfactory level.

By far the most detrimental effects on the child are produced by rejection. The rejection

of a child is not restricted to any one social class. The child may be rejected in upper class families as well as in families of lower class status. In the latter case rejection may be quite apparent and obvious; in the former case the rejection is no less real but may be disguised as overindulgence and overprivilege.

In its most direct form rejection may be seen as hostility, isolation, and indifference to the wants, needs, and desires of the child or even physical or psychological abuse. Children who are rejected may not always be readily identified as such since the behavioral symptoms they show—aggression, hostility, tension, apprehension, anxiety, and withdrawal—are not unlike those of other problems. Children who exhibit such behaviors should be investigated more thoroughly to determine the underlying causes.

Conversely, children who receive warmth, love, and acceptance accompanied by proper limits and guidance find themselves free from the stress and tension of rejection and are able to devote their full efforts to meeting head-on the problems of school and interpersonal relationships in living. The child who is free of the conviction that others do not like him is able to face new situations more easily and readily.

In general, evidence supports the concept that the most effective functioning for the child can be achieved in a home where stress, apprehension, and anxiety are minimized and where warmth, attention, and some degree of freedom, but with definite limits, are clearly recognized by the child.

Family size

Many studies in recent years have attempted to isolate pertinent factors with regard to family size. Under consideration have been the effects on development produced by the large family, the small family, and the single-parent family.

The problems facing the child in a very large family are numerous. One real problem is that there is often "not enough" of many material things to supply adequately the needs of all the family members. The child who must constantly share his toys and share his bedroom may feel that he has nothing of his very own. The child has little opportunity for privacy and quiet reflection without interruption. Conflicts arise when brothers and sisters feel they must compete with one another for parental recognition. Frequently responsibility falls on the older children to play parent substitute roles. Sometimes these arrangements are highly satisfactory in promoting a feeling of belonging and of importance in the older child as well as close interpersonal affection between an older and younger child. In other situations in which older children have been forced to take on excessive amounts of family responsibility, the results can be frustrating or even disastrous in preventing warm family relationships.

In the case of the only child parental attention often becomes fixed upon him so that he is not permitted to develop the independence and give-and-take necessary for adjusting in a world where his ideas, feelings, and thoughts will not receive the individualized recognition that he is accustomed to at home. This is not to say that the only child cannot grow up to be a well-adjusted, happy adult. In fact he may attain more self-confidence and ego strength than a child in a large family. Parents who set definite limits on the child's activities without being overly restrictive teach the child to expect some of the frustrations of life. By encouraging meaningful interactions with other children the parents can see to it that the child learns to recognize the needs of others. Frequently inviting children of the neighborhood in to play and making use of organizations such as scouts, Y.M.C.A. or Y.W.C.A., and the 4-H Club may provide the understanding of others of the same age that may be lacking in the home of the only child.

The rising rates of desertion and divorce in the United States have caused increasing concern over the behavioral development of the child in the single-parent family. The evidence suggests that the child who has both parents living together with love and acceptance of each other and of him is indeed fortunate. There are a number of detailed studies that report a wide range of adverse effects when a child grows up in a home in which one of his parents is absent.

Death is the most frequent cause of loss of the mother; desertion and divorce are more often the reasons why the father may be absent from the home. It is estimated that one out of every four marriages in the United States ends in divorce. At one time it was believed that an intolerable relationship between a husband and wife should be maintained at all costs "for the sake of the children" and that coming from a broken home would impose severe handicaps on the behavioral development of the child. It is now more widely believed that coming *from* a broken home may be less detrimental than living *in* a broken home. In other words, the effects of living in a single-parent family may be less harmful in the long run than those produced by a home in which civility is a guise for contempt, normal parent-child relationships are disrupted by antagonism, and the child feels that, if it were not for him, his parents could separate and be happy. Nevertheless, when the child is faced with a single-parent situation, whether from death, divorce, or desertion, some problems in development are inevitable.

Perhaps the most serious disadvantage to the child is the lack of appropriate role models. When a parent must be both mother and father to the child, it may be difficult for the child to distinguish between traditional masculine and feminine roles. This is particularly true for the little boy whose father is absent from the home. The result may be an overattachment and dependence on the mother that will conflict with the independence expected of him in later years.

There are differences between socioeconomic strata of society regarding the parent's attitude toward the child that may arise as the result of the parent's single status. The parent from upper socioeconomic strata may try to compensate for the personal gratifications usually provided in marriage by turning attention toward work. The parent may be so busy with social and business acquaintances in order to quell feelings of loneliness and inadequacy that emotional support and comfort for the child are lacking. The child may be seen as a detriment to social and occupational advancement. The parent may attempt to allay the sense of guilt arising from the dereliction of parental responsibility by showering the child with material gifts.

On the other hand, the single parent from a disadvantaged population is frequently unable to find employment that provides job satisfaction. As a result the parent may turn to the child for compensation and may have increased enjoyment in the child's company. This can be rewarding for both, but, conversely, the single parent may use the child as an outlet for his frustrations or reject him. (See p. 8 for more discussion of rejection.) Whatever the socioeconomic status, the single parent must face his responsibility without the benefit of a partner with whom he or she can share the problems of raising a child.

Family interrelationships

The way in which family members react to one another will establish the emotional climate of the home. As mentioned earlier, the manner in which parents behave toward one another can have long-term effects on the development of the child. Parents who love and accept one another are able to convey these feelings to the child. Conversely, when parents are having marital difficulties one of the parents might channel his aggression toward the child instead of forcing a direct confrontation between them that might disrupt the entire family. For example, if the husband constantly comes home to a messy house, he may unduly scold his daughter for not picking up her things and helping her mother cook, clean, and do the laundry. The mother may witness her husband's display of anger and hostility toward the child without coming to her defense because she sees the situation as a way of projecting the blame for her own problem of inadequacy in housekeeping onto the child. Further examples of such "scapegoating" of the child are provided by Vogel and Bell (1965). Such family pressures create conflict for the child and may lead to serious emotional disturbance.

Many of the behaviors the child acquires will be learned from his siblings rather than his parents. The child with a sibling of the opposite sex will learn something of the way in which he is expected to behave in relation to the opposite sex in other social situations. The child who comes from a family in which *all* of his siblings are of the opposite sex may even adopt the behaviors of that sex himself. The boy who comes from a family of girls may be branded by his peers as a "sissy"; the girl who comes from a family of boys may be considered a "tomboy." This stereotyping of sex roles, however, is recently being modified to the point that it is becoming less of a problem.

The position of the child in the family will also determine his behavior in relation to the other children. The child who is born first and claims the full attention of his parents in his younger years will have to relinquish some of this attention when the second child comes along. The older child may be resentful of this intrusion and may have difficulty adjusting to the idea of sharing, especially if the parents themselves tend to neglect him in their excitement over the new baby. On the other hand, the oldest child has a position of prestige as the firstborn. He tends to feel a strong sense of responsibility for carrying on the family traditions and is often reminded that the younger children are "looking up" to him.

The youngest child may be in a favored position because he is the baby of the family. Both parents and siblings may be oversolicitous to his needs. While this favored position may bring him an increased sense of security, it may also delay the development of self-reliance. There is some evidence that the middle child sometimes encounters more adjustive difficulties because there is nothing distinctive about his position in the family.

As a child enters adolescence, peer group associations become increasingly important, enlarging the sphere of influence. When values of the peer group differ from those of the family, conflicts may occur. To avoid putting the adolescent on the defensive, parents should not force him into an either-or position. They can discuss varying viewpoints objectively and explain the reasons they believe as they do. If a mutually acceptable compromise is made, the adolescent will feel that he is a participant in decision making. Decision making with parental guidance promotes a logical progression toward complete responsibility for one's own behavior. It is the lack of communication between adolescents and their parents that contributes to the adolescent's feelings of alienation, being unloved, and not being understood. Without communication with parents the adolescent may take an undesirable route to gain his own objectives.

Maternal care

The kind of maternal care the child receives influences him throughout his life. Through both human and animal studies, psychologists, psychiatrists, and other researchers have sought to link early experience with later behaviors. For many years there has been the conviction that early experience can account for many of the deviant or unusual adult behaviors. Years of collecting case histories pointed up situations that could not be explained away and that seemed to account for later behavior patterns. However, it was only after direct experimentation on animals and systematic observation over a period of years on the development of children in a variety of settings—orphanages, foster homes, "good" homes, and homes

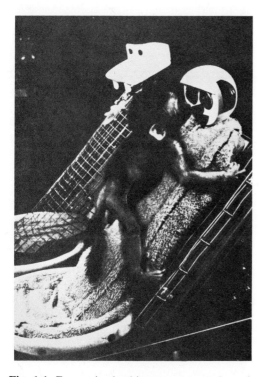

Fig. 1-1. Even animal subjects react to mother substitutes. In Harlow's work with monkeys he found that "soft" cloth mothers were preferred to wire models even though the wire model had a milk supply available. (Courtesy H. F. Harlow.)

showing different types of discipline—that any conclusive evidence has been brought forth in support of the early theories.

Most fascinating among these studies have been those conducted by Harry Harlow and his associates at the University of Wisconsin (Harlow and Zimmerman, 1949). In his work Harlow performed a variety of experiments in which infant monkeys were removed from their mothers at various stages of development and placed with a mother substitute. This substitute mother was made of wire (Fig. 1-1). In some cases the mother substitute was covered with a soft terry cloth material, whereas in other cases it was warm, provided milk, or even was provided with sharp projections that made claim by the infant monkey quite difficult. Those monkeys that were reared by the warm, soft "mother" developed more stability in their behavior than those reared with the less desirable forms. However, none of the monkeys raised under these conditions developed normal adult behaviors. Females were cold and indifferent sexually; males showed similar patterns with withdrawal and indifference to others of their species. The following is one hypothesis that has been advanced in explanation of this behavior: Not only did these monkeys lack a social model to follow in developing their behavior, but, in addition, a period of optimum learning of social behaviors had passed.

Lacking the normal emotional and affectional supports found in homes, institutionalized children frequently grow into adulthood lacking the ability to interact with warmth and affection with others. The results of studies conducted by René Spitz were striking (Spitz and Wolf, 1946). He made observations of children in institutional settings and used the term *anaclitic depression* in describing the behavior of infants separated from their mothers over a period of time. Although the infants cried at first on separation, later they were apathetic and showed little responsive behavior. They seemed less active and more withdrawn and showed little interest in objects around them. Their facial expressions were sad.

Bakwin (1949) described infants who had been maternally deprived in institutions as thin, pale, failing to grow and thrive, having febrile episodes, having a poor appetite, and looking unhappy.

The infants in the preceding situations were not only deprived of individual mothering and handling but also lacked sensory stimulation. Maternally deprived children may have difficulties in establishing effective relationships with others in later life.

An excellent summary of the many studies done in the area of maternal separation is provided in *Child Development Research* (Hoffman and Hoffman, 1964). In a chapter on separation from parents in early childhood, Yarrow points out that there are several variables that may affect the results of a separation. The child is most vulnerable at the time he is establishing stable affectional relationships (about 6 months to 2 years of age). Other variables contributing to effects of the child's separation from a loved one include the quality of the relationship with the mother prior to separation, the character of the relationship with the parents during temporary separation, the duration of the separation experience, subsequent reinforcing experiences, and the role of constitutional or congenital factors in personality.

No conclusive studies have been made on the effect of maternal employment on children. Here again there are variables that make direct correlations difficult to obtain, such as the kind of care the child has while his mother is working, the reason for the mother's working, and so on.

EFFECTS OF HOME ENVIRONMENT ON PHYSICAL HEALTH

The influences of the home environment that affect the behavioral development of the child are responsible for his social and emotional adjustment in society. They are major contributors to his mental health. Of no less importance are the effects of these same influences of the home environment on the physical health of the child as reflected by his physical growth and development, his susceptibility to disease, and his attitude and accessibility to health care. Such factors as housing conditions, sanitation, and nutrition have a bearing on the child's state of health.

Physical growth and development

Culture, community, subgroup membership, and the family—the major features of the child's home environment—are as relevant to the physical growth and development of the child as they are to his social development. In the following chapters normal patterns of physical growth and development of children will be outlined in detail. Although heredity is a factor in determining ultimate growth potential and the manner in which an individual child proceeds according to these defined patterns, it must be remembered that the environment in which a child grows can produce significant alterations in these processes. Indeed, the child's genetic heritage itself is influenced by the environment in that the social forces of culture, community, and subgroup membership have played a role in bringing together the two individuals who are his parents.

Human growth and development are complex biological processes that require sufficient inputs from the environment to maintain an optimum rate of cell proliferation and maturation. Among the most important environmental needs for proper growth are good nutrition and adequate protection from exposure to the natural elements. Features of the child's home will determine whether or not these basic requirements for food and shelter can be met. One thinks immediately of the socioeconomic status of the child's family as a significant factor in this respect; however, income is certainly not the only criterion. An examination of the influences of culture and subgroup membership in shaping the food habits of the child can illustrate the dynamic and interrelated effects of the home situation.

In primitive societies, food habits were established mainly on the basis of what nature itself could provide at a particular time and place. Since the ways of nature are capricious, food shortages were a real problem to survival. Modern man has learned to adapt nature to the scientific practice of agriculture so that today he exerts a considerable amount of control over his food supply; he has a wider variety of foods available to him than ever before. From a physiological point of view any substance that provides essential nutrients and can be ingested without toxic effects can be considered as food. Yet one only has to travel around the world to see that the foods eaten in one country may be unacceptable in another. Thus it is that culture determines what the individual will recognize as food and fit for him to eat, what he will recognize as food fit for others but unacceptable to him, and what he will refuse to recognize as food under any circumstance. It would be fortunate if every culture prescribed food patterns that provided precisely the right combination of nutrients for optimum growth and development, but this is not always the case. High rates of child mortality in some underdeveloped countries today can be partly ascribed to nutritionally inadequate cultural food habits. Nevertheless, child mortality has been decreasing because of increased knowledge, education, and better medical care with the result that populations are exploding. In many developing countries the burgeoning numbers of people to feed are offsetting or even reversing these benefits.

The culture not only dictates which foods are acceptable to its population as a whole, but it also determines which foods are appropriate for various subgroups within the population. For example, American culture promotes the idea that milk is an appropriate food for children and pregnant women. The basis for this belief is scientific data relating the nutrient composition of milk to optimum growth and development. In a native population of South Africa, milk is not considered an appropriate food for children and pregnant women. The basis for this belief is rooted in a complicated system of taboos derived from prestige and kinship relations within the group.

The community in which a child lives can have a significant influence on food availability. The migration of rural people to the city can result in a decrease in the quality of the diet. On the farm the family may have easy access to fresh fruits and vegetables grown in a backyard garden. Land in which to plant gardens is scarce in the city. Fruits and vegetables may be difficult to obtain. If families do not have enough money to purchase these foods at the grocery store, they may have to rely on cheaper, processed items of an inferior nutritional quality.

Subgroup associations play a considerable role in determining food habits. The church may set codes of food behavior—examples are the orthodox Jewish and Moslem avoidance of pork and the Hindu practice of vegetarianism. The most significant subgroup influence comes from socioeconomic status. Income and the availability of food are obvious correlations, but money is not always a guarantee of proper nutrition; surveys report that some degree of malnutrition exists among people of upper income status. Education may be a more important determinant. A young woman who knows none of the "principles of nutrition" may be unaware that the meals she serves her child are inadequate. If she lacks basic cooking skills, she may not know how to prepare a new food even if she has the money to buy it.

As the child grows older, peer group associations play an increasing role in the direction of his eating behavior. Pressures of the peer group not only prescribe what the child should eat to "be in" but also where and when he should eat. The group may have its popular "hangout" to which the child may go to eat in preference to eating at home with his family.

Endless examples of the manner in which the child's home environment influences the development of food habits, nutritional status, and growth can be cited. Those presented here are sufficient to illustrate that, although nutrition to meet the requirements for growth and development explains the child's primary need for food, the wide range of meanings that food holds for man in society are more likely to determine whether or not that need is met. They also provide a basis for understanding why the child's food habits, once established for better or worse, are difficult to change. Similar analogies can be drawn for every other aspect of the environment that has a significant input in the child's physical growth and development.

Attitude and accessibility to health care

Much of what accounts for the attitude of the parents and child concerning health care is explained by their perceptions of health and disease. The value of good health is almost universally accepted, but what actually constitutes good health may be a matter of debate. For some people good health may merely mean the absence of overt symptoms of disease; as long as he *feels* well and can perform everyday activities without interference from severe somatic distress, the individual perceives that he is in good health. He may see no value in preventive care.

Others regard health as being whatever is *normal* for them. This may be conditioned by the attitudes and situations of people around them. For example, in areas of poor environmental sanitation it is common for children to have parasitic infestation. All the children have it; it is nothing abnormal so the parent does not recognize worms as related to the child's health status.

Sociocultural influences may also determine what the individual *does* if he perceives that he is in ill health. For example, certain religions look upon illness as a punishment for sin—the individual is expected to bear it without complaint as the "will of God." Others stress personal strength, fortitude, and the power of positive thinking as appropriate cures of illness. People who have such beliefs may seek out a "faith healer" in preference to a qualified physician.

In other instances remedies suggested by neighbors, older relatives, parental family practices, respected authority figures, or advertising may be used, thus delaying or preventing diagnosis and treatment of sick children.

Individuals who have no sense of control over their own destinies may develop a fatalistic attitude toward health and disease. They may recognize illness when it occurs, may wish to seek proper care, but may believe that they are powerless in their ability to approach and deal with the complicated channels of authority encountered in a highly technical and bureaucratic health care system.

Educational background and intellectual ability of the parents also play a role in the success of the child's treatment when he is ill. Physicians may give specific orders regarding the child's care, but their directions may be unintelligible to the parents. They may misconstrue the order, forget about it, or simply not follow it because they are unsure exactly what the doctor meant. This kind of situation is especially common regarding drug prescriptions and dietary advice. Such possibilities suggest that frequent and continuous follow-up must be made to make sure that the child is actually receiving the treatment prescribed.

Part of the differential in health statistics, especially those related to infant and child morbidity and mortality, can be explained by inequities in the accessibility of health care. Rural and thinly populated areas in the United States are notorious for their lack of physicians, dentists, nurses, and other health personnel. Preventive health measures are often unattended because it is just too much trouble to get the child to the doctor's or dentist's office. Minor illnesses may go untreated for the same reason. Debilitating sequences of minor disease episodes may eventually lead to the child's becoming seriously ill. It may be only then that the child is brought to medical attention. By this time the condition may have progressed beyond the possibility of satisfactory cure.

The same situation is true of low income families in urban areas. A day's absence from work, even if it is to take the child to the doctor, may mean not merely the loss of a day's pay but also loss of the job for the parent. Agencies tend to schedule clinic services with the convenience of staff as a priority rather than the convenience and need of families for health services. Unstable incomes cannot afford payment of heavy physician's fees; therefore most low income families do not have their own private doctor who is thoroughly familiar with the child's medical history. Instead, they must rely on outpatient clinics or emergency hospital facilities where there is no guarantee that treatment will be prompt or personalized. Those whose work is sporadic and irregular may not be able to benefit from employee health insurance programs that cover the cost of hospitalization or extended health care. Since the child is the most expendable member of the family when it comes to its economic survival, his health needs may be the last to be met. Again, it may only be when a serious illness threatens his life that medical help is sought.

These conditions relative to the accessibility of health care are the subject of concerted investigation in the United States today. Attempts have been made to equalize medical attention to children in the lower strata of our population through maternity and infant care clinics, children and youth clinics, and well child conferences. Even at best these efforts reach only a small percentage of those needing care. Meanwhile, future efforts of members of the health professions will continue to focus on closing the accessibility gap and improving the quality of health care for those who can be reached.

SUMMARY

The nurse can better understand the child and promote his health if she understands his home environment and how it influences his behavior and health. Factors that have been discussed include culture, the community, subgroup membership, family relationships, maternal care, effect of the home on physical growth and development, and the attitude of the family toward health care. The child who comes from a home environment that promotes his health and happiness is one who better adjusts to new situations and can relate more easily to his peers and others in the environment.

REFERENCES

Altus, N. D.: Birth order and its sequelae, Int. J. Psychiatry **3:**23-39, 1967.

Bakwin, H.: Emotional deprivation in infants, J. Pediatr. **35:**512, 1949.

Beres, D., and Obers, S.: The effects of extreme deprivation in infancy on psychic structure in adolescence, Psychoanal. Study Child **5:**121, 1950.

Bowlby, J.: Separation anxiety; a critical review of the literature, J. Child Psychol. Psychiatry **1:**251, 1960.

Breckenridge, M. E., and Murphy, M. N.: Growth and development of the young child, ed. 8, Philadelphia, 1969, W. B. Saunders Co.

Crawford, C., editor: Health and the family, New York, 1971, The Macmillan Co.

Elam, H.: Malignant culture deprivation—its evolution, Pediatrics **44:**319, 1969.

Grimm, E.: Psychological and social factor in pregnancy, delivery and outcome. In Richardson, S., and Gutmacher, A., editors: Childbearing—its social and psychological aspects, Baltimore, 1967, The Williams & Wilkins Co.

Harlow, H. F., and Zimmermann, R. R.: Affectional responses in the infant monkey, Science **130:**421, 1959.

Herzog, E.: About the poor; some facts and some fictions, Children Bureau Pub. No. 451-1967, Washington, D.C., 1967, U.S. Department of Health, Education, and Welfare.

Hoffman, M. L., and Hoffman, L. W.: Review of child development research, New York, 1964, Russell Sage Foundation.

Irelan, L. M.: Low-income life styles, Welfare Administration Pub. No. 14, Washington, D.C., 1968, U.S. Department of Health, Education, and Welfare.

Kosa, J., Antonovsky, A., and Zola, I. K., editors: Poverty and health; a sociological analysis, Cambridge, Mass., 1969, Harvard University Press.

McKinley, D. G.: Social class and family life, London, 1964, Cassell & Collier Macmillan, Ltd.

Mussen, H. M., Conger, J. J., and Kagan, J.: Child development and personality, ed. 4, New York, 1974, Harper & Row, Publishers.

Prugh, D. G., and Harlow, R. G.: Masked deprivation in infants and young children. In Deprivation of maternal care, Public Health Papers No. 14, Geneva, 1962, World Health Organization.

Sarason, I. G.: Personality; an objective approach, New York, 1966, John Wiley & Sons, Inc.

Schoaler, C. Birth order effects; not here, not now! Psychol. Bull. **78:**161-175, 1972.

Spitz, R. A., and Wolf, K.: Anaclitic depression, Psychoanal. Study Child **2:**313, 1946.

Vogel, E. F., and Bell, N. W.: The emotionally disturbed child; a family scapegoat. In Rodman, H., editor: Marriage, family, and society, New York, 1965, Random House.

Yarrow, L.: Separation from parents during early childhood. In Hoffman, M. L., and Hoffman, L. W., editors: Review of child development research, Vol. 1, New York, 1964, Russell Sage Foundation.

2
TOWARD GOOD HEALTH
OF THE NEONATE

PRECONCEPTUAL INFLUENCES

Professionals dealing with the health of neonates, infants, and children have recognized the need for a healthy beginning. Toward this end emphasis has been placed on improvement in prenatal care to increase the probability of a healthy, well-developed neonate being delivered to a healthy, well-adjusted mother. Improvement in prenatal care and the wider acceptance of services have contributed to the decrease in infant mortality and morbidity. However, it must be recognized that many women seek prenatal care when they are 10, 12, even 16 or more weeks pregnant. Organogenesis is nearing completion before medical evaluation is made. Emphasis on prenatal care, which is vitally important, has overshadowed the influence of preconceptual care on the outcome of pregnancy. In the following pages education for family living, health of potential parents, and nutrition are discussed. Since parents may seek genetic counseling after the birth of a defective baby, a discussion of genetic counseling is included here.

Education for family living

More and more health professionals are coming to the realization that the time for preparation for parenthood is when the potential parents are children themselves. Education begins in infancy with the parents' acceptance of the sex of the child and continues with the manner in which they handle the infant, bathe him, diaper him, and act if and when the infant handles his genitalia. If either of the parents shows disgust when the infant soils himself or slaps the infant's hands if the latter plays with his genital organs, the child is likely to receive an impression that his body is not nice or that there is

something wrong with his body. This is true throughout the period of toilet training.

Receiving affection and love is important to the child in terms not only of his total well-being but also because as an adult he will find it difficult to give love to another if he has not received it himself. Feeling accepted, wanted, and loved as an infant and child affects the ability of the person to form and maintain lasting friendships or any relationship that involves depth of feeling.

The adult patterns his behavior as a parent on what he saw as a growing child. Thus it is based on childhood interpretations of the roles of his mother and father in the home as well as on observation of the parents of his friends. His opinion as to whether the father should play with a child, help care for an infant, assist with washing dishes, and be considerate and affectionate to the mother is influenced by childhood observation in his own or in a playmate's family. Respect for the elderly and protection of the young child are part of the observed patterns of family behavior. Also, values and standards of his family affect the child's philosophy as an adult.

Specific learnings in sex education associated with the preschool period are (1) names of parts of the body, (2) knowledge that babies come from the mother, and (3) information about the behavior of infants. Infants sleep a lot and do not talk or walk; they drink from a bottle or from the mother's breast. The early school period should include knowledge of the father's part in reproduction plus possibly a repetition of information given earlier but forgotten. In the preadolescent period (about fifth or sixth grade) children should be told about certain changes that will take place in their bodies during adolescence, such as change in body contours, rapid growth in height, menstruation in girls, seminal emissions in boys, and appearance of pubic and axillary hair. Each sex should know about changes in the other. This saves worry, embarrassment, and perhaps even fear at a later date.

The parents, the schools, or both should contribute to this information. Sometimes this is part of health education in schools. Excellent films are available as teaching aids in this field. Answers to specific questions of children should be given simply, truthfully, and in accordance with the child's curiosity and ability to understand.

During junior and senior high school, experiences in group living such as scouting, camping, playing team games, or participating in activities with a peer group are all means of furthering the art of getting along with others, which is so essential in marriage.

Health education in high school may include a course in family living that includes information about budgeting, marriage laws, human reproduction, dating, choosing a mate, sexuality, and other pertinent information. If the school that a particular teenager attends does not offer such a course, then it behooves parents to take more responsibility for discussing these matters with their children.

It is desirable to offer a course in child care in both junior and senior high school not only because children in junior high school babysit often but also because the majority of those young people will someday be parents.

Dating plays an important part in education for family living since only by knowing several different boys can a girl form judgments regarding a man with whom she would finally like to spend the remainder of her life. This is true of boys' dating also. To date only one girl gives little basis for judgment in choosing a mate.

In summary, attitudes toward sex are developed in early childhood. These may be changed later, but it is harder to reeducate than to educate. Specific knowledge varies with the interests of the growing child. At different stages of his growth he needs different kinds of information and group experiences. Sexual ad-

justment, budgeting, child care, and marriage laws are of paramount importance to the adolescent and to the engaged couple. Emotional problems and marital unhappiness can have their roots in misconceptions about sex and sexuality. The problem of rearing children when either father or mother is still in school needs discussion, as well as problems of the working mother. In some areas there are family planning clinics with available counseling.

Health of potential parents
Premarital examination

In addition to the blood test for syphilis that is required in most states for a license to marry an engaged couple should have a complete physical examination. If medical problems exist, they should be evaluated and treated prior to marriage. If chronic conditions or advanced debilitating diseases exist, their effect on the marriage and family life and the health of potential offspring must be seriously considered by the couple.

Evaluation of the female should include nutritional status since she is the potential childbearer. Nutritional deficiency in the fetus may be induced in utero when there is lack of either quantity or quality of the mother's nutritional intake. Deficiencies should be corrected prior to pregnancy if at all possible. A vaginal examination is indicated to determine the status of the organs of reproduction and the condition of the hymen. Resistant hymen can interfere with coital function due to pain on penetration. Minor surgery, hymenotomy, may be indicated prior to marriage to minimize the problem of initially painful coitus.

At the time of the examination the physician may take the opportunity to discuss family planning, giving the couple advice and information on the importance of planning a family. The couple will need time to discuss their needs and ask questions about specific contraceptive methods. If the couple has made the decision to adopt a method of contraception, the physician may implement the method at the time of the premarital examination. Family planning promotes dignity of the family as well as general family stability. Spacing of children contributes to the lowering of rates of perinatal and infant mortality and prematurity. This allows the family a chance to develop the potential of each child. It gives the youngest child in the family a chance to have his full share of "babying" as well as a chance to become somewhat independent so he is less apt to feel displaced.

Genetic counseling

Typically the couples who seek genetic counseling are parents who have a child with a genetic defect and who must make a decision about having other children. The counselor's role is to determine the risk of recurrence, to interpret the findings to the parents, and to assist them through guidance to make a responsible decision. The decision is a personal one between husband and wife and theirs alone. Less often a family history of abnormality or hereditary disease will prompt a couple to question a physician about the possibility that they may have a child with the anomaly or the disease. Fortunately young people are becoming more willing than their parents to discuss problems in the family.

Risk of having an affected offspring is most easily assessed when the condition is known to be controlled by a single gene. In autosomal dominant inheritance, for example, Huntington's disease, one of the parents would have the disease. In such an instance there is a 50% risk that any given offspring would be affected. More than 900 dominantly inherited disorders have been identified and described.

In recessive inheritance, for example, sickle cell disease, affected children may be born to outwardly normal parents each of whom carries the deleterious gene. Children of parents who are heterozygous for the recessive deleterious gene have a one in four chance of being normal, a one in four chance of having the disease, and a two in four chance of being a carrier of the trait. More than 750 disorders are transmitted by recessive inheritance.

Sex-linked recessive inheritance, for example, hemophilia, appears in the sons of normal fathers and normal but carrier mothers. If the father has the disease and the mother is normal, all of their sons will be normal and all of their daughters will be carriers of the trait.

If the father is normal and the mother is a carrier of the trait, their daughters will have a 50% risk of being carriers. Their sons will have a 50% risk of having the disease. One hundred and fifty sex-linked recessive disorders have been identified and described.

There is an unknown number of disorders classified as mixed inheritance or multifactorial in which a single gene cannot be identified as the causative factor, for example, diabetes mellitus. It is the result of interaction between two or more genes. Predicting risk or occurrence in multifactorial inheritance is based on studies of statistical tables or recurrence within families and the incidence of the disease in the general population.

In addition, there are genetic disorders produced by intergenic alteration in both chromosomal structure and number. One of the most discussed examples of alteration in chromosomal number is Down's syndrome, in which there is the equivalent of three chromosomes 21 instead of two. Genetic disorders of this kind are referred to as trisomies. (See Chapter 19.)

The counselor must be alert to the possibility that parents may misunderstand the risks since they are stated in percentages or fractions. For example, when parents have a child with a genetic disorder due to recessive inheritance, they may think that a one in four risk means that the next three children will be normal. This is clearly a misunderstanding since each pregnancy is an independent event; the risk is the same for every child of the same mother and father. In some instances of congenital defect as a result of chromosomal aberration the risk increases with each subsequent pregnancy.

Prenatal genetic diagnosis

Transabdominal amniocentesis has been used for many years for a variety of purposes. This procedure, in which amniotic fluid is withdrawn from the uterus of a pregnant woman, has been an effective tool in the management of pregnancies in women sensitized to the Rh antigen. Now prenatal genetic diagnoses are being made using the same technique for the collection of amniotic fluid for chromosomal studies. Amniocentesis is not attempted prior to 12 weeks of gestation. It has been estimated that the volume of amniotic fluid at 12 weeks is 50 ml. By 14 weeks the volume has increased to between 98 and 116 ml., and by 16 weeks it is between 200 and 285 ml. The procedure of amniocentesis is usually done between 14 and 16 weeks of gestation; between 10 and 20 ml. of amniotic fluid is withdrawn. The fluid contains sloughed cells from the respiratory and urinary tracts and from the skin of the fetus. A culture is prepared from the fluid, and cells can be harvested for analysis between 15 and 40 days following amniocentesis. Harvesting is dependent on the proliferation of cells in the culture. Cells can be examined directly without culture for sex chromatin bodies and fluorescent Y bodies. The fluid can be analyzed for metabolites and infective agents. Cultured cells can be analyzed for aberrations in chromosomal structure and number as well as for approximately 40 biochemical disorders.

As with all surgical procedures, there are some risks. There is the risk of infection and abortion for the mother, and for the fetus there is the risk of injury by the needle. The risk of hemorrhage from puncture of the placenta is minimized by localizing the placenta through ultrasonic techniques prior to the amniocentesis.

New dimensions have been added to genetic counseling through the use of amniocentesis for prenatal diagnosis. Definitive diagnosis can be made in some conditions, and the genetic counselor need not rely solely on statistical or mathematical probability.

PRENATAL INFLUENCES
Mental health in pregnancy

Many behavioral scientists have intepreted pregnancy as a period of crisis, although the time element is too long to fit the concept of crisis. An alternative approach might be to consider pregnancy as an example of normal stress in which physiological and psychological change occurs and is resolved through normal adaptation processes.

The reaction of the couple to the news of a confirmed pregnancy will be relative to each parent's developmental achievements and their desire to be parents. If the pregnancy has been planned, the news should be joyfully received; if unplanned, there still could be happy antici-

pation. The expectant mother's maturity, her attitudes toward sex, and her ability to identify herself with her own mother as a woman, wife, and mother influence her during this period. If she is not able to accept her own sex role, pregnancy is not apt to be a fulfilling experience. Also, the father's feelings about parenthood reflect his developmental experiences and his identification with male role models.

Pregnancy brings with it a more complex role. New familial developmental tasks have to be learned. With the first pregnancy the woman is moving from the wife role to the wife-mother role. The father moves from the husband role to the husband-father role. Economic and social planning must begin to move away from activities around young married couples to involvement with young couples with children. With each subsequent pregnancy there are further subtle role changes. This necessitates reevaluation and readjustment of the family lifestyle. Change brings about a state of disequilibrium and a need to reestablish homeostasis.

Mood swings and ambivalence during pregnancy can be attributed to an interaction of physiological and psychological factors. The potential father needs to be prepared for unexplained mood swings in his wife. She may show increased sensitivity; she cries more easily but is also quick to laugh. This "quicksilver" behavior must be recognized as a part of pregnancy and interpreted as being in the realm of normal. The husband should be encouraged to respond to such vacillation in behavior with increased tolerance, support, and affection. The extent that the mother herself has been and is loved and accepted will influence the way she in turn loves the child.

It is essential for the nurse to assess the emotional state of the pregnant woman because she is in a unique position to identify problems with which prospective parents must cope. Knowledge about a woman's response to pregnancy can indicate the need for intervention. Timely intervention may contribute to increased comfort for the mother. Anticipatory guidance can reduce some of the stress and fears of pregnancy and may prevent the development of a disordered mother-child relationship during the neonatal period. Animal studies on the effects of emotional stress and disturbances in pregnancy and the subsequent dysfunctional mother-child relationships have been reported in the literature. However, there is a lack of data supporting a cause-and-effect relation in women. Most studies of human subjects are carried out on a retrospective basis and it is difficult to measure the degree and duration of stress.

Parent prenatal education classes are most helpful in allaying fears and afford additional opportunities for guidance. Parents will easily discern that other couples have some of the same questions for which answers are needed. To be able to identify with other couples is important. Topics that are usually covered in parent education programs include physical changes in pregnancy, nutrition, hygiene, preparation for labor and delivery, and care of the neonate. There is little doubt that when parents are prepared with adequate information their experiences are less traumatic than when they are left to the fantasies of morbid imaginings.

In the early weeks of pregnancy the mother is interested in changes in her own body. A well-fitting brassiere plus a pretty maternity dress aid the expectant mother's morale as well as help her to feel more comfortable. Later, when she is more conscious of the growing fetus, she is interested in knowing about the development of the fetus, how the infant will be born, and what a neonate looks like.

The mother needs to decide whether she will breast- or bottle-feed the infant. If the mother does not wish to breast-feed the infant, she should not be urged to do so or made to feel guilty. If this is her choice, she needs to become familiar with the technique of bottle-feeding, formula making, and terminal sterilization. (See pp. 68 and 73.) If her choice is breast-feeding, then she needs instruction in breast care and breast-feeding. (See pp. 66 and 67.)

Supplies for the neonate (undershirts, diapers, blankets, and crib) and supplies for herself to take to the hospital need discussion. Planning needs to be done concerning the care of the older siblings when the mother is in the hospital as well as when she first returns home. In addition, the mother needs assistance herself on her return from the hospital. She will need additional rest and is not ready to fully assume a role of wife, housekeeper, and mother.

Sibling preparation

The preparation of the children in the family for the arrival of a new infant has a bearing on the future relationships of the siblings to the child. Whatever information is given to siblings should be in accord with their interest and ability to understand. For a 2-year-old, the explanation that he is going to have a new brother or sister has limited meaning. The explanation should not be given more than a few weeks prior to the event. The small child may like to put his hand on the mother's abdomen and feel the baby move. He can be shown supplies for the infant and be told that the infant will sleep a lot, has to be carried, and cannot talk yet. The young child needs to be prepared for the fact that his mother will be away for a few days in the hospital. If he is the only sibling, this could be particularly distressing. Before the new baby arrives, the young child (and/or other children in the family) should have the experience of being alone with the person who will care for them while the mother is away. Of course, if a sibling is sleeping in the same room with the parents, he should be moved into another room several months before the arrival of the new infant.

Older children may help in cleaning the baby bed, selection of supplies, and preparing the room. In this way the siblings will feel they are part of the big event and important to the little newcomer. So much has been written about the jealously of other siblings toward the infant that the nurse may need to be reminded that sometimes older children look forward and are excited about a new brother or sister. When the infant does arrive, sometimes they are so proud that they show him off to all their friends. They want them to see and admire the new family treasure. They like their new possession.

Sometimes a teenager may be embarrassed by the mother's appearance and, depending on his total attitude toward sex, may take a negative view of the process of pregnancy and birth. If the mother gives additional attention to her grooming and dressing, this may help her to be more attractive to her teen-ager. This may be an excellent period to reeducate the boy or girl in understanding sex and related matters. Books give knowledge, but only through discussion can attitudes be clarified or changed. The nurse may be a resource person for the mother, or she may talk with the teenager herself. Sometimes both courses may be advisable, depending on the situation. The pregnancy of the mother can be pointed out to the adolescent boy or girl as the outcome of love that should continue as long as the parents live. Young people who have seen demonstrations of affection between parents and signs of their mutual thoughtfulness may accept pregnancy of the mother in a more matter-of-fact way. The evidence that their parents are lovers does not come as a shock.

If the adolescent in the family is given specific responsibility in household tasks to help his mother as well as some responsibility in gathering equipment together for the baby it may make him feel important. This places him in the role of a responsible person.

Health supervision

The goal of prenatal care is a gestation during which emotional and physical discomfort are minimized, terminating with a healthy mother delivering a well-developed, healthy neonate under optimal conditions. Ancillary goals include the integration of sound health practices acquired during pregnancy into continuing family life.

To increase the probability of goal achievement, clinical prenatal care and medical supervision are essential. The following is simply a brief outline of what is included in such care. (For details consult a textbook on maternity nursing listed in the References.)

The number of visits made to a clinic or to a physician's office vary widely. However, there is agreement that the first visit should be made as soon as pregnancy is suspected. This visit will include a comprehensive health history, a complete physical examination, and laboratory diagnostic and screening procedures. Results of the examination and laboratory findings give direction for continuing care. Instructions are given regarding reportable signs and symptoms and information about the course of pregnancy as a point for anticipatory guidance. Plans are made for follow-up appointments and for enrolling in prenatal or expectant parents' classes.

Follow-up appointments are scheduled on a planned basis. The visits should incude, as a minimum, general physical assessment, determination of nutritional status, evaluation of fetal growth and activity, measurement of vital signs, and routine laboratory procedures. Informal interviewing techniques are used to identify intervening problems and make value judgments as to the need for referral to another medical service or to a social agency. During these visits the nurse should establish and maintain her role as a person with whom the pregnant woman can communicate.

The study of Lesser and Keane (1956) indicated that women were well satisfied with the technical care they received during pregnancy, labor, and delivery; however, their emotional and informational needs were not as well met. Progress has been made in the area of support functions of nursing personnel, but nurses have not developed the same level of competence in interpersonal skills as they have in technical skills. This is a goal toward which nursing practice is being directed.

Communication

Communication is more than the transmission of an idea. It involves the accurate interpretation of the message by a receiver. One usually thinks in terms of words, spoken and written, as the form of communication in the nurse-patient relationship; however, accurate perception may depend on nonverbal behavior. Body movements, posture, and facial expressions convey messages that sometimes contradict the verbal expression. The nurse who tells a patient that she is interested and has time to listen but keeps checking her watch is transmitting conflicting messages.

Open-ended comments and questions encourage expression and ask for description. Such a comment would be "Tell me about it." Sometimes a simple exclamation as "Oh" or the nodding of the head indicates attention or concern and encourages the patient to continue speaking. Reflective techniques are useful in promoting communication. Both content and feeling can be reflected. In reflecting content the nurse uses the patient's words. The patient may say, "I feel sick." The nurse seeks further elaboration by responding, "You feel sick?" If an emotional tone is discerned, the feeling may be reflected rather than the content. The statement "I feel sick" may be accompanied by behavior that indicates that the discomfort is not physical. The response may then be, "You seem upset; what happened?"

In an attempt to open communications the nurse may share her perceptions with the patient. After perceiving that a patient's hands are shaking the nurse may think the patient is cold, nervous, or agitated. She interprets the behavior in a way that may or may not be accurate. She may say to the patient, "Your hands are shaking; what is the matter?" If the patient does not respond, the nurse may follow up with her thoughts: "I thought you might be cold."

It must be remembered that communication techniques are tools, not ends in themselves. They are used in achieving the goals of the nurse-patient relationship.

One form of communication used frequently in nursing is the interview. It has been defined as conversation with a purpose and a direction. The uses of the interview are manifold. It is used to obtain information, to give information, to provide opportunity for expression of feelings, to identify needs, to clarify goals, to teach, and to counsel. Frequently these interviews are structured, particularly information-gathering interviews to obtain patient medical and social histories. Most agencies have forms printed for use so that all pertinent information will be sought. (For details on interviewing refer to a text on interviewing listed in the References.)

Drugs

Many drugs have been implicated in adverse outcomes of pregnancy. Although therapeutic substances are seldom administered directly to the fetus, there is a route of access through the placenta. Most drugs cross the placental barrier, and it is important for nurses to realize that most women take medication while they are pregnant. A large percentage of the medications are self-prescribed and are taken without medical supervision or knowledge. There are few innocuous drugs. Even aspirin in dosages of 20 gr. daily in the last weeks of pregnancy has been the causative agent of hemorrhagic problems in the neonate.

Certain drugs administered to pregnant women during the period of organogenesis have been proven to be teratogenic. The most widely publicized of these drugs is thalidomide, which induced phocomelia in the fetus. Therapeutic agents such as methotrexate, which is used in cancer therapy, distort the fetal growth pattern. Aminopterin, a folic acid antagonist used in the treatment of leukemia, induces abortion. During the fetal period, drugs administered to the mother may alter or modify the growth of a structurally intact fetus. Medications that are used in the treatment of thyroid dysfunction such as thiouracil and the iodides are responsible for neonates with hypothyroidism and neonatal goiter. Warfarin derivatives administered during pregnancy as anticoagulation therapy are associated with intrauterine hemorrhage and fetal loss. Thiazide diuretics are related to neonatal thrombocytopenia.

Some drugs administered during labor or immediately preceding labor may have little or no effect on the neonate. Other drugs produce serious effects. Drugs that can be hazardous to the neonate fall into numerous categories such as analgesics, anesthetics, antibiotics, hypnotics, muscle relaxants, antihypertensives, and chemotherapeutic agents.

It should be remembered that pregnancy does not confer immunity to medical diseases, and medications may be thoroughly indicated and their use unavoidable. These drugs are administered under strict medical supervision.

The preceding paragraphs give examples of drugs that produce adverse effects in the fetus. Nurses have the responsibility of keeping themselves informed as to the action, side effects, and limitations in use of all drugs that they are administering to patients. Nurses are referred to the American Medical Association drug evaluation texts, which are updated annually.

Infections

Maternal infections that affect the fetus in utero may be bacterial, protozoal, spirochetal, or viral. Transmission to the fetus may occur in either of two ways. First, the organism may be carried by the maternal bloodstream through the placenta to the fetus. Second, the organism may ascend through the cervix into the amniotic fluid.

Defense against infection in the fetus is dependent upon maternal IgG (immune globulin G) antibodies, which cross the placenta. Some IgM (immune globulin M) antibodies are produced by the fetus in the presence of infection. The maternal antibodies provide immunity to many infections, particularly those that are viral.

Rubella

Of the viral infections rubella has been given the most emphasis because of the teratogenic effects on the fetus when the disease is contracted by the mother prior to the sixteenth week of gestation. Different organs are vulnerable to infection at various times during early pregnancy, and there appears to be a relationship between anomalies and the time of organogenesis. Cardiac defects and eye lesions are found to be associated with maternal rubella during the first 8 weeks of pregnancy. Hearing defects are associated with the infection during the fifth to the twelfth weeks of pregnancy. There is an increased incidence of fetal loss, abortion, and stillbirth associated with maternal rubella. It may be well to remember that severe maternal infections of any type may result in fetal loss.

Cytomegalic inclusion virus

Cytomegalic inclusion virus infections are usually asymptomatic, and it is difficult to correlate fetal anomalies with such infections. In instances of known infections there is an increased incidence of neonates of low birth weight, microcephaly, mental retardation, hepatosplenomegaly, motor dysfunction, choroidoretinitis, and jaundice. Usually only some of the defects are present in each case.

Other viral diseases

Fetal loss and placental and fetal infection occur with influenza, poliomyelitis, herpes simplex, varicella, infection with coxsackievirus B, rubeola, variola, and vaccinia. Vari-

cella in the last days of pregnancy causes a high fetal mortality.

Syphilis

Treponema pallidum, the causative organism of syphilis, crosses the placenta and can affect the fetus. Seldom, if ever, can the fetus be affected prior to the fourth lunar month of gestation. Spirochetes have not been found in tissue of abortuses of less than 18 weeks gestation. A barrier to *T. pallidum* is created by the Langhans layer of the chorion, which disappears by the sixteenth week of pregnancy.

Adequate treatment of syphilis in the mother usually cures the disease, and since antibiotics cross the placenta the fetus is also cured. Even with the ability to detect and treat the disease, there is an alarming increase in the prevalence of untreated syphilis. Untreated syphilis in gravid women results in stillbirths at a rate of 30%. The other 70% will be liveborn neonates with the disease. Symptoms of congenital syphilis are manifested in only severe infections. Usually the neonate appears healthy at birth, and the symptoms of the disease appear between the second and sixth week of life. Onset of symptoms may be delayed for a year or longer with the disease remaining in a dormant or latent phase.

Radiation

In obstetrics the most common source of concentrated radiation is from diagnostic procedures, which include chest x-ray films and pelvimetry. Although medical use of radiological procedures may result in deleterious mutations, it does not mean that the use of x-ray procedures should be discouraged. It does mean that the dangers must be weighed against the need before a medical judgment is made. Chest x-ray films in pregnancy are a part of the routine protocol in many clinics. This procedure detects four times the incidence of lung pathology, particularly tuberculosis, that can be diagnosed by history and physical alone. Chest x-ray films should be delayed until the first trimester of pregnancy is completed. X-radiation interrupts the process of mitosis, and the first trimester is a period of rapid cell division and cell differentiation. Precautions should be taken to shield the maternal abdomen from large doses of x-rays, thereby protecting the gonads of both the mother and the fetus.

X-ray pelvimetry as a routine procedure has been discouraged, but it is indicated in many instances to reduce the hazards of traumatic labor and delivery for mothers and fetuses.

There is a trend toward the use of ultrasonic radiation in pregnancy. With the use of this technique there have been no deleterious effects on fetal development reported. However, it must be remembered that x-radiation was used for many years before some of the harmful effects were identified.

Complications of pregnancy

The complications of pregnancy may be categorized as those associated with pregnancy and those coincidental to pregnancy. A classification of conditions that place the fetus and the neonate at high risk can be found in Table 2-1. The brief descriptions of the complications of pregnancy will be directed toward their effects on the fetus and the neonate.

Toxemia

When the term *toxemia* is used it usually refers to preeclampsia, which may be mild to severe. Preeclampsia is a hypertensive disease that occurs after the twentieth week of pregnancy and in puerperal women. The disease is characterized by one or more of the following symptoms: sudden and rapid rise in blood pressure, edema, and proteinuria. The most severe form of the disease is termed eclampsia. In addition to the triad of hypertension, edema, and proteinuria there are convulsions and coma.

The outcome for the fetus is dependent on the

Table 2-1. High-risk infants*

Family history	*Present pregnancy—cont'd*
Presence of mutant genes	Anesthesia
Central nervous system disorders	Maternal rubella in first trimester
Low socioeconomic group	Diabetes
Previous defective sibling	Toxemia
Parental consanguinity	Fetal-maternal blood group incompatibility
Intrafamilial emotional disorder	*Labor and delivery*
Medical history of mother	Absence of prenatal care
Diabetes	Prematurity
Hypertension	Postmaturity or dysmaturity
Radiation	Precipitate, prolonged, or complicated delivery
Cardiovascular or renal disease	Low Apgar score—5 minutes
Thyroid disease	*Placenta*
Idiopathic thrombocytopenic purpura	Massive infarction
Previous obstetrical history of mother	Amnion nodosum
Toxemia	Placentitis
Miscarriage immediately preceding pregnancy	*Neonate*
Size of infants	Single umbilical artery
High parity	Jaundice
Prolonged infertility	Head size
Present pregnancy	Infection
Maternal age <16 or >35	Hypoxia
Multiple births	Severe dehydration, hyperosmolarity, and hypernatremia
Polyhydramnios	Convulsions
Pyelonephritis	Failure to regain birth weight by 10 days
Out-of-wedlock pregnancy	Manifest congenital defects
Oligohydramnios	Disproportion between weight or length and gestational age
Medications	Survival following meningitides, encephalopathies, and
Radiations	traumatic intracranial episodes

*Adapted from Proceedings of the White House Conference on Mental Retardation, Washington, D.C., 1963; from the American Medical Association: Mental retardation—a handbook for the primary physician, J.A.M.A. **191:**183, 1965.

period of pregnancy in which the disease appears and on its severity. Since the most effective treatment in severe preeclampsia and eclampsia is the termination of the pregnancy, much of the perinatal mortality is caused by prematurity. However, it must be recognized that a controlled external environment for the neonate is more conducive to survival than an intrauterine environment that may induce fetal distress.

Although the etiology of the disease is unknown, the magnitude of maternal and fetal loss can be diminished through conscientious and thorough prenatal supervision directed toward prevention, early detection, and intervention.

Hemorrhage

Hemorrhage in the second half of pregnancy is usually caused by abruptio placentae or placenta previa. Abruptio placentae is the premature separation of a normally implanted placenta from the uterine wall. In placenta previa the placenta is implanted in the lower uterine segment contiguous to or overlying the internal cervical os. As in toxemia, the fetal outcome is dependent upon the time of onset and the extent of the process. Premature delivery is often forced by the degree of hemorrhage. Delay in definitive treatment in the presence of extensive hemorrhage results in in impaired fetal circulation, fetal anoxia, and intrauterine fetal death.

Diabetes mellitus

Maternal diabetes has deleterious effects on pregnancy, the fetus, and the neonate. In addition to the problem of maintaining stability in the diabetic status of the mother, problems in the management of pregnancy occur. There is an increased incidence of preeclampsia, eclampsia, hydramnios, and cesarean section associated with diabetes in pregnancy. There is a high incidence of intrauterine fetal death after the thirty-sixth week of gestation and a high neonatal mortality. Birth injuries occur more frequently as a result of disproportion between fetal size and maternal pelvis due to fetal macrosomia. The neonate tends to be large and plump with plethoric facies. Fat rather than

fluid retention increases body weight. One theory for the increased size of the neonate born to the diabetic mother is that fetal hyperinsulinism is the response to maternal hyperglycemia. The hypoglycemia in the neonate is believed to be caused by inadequate stores of glycogen as a result of fetal hyperinsulinism. Constant observation must be maintained for cyanosis, respiratory distress, hypoglycemia, and convulsions, which are not uncommon in the neonate of the diabetic mother.

Heart disease

Maternal heart disease usually has little direct effect on the fetus. However, rheumatic heart disease is the fourth leading cause of maternal death following toxemia, hemorrhage, and infection. The incidence of this disease is decreasing, and with careful assessment of cardiac status early in pregnancy, together with sound medical management, the gestation can be uneventful. The risk to the mother is proportional to the gravity of the heart lesion.

NATAL INFLUENCES

A comprehensive presentation of the course of labor will not be undertaken here. The following paragraphs will be directed toward those intrapartum factors that have a direct effect on the neonate.

Labor

The average duration of labor in the primiparous patient is between 14 and 16 hours; in the multiparous patient this time is reduced to between 8 and 10 hours. Continuation of labor to 24 hours or longer is termed protracted or prolonged labor and may induce anoxia and asphyxia in the fetus. Rapid or precipitous labor and delivery can also have adverse effects on the neonate. The most common problem encountered as a result of precipitous delivery is intracranial hemorrhage. Frequently, in an attempt to delay delivery until the physician is prepared, undue pressure is exerted on the fetal head, which may result in fetal bradycardia and anoxia.

Stages of labor

Several theories have been proposed to explain the onset of labor, not one of which fully explains the phenomenon. Uterine distension and hydrostatic pressure, progesterone deprivation, increased oxytocin production, and localized progesterone activity have each been proposed as the initiating cause. Although the cause is still to be determined, the process or the pattern of labor can be described.

Labor is divided into three stages. The first stage is the stage of dilatation. It is defined as beginning with regular and rhythmical contractions of the uterus and ending with complete dilatation and effacement of the cervix. The second stage, the stage of expulsion, begins with complete dilatation and effacement of the cervix and ends with the delivery of the neonate. The third stage is the placental stage; it is defined as the time between the delivery of the neonate and the expulsion of the placenta.

Course of labor

The course of labor is influenced by the general health of the mother, the size of her pelvis, the size of the fetus, and fetal presentation and position. These factors can be determined and evaluated for their effects prior to the onset of active labor. Contributing factors that cannot readily be determined are pain threshold, interpretation of pain, fear, and tension. Without intervention that supports and promotes the comfort of the mother a vicious cycle of fear inducing tension, tension causing pain, and pain causing fear is established. This cycle can inhibit the progress of labor and evoke a negative response from the mother toward her husband, the fetus, and the care giver. Women in labor should not be left alone; they should have the attention of someone who is supportive and able to assist them to cope with labor. Fathers who are prepared and are able to cope with the stress of labor can provide much of the supportive care needed by the woman in labor.

Presentation and position

Presentation is a term used to designate that part of the fetus presenting at the internal cervical os. Cephalic presentations are the most common, occurring in approximately 97% of all term deliveries. Cephalic presentations may be grouped into three categories: vertex, face, and brow presentations. The vertex presentation is the most common, followed by face and then brow presentations. A brow presentation usually results in dysfunctional labor and an operative delivery (cesarean section).

Breech presentations are next in the order of frequency, occurring in about 3% of deliveries. Early and accurate pelvimetry is essential for the proper management of a breech delivery since a trial of labor cannot be permitted without assurance that the fetus can negotiate the maternal pelvis. The neonate delivered in the breech presentation is at higher risk of cerebral and liver damage.

Transverse or shoulder presentations are the least common and are relatively rare. They are associated with atonia or hypotonia of the abdominal musculature, pelvic contractions, and placenta previa. It is virtually impossible to deliver a fully developed fetus without an operative procedure.

Position is defined as the relationship of some predetermined, arbitrarily selected part of the fetus to the quadrants of the mother's pelvis. Position may be anterior, posterior, or transverse. The anterior positions usually pose no problems; however, the transverse and posterior positions associated with vertex presentations contribute to prolonged labor that increases the probability of intracranial hemorrhage and fetal anoxia.

Fetal size

Fetal size in relation to the mother's pelvis is important not only from the standpoint of duration of labor but also from the standpoint of increased probability of birth injuries as a result of dystocia. When the fetal head is large in proportion to the pelvis, traumatic intracranial hemorrhage and linear skull fractures may occur. There may be injuries to the spine, spinal cord, and peripheral nerves; fractures and dislocations of bones are not uncommon. Surgical intervention by cesarean section is the mode of delivery for cephalopelvic disproportion.

Fetal monitoring

Until recently the only means of monitoring the fetus was abdominal palpation and auscultation. Auscultation of fetal heart rate by the traditional method of a fetoscope, a head stethoscope, cannot be accomplished until about the twentieth week of gestation when the heart tones become audible. Even with the use of head stethoscope, it is sometimes difficult to differentiate fetal heart tones from the pulsation of the maternal abdominal aorta. Recently several instruments have been developed to detect fetal heart action as early as the end of the first trimester of pregnancy or thirteen weeks of gestation. Such instruments utilize the Doppler principles of ultrasound. The shift in the frequency of moving blood cells is detected by a receiving crystal, which is adjacent to a transmitting crystal. The sounds of fetal pulsation are audible, can be magnified, and can be differentiated from the pulsation of the mother. Commercial instruments such as the Doptone and the Ultradop are of value in monitoring fetal heart rates in pregnancies complicated by hydramnios and maternal obesity. External monitoring as currently practiced is usually sufficient for low-risk patients. Should fetal distress be anticipated, reliable electronic instruments have been developed to provide the physician with precise visual recordings of the pattern and intensity of uterine pressure during contractions and the effect of the pressure on the fetal heart rate patterns. Fetal membranes are ruptured, and a fetal blood sample may be taken to determine the acid-base balance. A scalp electrode is applied, and attachment of the electronic recording device provides permanent visual tracings of contractions and fetal heart beats for comparative study.

In addition to no change in heart rate and change that is coincidental to uterine contraction three patterns of heart rate change have been identified: early, late, and variable deceleration. Early deceleration shows fetal heart rate slowing before the onset of contraction and is thought to occur as a result of compression of the fetal head and does not signify fetal distress. In late deceleration patterns the slowing pattern persists after cessation of the contraction. Variable deceleration patterns are a combination of early and late patterns. Late and variable patterns are indicative of fetal distress, and fetal outcome can be correlated with the intensity and duration of the patterns.

Accurate interpretation of the monitoring will result in improvement in fetal morbidity and mortality. Fetal monitoring is becoming a necessary adjunct to the management of the high-risk patient.

Analgesia and anesthesia

Labor and delivery are usually painful, and since pain is unpleasant and undesirable there is need for relief. The use of narcotics, sedatives, and anesthetics in labor and delivery remains a controversial subject.

Analgesic drugs such as meperidine are used in labor. These drugs readily cross the placenta to the fetus, who may retain a significant proportion of the drug. There is a strong correlation between administration of narcotic drugs and depressed Apgar scores. Although there is controversy, some studies indicate that even with fetal depression there is no correlation of perinatal mortality with the administration of predelivery narcotics.

Until recently the most frequently used medication in labor was a combination of a narcotic drug for its analgesic effect and scopolomine for its amnesic effect. Scopolomine in the presence of pain causes varying degrees of restlessness, excitement, and oblivion. More recently, tranquilizing drugs such as promethazine (Phenergan), hydroxyzine (Vistaril), and diazepam (Valium) are being used in conjunction with a narcotic such as meperidine (Demerol). Once labor is established with progressive dilatation and effacement of the cervix associated with regularity in contractions, analgesia is indicated unless the mother has expressed the wish and is well prepared for natural childbirth methods.

A narcotic antagonist such as nalorphine administered to the mother in combination with the narcotic appears to have insufficient effect in preventing respiratory depression in the neonate. More effective use of narcotic antagonists is achieved when they are administered to the neonate.

Regional blocks with local anesthetic agents have become widely used in this country. They can provide adequate analgesia, do not affect the progress of labor, and in controlled dosages will not depress the mother or the fetus. Lumbar epidural and caudal anesthesia are usually administered by continuous method and are used during labor and in nonmanipulative deliveries. Once administered, saddle blocks or low spinal anesthesia are effective from 1 to 3 hours. The abdomen below the umbilicus and the lower extremities lose sensation. The mother is not able to use the voluntary muscles of the abdomen to assist in the expulsion of the fetus. Delivery is usually accomplished with the use of low forceps. Pudendal blocks are usually done immediately prior to delivery to produce anesthesia of the perineum in preparation for episiotomy. Injection of the pudendal nerve with the local anesthetic agent can be done either transvaginally or through the skin surfaces. Paracervical block is done in the later phase of the first stage of labor for its analgesic effects. Bradycardia in the fetus has been noted with the use of paracervical blocks.

Volatile anesthetics such as ether, chloroform, and trichlorethylene readily cross the placenta and are capable of producing narcosis in the fetus. Gaseous anesthetics such as nitrous oxide and cyclopropane are used in varying degrees. Nitrous oxide with oxygen is often used intermittently with contractions as a form of analgesia. Cyclopropane produces rapid relaxation of abdominal muscles and has been known to produce laryngospasm in the mother. Prolonged use of cyclopropane depresses the respiratory center of the fetus. A light, balanced general anesthetic of halothane and nitrous oxide is used in manipulative procedures for the duration of need for uterine relaxation.

Delivery

The technique employed in delivery has a direct bearing on the fetal outcome. Knowledge of the fetal position and presentation is essential in determining the type of delivery that is undertaken. Low forceps deliveries are done to shorten the second stage of labor, to protect the fetal head from pressure of a resistant perineum, and to protect the maternal perineum from injury by prolonged distension. An episiotomy is usually done in conjunction with the application of forceps and enhances the probability of achieving these goals.

Spontaneous delivery must be a controlled delivery to prevent "popping" of the head of the fetus. Rapid and sudden change of pressure on the head may result in intracranial hemorrhage. Undue manipulation of the body of the neonate during the delivery should be avoided to prevent skeletal and nerve injury. Recognition of signs of distress in either the mother or the fetus and rapid intervention may be the difference between the delivery of a healthy neonate and a brain-damaged one.

SUMMARY

Health workers in the area of maternal and child health must recognize that the health of infants and children is influenced even before they are conceived. Nurses in particular must be ready to assume leadership roles in stimulating action toward early and continued health supervision of children long before they are ready to assume the responsibilities of parenthood. Sound health practices must be instituted early and continue throughout life.

Once conception has occurred and health supervision is sought nurses have a unique opportunity to explore parents' feelings toward pregnancy and to give anticipatory guidance and information on the course of pregnancy, nutrition, labor, delivery, and child care. Pregnancy offers an opportunity to improve nutrition for the pregnant woman as well as her family through the incorporation of principles of sound nutrition into family living.

During the process of labor and delivery the nurse assumes the supportive role. She is ever conscious of the need to monitor the progress of the labor and the effects of labor on the fetus. The nurse is responsible for being well informed so that appropriate plans for nursing management can be carried out.

REFERENCES

Apgar, V.: Drugs in pregnancy, Am. J. Nurs. **65:**104, March, 1965.

Bermosk, L., and Mordan, M. J.: Interviewing in nursing, New York, 1964, The Macmillan Co.

Broderick, C., and Bernard, J., editors: The individual, sex and society, Baltimore, 1969, The Johns Hopkins University Press.

Buxton, C. L.: A study of psychophysical methods for relief of childbirth pain, Philadelphia, 1962, W. B. Saunders Co.

Caplan, G.: An approach to community mental health, New York, 1961, Grune & Stratton, Inc.

Caplan, G.: Concepts of mental health and consultation, Washington, D.C., 1969, U.S. Department of Health, Education, and Welfare.

Chinn, P.: Child health maintenance: Concepts in family centered care, St. Louis, 1974, The C. V. Mosby Co.

Clausen, J., et al.: Maternity nursing today, New York, 1973, McGraw-Hill Book Co.

Committee on Maternal Health of the National Research Council: Maternal nutrition and the course of human pregnancy, Washington, D.C., 1970, National Academy of Sciences.

Committee on Nutrition, American College of Obstetricians and Gynecologists: Nutrition in maternal health care, New York, 1974, American College of Obstetricians and Gynecologists.

Czalnecki, L.: The integration of sex education in pediatric nursing practice, Pediatr. Nurs. **2:**12, March-April, 1976.

Davis, E. M., and Rubin, R.: DeLee's obstetrics for nurses, ed. 18, Philadelphia, 1966, W. B. Saunders Co.

Fitzpatrick, E., et al.: Maternity nursing, ed. 12, Philadelphia, 1971, J. B. Lippincott Co.

Gadpaille, W.: Parent-school cooperation in sex-education. How can the professional help? Family Coordinator, **19:**30, October, 1970.

Garrett, A.: Interviewing: Its principles and methods, New York, 1970, Family Service Association of America.

Gifford, F. B., et al., editors: A handbook of prenatal paediatrics, Philadelphia, 1971, J. B. Lippincott Co.

Gordis, L., et al.: Adolescent pregnancy: A hospital-based program for primary prevention, Am. J. Public Health **58:**849, May, 1968.

Gordon, S.: The sexual adolescent: Communicating with teenagers about sex, N. Scituate, Mass., 1973, Duxbury Press.

Harter, C., and Parrish, V.: Maternal preference of socialization agent for sex education, J. Marriage Family **30:** 423, 1968.

Hellman, L., and Pritchard, J.: Williams' obstetrics, ed. 14, New York, 1971, Appleton-Century-Crofts.

Hillsman, G.: Genetics and the nurse, Nurs. Outlook **14:** 34, January, 1966.

Hoff, F.: Natural childbirth: How any nurse can help, Am. J. Nurs. **69:**1451, July, 1969.

Kahn, R., and Cannel, C.: The dynamics of interviewing, New York, 1964, John Wiley & Sons, Inc.

Kirkendall, L., and Cox, H.: Starting a sex-education program, Children **14:**136, August, 1967.

Lasater, C.: Electronic monitoring of mother and fetus, Am. J. Nurs. **72:**728, April, 1972.

Lesser, M., and Keane, V.: Nurse-patient relationship in hospital maternity service, St. Louis, 1956, The C. V. Mosby Co.

Lussier, R.: Health education and student needs, J. School Health **42:**618, December, 1972.

Masters, W. H., and Johnson, V. E.: Human sexual response, Boston, 1966, Little, Brown & Co.

McCarey, Y. L.: Human sexuality, New York, 1967, D. Van Nostrand Co.

Nitowsky, H.: Prenatal diagnosis of genetic abnormality, Am. J. Nurs. **71:**1551, August, 1971.

Reed, S.: Parenthood and heredity, New York, 1964, John Wiley & Sons, Inc.

Robinson, C.: Normal and therapeutic nutrition, ed. 14, New York, 1972, The Macmillan Co.

Sasmor, J. L.: The childbirth team during labor, Am. J. Nurs. **73:**444, March, 1973.

Shertzer, B., and Stone, S.: Fundamentals of counseling, Boston, 1968, Houghton-Mifflin Co.

Thompson, J., and Thompson, M.: Genetics in medicine, ed. 2., Philadelphia, 1973, W. B. Saunders Co.

Wallace, H., et al., editors: Maternal and child health practices, Springfield, Ill., 1973, Charles C Thomas, Publisher.

Wiedenbach, E.: Family-centered maternity nursing, New York, 1967, G. P. Putnam's Sons.

Wiedenbach, E.: Genetics and the nurse, Bull. Am. Coll. Nurse-Midwifery, **13:**8, May, 1968.

Williams, B., and Richards, S.: Fetal monitoring during labor, Am. J. Nurs. **70:**2384, November, 1970.

Woody, J.: Contemporary sex-education: Attitudes and implications for childrearing, J. School Health **43:**241, April, 1973.

Ziegel, E., and VanBlarcom, C.: Obstetric nursing, ed. 6, New York, 1972, The Macmillan Co.

3

NUTRITION DURING PREGNANCY AND LACTATION

JOYCE A. VERMEERSCH, Dr.P.H.

The aim of nutrition during pregnancy and lactation, like that of all maternal and infant care, is to provide all the advantages possible that will promote a normal course of pregnancy for the mother, produce a viable infant, and give him a healthy start in life. We will examine in this chapter some of the effects of nutrition on the outcome of pregnancy, nutrient needs and counseling principles for pregnant and lactating women, and some dietary implications of complicating conditions. Although the discussion is directed toward pregnancy and lactation, it should be kept in mind as you read subsequent chapters of this book that the underlying principles of the dietary recommendations we shall discuss apply throughout the life cycle. All people, regardless of age, sex, or physical condition, need the same nutrients to promote growth and optimum health—only the amounts of these nutrients differ from person to person and from time to time. Discovering how the nutrients function in growth, health, and disease is what the science of nutrition is all about.

As nurses move into expanded roles in obstetrical and pediatric care, they will have an increasing responsibility for nutritional guidance of their patients. Monitoring nutritional status, recognizing nutritional problems, and providing dietary advice are only a few of the many functions nurses perform, but they are among the most important where the patient's welfare is concerned. In many settings dietitians and nutritionists will be available to help the nurse, and the services of these persons should be freely used. Ideally the nurse should seek the assistance of the dietitian whenever a patient presents a potential nutritional risk.

Unfortunately dietitians are not always available; even where they are, the nurse is often the patient's first contact with the health care system, and she has a responsibility for coordinating his care. If the nurse is unable to recognize a nutritional problem, the condition may never receive the attention it requires. For these reasons it is essential that the nurse have a good understanding of the principles of nutrition and its importance in the maintenance of health.

NUTRITION AND THE OUTCOME OF PREGNANCY

What difference does nutrition make in the pregnant woman's obstetrical performance and the condition of her infant at birth? Answers to this question have frequently been contradictory and confusing. In the 1940's, when studies indicated that the difference was significant indeed, much attention and enthusiasm were accorded diet during pregnancy. Then in the 1950's, when more carefully controlled investigations tended to produce equivocal results, enthusiasm waned toward indifference and neglect.

Looking back we can now see that much of the confusion stemmed from methodological difficulties that are inevitable in studies designed for clinical trials. But, more important, we have learned how unreasonable it is to expect a simple, clear-cut answer to a question that is immeasurably complex.

Nonetheless, the studies are important for the light they shed on some of the misunderstandings that have surrounded dietary recommendations over the years. In general they fall into three categories: (1) studies of the effects of dietary intake during pregnancy, (2) studies of indirect nutritional indices such as maternal height, prepregnancy weight, and weight gain, and (3) most recently studies focusing on the effects of maternal and fetal nutrition at the cellular level.

Dietary intake

Many studies during the 1940's and early 1950's were concerned with the effects of diet on the immediate outcomes of pregnancy: the incidence of spontaneous abortions, stillbirths, prematurity, and maternal complications of labor and delivery. The factor that has received most of the attention has been low birth weight because of its association with increased risks of neonatal death, congenital malformations, and mental retardation. The questions that many of the studies sought to answer were: Do poor diets in pregnant women result in higher rates of low birth weight and other undesirable outcomes? and Can good diets prevent these problems and lower the rates?

The deprivations of war afforded researchers an opportunity to study the first of these questions under conditions that could not be duplicated in the laboratory. Throughout much of Europe at various times during World War II food shortages were commonplace. An 18-month period of acute starvation was experienced in Russia during the siege of Leningrad in 1942. By comparing statistics for infants born before and during the siege, Antonov (1947) was able to show a doubling of the fetal mortality rate and an increase in the number of infants weighing 2,500 gm. or less at birth during the famine period.

Similar findings were reported by Smith (1947) from Holland. Here the results are more provocative because the famine was sharply demarcated and limited to approximately 6 months during the winter of 1944 and 1945. It was not accompanied by other hardships as severe as those experienced during the siege of Leningrad, and the women of Holland were considered to have eaten fairly good diets prior to the food shortage. During the famine, however, calorie intake dropped to less than 1,000 per day and protein intake was between 30 and

40 gm. Since the famine lasted only 6 months, fetuses conceived before and during it were exposed for varying lengths of time but none were exposed for the entire course of gestation. Thus Smith was able to consider the question of *when* poor nutrition during pregnancy would produce its most adverse effects.

The statistics showed that average birth weights decreased about 10%. Weights were lowest for infants exposed to the famine during the entire last half of gestation. Added exposure prior to that time did not reduce birth weights further. In fact, infants who were exposed during the first 27 weeks but finished gestation after the famine ended had higher average birth weights than those who were only exposed during the last 3 weeks of gestation.

The data for other undesirable outcomes such as stillbirths and congenital malformations followed a different pattern. These rates were lowest for infants born during the famine and highest for those born after the famine ended.

Smith concluded that the effects of poor diet during pregnancy depend on the extent of poor intake and the period of gestation in which it occurs. Poor nutrition during the later part of pregnancy most likely affects fetal growth, whereas poor nutrition during the early months affects development of the fetus and its capacity to survive. Since an average 10% decrease in birth weight was not inordinately large, Smith thought that the preconceptional nutritional status of the mothers contributed significantly to the outcome of pregnancy.

It is interesting to note that in contrast to the experiences in Russia and Holland the perinatal mortality rate in Great Britain, which was fairly constant prior to 1939, actually declined during the war years 1940 to 1945 despite poor environmental conditions and no discernable changes in maternal care. One explanation is that pregnant and lactating women were accorded priority status under Britain's food rationing policy.

These and other wartime experiences lend support to what has long been known from animal studies, namely, that severe nutritional deficiencies during pregnancy will produce low birth weight and other abnormalities in the offspring. But they do not answer the more practical questions about the effects of poor nutrition short of outright starvation and short of the extreme physical and psychological adversities that accompany famine and war. In other words, what are the effects of nutrition under more normal circumstances?

The study of Burke et al. (1943) at the Boston Lying-In Hospital in the 1940's addressed the simple question of whether women who ate diets of different nutritional quality had different courses and outcomes of pregnancy. After obtaining dietary histories of 216 pregnant women, Burke and her associates rated the intakes as good, fair, poor, and very poor according to their conformity with the recommended dietary allowances. When the infants were born, obstetricians and pediatricians (without knowing the mothers' diet ratings) were asked to rate the course of pregnancy and the condition of the infants at birth. When the ratings were compared, there was a significant tendency for the rating of the mother's diet and the rating of her infant to correspond; that is, the higher the diet rating, the better the condition of the infant at birth. A similar but less striking correspondence was noted for diets and ratings of the course of pregnancy.

More recently, Higgins at the Montreal Diet Dispensary conducted a study of the effects of supplementing poor diets with foods and counseling during pregnancy. Knowing the risk of poor pregnancy performance associated with low income, Higgins selected the hospital handling the highest percentage of poor patients in Montreal. All patients from two of the hospital's public maternity clinics were enrolled in the study—a total of 1,544 between 1963 and 1970. A unique feature was that dietary requirements for calories and protein were individually calculated for each woman based on her body weight with adjustments for protein deficiency (as revealed by dietary histories), underweight, and other stress conditions. Women whose family incomes fell short of specified levels (70% of all women in the study) were supplied with milk, eggs, and oranges every 2 weeks. All women received dietary counseling at each clinic visit, and nutritionists visited all the patients at home at least once during their pregnancies.

Such intensive efforts to assure adequate nutrition resulted in both the supplemented group and the instruction-only group averaging over 90% of their caloric and protein requirements. Since both groups started out with large average daily deficits, they showed significant gains.

The payoff is indicated by the birth statistics. The prematurity rate in the study group was equal to the all-Canada rate and lower than the rate for Quebec province. (Remember, the study group consisted of low income patients whose prematurity rates are usually much higher than rates for the general population.) Stillbirths and neonatal and perinatal mortality were all lower than the Canada and Quebec rates. The frequency of spontaneous deliveries versus those requiring cesarean section was higher in the study group compared to private patients and public patients not included in the study who delivered at the same hospital.

Higgins also found a direct relationship between maternal weight gain (average 26 pounds) and birth weights. These factors were also directly related to the length of time the women had received Diet Dispensary service. No such relationship between birth weights and length of service was observed for other public patients who were not part of the study.

Not all studies have been able to show such positive associations between diet and the outcome of pregnancy. The Vanderbilt Cooperative Study of Maternal and Infant Nutrition in the 1950's (McGanity et al., 1955) was a very carefully controlled study that examined over 2,000 women and their infants. It included biochemical tests and clinical examinations as well as assessment of dietary intakes to determine nutritional status. The mothers of low birth weight babies tended to have slightly lower blood levels of vitamin C and were more frequently designated as "undernourished" on clinical examination, but the researchers could find no other association between low birth weight or other fetal or maternal abnormalities and any other biochemical or dietary parameters. Twenty-seven percent of the mothers were given vitamin supplements during their pregnancies, and these were not shown to produce any significant improvements in performance or outcome.

In spite of these findings, the Vanderbilt group did not deny the importance of nutrition to the outcome of pregnancy. Instead, they took a view similar to Smith's and conceded that women who enter pregnancy in good nutritional status are less at risk than those whose pregnancy is superimposed on a lifetime of nutritional inadequacy. They further concluded that, with the possible exception of iron, routine vitamin supplementation during pregnancy does not produce benefits beyond those achieved from a nutritionally balanced diet.

Maternal height, weight, and weight gain

The implications of dietary studies during pregnancy led researchers to suspect that the role of nutrition in outcome might involve more than the 9 short months of gestation.

Thomson, who originally set out to answer a question quite similar to Burke's, could find no relation between infant birth weights and the pregnancy diets of the mothers he studied in Aberdeen, Scotland (Thomson, 1959; Thomson et al., 1963). Even though fewer low birth weight infants were born to mothers who had the highest caloric intakes during pregnancy, Thomson considered the association spurious because these mothers came from a higher social class and were taller and heavier than women who ate fewer calories and delivered low birth weight babies. A relationship that held even when controlled for the mother's weight was birth weight and maternal height.

Several other researchers have provided evidence that taller women have fewer low birth weight babies and fewer problems of pregnancy than short women do. This raises the old question of nature versus nurture. While ultimate stature may be determined by genetics, it is certainly true that a woman's ability to achieve her full potential is a product of diet and other environmental circumstances. The fact that adult women have already reached their maximum height by the time they enter pregnancy should not cause us to take a fatalistic view of the importance of nutrition to outcome. Rather, short-statured women, particularly from deprived socioeconomic groups, should be designated as potential risks. They

and their infants should receive priority attention and the best diets possible to counteract the consequences of earlier malnutrition and to break the cycle of childhood malnutrition and pregnancy wastage in later life.

A similar recommendation can be made for pregnant women who are underweight. A number of studies have shown that women who enter pregnancy at 10% or more below their desirable weight for height are at higher risk (for themselves and their infants) than women of normal weight and even those who are overweight.

The findings with perhaps the most significant immediate implications for obstetrical care are those related to maternal weight gain. In the United States and in other countries, it has frequently been the practice to restrict weight gain during pregnancy in the belief that this would prevent toxemia and other complications. The notion seems to have originated around the turn of the century with a German obstetrician who advocated weight restriction to produce a smaller baby that would be easier to deliver. The idea began to find its way into medical textbooks after World War I when, without further investigation to confirm the relationship, it was observed that the incidence of eclampsia had declined in Austria and Germany where diets were poor in war-scarce meats and fats and pregnant women gained less.

When the question began to be studied seriously, it was most often found that the opposite was the case. Thomson (1959) reported that women who gained approximately 27.5 pounds over the course of gestation had the lowest incidence of preeclampsia. We have already cited the association found by Higgins between maternal weight gain and birth weight. Thomson observed a similar association, as did Singer et al. (1968) and Eastman and Jackson (1968). A recent report of factors associated with birth weights of infants in Harlem (New York City) concluded, "Birthweight sustains an association with mother's prepregnancy weight and weight gain in pregnancy at all levels of these two variables and in analyses that introduce all other control variables" (Jacobson, 1973). Thus, if we had to cite a nutritional index that consistently shows the most clear-cut relation to pregnancy outcome, adequate maternal weight gain would have to be it. This has prompted the Committee on Food and Nutrition of the National Research Council to state the following in its 1970 report, *Maternal Nutrition and the Course of Pregnancy:*

An average weight gain of 24 lbs. (range 20-25 lbs.) is commensurate with a better than average course and outcome of pregnancy. This would be a gain of 1.5 to 3.0 lbs. during the first trimester and a gain of 0.8 lb. per week during the remainder of pregnancy. There is no scientific justification for routine limitations of weight gains to lesser amounts.

Cellular effects

As strong as the clinical evidence is to support the role of nutrition in the outcome of pregnancy, a new area of research with much promise of importance is study of the effects of nutrition at the cellular and molecular levels. Of necessity much of this kind of work has to be done in animals, but recently two lines of investigation with implications for human nutrition have emerged.

Winick (1976) has been concerned with stages of growth in the number and size of cells. He has been able to discern a general pattern of growth, which has four phases: stage I, in which new cells of the same average size rapidly proliferate (hyperplasia); stage II, in which proliferation continues at a reduced rate and cells become larger (hyperplasia and hypertrophy); stage III, in which new cells are no longer produced but cells continue to grow larger (hypertrophy); and stage IV, in which cells are mature and all cell growth stops.

These four stages of cell growth appear to be typical of all cells of the body. The question now under consideration is What happens to the process of cell growth when malnutrition occurs? Postnatal studies in animals and humans have shown that malnutrition during the hyperplastic stage can result in a deficit in the number of cells produced. Malnutrition during the hypertrophic stage results in cells of smaller size.

These findings are critically important with respect to the number and size of brain cells; we know that, in contrast to those of most other systems of the body, cells of the central nervous system do not regenerate. It raises the specter of mental retardation as a consequence of malnutrition and limits the possibility of reversing the condition once the critical hyperplastic period is passed.

Research is under way all over the world to determine the effects of malnutrition on intellectual capacity and to delineate the critical periods of brain cell proliferation in humans. There are strong indications that one such period is pregnancy. For example, Winick (1976) examined infants who were full term and had normal birth weights but who died of marasmus in the first year of life and found a 15% to 20% reduction in numbers of brain cells. In infants who weighed less than 2,000 gm. at birth and who also died of malnutrition in infancy the reduction in brain cell number was a staggering 60%. At present researchers are not sure whether this represents the combined effects of prenatal and infant malnutrition or whether low birth weight merely makes infants more susceptible to malnutrition in the first year of life. Known effects of prenatal malnutrition in rats suggest that the first hypothesis is more likely correct.

A similar pattern of cell growth has been observed by Hirsch and others for adipose cells (Winick, 1974). Here the concern is not for a reduction in the number of fat cells but for an abnormal increase in them from overfeeding, which could program an individual for obesity in later life.

It is now generally recognized that there are really two kinds of obesity and that they have different responses to treatment. When the onset of obesity is in adulthood individuals usually have a normal number of large fat cells. When they reduce the loss is in cell size, not in cell number. In contrast, individuals who become obese in childhood usually have not only enlarged fat cells but nearly twice as many fat cells as persons of normal weight. When these people reduce the loss is also in cell size, not in cell number. Juvenile-onset obesity is therefore much more difficult to treat, and treatment is generally far less successful. The need to prevent juvenile-onset obesity is apparent.

Hirsch believes that the critical times are the last trimester of pregnancy, the first 3 years of life, and adolescence (Winick, 1974).

It seems as though the pregnant woman walks a line between undernutrition on the one hand and overnutrition on the other in respect to both short- and long-term effects on her infant. In some respects the cellular studies parallel and raise the same questions as the wartime experiences because for the most part they have been concerned with the consequences of gross malnutrition and have not yet provided evidence of the effects of malnutrition in its subclinical forms. They truly represent but the tip of the iceberg, and future research in this area will continue to influence our views of the importance of nutrition to the outcome of pregnancy for years to come.

NUTRIENT NEEDS
DURING PREGNANCY

The nutrients function during pregnancy in the same manner that they do in other periods of the life cycle, but, because it is a time of growth, requirements are generally increased above those of a nonpregnant woman. In addi-tion, maternal physiological adjustments and specific needs of the fetus determine how efficiently the nutrients are used. It was once believed that the fetus was a parasite that would automatically draw what it needed from the mother to maintain its own growth. The studies we reviewed in the previous section and other findings from fetal and maternal physiology have now shown that this is not always so.

While pregnancy is certainly not an abnormal or pathological state, there are many clinical and biochemical features that, if seen in a non-pregnant woman, would be causes for concern. The difficulties in setting nutrient requirements during pregnancy are related to our ability to separate what is normal from what is not. We now realize that the increased needs of the pregnant woman are not simply tacked on to those of a woman who is not pregnant. They are influenced by changes in endocrinology and general metabolism that accompany the pregnant state. The aim is to provide a diet that will take these changes into account and meet the needs of *both* the mother and the child.

Table 3-1 presents recommended dietary allowances set by the National Research Coun-

Table 3-1. Recommended dietary allowances for pregnant and lactating women*

	Nonpregnant adult women and women in first month of pregnancy	Pregnant adult women from second month to term	Lactating women
Calories	2,000	2,300 (at least 36 kcal./kg.)	2,500
Protein (gm.)	46	76 (at least 1.3 gm/kg.)	66
Vitamin A	800 R.E. (4,000 I.U.)	1,000 R.E. (5,000 I.U.)	1,000 R.E. (5,000 I.U.)
Vitamin D (I.U.)	—	400	400
Vitamin E (I.U.)	12	15	15
Ascorbic acid (mg.)	45	60	60
Folic acid (μg.)	400	800	600
Niacin (mg.)	13	15	17
Riboflavin (mg.)	1.2	1.5	1.7
Thiamin (mg.)	1.0	1.3	1.3
Vitamin B_6 (mg.)	2.0	2.5	2.5
Vitamin B_{12} (μg.)	3.0	4.0	4.0
Calcium (mg.)	800	1,200	1,200
Phosphorus (mg.)	800	1,200	1,200
Iodine (μg.)	100	125	150
Iron (mg.)	18	18+	18
Magnesium (mg.)	300	450	450
Zinc (mg.)	15	20	25

*From Recommended dietary allowances (revised 1974), Food and Nutrition Board, National Academy of Sciences–National Research Council.

cil for pregnant and lactating women compared to needs of nonpregnant women. The numbers in this table are based on the so-called ''reference'' woman who is 64 inches tall and weighs 128 pounds when conception occurs. Women may need more or less than these amounts depending on body size and general health status. It is a good idea to calculate individual caloric and protein allowances for pregnant women according to pregnant body weight. Allowances for vitamins and minerals provide sufficient room for individual variations so that they can generally be applied to all healthy pregnant women. They may not be adequate for women who enter pregnancy in poor nutritional status or who suffer from chronic diseases or other complicating conditions.

Energy

The evidence supporting the desirability of an adequate weight gain during pregnancy should come as no surprise. Much of the recommended 24-pound gain can be accounted for by the products of conception—weight of the fetus and placenta, enlargement of the uterus and breasts, expansion of the maternal blood volume, and the amnionic fluid. Pregnancy is therefore an anabolic period of growth, which requires additional energy. It is accompanied by an increase in the metabolic rate.

It has been estimated that the total energy cost of a full-term pregnancy in addition to the need for normal maintenance is 80,000 calories. This breaks down to an allowance of 300 calories per day more than a nonpregnant woman normally eats. For the average woman this means 2,300 calories per day. Energy requirements can vary above or below this level depending on the woman's body size, prepregnant weight, and activity, but *in no instance* should intakes be less than 36 calories per kg. of pregnant body weight. Intakes below this level cause body protein and fat to be broken down to supply energy needs. This robs the pregnant woman of vital stores for her own health maintenance. There is also evidence that ketosis (high blood concentrations of keto acids, which come from excessive breakdown of body fat) causes damage to the developing fetal nervous system.

Obviously pregnancy is no time for a woman to try to lose weight. Even obese women should be encouraged to gain about 20 pounds. The diet should provide a source of good quality protein at every meal and should be balanced by approximately equal calories from carbohydrates and fats. The woman's own appetite confirmed by a normal weight gain pattern (about 3 pounds during the first trimester and about 1 pound per week thereafter) is the best measure that caloric needs are being met. There will be slight variations, of course. Underweight women, primigravidas, and teenagers generally gain more, and the patterns may not always be steady. However, erratic, rapid weight gains over short periods should be considered an indication of excess fluid retention and a sign of potential danger. (See section on toxemia.)

Protein

Growth and development of new tissue in the mother and the fetus require adequate supplies of protein. Approximately 925 gm. of protein is deposited in the fetus and maternal tissues throughout the course of pregnancy.

Requirements for protein are based on nitrogen retention and the body's efficiency in using protein from foods. During periods of growth such as pregnancy the body is using protein and incorporating the nitrogen it contains into new tissue. Nitrogen intake is therefore greater than nitrogen excretion in the urine, and the body is said to be in positive nitrogen balance. Requirements for protein are derived by gradually increasing intakes until the body is in nitrogen equilibrium—intake equals output. This indicates that the body has all the nitrogen it needs and further intakes will merely be excreted. The requirements are then adjusted upward in consideration of the fact that only 70% to 75% of the nitrogen is completely available from average diets containing mixed sources of protein and to allow for individual variations in absorption, efficiency, and needs.

New evidence from studies of this type caused the National Research Council to make considerable changes in the 1974 recommended dietary allowance for protein. The recommended intake for nonpregnant women and women in their first month of pregnancy is 46 gm. or 0.8 gm. per kg. of body weight. This is a shift downward from previous allowances.

The allowance assumes that adequate calories will be derived from carbohydrates and fats to spare the body the need of using dietary protein to meet energy requirements. Preferably a third of the protein each day should come from foods of high biological value (foods that are complete and balanced sources of the eight essential amino acids) such as meats, fish, poultry, eggs, milk, and cheese or from complimentary combinations of legumes, cereals, nuts, seeds, and grains. (See section on vegetarian diets during pregnancy.)

If we calculated a diet that contained 46 gm. of protein and the remaining caloric requirement met by carbohydrates and fats, we could devise a meal plan that would meet the needs for these three nutrients but it would probably look rather strange compared to what most people usually eat. In the United States and other Western countries we consume diets in which 11% to 13% of calories come from protein. This means that we generally eat 75 to 100 gm. of protein or more each day. In addition to palatability, we rely on these foods for valuable nutrients such as B vitamins, iron, and trace minerals. In setting its new allowance the council was concerned with nitrogen retention and absolute protein requirements, and the implication is that we generally eat more protein than we need. But where pregnant women are concerned the council recognized the contribution of protein foods to vitamin and mineral intake as well as the possible consequences of inadequate protein consumption. They therefore recommended a generous allowance of 30 gm. more of protein each day from the second month to the end of gestation. This totals 76 gm. for the average pregnant woman or 1.3 gm. per kg. of pregnant body weight. An allowance of this amount is more in keeping with general dietary preferences. As for a nonpregnant woman, high-quality protein foods should make up one third of the intake, and the diet should provide sufficient calories from carbohydrates and fats.

Vitamins
Vitamin A

Vitamin A is provided by the diet in several forms. Vitamin A that is preformed in food is called retinol, and it is present mainly in animal products, usually in combination with fat. Good sources are organ meats, egg yolks, and milk. Vitamin A can also be derived from plant foods in the form of carotenes. These are pigments that give the deep orange and green colors to foods such as squash, sweet potatoes, carrots, tomatoes, cantaloupes, apricots, spinach, greens, and broccoli.

Previous editions of the *Recommended Dietary Allowances* specified vitamin A needs in terms of the international unit (I.U.). This standard has been confusing because the amount of vitamin A activity available from foods differs according to whether it comes from retionol or one of the several kinds of carotenes. In 1974 a new standard, the retinol equivalent (R.E.), was adopted. This standard allows a more uniform measurement based on the activity of retinol. One retinol equivalent equals 1 μg. of retinol, 6 μg. of beta carotene, and 12 μg. of other provitamin A substances. Retinol equivalents for foods can be calculated from the I.U. values listed in the food composition tables by dividing I.U. values from retinol by 3.33 and those from beta carotene by 10.

The recommended intake of Vitamin A during pregnancy is 1,000 R.E. (5,000 I.U.) per day. This is 200 R.E. (1,000 I.U.) more than the allowance for nonpregnant women to compensate for storage of vitamin A by the fetus and to promote tissue growth.

Vitamin C (ascorbic acid)

Recent claims for ascorbic acid in preventing the common cold have promoted controversy over dietary needs for this vitamin. We know that vitamin C is essential for the prevention of scurvy, a disease characterized by weakening of the collagenous structures of the body and subcutaneous hemorrhage. Yet as little as 10 mg. of ascorbic acid daily is effective in the prevention of scurvy, and an intake of 45 mg. per day will maintain adequate body pools in most adults. If vitamin C taken in doses as large as

10 gm. does produce an advantage with respect to colds, the action is probably due to a pharmacological effect and not to what we generally think of as a nutritional need.

A pregnant woman needs vitamin C in amounts of 60 mg. per day to promote absorption of iron and normal tissue growth in her own body and in that of the fetus. This need can be supplied by ½ cup orange juice or an average serving of other citrus fruits, strawberries, cantaloupe, broccoli, or green peppers. Other vegetables such as tomatoes, greens, cabbage, and potatoes also supply vitamin C but in smaller amounts. Prolonged cooking destroys vitamin C, so whenever possible these foods should be eaten fresh. When eaten in combination the fair sources can supply vitamin C as adequately as citrus fruits.

As desirable as it is to keep the pregnant woman free of infection, recommending large doses of vitamin C does not seem warranted and in some instances may be harmful. There are indications that excessive amounts of ascorbate can aggravate a prediabetic condition and may impair kidney function in susceptible individuals.

B vitamins

Thiamin, riboflavin, niacin, pyridoxine (B_6), folic acid, cobalamin (B_{12}), and pantothenic acid are all vitamins that are commonly grouped in the B complex. These vitamins function as coenzymes for many of the body's chemical reactions. Thiamin, niacin, and pantothenic acid are involved in the breakdown of carbohydrate and fat for the production of energy. Riboflavin and pyridoxine are intimately concerned with protein metabolism. The needs for these vitamins are therefore increased whenever caloric and protein requirements rise. Sources are widespread throughout an average balanced diet, but some foods are especially high in a particular B vitamin. Riboflavin in milk, thiamin in pork, niacin in chicken, and pyridoxine in wheat and corn products are a few examples.

Folic acid and vitamin B_{12} are essential coenzymes that operate in cell division and hence are important for the growth and development of all tissues of the body. Because of the rapid turnover in red blood cells, clinical symptoms of folic acid or B_{12} deficiency generally appear first as a specific type of anemia.

A good way to remember food sources of folic acid is the word from which its name is derived—foliage. Thus fresh green leafy vegetables are high in this vitamin. In contrast, vitamin B_{12} is found only in animal products such as meat, milk, eggs, poultry, and fish.

Other vitamins

Vitamins D and E are both needed by pregnant women in increased amounts.

Vitamin D promotes the absorption of calcium and its incorporation into teeth and bones. Adults can meet their need for vitamin D from its precursor, 7-dehydrocholesterol, which produces vitamin D activity when irradiated by sunlight on the skin. Increased needs for calcium, however, make a dietary allowance of 400 I.U. of vitamin D per day necessary during pregnancy.

Natural food sources of vitamin D are fatty fishes, eggs, and liver. Vitamin D is added to most milk sold in the United States in amounts of 400 I.U. per quart, and many margarines are also fortified. Most pregnant women have no need of vitamin D supplements if they consume these foods and enjoy the sunshine whenever possible.

Known functions of vitamin E in humans are related to the preservation of polyunsaturated fatty acids in body cells. Polyunsaturated fatty acids are part of the structural components of cells, and low levels of vitamin E induce the fats to peroxidize and the cells to degenerate. In red blood cells this can lead to hemolysis.

It has been observed that newborns, particularly low birth weight infants, have lower plasma vitamin E concentrations than adults. These levels gradually rise to normal within 1 month after birth. At present it is not known whether this self-adjusting phenomenon is normal for newborns or whether it represents inefficient placental transfer of vitamin E. The clinical significance is not clear either, but it raises a concern about the need to monitor the vitamin E content of infant formulas, especially those designed for low birth weight infants.

The recommended allowance for vitamin E

during pregnancy is 15 I.U. per day. Requirements for vitamin E parallel polyunsaturated fatty acid intake—the higher the intake of polyunsaturates, the greater the need for vitamin E. Fortunately, vegetable oils, which are primary sources of polyunsaturated fatty acids in the diet, are also among our best sources of vitamin E, so increased vitamin E intake is generally automatic with high polyunsaturate consumption. Other food sources of vitamin E include meats, eggs, fish, whole grain cereals, and leafy vegetables. Consumption of these foods will adequately supply the 15 I.U. of vitamin E needed during pregnancy, and supplements are not recommended.

Minerals
Iron

Iron requirements during pregnancy have been difficult to establish because of the fall in hemoglobin that accompanies expansion of the maternal blood volume. There has long been a question of whether this is normal and "physiological" or whether it represents true iron deficiency that can be prevented by increased intakes. Medical opinion now generally concedes that a slight drop in hemoglobin is a normal consequence of pregnancy that cannot be avoided. However, the full-term infant has about 246 mg. of iron in his blood and body stores, most of which is accumulated during the last 3 months of gestation. Additional iron is stored in the placenta, and about 290 mg. is taken up by expansion of the mother's blood. This iron must come from the mother, either from her diet or from her own body stores. Studies of women of child-bearing age in the United States and abroad have repeatedly shown that body stores of iron are low or completely absent in most cases. Thus, if the diet is not adequate in iron, the pregnant woman chances developing an anemia that is not simply physiological. The consequences could be an infant with reduced iron reserves or added risk to the mother in case of hemorrhage on delivery.

Working in favor of the increased maternal iron needs is the 120 mg. or more of iron that is saved by the cessation of menstruation during pregnancy. Furthermore, intestinal absorption of iron tends to increase, possibly to as much as 30% of intake compared to the usual 10% absorption of iron from the diet. Nevertheless, the National Research Council believes that an intake in excess of the 18 mg. per day recommended for nonpregnant women is desirable during pregnancy.

This amount could be supplied by the diet if the pregnant woman ate large amounts of high-iron foods each day. Unfortunately, such foods are limited to organ meats (liver, heart, kidney), oysters, clams, dried beans, and prune juice—foods that should be encouraged for pregnant women but cannot realistically be considered daily fare. From an average mixed diet approximately 6 mg. of iron will be obtained from each 1,000 calories of food. If a pregnant woman eats the recommended, 2,300 calories per day, she will fall more than 3 mg. short. Women who require fewer calories to support a normal weight gain will have an even larger deficit. The National Research Council therefore recommends a prophylactic supplement of 30 to 60 mg. of iron per day during the second and third trimesters of pregnancy. Dietary counseling should emphasize iron-rich foods as well as fair sources such as dried fruits (raisins, prunes, apricots), dark green leafy vegetables, and whole grain or enriched cereals and breads.

Calcium and phosphorus

There used to be an old saying, "For every child, a tooth." There is no evidence that pregnancy causes demineralization of teeth or increased susceptibility to tooth decay, but it is true that increased supplies of calcium and phosphorus are needed during pregnancy to maintain healthy teeth and bones and to promote fetal skeletal growth and development. A newborn has approximately 25 gm. of calcium in his body and, as in the case of iron, this amount must come from maternal stores if the diet is inadequate. In addition to its use in building teeth and bones, calcium is used by muscles in contraction, it plays a role in regulating the heartbeat, and it is necessary for blood coagulation and maintenance of the substances that cement cells of the body together.

Phosphorus is present in almost all body cells and is involved in many chemical reactions, particularly those needed for the production of energy. Many of the B vitamins cannot function properly if phosphorus is absent. It is present in almost all foods, however, so dietary deficiencies are rarely seen.

Balance studies show that the body is capable of adjusting to varying levels of calcium intake—a higher proportion is absorbed from the diet when intake is low—and pregnancy itself induces absorption to increase. Nonetheless, the National Research Council recommends a liberal allowance of 1,200 mg. per day for women in the second and third trimesters.

About 85% of this allowance can be met by three to four servings of milk or milk products with the remainder supplied by dark green vegetables, dried beans, breads, and cereals.

The needs of women who do not drink milk are difficult to meet. There is nearly 300 mg. of calcium in an 8-ounce glass of milk compared to 190 mg. in a ¾-cup serving of turnip greens, one of milk's nearest competitors. If calcium were the only nutrient milk supplied, recommending calcium tablets for pregnant women who do not drink milk might be advised. However, milk is also the best known food source of riboflavin, and it contains substantial amounts of other B vitamins and vitamins A and D. Incorporating some milk into the diet by way of puddings, custards, ice cream, and cheese or using it in liquid or powdered form to supplement meat dishes and casseroles is better than doing without it altogether.

Some women complain of leg cramps in the later months of pregnancy. This is sometimes blamed on an imbalance in the body's ratio of calcium to phosphorus caused by too much milk. There is little evidence to support this claim. Although milk is high in phosphorus, the body can tolerate varying ratios provided vitamin D is adequate.

Other mineral elements

There are 92 natural elements in the periodic table, and one of the newest thrusts in nutrition research is to determine which are required by humans. Carbon, hydrogen, oxygen, and nitrogen are basic to the structures of carbohydrates, fats, and proteins, and the functions of macroelements such as sodium, potassium, calcium,

phosphorus, and iodine have long been known. But new research has uncovered functions for elements we never dreamed were essential before. Zinc, fluorine, magnesium, manganese, molybdenum, tin, copper, vanadium, cobalt, silicon, selenium, and nickel have all been shown to be required in trace amounts. Even substances such as lead and arsenic, which are extremely toxic in large doses, are now known to produce benefits at very low levels.

It seems as though the human body is a veritable chemical storehouse, and one of the most consistent findings is that these trace elements play a significant role in growth. Except for zinc and magnesium, our knowledge of their functions at this time does not permit meaningful recommendations for dietary intakes to be made, but their importance in pregnancy is avowed. The implication is that we must rely on a wide variety of foods to provide complete and balanced nutrition. The need for trace minerals is the most important reason why we must not depend on vitamin pills to substitute for food during pregnancy or for that matter during any phase of the life cycle.

NUTRITIONAL GUIDANCE
General principles

Our concern for the nutritional well-being of the expectant mother and her infant makes dietary counseling one of the most important aspects of prenatal care. Efforts to set the mother on her way to good nutrition should begin with her first visit and should be followed up at every visit thereafter. With all the new things the mother has to learn and remember about her pregnancy, it is best not to overwhelm her with dietary recommendations on the first visit. If the mother can take home one or two new ideas *each* time she comes for care, there is a better chance that she will remember the advice and follow it.

While pregnancy is perhaps the most opportune time to intervene and correct nutritional misunderstandings and poor food habits, we should expect that something as long-standing and personal as eating behavior may sometimes be resistant to change. Occasionally in our anxious attempts to motivate a woman to accept dietary advice we have resorted to threats of dire consequences for the mother or her infant if she does not "eat right." Of course, when the predicted catastrophes do not occur the mother not only becomes suspicious of nutrition but of the nurse as well.

A better way is to approach the mother with understanding and sensitivity to her beliefs and needs. The public in general and women in particular are not only becoming more interested in nutrition but they are becoming better versed in its principles. Old-fashioned dictates about what people ought to eat simply do not work anymore. An uncomplicated but sound explanation of *why* nutrient needs are increased, tempered with an assurance that nutrition is but one of the many facets of a successful pregnancy, can tap the woman's interest and place nutrition in its proper and realsitic perspective.

Whether the nurse counsels mothers individually or in groups, she should always try to find out what they know about nutrition and what their concerns are about diet during pregnancy. In doing so the nurse will discover that food and eating take place in the context of family living. Day-to-day problems of money management, family tensions, and other distractions will influence what a woman eats as much as, if not more than, what she knows

about nutrition. Often the husband's food preferences are more important than the mother's in determining whether her needs are met since a pregnant woman cannot be expected to prepare special dishes for herself that other family members do not like. Diet during pregnancy is therefore a family affair, and whenever possible expectant fathers should be invited to attend prenatal classes when food needs of the mother and baby are discussed.

Food guides to meet nutrient needs

Suggested food patterns to meet nutritional requirements during pregnancy and lactation have been devised to assist in teaching, and they are available from hospital dietary departments and public health agencies. These guides, like the one in Table 3-2, usually recommend daily servings from the Basic Four food groups and reflect eating habits and food preferences that are traditional in the United States. When using these guides, the nurse should remember that it is the *nutrients,* not the foods per se, that are important and that not all people eat in the typical American way. The nurse should begin by investigating what kinds of foods the family usually eats and what the meal schedules are. This can be done by asking the mother to recall

Table 3-2. Food guide for pregnant and lactating women (servings per day)*

	Nonpregnant adult women and women in first month of pregnancy	Pregnant women from second month to term	Lactating women
Milk group Milk, cheese, ice cream, etc. for protein, calcium, phosphorus, B vitamins, and vitamins A and D	2	3-4	4
Meat group Meat, fish, poultry, eggs, dried peas, and beans for protein, B vitamins, iron, and vitamin A	2	3-4	3-4
Fruit and vegetable group Vitamin C–source citrus fruits, berries, melons, etc.	1	1	1
Dark orange and leafy green vegetables for vitamin A, vitamin C, calcium, and iron	1-2	2	2
Other fruits and vegetables for additional calories	1-2	2	2
Bread and cereal group Whole grain or enriched for B vitamins, calcium, and iron	3	4	4-5

*Food guides supply approximately 1,200, 1,500, and 1,800 calories respectively. Pregnant and lactating women can meet additional caloric needs from fats and oils, desserts, and other foods they like to eat.

what she and her family had to eat within the past 24 hours and then probing to discover how often other foods from the four groups are consumed. If the nurse encounters foods that are unfamiliar to her, she should not hesitate to look up their nutritional values in food composition tables such as the U.S. Department of Agriculture *Handbook 456: Nutritive Value of American Foods in Common Units.* Often food patterns that initially look strange to the nurse turn out to be perfectly adequate. In other cases poor diets can be improved with culturally preferred foods if the nurse knows what nutrients they contain. Expertise in judging the nutritional adequacy of nontypical food patterns will come from practice with the food composition tables and help from the dietitian.

Vegetarian diets

In many parts of the world, either out of economic necessity or out of increasing concern for ecology and the environment, more and more people are consuming vegetarian diets, and a few words need to be said about the use of these regimens during pregnancy. Of primary concern is the adequacy of protein derived mainly from plant sources. If the regimen allows liberal consumption of milk products and eggs, there is no danger, but a woman following a diet strictly limited to vegetable proteins chances an imbalance of essential amino acids that are necessary for proper growth. Since legumes, nuts, seeds, cereals, and grains are all deficient in one or more of the essential amino acids, they must be consumed *in combination at the same meal* and usually in larger amounts on a weight-for-weight basis than animal protein foods.

Calcium requirements can be met from soy products such as soy milk and tofu and from cereals and dark green vegetables, but these do not contain vitamin D, and therefore supplements may be in order. Since vitamin B_{12} is confined to animal products, the pregnant vegetarian woman risks a deficiency of this vitamin if she has eliminated milk and eggs from her diet over a period of time.

Nutritional needs during pregnancy can be met by vegetarian diets, but, because of the dangers inherent in food selection, they should be called to the attention of the physician and

nutritionist whenever they are encountered during growth periods such as pregnancy, lactation, childhood, and adolescence.

Programs for low income mothers

Expectant mothers from deprived socioeconomic groups should always be considered nutritionally at risk. Chances are they will not only enter pregnancy in poor nutritional status but they will also find it difficult to afford the good-quality food they need to meet their increased requirements.

Nurses can provide helpful hints on how to cut the food budget and maintain an adequate diet. Table 3-3 lists some inexpensive foods of high nutritional value. It is also usually cheaper

Table 3-3. Less expensive foods of high nutritional value

Milk group
    Nonfat dry milk
    Ice milk
    Cheddar cheese
    Cheese food
Meat and meat substitutes
    Good and standard grades
    Ground meats
    Stewing meats and other less tender cuts
    Pork liver
    Other variety meats: kidney, heart
    Fresh or frozen fish
    Soy-meat combination foods
    Whole chicken or wings, necks, and backs
    Dried beans (navy, kidney, pinto, lima, etc.)
    Lentils or dried peas (split peas, black-eyed peas, garbanzos, etc.)
    Peanut butter
Fruits and vegetables
    Fresh in season
    Frozen plain varieties (versus combinations or prepared with sauces)
    Greens (turnip, collard, kale, mustard)
Breads, cereals, and grains
    Day-old bread
    Rolled oats and rolled wheat
    Cracked wheat
    Bulgur
    Enriched farina
    Enriched grits
    Large packages of cereal (versus individual variety packs)
    Enriched pastas (macaroni, spaghetti, noodles)
    Regular bread and cereal varieties (versus ''natural,'' ''organic,'' or mixed grain varieties)

to purchase food in bulk quantities and fresh fruits and vegetables in season. Using meat extenders such as casseroles and making them from scratch are another way to cut food costs.

Although these tips can help, the nurse should know that they are not a panacea, and in some cases they may be impractical. A working mother with small children cannot spend hours toiling in the kitchen, and some women do not have the skill to make dishes from scratch even if they have the time. They have to rely on the more expensive convenience items to some extent. Lack of refrigeration and cramped living space may prevent mothers from buying food in bulk. There is therefore a limit to how much we can expect, and we must realize that all the good advice in the world cannot substitute for dollars to buy adequate food.

There are programs in the United States to assist mothers of low income families. Most counties operate the federally sponsored food stamp program. Food stamps are bought each month by the head of the household, and they entitle the recipient to a bonus in food purchasing power over the actual amount paid for the stamps. Eligibility is determined by family income and family size, and mothers do not have to be receiving welfare to participate. There are many people who are eligible for food stamps but do not know it; the nurse should be aware of the criteria in her county and work to get low income families on the program.

In some locations health or welfare agencies offer one of two other federal food programs especially designed for low income pregnant and lactating women and their children. The Supplemental Food Program offers surplus commodities from the U.S. Department of Agriculture to needy women and children at no

cost. The newer Special Supplemental Food Program for Women, Infants, and Children (WIC) provides food or vouchers that can be redeemed for food at local markets. The vouchers are free and provided on the basis of income and nutritional need.

NUTRITION AND COMPLICATING CONDITIONS
Teenage mothers

Since growth is not complete for most young women until they reach about 17 years of age, girls who become pregnant in their teens face the added burden of meeting their own growth and development needs as well as those of the fetus. Three nutrients that become particularly important for teenage mothers are calories, protein, and calcium. Allowances for these nutrients are higher in adolescence than they are at any other time in a woman's life. In pregnancy they are increased even more (Table 3-4).

The qualification cited earlier with respect to the 1974 recommended allowance for protein also applies to teenagers. The recommended intake supports a positive nitrogen balance, but recently King et al. (1972) have shown that levels in excess of this amount will continue to promote nitrogen retention in pregnant teenagers. In view of this and the practical difficulty of meeting the high caloric needs of teenage mothers, protein intake should be liberal and unrestricted. Because of the increased needs for calories and protein, allowances for thiamin, niacin, and riboflavin are also slightly higher for teenage mothers than for pregnant adult women.

The requirements can be met by adding an extra serving of milk to the pregnant woman's food guide and by encouraging slightly larger portions of the other Basic Four foods at mealtimes or as between-meal snacks.

Fashion-conscious adolescents may not always take readily to the idea of eating more during pregnancy. Surveys of teenage food habits and attitudes toward diet have shown that many girls think that they ought to lose weight even though they are not obese by nutritional standards. They are susceptible to diet fads and often have a poor understanding of the nutrient composition of foods. Many find it

Table 3-4. Recommended dietary allowances for teenagers (1974)

	Calories	Protein (g.)	Calcium (mg.)
Age 11 to 14 years	2400	44	1200
Age 15 to 18 years	2100	48	1200
Pregnancy	+300	+30	+400
Lactation	+500	+20	+400

much more "adult" to substitute coffee and other empty-calorie beverages for milk.

The nurse must approach the teenage mother with all the sympathy and understanding at her command. Pregnancy is bound to be a time of confusion for an adolescent who is still struggling with her own identity. Although society is adopting a more liberal attitude toward the teenage mother, she may still face ostracism from some adults and peers, especially if the pregnancy is out of wedlock, and she may even have to drop out of school. Harping on diet can only add to the troubles.

Nutrition should be emphasized as one of the positive aspects of pregnancy. Instead of treating the diet as something that must be restricted, the nurse should help the teenage mother see it as a vehicle of freedom and as an opportunity for self-control. Group sessions that allow teenage mothers to get together and talk about diet and other concerns is often a more successful method of education because it enables them to express their own ideas and places the nurse in a less authoritarian role.

Anemias
Iron deficiency anemia

The needs of the mother and fetus for increased iron for normal hematopoiesis make anemia a possible problem of pregnancy. Iron deficiency and acute blood loss are the most common causes. The condition is diagnosed by a reduction in hemoglobin concentration from the normal range of 12 to 15 gm. per 100 ml. or by a fall in the packed red cell volume per 100 ml. of blood.

A slight decrease in hemoglobin concentration can be expected in the later months of pregnancy due to expansion of the maternal blood volume, but significant deviations from normal values pose increased risks for the mother and infant, particularly if multiple births are anticipated.

Iron deficiency anemia cannot be corrected by dietary means alone. It requires daily doses of ferrous sulfate or ferrous gluconate to bring about a satisfactory response. Three 0.2 gm. tablets of ferrous sulfate or six 0.3 gm. tablets of ferrous gluconate supply 200 mg. of iron per day.

The unpleasant gastrointestinal effects of therapeutic iron seem to be related to the amount of iron absorbed rather than to the absolute amount of iron ingested. These symptoms can be minimized if the tablets are introduced gradually until the maximum dosage is reached and if they are spread out over the day and taken at mealtimes. Preparations that include substances such as ascorbic acid, other hematopoietic elements, liver, and bone marrow extracts are usually more expensive than simple iron compounds and do not relieve gastric symptoms or improve iron absorption to any significant extent. A good diet seems to be the best accompaniment to iron therapy for the improvement of iron deficiency anemia.

Pica. The ingestion of bizarre items such as laundry starch, clay, coffee grounds, and refrigerator frost is sometimes seen during pregnancy, particularly among low income patients from the southern and southwestern United States. There has been evidence that these practices are associated with an increased incidence of iron deficiency anemia.

Two theories are proposed for this association. One is that these items, especially certain kinds of clay, interfere with intestinal iron absorption. The other explanation is that ingestion of large amounts (and intakes by the pound are not uncommon) decreases appetite for food, thus reducing iron availability in the diet. This reasoning applies particularly to larundry starch and cornstarch, from which calories but no other nutrients are derived.

The practices usually stem from long-standing habits and cultural traditions. Sometimes pregnant women crave these things simply because they are expected to do so. The nurse should be on the alert for pica among susceptible women and use her good judgment in correcting beliefs associated with the practice.

Megaloblastic anemia

Pregnancy causes an increased need for folic acid and vitamin B_{12}. A deficiency of these nutrients produces red blood cells that are arrested in the megaloblastic stage of development. The cells are abnormally large and nucleated, and their oxygen-carrying capacity is reduced. Symptoms of megaloblastic anemia include fatigue, anorexia, and persistant nausea and vomiting that are more intense than the morning sickness commonly seen in the early months of pregnancy.

Megaloblastic anemia due to dietary deficiency is rarely seen as long as diets include fresh green leafy vegetables and animal products; however, low serum levels of folate have quite frequently been observed in the early months of pregnancy without other symptoms of megaloblastic anemia. Although the consequences are not yet proved, there are some researchers who have associated abnormally low serum folate levels with abruptio placentae and fetal malformations. Until more is known of the effects of low serum folate, the National Research Council recommends that a daily supplement of 200 to 400 μg. of folic acid be given routinely during pregnancy. Supplements in excess of this amount are not recommended. Extra folic acid is not advised for nonpregnant women because of the possibility of masking the hematological symptoms of addisonian (pernicious) anemia caused by inadequate absorption of vitamin B_{12}.

Toxemia

Historically many erroneous recommendations regarding diet during pregnancy can be traced to the poorly understood relationship between nutrition and toxemia. Confusion sometimes comes from differentiating the role of diet in *preventing* toxemia and its use in *treating* the condition once it has developed.

Etiology and prevention

There have been many theories about the role of diet in the cause and prevention of toxemia, but interest has tended to focus on calories, salt, and protein.

Because erratic, rapid gains in weight have been observed as preludes to preeclampsia, caloric restriction as a means of preventing weight gain in pregnancy has often been prescribed. The problem with this recommendation has been a failure to distinguish whether the added weight comes from too much fluid or excess fat. We have already cited evidence indicating that a weight gain of 20 to 25 pounds is associated with a better than average course

of pregnancy and that much of this gain can be accounted for by the products of conception. Overweight women and women who gain in excess of 30 pounds over the entire course of gestation do not show an increased incidence of toxemia. It is women who are underweight who pose the greatest risks. Thus high caloric consumption does not predispose women to toxemia, and restricting calories to induce weight loss will not prevent it.

Excessive fluid retention is one of the signs of toxemia. Since sodium retention is a factor in the accumulation of fluid in the tissues, intake has frequently been routinely restricted during pregnancy as a preventative measure. A mild degree of edema in the *absence* of hypertension and proteinuria is physiological and does not appear to be harmful. There is no evidence that the edema and hypertension of toxemia are caused by too much salt or that they will be prevented if sodium intake is automatically restricted. In fact, clinical experience has shown that low-sodium diets in combination with diuretics used routinely in normal pregnancy can produce sodium depletion and fluid and electrolyte imbalances that potentially prove more hazardous than modest degrees of edema. Routine restrictions of sodium intake are therefore unwarranted.

Since proteinuria is another symptom of toxemia, protein too has received its share of attention in theories regarding etiology. At one time it was held that the loss of protein in the urine of toxic women was caused by a defect in renal function. A low-protein diet was advocated to ''spare the kidneys'' and prevent preeclampsia. This theory is widely disavowed today, and a completely opposite view is now being investigated. For example, there is a hypothesis that hypoproteinemia is the cause of the edema of preeclampsia. Others have suggested that protein deficiency is a factor responsible for the liver's inability to deal with toxic substances.

That toxemia is more prevalent in women from the lower socioeconomic strata lends support to the idea that malnutrition may be involved, but whether it can be specifically traced to protein deficiency is still unknown. At best conclusions with respect to diet in the etiology and prevention of toxemia can only identify it as one potential factor in a puzzling and complex disease. A normally well-balanced diet that allows adequate weight gain seems to be the most reasonable recommendation that can be made at the present time.

Treatment

If toxemia develops, dietary changes may be necessary. Although sodium intake does not appear to cause edema and hypertension, excessive intakes can exacerbate them. The degree of sodium restriction depends on the severity of the symptoms. A moderate sodium restriction is most effectively achieved by advising the woman to do without the salt shaker and to avoid salty foods like processed meats, packaged snacks, and condiments. More progressive stages of the disease will require hospitalization, and 1,000 to 2,000 mg. sodium diets may be prescribed. On these regimens the amounts of milk, bread, and butter may be regulated or low-sodium products may be substituted.

Excessive proteinuria will call for liberal amounts of protein in the diet to restore serum protein levels and prevent further edema. In a minority of cases, however, renal function may be so seriously impaired that low-protein diets may have to be used.

Chronic diseases
Diabetes

The nutritional needs of a diabetic mother are no different from those of a healthy pregnant woman; however, changes in maternal physiology make careful dietary management imperative. Since metabolic rate and food intake increase during pregnancy, insulin dosages may have to be adjusted, and women who are usually maintained on oral hypoglycemic agents may be placed on insulin during gestation. Of prime importance is the maintenance of regular meal schedules to balance the action of insulin and to prevent acidosis.

Nausea and vomiting in the early months of pregnancy can be especially hazardous for the diabetic mother because of resultant depletion of glycogen reserves and disruptions in acid-base and fluid and electrolyte balance. Nausea and vomiting can be minimized if the woman is advised to take her meals dry and reserve liquids for between-meal feedings. Using the carbohydrate allowance for such things as dry toast and crackers can also help settle the stomach. If insulin action allows, breaking meals, particularly breakfast, into small, frequent feedings is better than eating all the food at one time.

Heart disease

The pregnant woman with congenital heart defect, rheumatic heart disease, or hypertension poses a special risk. Heart disease is the fourth leading cause of maternal death in the United States.

Management of the conditions may include a sodium-restricted diet. By far the most important consideration is that the diet be nutritionally adequate. A normal weight gain is desirable, but closer control of overweight should be maintained for women with heart problems than for healthy mothers.

Anemia can add to the risk of heart disease during pregnancy. Routine iron supplementation should be accompanied by dietary advice regarding iron-rich foods.

In severe cases adequate rest and avoidance of tension are especially important. Meals should be taken leisurely, they should not be unduly large or heavily laden with fatty foods, and, if possible, they should be broken into several small feedings during the day. The pregnant woman with heart disease should be advised to avoid foods that she knows give her indigestion or "heartburn."

Tuberculosis

Tuberculosis is an infectious condition that draws on the body's reserves of energy, protein, and vitamins to combat the disease and repair damaged tissue. The nutrient needs of a pregnant woman with tuberculosis are therefore higher than those of a woman who enters pregnancy in a healthy state. An allowance of 3,000 calories per day is not unusual for a woman who is in the active phase of tuberculosis. Vitamins A and C, which are used for the repair and maintenance of epithelial tissue, are important constituents of this increase, as is protein. Higher needs for calories and protein raise the requirements for thiamin, niacin, and riboflavin.

An obvious problem is getting the woman to eat all the food she requires, especially since the appetite may be poor. Encouraging foods the mother likes and offering her high calorie–high protein beverages such as milkshakes or proprietary formulas may help overcome this problem. Women who do not eat well may require vitamin and mineral supplements.

Isonicotinic acid hydrazide (isoniazid), a drug commonly used in the treatment of tuberculosis, increases the need for pyridoxine (vitamin B_6). In addition, several researchers have reported that the urinary excretion of pyridoxine metabolites is increased during normal pregnancy. This suggests an alteration of function and a higher requirement for the vitamin. Tuberculous mothers receiving isoniazid may require supplements of vitamin B_6.

NUTRITION DURING LACTATION
Nutrient needs

Preparation for lactation begins during pregnancy with the growth and development of mammary glands and deposition of fat to build energy reserves. After parturition the metabolic adjustments that sustained the mother during pregnancy will gradually revert to their normal course. Except for hormonal secretions that promote the synthesis of breast milk and an apparent tendency for the excretion of calcium in the urine to be reduced, there do not seem to be any other metabolic characteristics that markedly distinguish lactation from the normal nonpregnant state. This means that the lactating woman must rely heavily on her diet and on her own nutrient reserves to meet the demands of maintaining an adequate milk supply. Inadequate nutrition does not interfere with the quality of breast milk as much as it does with the amount of milk produced.

Breast milk has an energy content of between 67 and 77 calories per 100 ml. A normal production of about 850 ml. per day means that 600 to 700 calories of energy must be transferred from the mother to her milk. The efficiency of this conversion is about 80%. The total energy requirement for the mother is therefore between 700 and 800 extra calories per day.

Some of this energy can come from fat reserves laid down during pregnancy; the remainder must come from food. An allowance of 500 additional calories is recommended to maintain adequate milk production. If breast-feeding continues beyond 100 days, the caloric intake of normal and underweight women should be increased because the fat depots from pregnancy will be exhausted by this time.

A similar conversion from food to breast milk is made for protein. The average daily supply of breast milk contains about 1.2% protein, or 10 gm. in 850 ml. The conversion factor is 70%. To allow for this and for the fact that some women secrete as much as 1,200 ml. of milk per day the recommended dietary allowance for protein is an additional 20 gm.

Transfer of vitamins and minerals from the mother to her milk cannot be calculated as precisely as that of energy and protein. It is known, however, that dietary deficiencies of vitamins A and C can result in milk with reduced values.

The calcium content of breast milk is approximately 250 mg. per 850 ml. during the first two months of lactation and 300 mg. per 850 ml. after the third month. Women who secrete larger amounts of milk may lose as much as 1 gm. of calcium per day. Although urinary excretion indicates that lactating women conserve calcium better than pregnant women

Table 3-5. Energy and protein conversions in lactation

Energy (daily)	
850 ml. breast milk	600-700 calories
Adjustment for 80% conversion efficiency	+100 calories
Total energy requirement	700-800 calories
Maternal fat depots (100-day supply)	−200-300 calories
Recommended dietary allowance	500 calories*
Protein (daily)	
850-1,200 ml. breast milk	10-15 gm.
Adjustment for 70% conversion efficiency	+5 gm.
Recommended dietary allowance	20 gm.*

*Added to calorie and protein allowances for normal nonpregnant women. Calories: 2,000 + 500 = 2,500. Protein: 46 gm. + 20 gm. = 66 gm.

do, the dietary allowance is maintained at the pregnant level of 1,200 mg. per day.

As always when caloric and protein intakes increase, the allowances for thiamin, riboflavin, and niacin are raised above normal needs.

Nutritional guidance

Lactating women need an extra serving from the milk and meat groups and from the bread and cereal group to meet their increased caloric, calcium, and B vitamin needs. Additional calories can be obtained from fruits and vegetables, fats, desserts, or other foods they enjoy. The extra caloric needs make it advisable for the lactating woman to have nutritious between-meal snacks.

Since milk is a body secretion, the fluid needs of the mother are also important during lactation. This point is sometimes overlooked. The lactating mother should have from 2 to 3 liters of liquids each day to maintain fluid balance. The extra milk as well as juice, water, and other beverages can easily supply most of this amount. Foods, especially fruits and vegetables, contain water, and about 200 to 300 ml. is produced when the body oxidizes fats and carbohydrates for energy.

Things to avoid

Sometimes mothers have been told to avoid foods such as chocolate, spices, strong-flavored vegetables (cabbage, brussel sprouts, onions, etc.) and certain fruits such as strawberries during lactation. The reasoning is that constituents of these foods are secreted in the milk and cause gastrointestinal upsets for the infant. With the possible exception of rhubarb, there does not appear to be any justification for these restrictions. If the baby is having gastrointestinal problems (a rare thing for breast-fed infants), the mother's diet should be examined as a possible cause, but there is no reason to automatically eliminate foods from the diet unless they cause discomfort to the mother herself.

There are, however, many substances that can be passed to the infant through mother's milk. Pesticide residues are one such group of substances; therefore fresh fruits and vegetables should always be carefully washed. Many common drugs such as aspirin, tranquilizers, anti-biotics, and antihistamines are also secreted in breast milk. Mothers should be advised to adhere closely to the physician's orders regarding their use during lactation.

Abused drugs like alcohol, amphetamines, barbiturates, heroin, nicotine, and even caffeine also pass through breast milk. Women with histories of heavy usage of these substances should receive special counseling and be made aware of their dangers.

Counseling principles

The same general principles of nutrition counseling during pregnancy also apply during lactation. Frequently the mother's dietary needs are neglected in all the attention and excitement over the new baby. Once delivered of the baby the mother may feel she is also delivered of the need to watch her diet. But what the mother herself eats is the prime source of nutrition for her infant, and nutrition during lactation is just as important as it was during pregnancy if not more so. The nurse should not wait until the infant is born to discuss the mother's choice of infant feeding. This decision should be made early, and pregnancy counseling in the later months should begin to prepare the mother for breast-feeding and its unique nutritional demands.

The psychological state of the mother is often as influential as adequate nutrition in successful breast-feeding. Anxiety and tension do not reduce the production of breast milk, but they can hold back its flow. The nurse has a role to play in making the mother comfortable and confident about her ability to breast-feed. Mothers, particularly those who are breast-feeding for the first time, need a quiet, peaceful atmosphere for themselves and their infants to become acquainted with the technique.

NUTRITION AND FAMILY PLANNING
General importance

Comprehensive family planning services are not intended solely for the distribution of contraceptives; their aim includes the preparation of women for future pregnancies and assurance of a healthy beginning for the children they choose to have. Since we know that the preconceptional nutritional status of women influences the course and outcome of pregnancy, nutritional guidance in family planning has an important role to play in achieving this aim.

Assessment of nutritional status and dietary counseling should be a routine part of family planning care; it can help to head off problems that complicate pregnancy later on. Teenagers, low income women, and women who are underweight or who suffer from chronic diseases all have been shown to be especially at risk. Giving them a nutritional head start when planning their families will not only improve their capacity for childbearing but it will also make dietary advising more successful during pregnancy itself.

The interconceptional period is also a good time for women to attack problems of overweight. Weight reduction programs in family planning clinics are effective means of teaching women the principles of food and nutrition and the importance of diet in health maintenance for themselves and for their families.

Nutrition and the pill

Most oral contraceptive agents contain estrogen and progesterone analogues that stimulate certain metabolic and physiologic adjustments characteristic of pregnancy. It is therefore not unusual to expect some nutritional consequences.

A tendency to gain weight may be a source of dismay for some users of oral contraceptives. A few women will also become hypertensive and retain fluid. In others blood lipids may undergo a modest increase.

On the positive side, oral contraceptives, depending on the type used, can improve nitrogen retention and the intestinal absorption of iron.

Two nutrients have recently received special attention because of the possibility of deficiencies associated with use of oral contraceptive agents. Several metabolic studies have discovered alterations in tryptophan metabolism (an essential amino acid that the body can convert to the B vitamin niacin) that are suggestive of an induced deficiency of vitamin B_6. One such investigation reported that as many as 75% of oral contraceptive users studied had abnormal urinary excretions of tryptophan metab-

olites (Luhby et al., 1972). Some clinicians have observed that the headaches, depression, and nausea that frequently accompany use of oral contraceptives are relieved with vitamin B_6 supplements.

The other nutrient undergoing scrutiny is folic acid. Biochemical evidence of folic acid deficiency has been cited by several investigators (Butterworth, 1973; Hodges, 1971). Some suspect that this may be related to the reduced serum folate levels seen later during pregnancy.

Although preliminary, these findings suggest a need to monitor the nutritional status of women who use oral contraceptive agents and to provide them with counseling to help them maintain nutritionally adequate diets.

SUMMARY

The preconceptional nutritional status and diet of the mother during pregnancy have been shown to influence the course of gestation and its outcome. A new area of research suggests that malnutrition during prenatal life can adversely affect the number and size of body cells. The immediate consequence of these effects may be an infant of low birth weight. They could furthermore subject the child to developmental disabilities that may be impossible to reverse.

Dietary restrictions of calories, sodium, and specific foods that were often routinely prescribed in the past have no place in the management of normal pregnant and lactating women today. A well-balanced diet that allows an average weight gain of 24 pounds results in a better than average course and outcome of pregnancy. During lactation the needs for calories, protein, calcium, and B vitamins are increased to maintain an adequate milk supply.

The nurse's role includes the identification of mothers at nutritional risk, monitoring nutritional status and adequacy of the diet during pregnancy and lactation, and counseling women to help them meet their food and nutrition needs. Teenage mothers, low income women, women who are undernourished, and those who suffer from chronic conditions are especially in need of nutritional guidance. The nurse can help improve their chances for successful childbearing by making dietary counseling a routine part of family planning and prenatal care.

REFERENCES

Antonov, A. N.: Children born during the siege of Leningrad in 1942, J. Pediatr. **30:**250, 1947.

Arena, J. M.: Contamination of the ideal food, Nutr. Today **5:**2, Winter, 1970.

Bergen, I..., and Susser, M. W.: Low birth weight and prenatal nutrition: An interpretive review, Pediatrics **46:**946, 1970.

Burke, B. S., et al.: Nutrition studies during pregnancy, Am. J. Obstet. Gynecol. **46:**38, 1943.

Butterworth, C. E., Jr.: Interactions of nutrients with oral contraceptives and other drugs, J. Am. Diet. Assoc. **62:**510, 1973.

Committee on Food and Nutrition, Food and Nutrition Board, National Academy of Sciences–National Research Council: Maternal nutrition and the course of pregnancy, Washington, D.C., 1970, U.S. Government Printing Office.

Eastman, N. J., and Jackson, E.: Weight relationships in pregnancy, Obstet. Gynecol. Surv. **23:**1003, 1968.

Food and Nutrition Board, National Academy of Sciences–National Research Council: Recommended Dietary Allowances, ed. 8, Washington, D.C., 1974, U.S. Government Printing Office.

Higgins, A.: A preliminary report of a nutrition study on public maternity patients, Montreal Diet Dispensary. (Unpublished.)

Hodges, R. E.: Nutrition and "the pill", J. Am. Diet. Assoc. **59:**212, 1971.

Jacobson, H. E.: Nutrition and pregnancy. In Wallace, H. M., Gold, E. A., and Lis, E. F., editors: Maternal and child health practices, Springfield, Ill., 1973, Charles C Thomas, Publisher, p. 311.

King, J. C., et al.: Nitrogen retention, total body ^{40}K and weight gain in teenage pregnant girls, J. Obstet. Gynecol. **79:**777, 1972.

Luhby, L., et al.: Nutrition in users of oral contraceptive agents. In Proceedings of Western Hemisphere Nutrition Congress III, Mount Kisco, N.Y., 1972, Futura Publishing Co., p. 384.

McGanity, W. J., et al.: The Vanderbilt cooperative study of maternal and infant nutrition. VII. Some nutritional implications, J. Am. Diet. Assoc. **3:**582, 1955.

Nutrition in pregnancy—A symposium, J. Reprod. Med. **7:**199, 1971.

Nutrition in pregnancy and lactation, WHO Tech. Rep. Ser. No. 302, Geneva, World Health Organization, 1965.

Singer, J. E., et al.: Relationship of weight gain during pregnancy to birth weight and infant growth and development in first year of life (Report from collaborative study of cerebral palsy), Obstet. Gynecol. **31:**417, 1968.

Smith, C. A.: The effect of wartime starvation in Holland upon pregnancy and its outcome, Am. J. Obstet. Gynecol. **53:**599, 1947.

Thomson, A. M.: Diet in relation to the course and outcome of pregnancy, Br. J. Nutr. **13:**509, 1959.

Thomson, A. M., et al.: Nutritional status, maternal physique, and reproductive efficiency, Proc. Nutr. Soc. **22:**55, 1963.

Winick, M.: Childhood obesity, Nutr. Today **9:**6, May-June, 1974.

Winick, M.: Malnutrition and brain development, New York, 1976, Oxford University Press.

4

PHYSICAL ASSESSMENT AND CARE
OF THE NEONATE

IMMEDIATE CARE

All modern delivery rooms are equipped to provide for the immediate care of the neonate. It is the responsibility of the nurse to determine the adequacy of supplies and the working condition of all equipment.

As soon as the neonate is delivered the nose and the mouth are aspirated to provide a clear air passage before the onset of respirations. The neonate should be maintained in a position with the head lower than the thorax to promote drainage of mucus and fluid and to prevent aspiration. A small rubber ear syringe or a soft rubber catheter with a mucous trap is used to aspirate the nose and the oropharynx. If respiration is not initiated with the aspiration of the nose and the mouth, direct laryngoscopy may be done by the physician to aspirate deep secretions and to establish an open airway. Oxygen may be administered by mask to alleviate anoxia.

The physician clamps and cuts the umbilical cord and places the neonate in a sterile receiving blanket in a heated crib or resuscitator. Care must be taken to avoid additional chilling of the neonate, who rapidly loses body heat through adaptation to a cooler environment and evaporation of the amniotic fluid with which he is covered.

Circulatory adaptation

At birth the neonate experiences the loss of blood flow through the placenta and a loss of metabolic support from the mother. In the unexpanded lungs of the fetus blood vessels are compressed. In addition, hypoxia and hypercapnea cause vasoconstriction of the blood vessels of the lungs. With the expansion of the lungs through respiration, the compression of the blood vessels is relieved, and with aeration of the lungs there is vasodilatation and resistance to blood flow is decreased.

With alteration in vascular pressure there is a low right atrial pressure and a high left atrial pressure, creating a tendency for blood to backflow from the left atrium into the right atrium. As a result the small valve that lies over the foramen ovale on the left side of the atrial septum closes over the opening. Functional closure occurs within minutes of birth, but permanent anatomical closure is not complete until about 1 year of age. Approximately 25% of all adults never have total anatomical closure of the foramen ovale, a condition classified as an interatrial septal defect.

In fetal circulation blood flows from the pulmonary artery through the ductus arteriosus into the aorta. The ductus arteriosus, which is patent during the fetal period, closes with alteration in vascular pressure as a result of expansion of the lungs. The increased aortic pressure and the decreased pulmonary arterial pressure cause blood to flow backward from the aorta into the pulmonary artery. Within 3 to 4 days of birth functional occlusion of the ductus arteriosus occurs as a result of constriction of the muscular wall of the vessel. During the second or third month of life the lumen of the ductus becomes anatomically occluded and permanently closed by fibrous tissue. The mechanism of closure of the ductus arteriosus is not understood. Proliferation of cells as a result of increased flow of oxygenated blood through the ductus arteriosus contributes to the closure. The degree of constriction of the ductus arteriosus is correlated with the availability of oxygen. Functional heart

COLR-3004-1
REV. 1/61
3

DELIVERY ROOM OBSERVATION OF THE NEONATE

1. PATIENT IDENTIFICATION

2. OBSERVED BY | 3. TITLE OR POSITION

4. DATE OF BIRTH Mo. | Day | Year | 5. TIME OF BIRTH (24-hr clock)

Time all events below as age before or after delivery

6. CORD CLAMPED (Age) Min. | Sec. ☐ Before Delivery ☐ After Delivery

7. FIRST BREATH (Age) Min. | Sec. ☐ Before Delivery ☐ After Delivery

8. FIRST CRY (Age) Min. | Sec. ☐ Before Delivery ☐ After Delivery

9. PROCEDURES (*Omit uncomplicated oral-pharyngeal suction*)

		Age Begun	Age Ended
☐ None 0	☐ Open Oxygen 4	Min.	Min.
☐ Gastric Suction 1	☐ Positive Pressure Oxygen or Air 5	Min.	Min.
☐ Tracheal Suction 2	☐ Intubation 6	Min.	Min.
☐ Drugs (*Give type & Dose*) 3	☐ Other (*Specify*) 8	Min.	Min.

10. APGAR SCORE (*Score infant at 1, 2 and 5 minutes of age. If score of 8 is not attained, score at 10, 15 and 20 minutes.*)

				11.	12.	13.	14.	15.	16.
1) AGE AT TIME OF SCORING				Min. | Sec.	Min. | Sec.	Min. | Sec.	Min. | Sec.	Min. | Sec.	Min. | Sec.
2) HEART RATE	0 – Absent	1 – Slow – Less Than 100	2 – 100 or over						
3) RESPIRATORY EFFORT	0 – Absent	1 – Weak Cry Hypoventilation	2 – Crying Lustily						
4) MUSCLE TONE	0 – Flaccid	1 – Some Flexion Extremities	2 – Well Flexed						
5) REFLEX IRRITABILITY	0 – No Response	1 – Some Motion	2 – Cry						
6) COLOR	0 – Blue Pale	1 – Blue Hands and Feet	2 – Entirely Pink						
			7) TOTAL						

PHYSICAL EXAMINATION | 17. Begun at_______ min. of age | 18. EXAMINED BY | 19. TITLE OR POSITION

20. RESPIRATION ☐ Normal 0 ☐ Other 8

21. MOTOR ACTIVITY AND TONE ☐ Normal and Symmetrical 0 ☐ Other 8

22. TONE OF NECK ☐ Normal and Symmetrical 0 ☐ Other 8

23. MOLDING ☐ Absent or Minimal 0 ☐ Moderate or Marked 1

24. FORCEPS MARKS ☐ Absent 0 ☐ Present 1

25. UMBILICAL CORD ☐ Unstained 0 ☐ Stained 1

26. LENGTH OF CORD (*Include all segments*)

On Body_______ Cm. Other_______ Cm.

On Placenta_______ Cm. Total_______ Cm.

27. SKIN (*Acute or transient findings*)
☐ Normal (*Including peripheral cyanosis*) 0
☐ Pallor 1 ☐ Petechiae 3
☐ General Cyanosis 2 ☐ Stained 4
☐ Other 8

28. CRY
☐ Present 0
☐ Present, Abnormal 1
☐ Absent After Maximal Stimulation 2

29. MORO REFLEX
☐ Flexor and Extensor Components Present and Symmetrical 0
☐ Other Pattern 8
☐ Not Evaluated 9

30. COMMENTS AND OTHER FINDINGS

(*Continue on CP-5, Continuation Sheet*)

31. RACE (*Copy from AR-1. Optional*) ☐ W 1 ☐ N 2 ☐ Or 3 ☐ PR 4 ☐ Other 8

32. SEX ☐ Male 1 ☐ Female 2 ☐ Undetermined 9

33. BIRTH WEIGHT

Collaborative Research
Perinatal Research Branch, NINDB, NIH
Bethesda 14, Md.

(PED-1) (Rev. 1-61)

Fig. 4-1. PED-1 form for immediate recording of observations and certain procedures on newborn infants in the delivery room. (Reprinted from The collaborative study on cerebral palsy, mental retardation, and other neurological and sensory disorders of infancy and childhood, National Institute of Neurological Diseases and Blindness, National Institutes of Health, Bethesda, Md.)

murmurs are detected frequently in the neonate as a result of incomplete closure of the ductus arteriosus and the foramen ovale.

The intra-abdominal remnant of the umbilical vein atrophies and obliterates within 3 to 4 days after birth, and the ductus venosus is anatomically occluded during the first week of life. The hypogastric arteries carry no blood after the umbilical cord ceases to pulsate. The distal portions of the hypogastric arteries consist of the umbilical arteries, which atrophy and become obliterated 3 to 4 days after birth to become the umbilical ligaments.

Assessment in the delivery room

Once the physician has placed the neonate in the heated crib and has determined that respirations are established, he returns to the mother to complete the delivery. He delegates the care of the neonate to the professional nurse.

Assessment begins with the observation and notation of spontaneous respiration and cry. Fig. 4-1 shows a form for use in evaluation in the delivery room. The most widely used tool in appraising the general condition of the neonate is the Apgar scoring system (Table 4-1). The system is based on the evaluation of five signs, which are ranked in order of importance: heart rate, respiratory effort, muscle tone, reflex irritability, and color. Each of the five signs is graded on a 3-point scale indicating the degree of response. The scores for each sign are added together to give a total score with 10 as a maximum. The scoring procedure is carried out at 1 and 5 minutes after delivery, and the results of these evaluations are used as indi-cators of present condition and as predictors of future adaptation and development.

Heart rate

Heart rate is the first and most important sign in the sequence. Rate is most accurately evaluated by using a stethoscope on the chest. A heart rate above 100 per minute is assigned a value of 2, a heart rate below 100 per minute is assigned 1, and absence of beat is scored 0. Tachycardia, a heart rate above 160, is indicative of recent anoxia; bradycardia, a heart rate below 100, is indicative of anoxia of longer standing.

Respiratory effort

Next in order of importance is respiratory effort. In the presence of a clear airway a score of 2 is given to the neonate with vigorous respirations and bilateral symmetry in the rise and fall of the chest. A score of 1 is assigned to the neonate when respirations are slow and irregular and fail to expand the chest. Zero is assigned when respirations are absent. Slow, irregular respirations or apnea is an indication of the need for prompt resuscitative intervention.

Muscle tone

Active flexion of the extremities with resistance to extension is given a score of 2. A score of 1 is given when the neonate moves and flexes the extremities but does not resist extension. Limp and flaccid neonates are given a score of 0.

Reflex irritability

Response of the neonate to any form of stimulation is used to grade or score reflex irritability. A neonate who cries vigorously in response to nasopharyngeal suction receives a score of 2. Frequently a slap on the neonate's foot with the palm of the hand is used to elicit a response that can be scored. If the cry is weak or if there is only a grimace, the neonate is given a score of 1. Zero is assigned if there is no response.

Color

Cyanosis is in evidence in all neonates. With the establishment of respirations and the adap-

Table 4-1. Apgar scoring chart for evaluating the neonate at delivery

Sign	0	1	2
Heart rate	Absent	Below 100	Above 100
Respiratory effort	Absent	Slow, irregular	Good crying
Muscle tone	Flaccid, limp	Some flexion of extremities	Active motion
Reflex irritability	No response	Grimace	Vigorous cry
Color	Pale, blue	Body pink, extremities blue	Completely pink

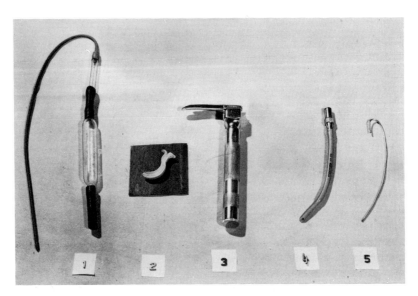

Fig. 4-2. Resuscitation apparatus. **1,** Pharyngeal suction catheter, No. 12 Rausch; **2,** plastic pharyngeal airway; **3,** pencil-handled laryngoscope with premature infant blade; **4,** plastic endotracheal tube, No. 12 Cole; **5,** stylet for endotracheal tube. (From Abramson, H., editor: Resuscitation of the newborn infant, ed. 2, St. Louis, 1966, The C. V. Mosby Co.)

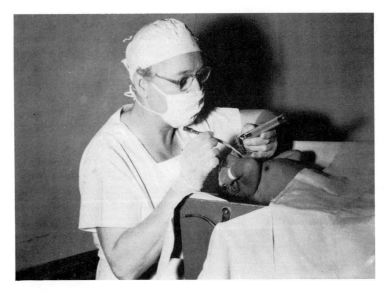

Fig. 4-3. Direct laryngoscopy with pencil-handled laryngoscope and premature infant blade, and tracheal intubation with No. 12 Cole tube. (From exhibit on Resuscitation of Newborn Infants, prepared by the Special Committee on Infant Mortality of the Medical Society of the County of New York, courtesy Association for the Aid of Crippled Children.)

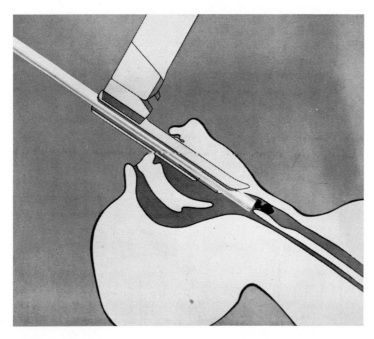

Fig. 4-4. Aspiration of foreign material with laryngoscope and premature blade in situ. (From "Resuscitation of the Newborn," motion picture by Smith, Kline & French Laboratories, Philadelphia, Pa.)

tation of circulation to extrauterine life, the body of the neonate takes on a pink hue. Since acrocyanosis is present in all neonates, even those considered to be in excellent condition, a score of 1 is frequently given for color. A score of 0 is assigned to the neonate who is blue or pale.

A neonate with an Apgar score of 7 to 10 is considered to be in good condition and requires no intervention but does require close observation. A score of 4 to 6 indicates that the neonate is in fair condition and needs to have an open airway maintained and oxygen administered. The body of the neonate should be dried to prevent further loss of body heat through evaporation. The neonate with an Apgar score of 0 to 3 is in acute distress, and active resuscitation must be undertaken to establish and maintain respirations and free oxygen–carbon dioxide gas exchange (Figs. 4-2 to 4-4).

Care of umbilical stump

Various techniques are used to occlude the blood vessels of the umbilical cord. The cord may be ligated using a braided tape, or it may be clamped with one of a variety of plastic or metal umbilical cord clamps. Regardless of the technique, the umbilical cord must be observed for bleeding. Dressings are usually not applied. The cord will dry and separate faster when exposed rather than covered. In addition, there is less chance of the cord being pulled and traumatically separated from its abdominal insertion if it is visible. Strict aseptic precautions must be used in handling the remnants of the cord to prevent the introduction of infection.

Prophylactic procedures

Prophylactic treatment of the eyes of the neonate to prevent gonorrheal infection (ophthalmia neonatorum) is regulated by state law. Most statutes require that a 1% solution of silver nitrate or an equally efficacious medicinal agent be instilled in the eyes of the neonate at birth to prevent such infections. Untreated gonorrheal infections of the eyes of the neonate may produce blindness. Instillation of medication is more easily accomplished if the head of the neonate is lowered and the eyes shaded from light. If silver nitrate is used, 2 drops of the solution is instilled in the conjunctival sac of each eye. Care must be taken to avoid dropping the solution on the cornea. In addition, prompt irrigation of the eyes with distilled water is necessary to prevent chemical conjunctivitis, which is manifested by redness, edema, and purulent discharge from the eyes.

Policies adopted by the hospital or by the physician determine whether or not vitamin K (phytonadione [Mephyton]) is to be administered to the neonate. Vitamin K, 1 mg. in 0.5 ml. given by intramuscular injection, may be administered by the nurse in either the delivery room or the nursery as prophylaxis against hemorrhagic problems in the neonate.

Identification

The neonate must have some form of identification applied before leaving the delivery room. The form of identification is prescribed by the institution in which the delivery takes place. A prenumbered dual identification system in which both the mother and the neonate are identified with bracelets bearing identical numbers is recommended to prevent the possibility of confused identity.

A footprint or palm print of the neonate and thumbprint of the mother are usually made on a permanent record of the neonate. This procedure should be an adjunct to identification and should never be the sole method employed.

Positioning

To facilitate drainage and to prevent aspiration of mucus, the neonate should be placed in a modified Trendelenburg position and propped on his side. An exaggerated Trendelenburg position, greater than 30 degrees, should be avoided because the abdominal organs can exert pressure on the diaphragm and impede full expansion of the lungs. Frequently the neonate is placed on his abdomen with knees flexed and thighs partially flexed toward the abdomen. The head is turned to the side. This type of positioning promotes drainage, prevents aspiration, and limits the possibility of an increase in intracranial pressure.

Introduction to parents

When the mother is awake she should be given the opportunity to see, examine, and hold

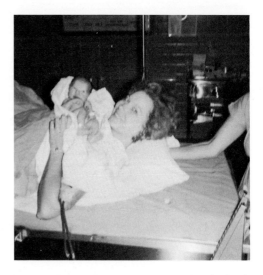

Fig. 4-5. This mother first saw her infant in the delivery room.

her neonate. The first question that is usually asked is "Is he all right?" This anxiety, now expressed, can be alleviated by seeing and handling the neonate, who until this time was a phantom or a dream child. The sex of the child should be emphasized. Many institutions allow fathers to participate in the delivery process. When this is allowed he should also be encouraged to examine and hold the neonate. The birth of the infant may be a high point in both parent's lives. (See Fig. 4-5.) Indeed, childbirth has been called the greatest experience a woman ever has. Further acquaintance with the neonate is discussed later in this chapter.

Anomalies and neonatal distress cannot be hidden. The question "Is he all right?" must be answered simply and honestly. Parents are better able to mourn the birth of a defective neonate than they are to cope with anxiety, fear, and suspicion of unanswered questions.

Neonatal record

The medical record of the neonate is initiated in the delivery room. Many forms have been designed specifically to transmit information from the delivery room to the nursery. Recognition of the importance of maternal history of disease, pregnancy, labor, and delivery has led many institutions to the practice of incorporating a copy of the maternity record into the chart of the neonate. This history is important in giving direction to observations and care of the neonate during adaptation to extrauterine life.

Neonates born to mothers with diabetes mellitus, for example, must be observed closely for tremors and convulsions resulting from hypoglycemia and hypocalcemia. A premature rupture of the fetal membranes alerts the nurse that the neonate must be observed for signs of infection. The neonate delivered in a breech presentation, by forceps, or after a prolonged labor must be observed for evidence of increased intracranial pressure, intracranial hemorrhage, and birth trauma. The signs may include a high, shrill cry, irritability, spasticity, apnea, cyanosis, bulging anterior fontanel, convulsions, vomiting, and failure to move an extremity. Maternal sensitization to the Rh antigen indicates a need for blood typing and possible Coombs' testing for levels of bilirubin in the neonate.

The assessment of the status of the neonate at birth provides the baseline data for evaluating change in behavior. The Apgar score is correlated with the ability of the neonate to adapt to extrauterine existence.

Transfer to the nursery

The neonate and his record initiated in the delivery room are transferred to the nursery by the delivery room nurse. It is recommended that the neonate be transported in an incubator to the nursery. The incubator provides a controlled environment and limits the possibility of injury as a result of being dropped or of the nurse falling while carrying the neonate.

PHYSICAL ASSESSMENT
General appearance

The neonate at birth is between 48 and 50 cm. (19 and 21½ inches) in length. The average male is 50 cm. long and weighs 3,400 gm. (approximately 7½ pounds). The average female is approximately 1.27 cm. (½ inch) shorter than the male and approximately 227 gm. (½ pound) lighter. The skin is pink to red in color and is wrinkled. A thick white cheese-like substance, vernix caseosa, may cover some or all of the body. The vernix disappears spon-

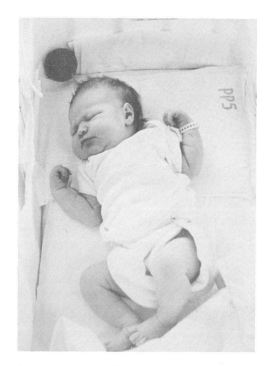

Fig. 4-6. A neonate sleeps much of the time, waking at short intervals, and responds to his environment through his senses.

taneously within the first few days of life. A soft, downy hair, lanugo, may be present on the upper arms, the back, and the forehead. The head, which is the largest circumference of the neonate, may be asymmetrical. It may be molded immediately after birth as a result of adapting to the maternal pelvis during delivery. The amount of hair on the head varies widely. The eyes are closed, and there are eyebrows and eyelashes. The hands are clenched into fists and are held at the level of the head. The legs are flexed and are externally rotated at the hips; the soles of the feet almost touch. When the neonate is awake the cry is lusty; movements are rapid and uncoordinated. The neonate will suck on anything that is placed in his mouth.

Skin

The skin is observed for color, hydration, texture, hemorrhage, and tumors. Acrocyanosis is usually present and is caused by sluggish peripheral blood flow and cool surface temperature. This condition normally persists for about

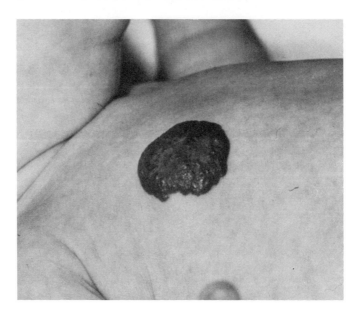

Fig. 4-7. Vascular nevus (strawberry type) on chest of newborn. Complete spontaneous progressive involution occurred by the age of 12 months.

4 to 6 hours, gradually diminishing first from the hands and then from the feet. Circumoral cyanosis is indicative of a pathological condition. Pallor in the neonate is usually associated with cardiac dysfunction.

Jaundice occurring in the neonate after 48 hours of life usually has a physiological basis; jaundice occurring in the first 48 hours usually has a pathological basis, particularly when there is a history of blood dyscrasias in the parents. Icteric coloring should be looked for in the skin, sclera, mucous membranes, and nail beds. Hereditary coloring may mask early detection of jaundice. With darker skinned neonates, jaundice may be detected by blanching the skin through the application of digital pressure on a body surface with minimal fat deposition, such as over the scapula or the tip of the nose.

White papillae, milia, appear on the nose and chin and are due to obstruction of sebaceous glands. These blemishes disappear in the first 2 weeks of life. There may be scratches, abrasions, petechiae, and ecchymosis on any part of the neonate's body as a result of trauma during the process of labor and delivery. All such observations should be recorded. Transient skin markings, nevus flammeus, can be found as dark pink spots between the eyebrows or on

the eyelids, the nose, the upper lip, or the back of the neck. These markings are commonly referred to as "stork bites." Mongolian spots are another type of mark found on the neonate. They are slate blue, well-demarcated areas of pigmentation over the buttocks and back. These kinds of marking can be found in about 50% of black neonates and occasionally in white neonates. They have no clinical significance, and it has been stated that there is no anthropological significance. These markings tend to disappear in the first year of life.

Transient localized edema over the presenting part and on the genitalia of both female and male neonates is not unusual; however, generalized edema is seen in neonates of diabetic mothers, neonates born prior to the thirty-eighth week of gestation, and neonates with erythroblastosis due to Rh incompatibility.

Head

The head of the neonate is proportionately large, averaging between 34 and 35 cm. with a range of 32 to 37 cm. The measurement of the head circumference provides the basis for evaluating skull growth, which in turn gives an indication of brain development.

The fontanels are open at the points of union

of the bones of the skull. The anterior fontanel is diamond shaped and is located at the junction of the two frontal and two parietal bones. The size of the fontanel varies. If it is small in size at birth, there is a tendency to increase in size during the first few months of life. This anterior fontanel, commonly referred to as the "soft spot," closes by the time the child is 18 months of age. The posterior fontanel is triangular in shape and is located at the junction of the parietal bones and the occipital bone. This fontanel usually closes by 3 months of age. The fontanels must be evaluated for both size and tension. Increased intracranial pressure due to intracranial hemorrhage, hydrocephalus, or meningitis causes the fontanels to bulge. Dehydration and fetal malnutrition are common causes of depressed fontanels.

Soft areas may be found in the parietal bones. If present, these soft spots, craniotabes, can be palpated by pressing the scalp firmly just behind and above the ears. A crackling sound is heard, a sound much like that heard when a Ping-Pong ball is compressed. Tabies are usually transient and inconsequential in premature neonates and in some normal infants under 6 months of age. There are pathological conditions in which craniotabes are found, such as syphilis, hydrocephalus, and osteogenesis imperfecta.

Asymmetry of the head may be noted particularly in neonates of primiparous mothers. The parietal bones tend to override the frontal and occipital bones as a result of adapting to the configuration of the maternal pelvis. The head of the neonate delivered in a breech presentation or by cesarean section has a characteristic roundness. In addition to the molding of the head, there may be edema of the scalp over the part of the head that presented during labor. This edema, caput succedaneum, is a soft, ill-defined enlargement that crosses the suture lines. It usually disappears by the third day of life. Occasionally the forces of labor cause the rupture of small blood vessels in the periosteum and a flat bone of the skull. This accumulation of blood is termed cephalhematoma. It is a soft, fluctuant, and irreducible mass that is confined to one bone and does not cross suture lines. Cephalhematomas may occur unilaterally or bilaterally. The duration is relative to size,

and it can be anticipated that it will be several weeks before resorption occurs. Although caput succedaneum and cephalhematoma are manifestations of birth trauma, in the absence of neurological signs there is no cause for alarm. No treatment is indicated.

Transillumination of the skull of the neonate can be done in a darkened room with a standard flashlight fitted with a soft rubber collar. The lighted end of the flashlight is placed flush against the skull. There is transillumination in partial absence of cerebral cortex, prosencephaly, or in displacement of the cortex by extra fluid as in hydrocephaly.

Ears

The ears of the neonate are evaluated as to position and structure. Small, low-set ears have been associated with congenital anomalies of the renal system and with chromosomal aberrations such as Down's syndrome. Normally the upper tip of the ear should be on a line with the inner and outer canthus of the eye. Examination of the ear of the neonate can best be accomplished by gently pulling downward on the pinna since the auditory canal is directed upward from the inside. The tympanic membrane is covered with vernix caseosa during the first 2 to 3 days of life and cannot be visualized. Early examination is done to determine the patency of the external auditory canal. Hearing in the neonate may be tested by observing for eye blink in response to a sharp sound such as snapping the fingers or clapping the hands. The acoustic blink reflex is difficult to elicit during the first 2 to 3 days of life and even after that time the blinking response to sound does not assure normal hearing. Nor is the absence of blinking response diagnostic of deafness.

Eyes

The eyes of the neonate are difficult to examine since the lids are usually tightly closed and attempts to separate them usually result in increased resistance. Eye structure should be noted. An Oriental slant characterized by a lateral upward slope with an inner epicanthal fold in neonates of non-Asian races may be indicative of chromosomal aberration.

Discharge from the eyes may be seen soon

after birth as a result of chemical irritation of the conjunctivae. Drainage from the eyes during the first week of life is commonly gonococcal in origin. Later conjunctivitis with drainage is usually viral in origin.

Eye movements are usually uncoordinated at birth. If this nystagmus persists after a few days of life, it may be indicative of blindness. Although absence of pupillary reflex is common in the neonate, unilateral constriction or dilation may be a sign of pathology. Small conjunctival, scleral, and retinal hemorrhages are common in the neonate and are rarely significant.

Nose

Almost all neonates are nasal breathers, and patency of the nasal passages may be determined by holding the mouth closed and occluding first one side and then the other side of the nose. If each side is patent, there will be no distress. Obstruction of the nasal passages occurs with displacement of the cartilage of the vomer during delivery and in choanal atresia. The passage of a soft rubber catheter through each nostril into the nasopharynx immediately after birth confirms the patency of the nasal passages.

Mouth

The mouth should be inspected for cleft lip, cleft palate, tumors, and cysts. Occasionally white pearllike cysts are seen along the ridges of the gums and are often mistaken for teeth. These cysts disappear spontaneously. Neonates are edentulous; however, teeth have been found in some neonates. They are without enamel and are usually shed within a few days of life. Frequently small yellow or white rounded elevations are seen on the hard palate. These are called Epstein's pearls and may persist in the mouth for several months. Oral moniliasis, thrush, is seen as flat, lacey, white curds on the mucous membrane of the mouth. There is an erythematous base that causes the neonate discomfort and can interfere with his sucking and swallowing. Moniliasis can be distinguished from milk curd in that it cannot be removed; milk curds can be wiped away easily.

There is little activity by the salivary glands during the first 3 months of life. The presence of large amounts of saliva in the mouth of the neonate is suggestive of tracheoesophageal fistula.

Neck

The neck of the neonate is short, creased, symmetrical, and supple. It should be possible to rotate the head from side to side. The neck may be observed by placing a hand behind the upper back and allowing the head to gently fall into extension. It is best examined with the thumb and the first two fingers while the neonate is held in this position. Injury to the sternomastoid muscle with bleeding into the muscle tissue due to stretching of the neck during delivery results in torticollis (wry neck). The neonate tilts the head toward the affected side and a palpable, firm, fibrous mass in the muscle develops before the end of the neonatal period.

Chest

The chest is bell shaped and is approximately the same circumference as the abdomen, approximately 0.5 cm. smaller than the head. The thorax is almost circular, with the anterior-posterior diameter equal to the bilateral diameter as a result of the pressure of the arms on the lateral walls of the chest during intrauterine life. Breathing is accomplished through the use of abdominal muscles and the diaphragm. Vibratory tremors can be palpated through the chest wall when the neonate cries. Changes in the transmission of sound through the lungs, pleura, and chest wall can be detected by placing the whole hand over the anterior, posterior, or lateral thorax of the neonate.

Respirations in the neonate range from 30 to 50 per minute. They are irregular in both rate and depth, intermittently shallow and slow, then rapid and deep. Crying will enhance auscultation by stimulating deep inspiration, and fortunately most neonates cry only on expiration.

The breasts of both male and female neonates may be enlarged, and a thin milky exudate can be expressed from the breasts (witch's milk). The mastitis, which is due to the influence of maternal hormones, may persist for 2 to 4 weeks. Because of the sensitivity of the breasts, they should be touched only as necessary.

Heart rate at birth varies from 100 to 160 beats per minute and stabilizes very shortly after birth to between 120 and 140 beats per minute. The rhythm is usually regular. Varying rhythm is associated with anoxia, cerebral defects, or increased intracranial pressure. Bradycardia is associated with anoxia and tachycardia with anemia. The heart percusses relatively large because of its more horizontal position. Murmurs are noted for loudness, quality, location, and timing, but their relative significance is usually not determined at this time since functional murmurs are frequently present in the normal neonate.

Abdomen

The abdomen of the neonate appears large and flabby due to the size of internal organs and to weak abdominal muscles. A neonate with a concave abdomen should be examined immediately for diaphragmatic hernia with displacement of abdominal organs.

The umbilical cord should be examined at birth to determine the presence of three blood vessels, one vein and two arteries. A single umbilical artery is one of the criteria used in designating a neonate at high risk. There is a high correlation between single arteries and congenital defects. The umbilical stump usually dries and drops from its insertion between 5 and 10 days. The skin retracts and becomes flush with the abdominal wall during this time. Neonates are prone to umbilical hernias and diastasis recti. These become apparent after 2 to 3 weeks of life and are easily detected when the neonate cries. Most umbilical hernias disappear by 1 year of life. Diastasis recti usually disappears in early childhood. Persistence may be due to congenital muscle weakness.

Auscultation of the abdomen for bowel sounds should be done before palpation since palpation usually induces crying. Palpation of the abdomen of the neonate is relatively easy. Relaxation can be achieved by flexing the legs at the knees and the hips. The liver edge can be felt 2 to 3 cm. below the right costal margin and the spleen tip under the left costal margin. The bladder can be felt and percussed up to the level of the umbilicus. For palpation of the kidneys, the neonate should be held at a 45-degree angle. The lower half of the right and the tip of the left kidney can normally be felt in the neonate. Masses in the flank are usually renal in origin, such as congenital hydronephrosis and Wilms' tumor.

The descending colon is felt as a sausage-like mass in the left lower quadrant. A midline suprapublic mass is often found in Hirschsprung's disease (congenital megacolon). Spasm and rigidity may be avoided by giving a bottle feeding during the palpation of the abdomen.

Genitalia

Assessment of the male genitalia presents little difficulty. The prepuce or foreskin adheres to the glans penis, covering it completely, with a small orifice at the distal end. The foreskin should be retracted, allowing for inspection of the urinary meatus for patency and position. Hypospadias is present when the position of the meatus is found at some point along the ventral surface of the glans or on the shaft of the penis. The testes should be palpable in the scrotum. If the testes are not found in the scrotum, they may take several months or even years to descend. Surgical intervention may be indicated in some instances. Hydroceles of the testes and the spermatic cord are not uncommon in the neonate and can be differentiated from hernias by transillumination: hydroceles transilluminate.

In the female neonate the labia minora are prominent. There may be blood-tinged mucous discharge, pseudomenstruation, through the vagina as a result of maternal hormonal influence. The hymenal ring generally protrudes through the introitus. The perineal structures can be visualized by separating the labia with the thumb and forefinger. A number of malformations may affect the genitalia. An unusually large clitoris in the female could be confused with a small penis in the male. Identification of the meatus in such instances is essential.

Rectum

Rectal temperatures in the neonate must be approached with caution because of the possibility of an imperforate anus. If large amounts of meconium have been passed, there is no need to question the patency of the rectum. The purpose of the rectal examination in the neonate is to determine the patency of the anus. The neonate is placed in a supine position with the legs flexed at the knees and the hips. The finger is then gently introduced into the rectum. The rectal examination of the neonate is usually followed by some bleeding from the rectum.

Back

With the neonate on the abdomen, the back should be inspected and palpated for deviations in alignment such as scoliosis and for spinal closure defects such as spina bifida occulta (defect of one or more vertebrae) and pilonidal sinus. Spina bifida with herniation (meningocele or meningomylocele) is a serious defect and requires immediate and constant attention.

Extremities

The hands and the feet should be examined for polydactyly (extra fingers or toes) and for syndactyly (fused fingers or toes). All of the major joints should be put through a complete range of motion. The position of the arms should be observed for evidence of fracture. The arms are normally flexed with the hands at the level of the head. An arm that is extended at a right angle to the body may indicate a brachial plexus injury or a fractured clavicle.

The feet of the neonate may appear deformed as a result of intrauterine position. If the foot can be passively brought into the opposite position, overcorrected, the apparent deformity is usually positional and requires only exercise for correction. True deformity resists placement in the neutral or opposite position, and orthopedic treatment may be indicated. With the neonate in the prone position with the legs extended the skin folds and creases of the buttocks and thighs should be inspected for symmetry. Asymmetrical creases and folds warrant further study for dislocation of the hip or hip deformity. The hips of the neonate should be examined for dislocation. With the neonate in the supine position the legs are flexed at right angles at the hip and the knee abducted until it touches the table. If the head of the femur is seen and felt, a dislocation is present. Subluxation of the femur may result in resistance to complete abduction.

NEUROLOGICAL ASSESSMENT

The general appearance, activity, cry, and position of the neonate are important observations in neurological assessment. Activities of the neonate are limited for the most part to sleeping for 20 of the 24 hours, crying to communicate discomfort, and feeding. Movements are rapid and uncoordinated and for the most part are reflexive responses to stimuli. Muscle tone, spasticity, or flaccidity can be determined by putting each major joint through its range of motion, testing for motor function.

Reflexes associated with feeding

Several reflexes are associated with feeding and are present at birth. The rooting reflex can be elicited by stroking the cheek, the upper lip, or the lower lip. The neonate will turn his head toward the area that is being stroked. This reflex helps the neonate to locate the nipple when the mother's breast touches the cheek. The rooting reflex disappears at about 3 to 4 months of age. The sucking reflex stimulates sucking movements of the mouth whenever anything thouches the lips of the neonate. This reflex can be demonstrated at birth. The sucking reflex is accompanied by the swallowing and gag reflexes. The gag reflex is stimulated by an excessive amount of liquid sucked into the mouth, which the neonate is unable to swallow.

Blinking reflex

The blinking reflex, in which the neonate closes the eyelids in response to light, is present at birth and usually disappears after the first year of life. Failure to respond to light may indicate blindness in the neonate.

Acoustic blink reflex

The acoustic blink reflex can be observed after the first 2 to 3 days of life. The time at which it disappears varies. The eyes of the neonate blink in response to a sharp sound such as the snapping of the fingers or the clapping of the hands at a distance of about 12 inches from the ears. Failure to respond may be indicative of impaired hearing.

Palmar grasp reflex

The grasp reflex is present at birth and disappears after 3 to 4 months of life. With the neonate in a supine position and the head aligned with the midline of the body, a finger is placed touching the palm of the hand or the foot of the neonate. The neonate will flex all of his fingers around the finger of the examiner. If the finger is placed on the foot, the toes will curl in an attempt to grasp the finger. Failure to respond may be indicative of cerebral dysfunction. Normally the neonate holds his hands clenched during the first month of life.

Trunk incurvation reflex

The trunk incurvation reflex is present at birth and disappears at about 2 months of age. The neonate is held in the prone position in the examiner's hand. The back of the neonate is stimulated by running the forefinger of the examiner's hand down the back in a line with and about 3 cm. from the spine. The back is stimulated from the shoulder to the buttocks. The neonate will respond by curving the trunk, the shoulder and the pelvis moving toward the side stimulated. Failure to elicit the response may be indicative of a spinal cord lesion.

Vertical suspension positioning

Vertical suspension positioning is present at birth and disappears after about 4 months of age. The neonate is held upright with the hands of the examiner under the axillae, the head aligned with the midline, and the legs flexed at the knees and hips. Normally the neonate will not change this position. If there is extension of the legs with crossing at the ankles, spastic paraplegia is suspected.

Placing response

The placing response is evident after 4 days of life and disappears in early infancy. The neonate is held upright with the dorsal surface of one foot touching the underside of a table. The neonate will respond by flexing the hip and knee and lifting the stimulated foot onto the table top. With one foot touching the table top the neonate will attempt stepping movements. This is sometimes called the dancing reflex. It is usually absent in the neonate born in the breech presentation and in neonates with paralysis.

Tonic neck reflex

The tonic neck reflex, commonly called the fencing position, may be present at birth but usually appears around 2 months of age and disappears at about 6 months. It can be seen when the neonate is positioned on the back with the head turned to the side and the jaw held over the shoulder. The arm and the leg on the side to which the head is turned are extended at right angles to the body. This reflex does not occur at all times; when it does or if it persists beyond 6 months of age, cerebral damage should be suspected.

Perez reflex

The Perez reflex is present at birth and disappears at varying times. The neonate is held in the prone position in the examiner's hand. The thumb of the other hand is placed on the sacrum of the neonate and is moved firmly up the spine toward the head. The neonate will respond by crying, extending his head, straightening his spine, flexing his legs, and voiding. This reflex has been found useful in collecting urine specimens from neonates.

Moro reflex

The Moro reflex, commonly called the startle reflex, is present at birth and disappears around the fourth month of life. With the neonate in the supine position the crib is jarred, or, if the neonate is held in the supine position, the head is allowed to fall back gently. The neonate will respond by drawing up the legs and extending the arms in an embracing motion followed by a short period of rigid and fixed position. Persistence of the Moro reflex beyond 4 months of age is indicative of neurological damage. Asymmetrical response in the upper extremities may indicate injury to the brachial nerve plexus or fracture of the clavical. Asymmetry or absence of response in the lower extremities may indicate dislocation of the hip or low spinal cord injury.

CARE IN THE NURSERY

Upon admission to the nursery excess blood and vernix are wiped from the head and body of the neonate. The nurse appraises the general condition, observing cry, color, respirations, and any anomalies present. After the neonate is dressed and wrapped in a blanket, he is placed in a warm crib on his abdomen or propped on his side. Close observation must be maintained for any signs of neonatal distress.

The routine daily care of the neonate should conform to the *Standards and Recommendations for the Hospital Care of Newborn Infants* (1971) prepared by the Committee on the Fetus and Newborn of the American Academy of Pediatrics.

Objectives in the care of the neonate are *maintaining respirations, preventing infection, providing adequate nutrition, maintaining normal body temperature, recognizing and reporting illnesses and deviations from normal response, meeting the emotional needs of the neonate,* and *educating the mother in his care.*

To meet these objectives the nurse must be committed to the care of the neonate and to be his advocate; develop her observational, technical, and teaching skills; understand the range of normal variation in the characteristics of the neonate; recognize and capitalize on all opportunities to teach; and be alert to signs of illness and distress in the neonate. What the nurse must not be is rigid, regimented, outdated, and outmoded in her approach to the care of the neonate.

Neonatal mortality statistics for the United States indicate that the mortality is decreasing; however, it must be pointed out that in spite of technical advances and improved obstetric and neonatal care approximately 73% of deaths in infants under 1 year of age occur during the first 28 days of life, and 65% of the deaths occur in the first 7 days of life (Table 4-2). The mortality is due to conditions present prior to birth, at birth, or shortly after birth. These conditions include immaturity, congenital anomalies, asphyxia, respiratory disease, birth injury, septicemia, and complications of pregnancy, labor, and delivery (Table 4-3). These statistics indicate the need for astute observation and meticulous care of the neonate by the nurse in the hospital and the need to educationally prepare mothers to give optimum care in the home.

Positioning

Frequently neonates in nurseries are positioned primarily on their abdomens to facilitate drainge and prevent aspiration. However, the well-developed neonate does not maintain a stationary position; he turns his head from side

Table 4-2. Neonatal deaths classified by age and sex*

Age	Male	Female	Total
1 hour	2,832	2,222	5,054
1-23 hours	10,321	7,268	17,589
1 day	3,153	2,295	5,448
2 days	2,129	1,423	3,552
3 days	1,007	719	1,726
4 days	601	433	1,034
5 days	480	348	828
6 days	345	283	628
7-13 days	1,362	1,062	2,424
14-20 days	712	599	1,311
21-27 days	593	477	1,070
TOTAL	23,535	17,129	40,664

*Based on 1973 statistical data from the Mortality Statistics Branch, Division of Vital Statistics of the National Center for Health Statistics, Department of Health, Education, and Welfare.

Table 4-3. Ten leading causes of neonatal deaths classified by sex*

Cause of death	Male	Female	Total
Congenital anomalies	3,448	2,694	6,142
Asphyxia (unspecified)	3,135	2,229	5,364
Complications of pregnancy, labor, and delivery	2,524	1,980	4,504
Hyaline membrane disease	2,739	1,670	4,409
Respiratory distress syndrome	2,559	1,465	4,024
Birth injury	1,084	754	1,838
Conditions of the placenta	745	567	1,312
Influenza and pneumonia	577	411	988
Septicemia	342	243	585

*Based on 1973 statistical data from the Mortality Statistics Branch, Division of Vital Statistics of the National Center for Health Statistics, Department of Health, Education, and Welfare.

to side and creeps up to the top of the crib. In carrying out these activities he rubs his chin, nose, cheeks, and knees over the sheets, and it is not uncommon to find excoriation of the skin over these areas. The position of the neonate should be changed from the abdomen to the side at frequent intervals, at least every 2 hours, to prevent hypostatic pneumonia, atelectasis, and areas of excoriation.

Control of infection

One of the most effective means of preventing infection in the neonate in the nursery or in the home is meticulous handwashing before handling the neonate or any materials and equipment used in his care. The importance of handwashing cannot be overemphasized. In addition, the probability of infection can be lowered by limiting the number of people permitted in the nursery or coming in contact with the neonate. To facilitate the control of the number of personnel giving care to the neonate, small units of 8 to 10 bassinets are recommended. The American Academy of Pediatrics advocates that there should be a minimum of 30 square feet allocated to each neonate with no less than 2 feet between bassinets. Personnel with infections or suspected infections should be barred from all contact with the neonate. There must be early recognition and isolation of neonates with infections.

Temperature

At delivery the temperature of the neonate approximates that of the mother but rapidly drops approximately 5° F. as a result of transfer from an intrauterine environment of approximately 100° F. to the cool ambient temperature of the delivery unit. Upon admission to the nursery the temperature of the neonate is between 95° and 96° F. Homeostasis is usually achieved at about 8 hours of life with a temperature between 98° and 99° F. Stabilization is achieved through increase in metabolic rates, increase in activity including crying, stimulation of the skin receptors through handling, prevention of heat loss by wrapping warmly, and maintenance of a stable ambient temperature of approximately 75° F. in the nursery. Wrappings should be adjusted to the climatic conditions in the nursery once stabilization in body temperature has been achieved. Persistent temperature of 96° F. or below may be indicative of birth trauma. Undue exposure of skin surfaces to cool environments should be avoided. A gross indicator of temperature in the normal neonate is the skin color of the face. If the face is pale, the neonate is cold and additional covering is indicated. If the face is flushed, the neonate is warm and some covering should be removed. Since peripheral circulation is not well developed at birth, the temperature of the hands and feet are poor indicators of true body temperature.

Skin care

The skin requires little or no care upon admission to the nursery. Blood and excess vernix may be wiped away from the face and head for aesthetic reasons. The time for first bathing is established by nursery policy of the institution. Bathing of the neonate on admission to the nursery tends to cause a further drop in body temperature, but the tactile stimulation of the skin through handling seems to shorten the time required for stabilization of temperature at a more normal level. Regardless of whether the bath is given on admission or 12 hours following birth, the procedure should be carried out as rapidly as possible to prevent undue exposure and loss of body heat.

Before undressing the neonate the head is washed with a mild soap and warm water and dried thoroughly. The face is washed with warm water. The eyes should be washed from the inner to the outer canthus. Care must be taken to remove debris from behind and over the ears. Once the head and face of the neonate are washed and dried, his clothing is removed and his body and extremities are washed with warm water and a mild soap. Particular attention is given to cleaning and drying skin creases and folds. The neonate is then dressed and wrapped warmly and placed on his abdomen or side in his crib. The skin over the genitals and the buttocks should be cleaned with warm water after each voiding and defecation. Oils and powders are not used on the skin of the neonate during the time he is in the nursery unless they are specifically ordered by the physician.

Emotional support

The neonate gains his initial impression of the world into which he has been born through contact with others in the satisfaction of his needs. Some of the elements that are important in meeting the emotional needs of the neonate are gentle physical contact; sounds of pleasant and varying tones of voice; feeding when he is hungry; soft, dry clothing; and a quiet, comfortable place to sleep. Restlessness and crying can be elicited from the neonate by any intense and noxious form of stimulation although there is no constant pattern of response. Responses that have been identified as fear in the neonate are more accurately labeled the Moro reflex, the neonate's response to being startled by a loud noise or an abrupt movement. The reaction is a result of sensory stimulation rather than the emotional response of fear. The neonate is not capable of anger; he responds to sufficiently dissatisfying stimuli by his only means of communication, crying. The neonate achieves a state of equilibrium when his needs are satisfied.

Nurses need to be aware of the importance of meeting the emotional needs of the neonate. Firm but gentle handling during all procedures is essential. Efforts should be directed toward prevention of exhaustion of the neonate, prompt relief of distress, promotion of comfort, and satisfaction through holding and feeding of the neonate.

Feeding

The neonate is not usually given feedings for the first 8 to 12 hours. He has more extracellular fluid than young children and does not need fluid immediately.

First feeding

The first feeding is usually a 5% glucose solution in water since if the neonate has an abnormality such as esophageal atresia or tracheoesophageal fistula (Chapter 12), it is less harmful for water to get in the lungs or bronchi than milk. It is best for the infant's first feeding to be given by the nurse. She can note how he sucks—whether poorly or vigorously—or whether he is indifferent to the feeding. She can see if the effort of sucking tires the infant quickly. If the infant coughs, vomits, or shows signs of respiratory distress, the nurse should stop the feeding at once and notify the doctor.

Breast-feeding

The decision to bottle-feed or breast-feed the infant is usually made before the birth of the baby. It is a decision the mother makes herself without any pressure from anyone. Because the mother may wish to discuss breast-feeding with the nurse in the prenatal clinic or elsewhere, a discussion of advantages and contraindications is given here as well as techniques of breast-feeding, care of breasts, and maintenance of a supply of breast milk.

Among the advantages of breast-feeding is the fact that breast milk is a natural food for human infants. It contains more vitamin A, niacin, and ascorbic acid than does cow's milk. Because the ratio of calcium to phosphorus is high, the possibility of neonatal tetany is lessened or eliminated. The protein constituent of breast milk (predominately lactalbumin) forms a soft curd that is easily digested; this in turn facilitates the action of digestive enzymes. Lactose is converted into lactic acid, which hinders the growth of pathogens.

In the last part of pregnancy colostrum may come from the nipple. It is a precursor of milk. It is present in sufficient amounts to nourish the neonate for several days until it is replaced by a transitory form of milk, which gradually becomes mature breast milk. Colostrum has a higher protein and mineral content than true breast milk and a slightly lower carbohydrate content. Breast-fed babies are rarely constipated and tend to be less susceptible to colic, skin disorders, and respiratory infections.

For the nursing mother there are also advantages. Sucking at the breast stimulates involution of the uterus after delivery. It has been theorized that early breast-feeding stimulates the evacuation of meconium, promotes an increase in the neonate's nutritional intake, and decreases the initial weight loss of the neonate. Breast-feeding encourages intimacy between mother and infant and gives physical enjoyment to both the mother and infant. It brings oral pleasure to the infant. It brings to the mother a sense of accomplishment and being important to her infant.

There are both temporary and permanent contraindications to breast-feeding. Permanent contraindications are septicemia, nephritis, eclampsia, profuse hemorrhage, active tuberculosis, typhoid fever, and malaria. Other conditions in the mother that contraindicate breast-feeding are chronic malnutrition, general debility, psychoses, severe neuroses, and known malignancy. Sore or cracked nipples that produce extreme pain when sucked may be an indication for temporary stopping of breast-feeding until the nipples heal. Maternal mastitis may be a temporary contraindication if the condition can be treated and relieved in a relatively short period of time.

The main factors in the secretion of true breast milk are the emptying of the breast and the influence of the hormone prolactin, which is produced by the anterior pituitary gland. (Estrogen and progesterone are both inhibited after the placenta is delivered or a short time later). Prolactin aids the alveoli in the breast to secrete milk. Myoepithelial cells surround the alveoli. They are contractile tissue. When the infant sucks, the cells act as a band, contracting and squeezing milk from the alveoli into the duct system. Oxytocin from the posterior lobe of the pituitary gland influences this and helps to explain why the uterus contracts when the baby nurses. Oxytocin acts on smooth muscle tissue. The action of the myoepithelial cells is known as "ejection" reflex, "let-down" reflex, or "draught" reflex. Psychological factors also are believed to influence the milk ejection reflex, such as pain, anxiety, fatigue, tension, and fear.

In addition to prolactin, the production of milk is aided by the emptying of the breasts, as mentioned. It is desirable to put the neonate to breast as soon as possible after delivery; indeed, some advocate that the neonate nurse immediately after delivery.

Although infants vary in the emptying time of their stomachs and thus the feeling of hunger, in general a 3-hour feeding is considered best for both infant and mother. Frequent nursing helps prevent engorgement and helps the "let-down" reflex. Also, the neonate tires easily and probably may suck less vigorously to receive milk. It is suggested that the infant nurse on *each* breast for 5 minutes the first day, 10 minutes the second day, and 15 minutes the third day. Both breasts are used at each feeding. At the next feeding the mother should place the baby on the last breast from which the infant nursed; thus this breast will be emptied of the residual milk from the prior feeding. This in turn stimulates further milk secretion.

When the nurse takes the infant to the mother for feedings, she should see that the mother is comfortably positioned. If the mother has had an episiotomy, it will be easier for her to nurse the infant if the head of the bed is lowered (but not completely flat). The infant can be placed on the bed. The mother can be instructed to turn on her side to nurse. She can place her second and third fingers around her breast and direct the nipple in a stroking position across the infant's mouth. This will stimulate the rooting reflex. The nurse and the mother need to be patient until the infant finally gets the nipple and areola into his mouth. If the nurse or mother tries to push the infant's head to the nipple, the infant will turn his head toward her hand instead of the nipple. When the infant does get the nipple into his mouth, the mother should hold the upper part of her breast away from his nose so he can breathe easily. The neonate can then place his mouth on the skin covering the areola of the breast, thus avoiding undue pressure on the nipple.

The nurse needs to demonstrate to the mother how to "burp" the neonate halfway through the feeding and again at the end of the feeding to expel swallowed air from the stomach. He can be turned on his abdomen for a few minutes, held over the mother's shoulder, or supported in a sitting position while the mother rubs his back. Discomfort from her stitches is a factor that will influence the mother's choice of method in "burping" her infant.

Discomfort of the mother as a result of overdistention or engorgement may be relieved by manually expressing milk from the breast. Manual expression of milk from the breasts is accomplished through two movements of the hands. The first movement is intended to move the milk into the lacteal sinuses. Starting at the base of the breast and continuing toward the areola, the whole breast is compressed between the hands. Firm pressure should be maintained while this movement is repeated several times. The second movement is intended to evacuate milk from the breast. The breast is supported with one hand and the thumb and forefinger of the other hand compress the tissue just behind the areola.

The baby does not need water or milk from a bottle while breast-feeding. Supplementary feedings are seldom necessary. He should be hungry when he comes to nurse and ready to suck vigorously. Actually it is easier to suck from a bottle than breast. Sucking the bottle is more of a tugging response, whereas sucking the nipple of the breast is more of a compression action of the lips, gums, and cheek muscles.

Lactation imposes a physical strain on the mother, an output of energy, so both her rest and her nutrition need attention. When the infant sleeps, the mother can rest. For dietary requirements of the lactating mother see Chapter 3. Sufficient to note, the quantity and quality of milk will be influenced by the mother's diet. A mother on an inadequate diet may become excessively fatigued and as a result be sometimes cross and irritable. Instead of feeding time being a pleasant and loving experience, it may become a source of tension from which neither the mother nor the infant derives any benefit. A well-fed, well-rested mother makes for a more contented breast-fed baby.

When the mother takes the neonate home, she should be cautioned that it takes the new infant awhile to adjust to a feeding schedule. He may be hungry at 3 hours one time, at 4 hours another time, and maybe 3½ hours at another time. By 2 to 3 weeks he wakens for feedings at a fairly regular time. Also, sometimes he seems hungrier than other times. This is normal; when he is hungry he will nurse well.

Bottle-feeding technique

Infant feeding technique deserves attention. Both the nurse and the infant need to be comfortable. The upper part of the infant's body should be higher than his abdomen to avoid possible aspiration at feeding. The bottle should be tilted so that the neck of the bottle is filled with solution (either water or formula); otherwise the infant sucks air and milk together. At the end of half the feeding the nurse should burp the infant and again at the end of the entire feeding. A nurse may like to put the infant over her shoulder to do this, but it is better for the nurse to hold him in a sitting position in her lap. One hand of the nurse should support the infant while the other hand is used to stroke his back from the center of the back upward. This facilitates burping. This method is suggested both for nurses on the pediatric hospital unit and for nurses in the newborn nursery, since infants are more susceptible to infection than older chil-

dren. The farther the infant can be kept from the nose and mouth of the nurse the better. The nurse may be harboring organisms that are not harmful to her but are to the infant.

The infant usually takes his feeding in 20 minutes. If he has not, then he has been offered too much milk, he is too weak or tired to suck, the milk is not coming out of the bottle, or he has an inadequate sucking reflex.

After feeding, the infant should usually be placed on his abdomen, although some authorities suggest that he be placed on his right side to facilitate emptying of the stomach into the intestines. If he is placed on his side, he needs to be very firmly propped or he may wiggle and turn onto his back with the resultant possibility of aspiration if he regurgitates or vomits part of the feeding. Placing the infant on his abdomen lessens the possibility of aspiration.

Regulation of feedings

The infant should be allowed to take what he wants from the bottle or breast. He may take part of the bottle or all of it. When an infant is satisfied, he is usually drowsy and quiet. If he is still hungry after the feeding, he fusses and/or sucks his lips. Sometimes he cries. If hungry, he should be offered more feeding. The infant tends to regulate his own feeding and does not necessarily take the same amount at each feeding. If he is on a 4-hour schedule and acts hungry before it is feeding time again, he should be fed. If he continually acts hungry, this information should be passed to the physician. The feeding schedule can be adjusted. In general, small babies are on 3-hour schedules and the larger ones on 4-hour schedules. The individual needs of the infant should be considered and the feedings should be on self-demand—the infant being fed whenever he is hungry. Infants should not be awakened at night for feedings if they are sleeping, nor should they be allowed to cry for long periods of time if they are hungry. Crying is the signal to the nurse that something is wrong.

Formula calculation

The formula for the infant is designed to meet his nutritional requirements. Since infancy is a period of rapid growth and development, calories and protein needs for the infant are high relative to his body weight. The infant needs from 50 to 55 calories and 1.5 to 2 gm. of protein per pound of body weight per day. The need for fluid is also high since the baby has a large surface area through which water may be lost. The kidneys also need extra fluid to clear out large amounts of metabolic waste products. The infant should receive from 2½ to 3 ounces of fluid per pound of body weight per day.

Human breast milk adequately meets these nutritional requirements. Since the composition of cow's milk differs from that of human milk, certain modifications for the infant's formula must be made. Cow's milk contains a higher total protein and mineral content than human milk and a slightly lower carbohydrate content. Whereas older children can tolerate these differences, the young infant has difficulty utilizing this concentrated protein; thus the cow's milk must be diluted with water. To account for the calories lost through dilution and to approximate the carbohydrate composition of human milk, some form of sugar is added. With these adjustments both human milk and cow's milk formula supply approximately 20 calories per ounce.

The amount of milk used in the formula is determined by the infant's protein requirement. For example, a neonate weighing 7 pounds would need from 10 to 14 gm. of protein a day. Several types of milk can be used. Fresh whole milk supplies 1 gm. of protein and 20 calories per ounce. If fresh whole milk is used, it should be pasteurized and homogenized. Canned evaporated milk has advantages over fresh whole milk in that it can be stored without refrigeration and it is generally less expensive. It supplies 2 gm. of protein and 40 calories per ounce. Mothers should be cautioned against using sweetened condensed milk. This milk has a high sugar content, which is poorly tolerated by the infant. Likewise mothers should not use nonfat milk unless it is prescribed by the physician. Although specific fat requirements for the infant have not been set, infants do require a supply of essential fatty acids for normal growth and development. These would not be provided in nonfat milk.

Seven ounces of evaporated milk would be needed in the example for calculating a formula for a 7-pound infant (14 gm. protein requirement ÷ 2 gm. per ounce of evaporated milk = 7 ounces).

The amount of carbohydrate to be added is determined by the infant's total calories requirement. The 7-pound infant would need approximately 385 calories per day. (55 calories per pound × 7 pounds = 385 calories.) The milk in the formula will supply 280 of these calories. (7 ounces evaporated milk × 40 calories per ounce = 280 calories.) The remaining calories must come from the added carbohydrate. Granulated cane sugar, liquid corn syrup, or mixtures of Dextri-maltose may be used. Each of these supplies approximately 120 calories per ounce. The liquid corn syrup seems to be tolerated best by most infants. Starch has also been used, but since the infant's starch-splitting enzymes are immature at birth, it is seldom recommended. If corn syrup were used, the amount needed for this example formula would be 1 ounce. The formula would then be diluted with water to meet the infant's total fluid requirement. (7 pounds × 3 ounces per pound = 21 ounces; 21 ounces − 7 ounces milk = 14 ounces water to be added.) A formula prescription for this infant written out for the mother might read as follows:

Evaporated milk	7 ounces
Corn syrup	1 ounce
Water	14 ounces
Total volume of formula	21 ounces

This is the infant's total feeding for 1 day. The formula may be divided into six or eight bottles of 3½ ounces or 2½ ounces each, depending on whether the infant demands a 4- or 3-hour feeding schedule.

Observation and recording

The condition of the neonate should be monitored on a continuing basis, and pertinent observations should be recorded. The quality and rate of respirations, color, activity, cry, and condition of the skin and cord should be noted. It is important to observe for voiding and defecation. Of particular importance is the first stool of the neonate, meconium, which is composed of salts, bile, epithelial cells, and amniotic fluid

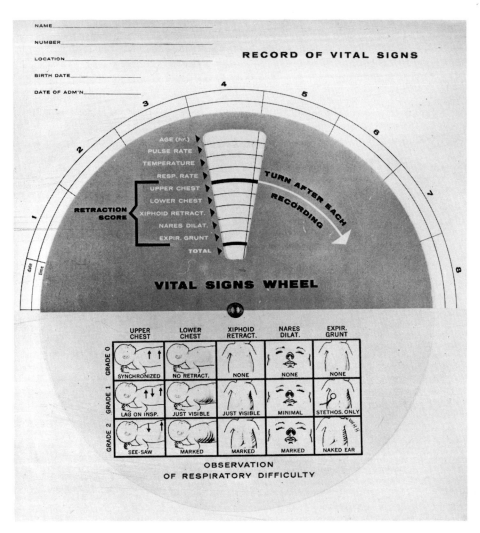

Fig. 4-8. Vital signs wheel that was developed at Babies Hospital, Columbia-Presbyterian Medical Center, New York, N.Y. Pulse rate, body temperature, respiratory rate, and respiratory performance (Silverman-Anderson score) are recorded on a data sheet at 6-hour intervals. To encourage the examiner to make each observation without knowledge of prior judgments, the preceding record is masked with the wheel. In scoring of retraction, four of the recorded criteria are inspiratory: (1) movement of upper chest and abdomen, (2) intercostal movement, (3) xiphoid movement, and (4) movement of nares. One recorded criterion is expiratory: (5) presence or absence of grunting. The retraction score that gives an index of respiratory distress is determined by grading each of the five arbitrary criteria as follows: grade 0 indicates no difficulty, grade 1 indicates moderate difficulty, and grade 2 indicates maximum respiratory difficulty. A retraction score of 0 indicates no retraction, and a score of 10 indicates maximum respiratory retraction and distress. (Courtesy Mead Johnson & Co., Evansville, Ind.; from Silverman, W. A., editor: Dunham's premature infants, ed. 3, New York, 1961, Harper & Row, Publishers.)

ingested during intrauterine life. These stools vary in color from dark greenish black to brown and are viscous, tenacious, and tarlike in consistency. Some meconium is usually passed during the first 12 hours after birth. Care must be taken to promptly remove the meconium from the buttocks of the neonate. If it is allowed to dry on the skin, removal presents a problem. Vigorous efforts to remove the dried meconium result in irritation of the skin over the buttocks.

Failure of the neonate to have a stool after 48 hours of life may indicate an imperforate anus that was not readily apparent on admission examination. After meconium has been passed and feedings have begun the stool will become soft and smooth in consistency and the color will gradually change to a greenish yellow and then to yellow. Frequency, color, and consistency of stools depend on the type of feedings given. Neonates who are breast-fed have softer and more frequent stools than do bottle-fed neonates. After the first 2 or 3 days of life the neonate will defecate between 3 and 6 times a day.

Observations made during the time the neonate is being fed should be recorded. Attention should be directed toward the vigor with which the feeding was taken. If the neonate is bottle-fed, the amount of the feeding taken should be recorded. Following feeding the neonate must be observed carefully for vomiting and regurgitation. Weighing the neonate before and after breast-feeding is a poor means at best for determining nutritional intake.

The neonate is relatively well supplied with body fluid at the time of birth. This fluid may constitute up to 35% of the total body weight. During the first few days of life there will be loss of body fluid with a reduction of 6% to 10% in body weight. Observations must be made for evidence of excessive loss of fluid resulting in dehydration as evidenced in dryness of the skin and poor skin turgor. With a daily intake of between 120 and 150 ml. of fluid and 100 calories per kg. of body weight, the neonate should regain his birth weight by the tenth day of life.

Crying is the neonate's means of communicating discomfort or distress. The pattern and quality of crying should be noted. A clean, dry, well-fed neonate usually sleeps without fretting and cries little. A high-pitched shrill cry may be indicative of increased intracranial pressure, and a low-pitched hoarse cry may indicate an anomaly of the throat. Personnel routinely caring for neonates become adept at detecting any deviation from the normal cry.

Any deviations from the normal behavior pattern and any evidence of illness or distress should be brought to the attention of the physician.

FURTHER ACQUAINTANCE OF PARENTS AND NEONATE

The first time the neonate is taken to the mother's bedside it should not be for feeding but to give her further opportunity to become acquainted with her new son or daughter. The mother may have seen her little one in the delivery room, but now she has a chance to really examine and touch her new infant.

After the nurse gives the neonate to the mother, she may wish to sit down and be unobstrusive. If it is the mother's first infant, the mother does not necessarily know how to handle the infant, and the nurse should remain for the neonate's sake. The mother may just wish to look at her neonate or she may wish to unwrap him and count his fingers and toes to see and "take in" this new person, the person about whom she has dreamed for so long. The mother may wish to touch and feel the infant. She may hold the infant close or keep him at a distance and just look at him.

What the mother does with the neonate helps indicate to the nurse how the mother feels about her infant. This is true not only the first time the neonate is brought to the mother but on succeeding times. The nurse needs to listen for cues from the mother as to instructions or assistance the mother needs. If the mother comments on how little the infant is, she may wish to further talk about the appearance of the neonate. If the mother touches the anterior fontanel of the infant and looks questioningly at the nurse, the nurse might explain what it is and care of the scalp in general.

Each time the infant is taken to the mother there may be a difference in the way the mother greets and holds her infant. The next time the infant is brought to the mother she may hold

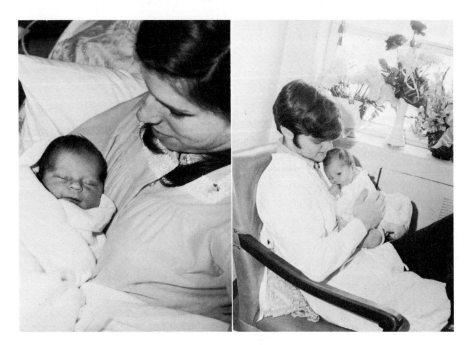

Fig. 4-9. Parents and infant become acquainted in the hospital.

him to feed him but not hold him close, that is, enfold him to her. It takes the new mother time to get used to and know her son or daughter. Even if this is a second child, the mother needs to become acquainted since no two infants are alike. Also each one may have a different meaning for her.

The mother needs positive reinforcement in any care she gives the neonate. If the mother comments that the infant took the breast or bottle well, the nurse should compliment her. This makes the mother feel more adequate. On the other hand, if the infant takes his feeding poorly, she may believe the infant is rejecting her. A hungry neonate nurses well. If the nursery nurse and the nurse on the postpartum unit watch for cues from the mother, it helps to determine her readiness for learning about the neonate's care and her own care. Of necessity much teaching is really individual, depending on the mother's interest and needs. When the mother walks to the nursery, she watches the nurse handle the infant; the nurse should be very sure to set a good example.

It is ideal if the father can put on a gown and hold the neonate. It not only makes him feel an important member of the family but it gives him an opportunity to practice holding the infant while there is supervision for safety's sake. The infant is the joint responsibility of both parents. Again, the nurse needs to watch for cues as to the father's needs for teaching or his need to express his feelings about his wife's pregnancy and delivery. What has this meant to him? Perhaps he has dreams for his child when he grows up.

Reuben (1961) has alluded to three phases of mother-child relationship: the taking-in phase, the taking-on, and the letting-go. If the mother leaves the hospital at the end of three days and this is her first child, then she is probably still in the phase of trying to get used to the infant. She is still concerned with her needs. It will be a while before she is ready to take on responsibilities for the care of the infant and later "let go" of her former role and see the baby as separate from her and a new person in the home with an individuality all his own.

PARENT EDUCATION

More and more frequently parents are attending programs of instruction on child care that are integrated into the concept of preparation for parenthood. During the course of instruction they may have been afforded an opportunity to develop some manual skills in the preparation of formulas, feeding, clothing, and bathing neonates. The hospital nurse should build her instructions on previous instructions. Just as needs for physical and emotional care differ among mothers, educational needs differ. It is the responsibility of the nurse to identify areas of instructional need. Instructions must meet the need as perceived by the mother if they are to be effective. After the mother's perceived need is met attention can be directed toward meeting the educational needs as perceived by the nurse.

Nurses are cautioned that previous experience in caring for neonates and educational achievement are not always reliable predictors of need for instruction. To assume that a woman does not need instructions because she has had previous children is erroneous. Her understanding of the requirements of this neonate is equally as important as that of the new mother. A sound understanding of the requirements for care of the neonate together with knowledge of how to meet the requirements promote in the mother a sense of confidence in her ability to assume the mothering role. In addition, mothers should understand that it is essential to carress and talk to the neonate, to investigate possible reasons for his crying, and to feed him promptly when he is hungry.

Teaching and demonstrations of each aspect of care is important. This should include feeding, bathing, handling, dressing, and meeting the emotional needs of the neonate. Both mothers and fathers should be oriented to the characteristics and the behavior of the neonate.

Specific written instructions on all aspects of care have been developed for the use of parents in giving care to their neonates. Nurses should make available to parents appropriate written instructions that will reinforce the information given to them in parents classes and in the hospital.

Meeting emotional needs

The *new* mother especially needs interpretation of the emotional needs of the neonate. She should be told that not only is cuddling the infant all right but that it is essential for his health. The way the neonate is handled influences whether he is tense or relaxed. He needs to be caressed and cuddled, to hear soothing tones of voice. He enjoys being rocked and sung to. A healthy infant cries little; when he does the possible cause should be investigated promptly and remedied. Feeding and bathing experiences should be pleasant. If allowed to cry for a prolonged period of time before nursing, he may be too tired to nurse well.

Feeding

Throughout the hospital experience the mother is taught the basic principles of feeding the neonate. (See the previous discussions of breast-feeding and bottle-feeding.) She will, however, need instructions on formula sterilization.

Sterilization

There are two methods of formula sterilization: terminal sterilization and the aseptic method.

Terminal sterilization is the method most often used in hospitals and homes. In this method the formula is made with clean but not sterile equipment. Tap water is mixed with the sugar and milk, and the mixture is poured directly into the bottles. The bottles with inverted nipples and slightly *loosened* caps are placed in a covered pan with water. The water is boiled for 25 minutes; then the unopened pan is allowed to cool. The bottles are then removed, the caps are tightened, and the bottles are refrigerated until ready for use.

If the mother does not have enough nursing bottles for each feeding, the number she does have can be utilized and the remainder of the formula can be sterilized in a clean glass jar or milk bottle. If the mother cannot afford to buy any calibrated baby bottles, a sterilized 6-ounce soda pop bottle fitted with a nipple may do just as well.

In the *aseptic method* all equipment to be used in making the formula, including bottles, nipples, caps, measuring cups, spoons, and can opener, are first washed thoroughly and then placed in a covered pan and sterilized in boiling water for 10 minutes. Water for the formula is boiled and measured in the sterile measuring cup; then the milk and sugar are measured and mixed into the water. If evaporated milk is used, the top of the can should be washed before it is opened. The mixture is poured into the sterile bottles, the nipples are inverted on top, and the caps are tightened. The bottles are allowed to cool and then are refrigerated. When it is time to feed the baby a bottle is removed from the refrigerator, the nipple is placed in its upright position, and the bottle is heated in warm water to body temperature.

Commercially prepared formulas

Many commercially prepared infant formulas are available in either liquid or powdered form. Most require only dilution with water and proper sterilization before giving them to the infant. These formulas, like evaporated milk, can be stored without refrigeration. Most have extra vitamins and minerals added, making further supplementation unnecessary. Specific nutrient compositions of these formulas must be printed on the labels.

Formulas that require no dilution or prior sterilization are also available; some come premeasured in disposable bottles. If the mother wishes to use one of these formulas, her physician will recommend the one that best meets her infant's needs.

Infants who are allergic to cow's milk or who have a metabolic defect that prevents them from tolerating human milk or cow's milk may be given special formulas in which the protein, carbohydrate, or fat content has been modified. Such infants accept these formulas well and can thrive normally on them. Some of these special formulas such as Lofenalac (used in the treatment of phenylketonuria) can be purchased only with a physician's prescription.

Bathing the neonate at home

If the mother has had experience in bathing neonates or has been taught the procedure in child care class, the nurse may just review the steps in the procedure. The nurse should give a demonstration of the procedure for the mother who has not been taught nor has had previous experience. The demonstration should be accompanied by verbal instructions and followed by written and illustrated instructions. All mothers should be told that the complete bath of the neonate may be delayed for 2 or 3 days if they are not feeling well. Washing of the face, hands, genitals, and buttocks of the neonate is sufficient for this short interval. A sponge bath is given until the cord stump has dropped off. After that time a tub bath may be given. The mother should select a time for the bath that will be most convenient for her and will fit into the family life-style.

The room in which the bath is given should be warm and free of drafts. All materials needed for the bath and fresh clothing should be assembled and placed in easy reach of the mother. A large dishpan may be used as a tub for the first few weeks of life. Before the neonate is undressed the face is washed with clear warm water and then dried. The head is then shampooed with a mild soap, using the palm of the hand rather than the fingertips. The ears are washed at this time. The head must be rinsed thoroughly to prevent a residue of soap from forming on the scalp. The head is gently dried before the neonate is undressed for the rest of the bath. The mother may find it easier to hold the neonate in one arm with his head over the tub for washing and rinsing. The important thing is that the neonate is held securely. A modified football carry position is recommended in which the neonate is held in the supine position along the forearm of the mother. The head is supported by the hand and the hips and legs of the neonate are supported against the mother by her elbow. After the head has been dried the neonate is undressed, and his body is washed with particular attention given to creases. He is then placed in the tub to be rinsed; while being held securely he may kick and move about in the water. The neonate is removed from the water and is patted dry. He is then dressed comfortably.

Mothers must be cautioned against leaving the neonate unattended on a table because neonates move, may roll over, and may fall. They should also be cautioned against using cotton applicators with inflexible sticks to clean the ears and nose of the neonate. Sudden unexpected movement of the neonate could result in injury if applicators are used.

Clothing

General characteristics of infant clothing are discussed in Chapter 5. Two areas of instruction related to the neonate's clothing should be emphasized in teaching the mother. First, the neonate responds to the environment and should be dressed appropriately. Since peripheral circulation is not well established and stabilized, the hands and feet are not the best indicators for the amount of clothing and covering needed by the neonate. The mother should be taught to feel the legs and the arms of the neonate to determine the need for covering. Second, the clothing, sheets, and blankets used by the neonate should be washed in a mild soap or detergent and rinsed thoroughly. The skin of the neonate is thin and sensitive and will react to residue of soap left in clothing and wraps. Particular emphasis should be placed on the care of diapers. Soiled diapers should be removed from the neonate immediately to prevent diaper rash and excoriation of the buttocks. Soiled diapers should be placed in a container of cold water until they are washed. As stated, only mild soaps or detergents should be used, and diapers should be rinsed three times in clear water. After washing and rinsing, diapers should be hung outdoors in the sunshine to dry if at all possible.

Medical supervision

The nurse should determine through conversation with the mother the plans that have been made for continued medical supervision of the neonate. If the mother has not planned for this care, she should be given instructions on the importance of medical supervision and early, periodic screening and examination to evaluate the health status, growth, and development of the infant. The first visit is usually made about 4 weeks following delivery, at which time immunizations will be started. If the mother indicates that she will not have a private doctor but will seek medical supervision through her local health department, the nurse should make a written referral of the neonate to the appropriate public health unit.

Fitting the neonate into the family

Most parents have made some plans for the addition to the family sometime prior to birth.

However, the advent of the firstborn changes the family structure from husband-wife to husband/father–wife/mother. There must be a realization that attention will now have to be shared. Anticipatory guidance is important during the first weeks of life. Parents should recognize that adjustments in life-style will of necessity have to be made; however, it is also important that they understand that the neonate will adjust to family living and that family members need not make all of the adjustments to the neonate.

The first few weeks are a time of concentrated learning experiences for parents. A more meaningful relationship can be developed by sharing experiences in caring for the neonate. One way of dispelling the left-out feelings of fathers is by including them in the care. Feelings of inadequacy are overcome by successful outcomes of the care given. Gradually the newness of parenthood wears off; bathing, clothing, and feeding of the neonate become routine, and mothers and fathers become comfortable in their roles.

Mothers should be cautioned to organize their activities so that some time can be devoted to their husbands. The father should not be made to feel that he is always second in line for consideration and attention. Also, he needs to be aware of the mother's need for emotional support during the period of adjustment to increased responsibility. Each parent must be aware of the need to share attention with the neonate. Adequate preparation for parenthood can reduce the jealousy and competition for attention that could arise.

To avoid jealousy and to promote good sibling relationships, older siblings should be prepared for the homecoming of the neonate (p. 20). When the neonate arrives older siblings, especially those of school age, may wish to bring their friends to see the infant. The children should be encouraged to do this; however, this does not mean that the neonate should be awakened if he is asleep or that the neonate should be passed around from one person's arms to the next.

Older children often like to share the care of the infant. They should be allowed to do so in accord with their age and their ability. Of course, the neonate's psychological needs (affection, relief from tension, and sensory stimulation) must be considered and met. Siblings are increasingly important to the infant as he grows older. The feeling that brothers and sisters belong to each other gives each sibling a certain amount of security.

If the mother and father continue to meet the siblings' needs and exhibit to them their love and concern, regression in children's behavior is less apt to be seen, especially if the children have been prepared for the new arrival. Each sibling needs to understand or feel that he will not lose the love and attention of his parents, that his is a unique role that only he can fill. If any regression of sibling behavior does occur, it should be met with love and understanding. The neonate has to fit into the family, and the family life should not revolve around the infant; nevertheless, the presence of one more person in the family does make life different for everyone concerned, no matter how welcome the newcomer is.

REFERENCES

Apgar, V.: Proposal for a new method of evaluation of the newborn infant, Anesth. Analg. **32:**4, 1953.

Barness, L.: Manual of pediatric physical diagnosis, ed. 4, Chicago, 1972, Year Book Medical Publishers, Inc.

Barnett, C. R., et al.: Neonatal separation: Maternal side of intervention, Pediatrics **45:**197, 1970.

Bates, B.: A guide to physical examination, Philadelphia, 1974, J. B. Lippincott Co.

Brody, S.: Patterns of mothering, New York, 1956, International Universities Press.

Committee on the Fetus and Newborn: Standards and recommendations for hospital care of newborn infants, ed. 5, Evanston, Ill., 1971, American Academy of Pediatrics.

Countryman, B.: Hospital care of the breast fed newborn, Am. J. Nurs. **71:**2365, December, 1971.

Fomon, S.: Infant nutrition, Philadelphia, 1967, W. B. Saunders Co.

Gezon, H.: Should nursery environmental control measures be reexamined? Pediatrics **44:**637, 1969.

Keaveny, M. E.: Breastfeeding, Nursing 72, **2:**31, 1972.

Keay, A., and Morgan, D.: Craig's care of the newly born infant, ed. 5, London: 1971, Churchill Livingstone.

Latham, H.: How does your nursery rate? Part 1, Mod. Hosp. **81:**77, September, 1953.

Latham, H.: How does your nursery rate? Part 2, Mod. Hosp. **81:**81, October, 1953.

Laupus, W.: Feeding of infants. In Vaughn, V., III, and McKay, R. J., editors: Nelson's textbook of pediatrics, ed. 10, Philadelphia, 1975, W. B. Saunders Co.

Rubin, R.: Puerperal change, Nurs. Outlook **9**(12):753, December, 1961.

Thompson, L. R.: Nursery infections, apparent and inapparent, Am. J. Nurs. **65:**80, November, 1965.

Vaughn, V., III: The newborn infant. In Vaughn, V., III, and McKay, R. J., editors: Nelson's textbook of pediatrics, ed. 10, Philadelphia, 1975, W. B. Saunders Co.

Whitner, W., and Thompson, M.: The influence of bathing on the newborn infant's body temperature, Nurs. Res. **19:**30, January-February 1970.

5
INFANCY

For a description of the appearance and behavior of the neonate refer to Chapter 4. In this chapter we will discuss the period of later infancy.

PHYSICAL DEVELOPMENT

Changes during the first year of life are tremendous. Yet for all their scope they are not as great as the changes that occurred during the prenatal period, in which the microscopic organism had its conception and in 9 months grew to be infinitely larger—perhaps to a birth weight of 7.5 pounds and a length of 19.9 inches. Through use of Figs. 5-3 and 5-4, showing height, weight, and head circumference, the normal growth patterns for infant boys and girls can be observed. Charts show that there is a normal variability in weight and height of infants at birth. Those children whose measure-

ments are below the tenth percentile or above the ninetieth percentile are unusual. Boys are born at a weight within the normal range of 6.3 to 9.1 pounds and with a height of 18.9 to 21 inches. Yet each nurse will encounter infants who fall outside these normal limits. Premature children who were born weighing less than 2 pounds have survived, whereas some infants have weighed as much as 11 pounds. Height variations are usually less spectacular, although unusual height records have been obtained as well. Figs. 5-3 and 5-4 show the slight variations between boys and girls in height and weight at birth. These slight consistent differences are maintained throughout the first year of development. Because of weight gains, the child is usually three times his birth weight by 1 year of age. In height the gain is an increase of 50%.

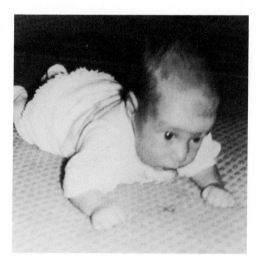

Fig. 5-1. This infant is 2 months old, but even at birth an infant can lift her head momentarily when prone.

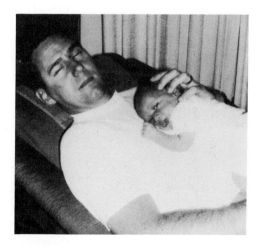

Fig. 5-2. Father and infant rest together.

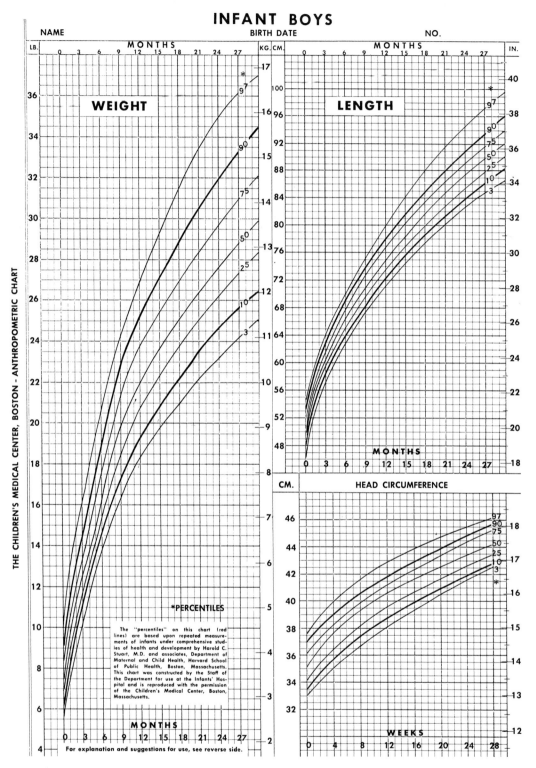

Fig. 5-3. Percentile chart for measurements of infant boys. (Courtesy The Children's Medical Center, Boston, Mass.)

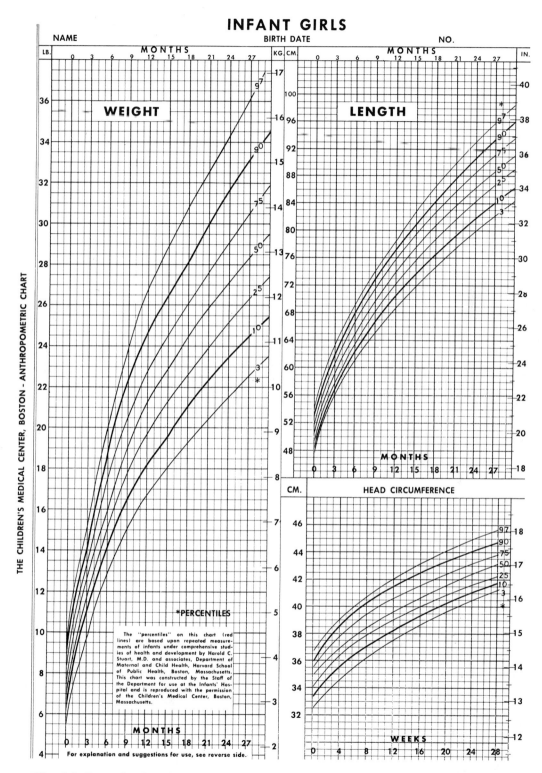

Fig. 5-4. Percentile chart for measurements of infant girls. (Courtesy The Children's Medical Center, Boston, Mass.)

Skeletal changes

From the time of conception and continuing through the first year of life there are differential changes in the size of various body parts. If we were to go back to the second month of fetal development, we would find that the head comprises one half of the fetus. This has changed by the fifth month, so one third of the fetus is head and two thirds is body. By the time of birth the head is one fourth of the body size and the body is the remaining three fourths. When the individual reaches adulthood his head is only about one eighth of his total body length. Legs, very short and stubby during the fetal period, increase in length until adulthood, when nearly one half of the body length is accounted for by the legs.

At birth the circumference of the head is larger than the circumference of the chest or the abdomen; yet at 6 months the circumferences of all three are about the same. At 1 year of age the circumference of the chest exceeds that of the head. During the first year of life the brain grows and develops more than at any other period during life. The head expands about 4 inches in circumference. Expansion takes place easily because the newborn has six fontanels, or soft spots. The most important of these are the posterior fontanel, which closes at 4 to 8 weeks, and the anterior fontanel, which may not close until 18 months, although in some infants the anterior fontanel is closed by 1 year. Anything that interferes with expansion of the skull is serious since it affects the growth of the brain as microcephalus or craniosynostosis (Chapter 19).

Growth and expansion of other bones in the body follow a varying pattern of development. Emphasis on various portions is increased or lessened, depending upon the particular stage of development involved. During adolescence, for example, emphasis is placed on the elongation of limbs during the early stages, whereas later stages are marked by thickening of bones and expansion of chest in boys and broadening of hips in girls.

Progression of development in bony structures follows a consistent and orderly course. All are formed first by cartilaginous material that later becomes calcified. As the infant matures, more and more development takes place in the change of cartilage into bone.

One of the most popular measures of skeletal development is through use of x-ray films, or roentgenograms. Since cartilage does not show up clearly on x-ray film and bone does, it is possible by making x-ray studies of certain portions of the body to judge the maturity of skeletal development in an individual. Commonly used are the hand and wrist bones. The evolution of the ossification centers of the hand and wrist has been studied, and results are available in the form of an atlas (Greulich and Pyle, 1959). An infant's x-ray films can be compared with this atlas for an accurate assessment of the infant's bone age.

Dentition

Dentition begins early during fetal development. Evidence suggests that deciduous teeth are already partially formed by the twelfth fetal week. Final eruption of the teeth is variable, but in general the first tooth (the lower central incisor) usually appears between 5 and 9 months of age. Girls may show a slightly earlier eruption than boys. The deciduous, or baby, teeth are 20 in number and are usually present by 2½ years of age. In addition to the central incisors, they include the lateral incisors, cuspids, and first and second molars.

Neuromuscular development

In our study of neuromuscular development we will concentrate on two major areas: the development and evolution of the sensory apparatus and the development of coordinated motor activities. In a later section we will also investigate the emergence of complex skills such as speech and intellectual capabilities.

Motor development

It is from reflexive actions and random uncoordinated movements, already mentioned, that many of the complex behaviors of a child emerge. Development follows a cephalocaudal order; that is, it proceeds from the head and neck through the torso and finally to the extremities.

Even though the newborn has little voluntary muscular control, he is able to elevate his head

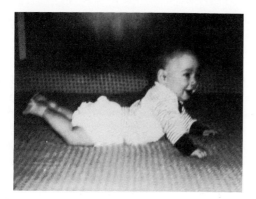

Fig. 5-5. At 4 months of age an infant can elevate head and shoulders when prone.

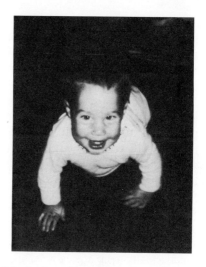

Fig. 5-6. At 9 or 10 months of age an infant can crawl.

when prone. Gradually the infant gains control of his head and neck, and by the third to fourth month he can keep it steady when held in an erect position. When placed in a prone position in the fourth month, the baby can lift his head and chest by pushing down on the surface with his hands (Fig. 5-5). The typical infant can hold this position for several seconds at a time.

The next major event in the motor development of the infant is sitting alone unsupported. The average infant can do this at 7 months.

Locomotion. Almost from birth there are many reflexive actions in the newborn that bear a striking similarity to the necessary components of creeping, crawling, or walking behavior. At this period of development the musculature is insufficiently developed and the organism far too weak to make any effective use of arms and legs. By the time he is 3 or 4 months old the random movements have resulted in strengthening to the point that the infant can turn from resting on his side to either his back or front. A little later, by the sixth or seventh month, he may completely reverse himself from lying on his back to a prone position. With these actions the child has broken through the barrier into mobility. No longer is he limited to the confines of space based on where his mother has placed him. In the succeeding months he will learn the rudiments of locomotion through a crawling or hitching motion either on his stomach or on his back. This evolves in relatively short order into a creeping movement. There are many variations on this form of locomotion. Some children combine a sitting position with a combined hitch-creep in which the child propels himself in a fashion that resembles a person paddling a canoe. Each step in development brings him closer to readiness for walking.

Walking. Most of us have heard the old truism, "You must crawl before you can walk." Although not absolutely true, it represents the general evolution of motor development for most persons. During the period of time when the individual is showing creeping and crawling behavior his musculature is too weak and unsteady to support and control his body weight. Coordination is not sufficient to provide the complex interactions necessary to permit him to walk. While supported, he may make many of the walking motions; yet when anything approaching his total body weight is placed on his legs, they do not respond properly, and if released he would fall. Prior to maturation of the neuromusculature walking cannot occur. There is a wide range of individual differences in this behavior, some of which are inherent; others are dependent upon the nutritional and experiential factors to which the infant is exposed. Many studies have shown that early practice does not help walking, sitting, or a number of other behaviors if the neural and muscular systems have not matured sufficiently to permit these activities. However, they have demonstrated also that, once sufficient maturation has taken place, experience and practice may perfect these behaviors to a higher level than is possible in children who have more restricted experiences.

In general the evolution of walking with help, pulling up to a standing position, and in a few instances negotiating a few steps can occur early, but the average child does not walk without support until the fifteenth month, in what is appropriately termed the toddler period. Children who do not walk until after 18 months of age are considered late in walking. In some instances the age of walking is affected by intellectual and emotional factors. Children who are slow intellectually tend to show in many instances a slightly slower development of motor skills. Exceptionally bright children often are precocious not only in intellectual skills but also in a wide variety of motor and sensory skills. The effect of emotional factors on the age of walking is less certain.

Traumatic experiences such as severe falls may cause the child to be inhibited and frightened with regard to walking. Fearing injury to the child, parents sometimes will inhibit his attempting to walk until well beyond the age at which he might be able to undertake the activities involved. The parents may physically restrain the child from walking activities, or they may implant fears and concerns in the child through a series of "Dont's." Children are not the logical creatures their parents are, and they frequently will learn to walk at about the normal time in spite of parental fears and anxieties. However, they may be prevented from developing the finer motor controls possible with the more extensive experience available to children who live in a freer environment.

Manual dexterity. Manual dexterity, like walking, is the result of a combination of maturation, experience, and a delicate balance between muscles and sensory apparatus.

In the early stages of development of manual dexterity, hand-eye coordination does not exist. The infant may follow objects with his eyes but be unable to make appropriate motor movements in the direction of perceived objects.

Illingworth and Ames have made an extensive study of the infant's use of hands for grasping or holding, sometimes called prehension (Illingworth, 1962). At birth and through the first 3 to 4 months few infants have gained any real control over the use of hands and fingers. The grasping and retention of objects is usually on a random and chance basis. The child has not yet learned the connection between the retention of objects and the action of muscles in the hand and fingers, or, if he is aware, he is unable to control action sufficiently. At 1 month of age the infant's hands are usually closed. By the third month hands are usually open, but movements are still random and only limited in control. By the third month development has progressed so that objects placed in the child's hand, such as a rattle or other small object, are retained. Infants at this age are able to pull at objects placed near them. In the third month the infant may play with his fingers (Fig. 5-7) and reach for an object using both hands in a wavering motion. During the sixth month the infant reaches directly and purposefully. He can hold a bottle and grasp objects, although only one at a time. He may transfer small objects from one hand to the other, bang them on tables or objects near-

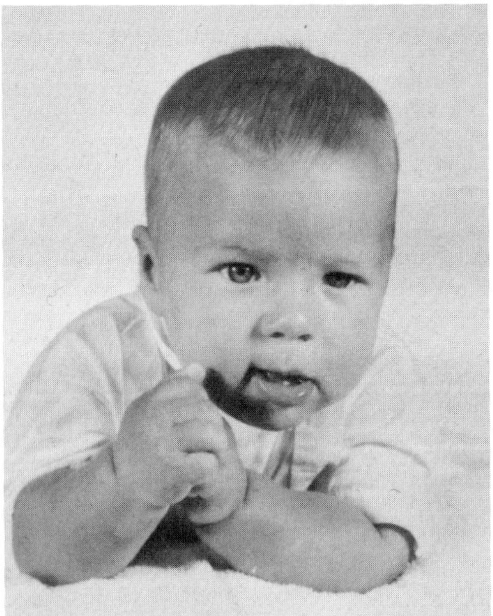

Fig. 5-7. A 4-month-old infant plays with his fingers.

by, and even hold objects in both hands simultaneously.

In the remaining months of the first year, starting with the tenth month, the child demonstrates finger-thumb apposition, which allows him to pick up small or delicate objects between his finger and thumb. He may place objects into a box, whereas earlier he was only able to remove them. His coordination is well enough developed that he can give objects to other people, throw them with some skill, and demonstrate a mature grasping and holding of cubes and other small objects. The thumb, as we have indicated, takes on increasing importance during the later stages of development of infant coordination. Prehension follows an orderly course from the palmar grasping of objects at 3 or 4 months to the coordinated use of thumb and forefinger in tweezerlike action by 1 year. (See Fig. 5-8.)

Sensory development

The development and emergence of sensory skills is of vital importance to the developing infant. It is through his senses that he is able to learn of the world around him. Sight, hearing, taste, smell, and tactile sensitivity supply a whole array of new experiences for the child. When difficulties or problems exist or deficits are found in any one area, the infant's capacity for learning is greatly reduced. To be sure, there are methods of compensating for these deficits, but the results in later life invariably show that sensory handicaps cannot be completely overcome.

Because we are unable to receive accurate reports from infants about their sensory experiences, we are still lacking in some of the factual material relating to the emergence and maturation of sensory abilities. In spite of these limitations much is known about the growth aspects

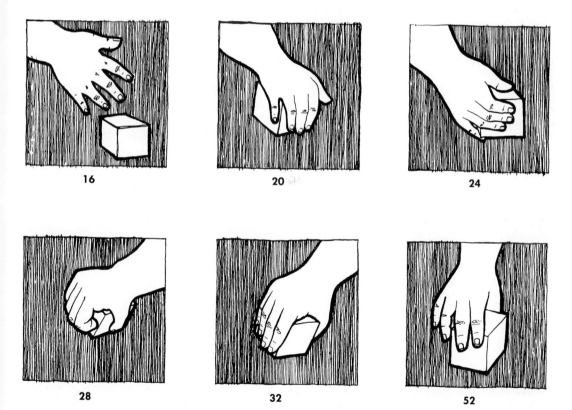

Fig. 5-8. The development of prehension. This illustration, with weeks of development indicated, reflects the evolution and development of manipulative ability.

of sensory experience. Our discussion will center on currently available facts related to abilities that exist during the first year.

Sight. Infants at birth do not have a fully developed visual apparatus. What they are able to respond to is not clearly understood, but work by Fantz (1965) indicates that newborns respond differentially to plain surfaces and black-and-white patterns. Other studies suggest that, even as early as the first 5 days, they have developed sufficient visual acuity to respond to complex visual patterns in preference to plain surfaces.

At birth the pupillary reflex is present. This is true even in the case of prematurely born infants. Reaction of pupils is initially rather slow but within the first few weeks of life becomes more rapid and can be elicited with small intensities of stimulation.

By the second month of life the infant is able to focus on an object such as his mother's face. Next he follows a moving object (3 months); then, as already stated, by 4 months he reaches with both hands to grasp an object seen. His movements are wavering, but he sees an object and tries to get it. At 6 months he reaches directly for an object with one hand. At the seventh month the infant's perceptual skills are sufficiently developed so that he is able to respond to reflections in a mirror.

Some of the more complex visual operations involving both learning and experience take a longer period of time to emerge. Such qualities as the perception of depth and recognition of an object's size, shape, color, texture, weight, and volume require additional experience and training. Many of these characteristics do require months or even years of experience to become fully developed. In a series of fascinating experiments Gibson and Walk (1960) have found that quite early in their development infants are sensitive to what appears to be a sudden increase in depth. Their studies involved placing infants on a flat surface with a textured pattern of a checkerboard design. At the midpoint the flat surface was extended by a sheet of strong glass. The same textured pattern used under the flat surface was placed beneath the glass at some distance, providing the illusion of depth. Gibson and Walk labeled this the "vi-

sual cliff.'' Infants as young as 6 months were able to perceive the drop and would not venture beyond the flat-textured surface onto the clear glass. In an attempt to test the fixed nature of this behavior, Gibson and Walk had mothers of infants stand on the other side of the cliff and attempt to draw the infants toward them. In spite of this lure, children would not venture onto the plain glass surface.

Other studies have revealed that, at least in animals, depth perception appears to be an unlearned response. The evidence regarding human infants is less conclusive. Generalization from Gibson and Walk's experiment is dangerous. Infants of this age will fall from the crib or bed when sides are not up without apparently perceiving the depth differentiation.

Other perceptual skills are less well developed during the first year. Since they are poorly formed during infancy, we will examine them in greater detail in the section on the toddler and preschool child.

Hearing. Experimental evaluation of infant hearing suggests that it is well developed and fully functioning at birth. As noted on p. 59, newborns characteristically have poor hearing during the first few days because of mucus or other liquid accumulations in the auditory canal or in the middle ear. These fluids dissipate rather rapidly, and hearing is fully functional thereafter. Even at birth the infant is able to respond to high intensities of sound. Reaction to sounds such as the human voice or low noises are readily noted. Studies of auditory discrimination reveal that infants are capable of tonal discrimination, although of course their ability to respond is somewhat limited. Researchers were able to establish a differential response to various tones in infants of this age by taking physiological measures such as activity level and the heart rate, which was found to be different when different tones were presented. As with vision, adequate auditory discrimination is possible only when extensive learning experiences have taken place. Sounds take a special meaning only after the child has had the time and opportunity to form associations between specific sounds and the objects to which they refer. This is a process of conditioning.

Smell. As is true also for the sense of hearing, the newborn's olfactory thresholds are high and almost nonexistent because of the presence of amniotic fluid or mucus, which blocks proper functioning of the sense organs. Once this material has been cleared the sensitivity to olfactory stimulation improves dramatically. This often takes place within the first few days of life. In young infants some differential response to olfactory stimulation is noted; yet it will be several years before the child has learned sufficiently to make accurate and meaningful discriminations among the many stimuli that will reach him. During the first months it is only the more pungent or noxious odors that cause a response in the infant. Less intense levels of olfactory stimulation may be recognized, but they do not produce a behavioral change that can be observed. Since researchers in this field rely on dramatic responses, it may well be that they find reaction to only those pungent or noxious odors able to produce measurable changes in behavior, such as movements of the head or limbs.

Taste. Infants react to sweet, salt, bitter, and sour flavors. Taste buds are not developed for bland flavors until children are in the preschool period.

When offered solid foods at the age of 2 or 3 months, the infant reacts to the consistency of the food rather than the taste.

One problem in studying taste in infants is the fact that they do not attach social value to a number of kinds of taste. Until they have had the opportunity to observe adult reactions and responses to a number of substances, they may not react negatively to substances that adults find unpleasant. Although there are definite limits to how much of a particular type of taste (sweet, salty, sour, or bitter) individuals can tolerate, the culture will play an important part in determining which substances are viewed as pleasant and which are rejected as unpleasant.

Temperature sensitivity. Anyone who has given a bottle that was too warm or too cold to an infant can attest to their sensitivity to temperature changes. Differences may exist in the temperatures preferred for milk and other foods. Infants reflect displeasure by squirming, twisting, and other actions when food items fail to fall within suitable ranges. Similarly, when warm or cold objects are placed on the infant, he may react with movement of limbs, twisting and turning of head, or variations in breathing and pulse rate.

When subjected to coolness or warmth infants generally show increased activity with cooler temperatures and are more quiescent when temperatures are high. Extreme temperatures in either direction result in many symptoms of stress, exaggerations of some of the previously mentioned response patterns.

Touch and pain. Although the sensation of touch seems highly developed at birth, reaction to pain is slower and not as intense. Experimenters testing for the presence of pain have found that it is difficult to elicit a response in the newborn infant with pinpricks, but withdrawal of the limb and movement occur by the eighth or tenth day. On the other hand, nurses have heard infants cry hard following circumcision when the infant was only a few days old.

Reaction to internal discomfort such as in colic is registered in most children by 6 or 8 weeks. As the infant continues to develop, further elaborations are made of his response mechanisms to touch and pain. The nurse can observe and interpret pain sensations in the infant not only from the kind of cry but also from vocalizations, muscle tension, posture, movement, and facial expression.

The sensation of touch will play a vital role in the learning experiences of the infant. The infant uses his fingers, tongue, and lips to explore nearly every aspect of his environment. As his motor coordination develops, he is increasingly able to incorporate additional features of his environment, which he thoroughly explores. When combined with visual and auditory experiences, learning progresses at a rapid pace.

Kinesthetic and vestibular senses. The sensory apparatus dealing with position, movement, and balance are imperfectly developed in the newborn and in the early stages of infancy. However, even the very young infant will make random or poorly controlled motor movements in an attempt to compensate for the postural changes when held or moved into different positions. Those mechanisms are centered in the semicircular canals of the ear and in brain

Table 5-1. Developmental norms of young children*

Age	Motor	Adaptive	Language	Personal-social
4 wk.	Lifts head momentarily when prone. Can turn head side to side when prone. Flexed position, but legs more extended than in neonatal period. Head lags when pulled to sitting position.	Has brief eye following. Drops toys immediately.	Makes small throaty sounds.	Stares at surroundings. "Listens" to sounds.
16 wk.	Can hold head steady when supported in sitting position or held to adult's shoulder. Lifts head and chest when prone. No head lag when pulled to sitting position. Pushes down with feet if held erect on flat surface.	Reaches and grasps object with two hands and brings object to mouth (incipient approach).	Vocalizes in response to adults talking to him.	Has spontaneous social smile. Plays with fingers. Is displeased when social contact broken.
28 wk.	Can turn from supine to prone position. May pivot when prone. Can sit alone briefly.	Reaches directly with one hand to grasp object. Transfers object from one hand to other. Can shake rattle.	Vocalizes actively and expressively. Uses polysyllabic vowel sounds.	Pats images in mirror. In supine position can bring feet up to mouth. Differentiates between strangers and familiar persons.
40 wk.	Sits well without support. Creeps or crawls. Pulls self to feet by holding onto object such as chair or playpen	Grasps objects with thumb and index finger. Tends to retrieve dropped object. Likes to poke at objects with index finger.	Makes repetitive consonant sounds (ma, da-da).	Plays peek-a-boo and pat-a-cake, waves bye-bye. Feeds self cracker.
52 wk. (1 yr.)	Walks with one hand held.	Puts cube into cup. Tries tower of 2 cubes.	Responds to "Give it to me" (releases object). Says two or more words	Cooperates in dressing. Plays simple ball game (rolls ball to another person).
15 mo.	Walks alone, toddles. Crawls upstairs.	Builds tower of 2 cubes. Puts 6 cubes into cup.	Says 4 to 6 words.	Points, vocalizes wants. Casts toys.
18 mo.	Walks well alone. Seats self in small chair. Climbs into adult chair. Walks upstairs with one hand held.	Builds tower of 3 to 4 cubes. Imitates vertical stroke.	Uses expressive jargon. Says 10 words.	Carries and hugs doll. Feeds self with help. May indicate or complain when wet.
2 yr.	Runs well. Walks up and down stairs one step at a time.	Builds tower of 6 cubes. Imitates circular scribbling.	Joins 2 to 3 words. Names 3 to 5 pictures (if familiar).	Puts doll to bed. Likes to open doors. Helps undress. Looks at picture books. Feeds self well.

*Modified from Vaughn, V. C., III: Growth and development. In Vaughn, V. C., III, and McKay, R. J., editors: Nelson's textbook of pediatrics, ed. 10, Philadelphia, 1975, W. B. Saunders Co., p. 49; and Gesell, A., and Amatruda, C.: Developmental diagnosis, New York, 1941, Paul B. Hoeber, Inc.

Table 5-1. Developmental norms of young children—cont'd

Age	Motor	Adaptive	Language	Personal-social
3 yr.	Walks up and down stairs alone with alternating feet. Rides tricycle. Stands on one foot momentarily.	Builds tower of 9 cubes. Imitates "house" of cubes. Imitates cross and circle.	Gives full name and sex. Counts 3 objects. Makes sentences.	"Parallel" play with another child. Washes hands, helps in bath. Asks to go to toilet. Puts on socks, helps undressing and unbuttoning. Manages "training" pants.

centers that receive information from the muscles of the body. They develop a coordination and information processing during infancy. Thus the child will have all the necessary mechanisms operating that will permit him to sit, stand, move in an upright position, and be fully aware of the location and position of each portion of his body. As adults we take these processes for granted. For the infant, however, it involves a complex process of maturation, learning, and muscular coordination.

SPEECH DEVELOPMENT

The development of speech and language is the most important characteristic distinguishing humans from lower animals. It represents an intellectual maturity beyond that found in other members of the animal kingdom.

Language is important to express needs as well as to communicate with others. Adults use language to initiate contact with others, but small children more often use language to maintain contact with others. Language is used as a means of self-expression in songs, poems, plays, and stories. The development of language appears to be a result of combining imitation and the reinforcement of word usage. All children in infancy produce the sounds that are essential to language in any form (providing there are no physical impairments in hearing). For example, vocalizations of infants of deaf parents are the same as those of infants of hearing parents. Infants from non-English-speaking countries utter the same sounds as English-speaking infants. As the infant hears, is talked to and is socialized with, he begins to lose those sounds that are nonexistent in his native language. The interaction with others provides the impetus for further continuance of a specific sound. When a child accidentally produces a sound that in our language has a symbol, we react. The child notices our reaction and tries to repeat the sound so that he can again be reinforced positively by the adult reaction. Gradually the child learns that this sound, which produces the pleasant actions of adults, is associated with a person or item or event. It is in this manner that the child builds his vocabulary and eliminates those sounds that are nonexistent in his language.

There are certain milestones in the language development of the infant and toddler. The infant in the second month of life has differential cries for hunger, pain, and discomfort. By 4 months of age he responds vocally if an adult talks to him and then pauses so the infant has a chance to answer. When happy and content the infant actively vocalizes in an expressive manner at 6 months. Vocalizing should be encouraged since it is a means of gaining control of the vocal mechanism for articulate speech. Talking to the infant, keeping him comfortable, and giving him play materials all help to stimulate vocalization.

After the early language expressions the next important step is comprehension. The infant understands what is said to him before he can say a definite word. By 1 year of age the toddler can say two or more words. At this stage the adults caring for the infant (parents, relatives, baby-sitters, nurses) should say the names of objects the infant uses: "spoon," "doll," "chair," "car," etc. The infant learns words in association with objects. The fact that at 15 months the toddler still points to objects shows his need of more vocabulary. Nouns account for a large part of the child's vocabulary during the second year of life.

The single-word sentence such as "Bye-bye" is next. Depending on the situation, "bye-bye" may mean that the infant is going riding of that he is saying good-bye to people around him. By 2 years of age children put two or more words together in a short phrase.

If a child is not talking by 2 years of age, any one of several reasons may be the cause: deafness, lack of necessity, prolonged illness, mental retardation, or environmental deprivation.

SOCIAL AND EMOTIONAL DEVELOPMENT
Stages in development

The social and emotional aspects in an infant's development are closely related, the social experiences being influenced by his emotional experiences. The infant's social development is an outgrowth of his experiences with other people.

At birth the infant is neither social nor antisocial—just nonsocial. The first social reaction of an infant is a smile in response to an adult smile. This occurs in the second month of life. When the infant smiles there is a difference in the expression of his eyes.

Physical comfort, soothing music, lullabies, stroking, and rocking will calm and relax the infant, while loud or banging noises, angry voices, or sudden outbursts produce tension and unhappiness. At 4 months the infant will try to make an adjustment to being lifted. If the adult smiles and holds out her hands, the infant puts out his arms and tries to raise himself. By 5 months the infant is sufficiently sensitive that he may cry at a scolding voice or reflect a friendly or angry facial expression.

A big milestone is reached at 6 months of

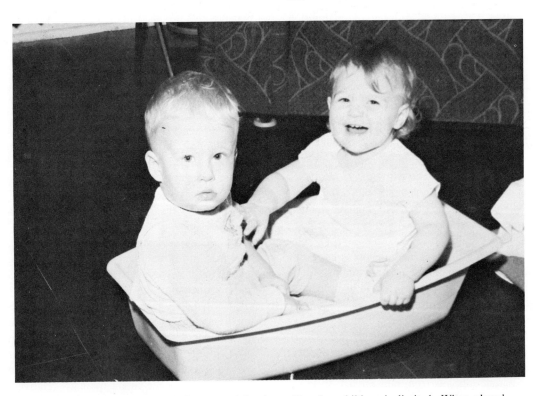

Fig. 5-9. Socialization. In infancy, socialization with other children is limited. When placed together each may be aware of the other's presence, but they do not interact meaningfully. The 9-month-old children shown here are much more interested in the adult (the father) who is taking the picture.

age. The infant can differentiate between strangers and people familiar to him. The infant is sociable with those that he knows and tries actively to seek contact with them. With strangers, he may be shy and afraid. His motor and language development assist him. He may gain attention through vocalization or by reaching out to touch someone. By 9 months, when he has some form of locomotion, he can be even more social by crawling over to the person whose attention he wishes.

The 9-month-old infant delights in playing peekaboo. To see people disappear and then appear again is fascinating to him. The fact that at 1 year of age he can understand a simple command makes the infant increasingly adaptive in his socialization.

Social interaction and care

To develop a healthy social interaction the infant needs warm relations with his family. His world revolves around parents and siblings, but friends and relatives should come and go as usual so that the child may become accustomed to others outside his immediate family. These others are usually grandparents or neighbors who are interested in and concerned with the well-being of the child. In addition to pleasant experiences playing with adults and older siblings, the infant needs to be taught early not to be too socially dependent. At times the infant should learn to be happy playing by himself.

When the nurse sees an infant in the hospital who smiles when she comes toward him and is playful and responsive during her contacts with him, she can be certain that the baby has had pleasant, meaningful experiences with other friendly adults.

A happy environment and a happy infant lay the foundations for a happy adult. The importance of maintaining this atmosphere for the infant cannot be stressed too strongly. A child reared in an atmosphere of rejection becomes lethargic. He withdraws to the point of not caring about life. A state of depression sets in, and it is most difficult to pull such a child out of the doldrums. Even if the environment changes to one of acceptance, it is difficult to know just how much damage has been done. In fact, we do not know if he ever recovers from this de-pression. The early months leave a lasting impression that carries over into adult life.

A sense of security is essential in building a happy foundation for the infant. Consistency is also important in the development of a supportive relationship between infant and environment. Routines should be adhered to. The child needs to know what to expect and approximately when to expect it. Routines such as bedtime and getting ready for bed, meals at the same time, knowing where his place is at the table, and knowing his room and his house are all important facets of the process of knowing that he belongs and is wanted. Infants have a hard time adjusting to new situations; therefore it is important that the status quo remain as much as is possible. New surroundings, for example, may be threatening to the young child. Moves are sometimes disrupting.

Pleasure in daily activities provides the basis for a healthy and happy relationship between parent and child. A happy infant cries much less than an unhappy one. Negative emotions are expressed in crying, and it becomes a sign of displeasure and unhappiness. Good health physically is also related to the overall development. Good physical health influences emotional stability and visa versa. If the infant is not emotionally secure, he will not be physically healthy. If the infant is not healthy physically, he may develop emotional illnesses. Frequently they go hand in hand.

How the infant views himself is important. He forms ideas of how others feel about him, and this is the basis for his self-concept. The manner in which the parents hold the child and how they talk to him are clues to the infant of how they feel toward him. The infant needs to be cuddled and talked to in a pleasing manner; he needs to feel the warmth of the parents' body and to be petted. The only way he has of knowing if he is accepted is in the physical handling of him. He learns through his senses at this time. The interaction between infant and parent needs to be stressed.

The mental health of the parent affects the infant. This relationship operates with any person working with children, not only the parent. The mother particularly needs to feel that her entire life is not surrounded with infants and their care. She needs outside diversions. It is particularly helpful if both parents have an occasional night out away from the family. An outside interest or hobby does wonders to enhance good mental health. Recreation for parents makes them better parents when they are with their children.

Oral phase

The first phase of the social interaction with parental figures has been described as the oral phase. In cases in which the mother breast-feeds the child this contact is quite intense for both the child and the mother. For the infant the major forms of pleasure are those gained through oral activity. Feeding experiences during this stage seem related to development in later years.

The interactions with the mother set the stage for much of the later social development of the infant. Because of the learning principal of generalization, the ways of responding to other persons are very likely to be a reflection of the experiences with the primary figure in the child's life.

Some of the chief socializing experiences for the child come as the result of the adequacy or inadequacy of handling by parental figures and of problems growing out of the feeding situation. In essence, the majority of studies reveal that neglect, disinterest, or lack of adequate handling during the period of infancy may act to limit severely future intellectual, social, and emotional development.

Special problems

Also germane to our discussion of infant development are emotional and social problems that are an outgrowth of feeding problems or related routine. Since hunger is one of the most important factors operating in the early development of the infant, it becomes the center of concern to parents and quite obviously to the infant. Some of the important variables that have been considered by researchers have been bottle-feeding versus breast-feeding, demand feeding versus adherence to a schedule, influences from which the culture, and attitudes of individual mothers in regard to feeding and dealing with the child. Other questions exist

with regard to feeding, but the foregoing appear to be the principal areas that have been thoroughly researched and investigated.

Much has been written about the necessity of breast-feeding, implying that it is only through the breast that a close personal relationship is established between the mother and child. Some writers have suggested that mothers who are unable to nurse children fail to do so because of an emotional block or rejection of the child. They cite an analogy wherein the withholding of milk is equivalent to the withholding of love. That this does not apply universally is obvious. Some mothers, for a variety of reasons, do not nurse children. Sometimes the physiological capacity to produce milk is limited. It is even possible that a mother may supply adequate amounts of milk to her infant, yet have feelings of rejection because of being forced to conform to a pattern of nursing that she does not particularly care for. Thus there is no uniform statement we can make on this particular issue. It does appear that in some cases failure to nurse an infant may be part of a general pattern of maternal rejection. However, this cannot be used to predict accurately for any single case. More important would appear to be the handling of the child during the feeding process. The handling and cuddling of a child during the period, whether he is being bottle-fed or breast-fed, seem to have far greater significance for the development of feelings of contentment and ease in the child than does the source of the supply of milk.

There have been great variations in opinion regarding the adoption of a schedule for feeding. In some generations it has been emphasized that a strict schedule should be set up and never varied. In other instances there has been a strong declaration that demand feeding is the only proper way. The results learned from these situations have been inconclusive. Generations growing up under either condition have managed to survive and grow into reasonably healthy adults.

One problem frequently encountered is the complete sacrifice of all other parental activities to the care of the young child. This usually takes place only with the first child, although there are parents who persist in such behavior through a succession of infants within the family. It is only when there is a mutual recognition of the rights of both mother and child that a stress-free and warm relationship can be successfully maintained.

Other cultures show wide varieties of different practices with regard to the subject of feeding. Some cultures permit breast-feeding well past the first year, whereas others allow nursing for only a part of the first year. Some groups allow their children to nurse until their fifth or sixth year. These and other cultural practices are reported by Whiting and Child (1953).

In our own country there are social class differences that appear from time to time in feeding and child-rearing practices. These variations are quite frequently altered by popular concepts on child rearing or ideas that are advanced by prominent individuals in pediatrics, such as in Spock's book, *Baby and Child Care.*

Rigidity of scheduling on the part of the mother undoubtedly will result in later years in the child's feeling guilty or anxious when he is unable to or does not want to adhere to rigid scueduling. The groundwork is laid for compulsive, conforming behavior in such instances. In other cases the more relaxed, easygoing mother may establish a greater freedom for her child and thus permit his later behaviors a greater freedom of expression and ease in the process of socialization.

Of greatest importance—far greater than scheduling, either rigid or lax—is the attitude of the parents toward the child. If it is a warm, giving, and sharing relationship, a positive social relationship is usually the result. If this attitude is positive early in the life of the infant, it is the basis for building a deeper and long-lasting positive relationship with the parents. Behaviors that may be irritating to rejecting parents may be the very ones that reinforce a positive relationship between a child and accepting parents. Their ability to cope with many of the child's problems in growing, exploring, and developing aid greatly in his normal development.

SUMMARY

The small infant is a helpless person depending entirely on other people for his care. He is able to suck and therefore can get food from his mother's breast or from a bottle, and he can cry to let others know he is unhappy. He makes random, uncoordinated movements, but for the most part he sleeps a great deal. The world around him is an unknown place, and all people are strangers. At birth the infant is 20 to 21 inches long and weighs 7 to 7½ pounds.

At 1 year of age he has tripled his birth weight, added 10 inches to his height (now about 30 inches), has acquired about six teeth, knows his immediate family, and recognizes familiar faces. He can vocalize actively and say three or more words. He can even walk when one hand is held. True, his gait is unsteady, and he drops to all fours and crawls at times. He enjoys poking his finger into small places and plays with toys. He likes to touch, taste, and feel objects. A toy that makes a noise is especially attractive to him. Going out in the stroller is a pleasure to him. At 1 year the child likes to try to feed himself. Milk is taken from a cup, except possibly for his bottle at nap time and nighttime. He usually takes an afternoon and morning nap.

Those caring for the infant must have their own physical, psychological, and intellectual needs met so that they are free to have a desirable relationship with the infant. If the infant has had parents and/or caretakers who have maintained a warm and loving relationship with him, are sensitive to his needs for affection and sensory stimulation, and have provided relief from tension, then he will be a happy infant ready for the next stage of development. According to Erickson, infancy is the period when a feeling of trust in others is acquired.

REFERENCES

Bellam, G.: The first year of life, Am. J. Nurs. **69:**1244, June, 1969.

Caldwell, B. M., et al.: Infant day care and attachment, Am. J. Orthopsychiatry **40:**397, 1970.

Cameron, J., et al.: Infant vocalizations and their relationship to mature intelligence, Science, **157:**331, 1967.

Cazden, D. B.: Child language and education, New York, 1972, Holt, Rinehart & Winston, Inc.

Coleman, R., Kris, E., and Provence, S.: The study of variations of early parental attitudes, Psychoanal. Study Child **8:**20, 1953.

Fantz, R. L.: Visual perception from birth as shown by patterns selectivity, Ann. N.Y. Acad. Sci. **118:**173, 1965.

Flavell, J. H.: The developmental psychology of Jean Piaget, New York, 1963, D. Van Nostrand Co.

Fries, M.: The child's ego development and the training of adults in his environment, Psycholoanal. Study Child **2:**85, 1946.

Gibson, E. J., and Walk, R. R.: The "visual cliff," Sci. Am. **202:**64, 1960.

Gruelich, W. W., and Pyle, S. I.: Radiographic atlas of skelctal development of the hand and wrist, Stanford, Calif., 1959, Stanford University Press.

Heseltine, M., and Pitts, J.: Economy in nutrition and feeding of infants, Am. J. Public Health, **56:**1756, 1966.

Hurlock, E.: Developmental psychology, New York, 1975, McGraw-Hill Book Co.

Illingworth, R. S.: An introduction to developmental assessment in the first year, London, 1962, National Spastics Society.

Kagan, J.: Change and continuity in infancy, New York, 1971, John Wiley & Sons, Inc.

Kagan, J.: Do infants think? Sci. Am. **226**(3):74, 1972.

Kessen, W.: The Child, New York, 1965, John Wiley & Sons, Inc.

Longstretch, L. E.: Psychological development of the child, New York, 1968, The Ronald Press Co.

Mussen, P., Conger, J., and Kagan, J.: Child development and personality, ed. 4, New York, 1974, Harper & Row, Publishers.

Peterson, C.: A child grows up, Port Washington, N.Y., 1974, Alfred Publishing Co., Inc.

Robertson, J.: Mothering as an influence in early development, Psychoanal. Study Child **17:**245, 1962.

Rubin, R.: Basic maternal behavior, Nurs. Outlook **9:**753, December, 1961.

Stroufe, L. A., and Wunsch, J. P.: The development of laughter in the first year of life, Child Dev. **43:**1326, 1972.

Thomas, A., Chess, S., and Birch, H. G.: The origin of personality, Sci. Am. **223:**102, 1970.

Trehub, S. E., and Robinovitch, M. S.: Auditory and linguistic sensitivity in early infancy, Dev. Psychol. **6:**74, 1972.

Tulkin, S. R., and Kagan, J.: Mother-child interaction in the first year of life, Child Dev. **43:**31, 1972.

Vaughan, V. C., III: Growth and development. In Vaughan, V., III, and McKay, J., (editors): Nelson's textbook of pediatrics, ed. 10, Philadelphia 1975, W. B. Saunders Co.

Whiting, G. W., and Child, I. L.: Child training and personality, New Haven, 1953, Yale University Press.

Zelazo, N. A., Zelazo, P. R., and Kolb, S.: Walking in the newborn, Science **176:**314, 1972.

6

TODDLER AND PRESCHOOL PERIOD

When two such extensive periods of development as the toddler and the preschool years are placed in a single chapter, a question may be raised as to justification for their combination. It is our belief that this grouping is warranted because in these two periods there are no distinct emergent qualities whose elaboration and amplification would require a separation. Motor skills, social behaviors, language development, and other qualities are already present in rudimentary form. During both of these phases of development they simply undergo expansion and elaboration. The break between infancy and the toddler stage is marked by the appearance of upright locomotion. It is also a time of breakthrough in verbal communication. The next major landmark for the child will be the advent of school, where socialization factors and separation from family provide the major point of demarkation. Preparation for these changes plays a large part in the training and education during the toddler and preschool years.

PHYSICAL DEVELOPMENT

Inspection of the height-weight tables (Figs. 6-1 and 6-2) for this period reveals that by the second year there is some deceleration in the rapid growth rate of the child. After the second year development follows a slow, relatively orderly process in the increase of both height and weight. Let us now look more closely at the specific areas of development and their changes during this period.

Height

The average increase in height for boys and girls is approximately 5 inches between the first and second years of life. In the ensuing years the rate of growth in height is much smaller. It averages a little less than 2 inches per year throughout this period. Boys maintain a very slight superiority in height during the early toddler and preschool years, but by the age of 4½ years girls have caught up to boys, and by 5 years they are slightly ahead. This slight superiority in height will continue until the onset of adolescence. It should be noted that individual variations are extensive, and the advantage maintained by girls is very, very slight, at least during the toddler and preschool period. The portions of the child's body undergoing most rapid growth during the toddler and preschool period are the legs. They contribute an increasing proportion of the child's total height. By the time he enters first grade an average of 45% of his height will be legs.

Weight

The rapid gain in weight found during the first year also undergoes a decline during the second year and the succeeding years of the toddler and preschool period. Whereas both boys and girls average a gain of 5 pounds between first and second years, subsequent weight gain is slightly less than 5 pounds between the second and third years and about 4 pounds from the third to fourth year and from the fourth to fifth year. Between the fifth and sixth years there is an increase in weight gain that is greater than in any period since infancy. By the time the child enters school he will weigh about 48 pounds (boys) or 46 pounds (girls). Even though girls are slightly taller during the later stages, their general body build is such that they show a lower percentage of muscle and thus a lower weight than boys.

Body proportions

In infancy, you will recall, bodily proportions are quite different from those of the adult. The head seems too large, the trunk too long, and the legs too short. As a result the child ap-

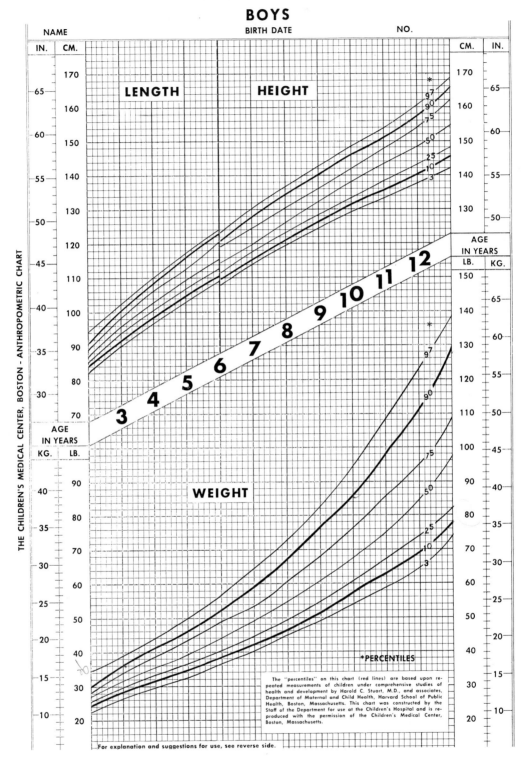

Fig. 6-1. Percentile chart for measurements of boys. (Courtesy The Children's Medical Center, Boston, Mass.)

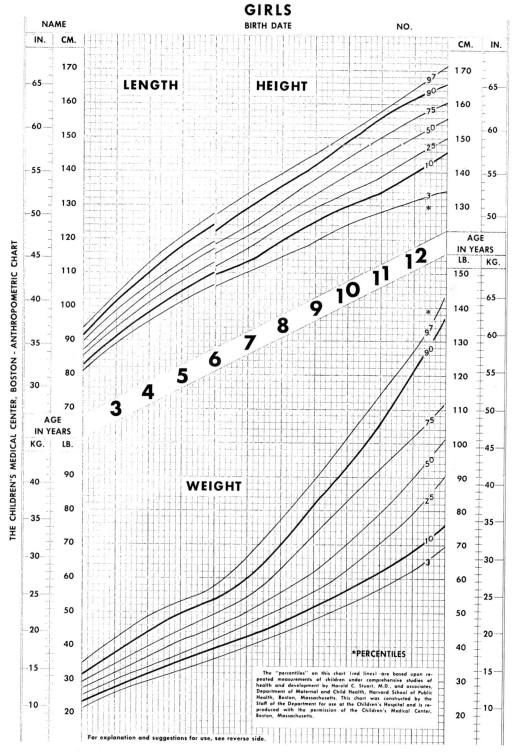

Fig. 6-2. Percentile chart for measurements of girls. (Courtesy The Children's Medical Center, Boston, Mass.)

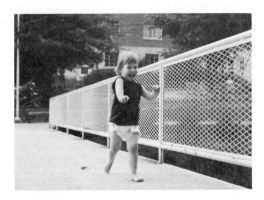

Fig. 6-3. The toddler. Walking upright is at first an uncertain and unsteady process.

pears unsteady and top-heavy when he makes his first halting attempts at locomotion. As development continues throughout the toddler and preschool period, the conformation of the body becomes increasingly like the form found in adults. During this period the head, so out of proportion during the first year, grows more slowly, whereas legs and arms undergo much more rapid growth.

Other less visible changes are also taking place. The anterior fontanel in the skull is closed by the eighteenth month, a high percentage of cartilage is replaced by bone, and there is a broadening and deepening of the chest.

Dentition

During the first year the first teeth appear. Most often these are the central incisors and in some instances the lateral incisors as well. The lower lateral incisors do not ordinarily erupt during the first year. They make their appearance early in the second year and are followed in rapid succession during the period from 2 to 2½ years by the cuspids, first molars, and second molars. In most cases all 20 deciduous teeth are present midway in the third year. There will then be no further major changes in dentition during the toddler and preschool period. Permanent teeth usually begin to make their appearance during the first year of school.

Other body systems

Some physical changes will have particular importance in the maintainance of health. Growth in such tissues as the adenoids and ton-

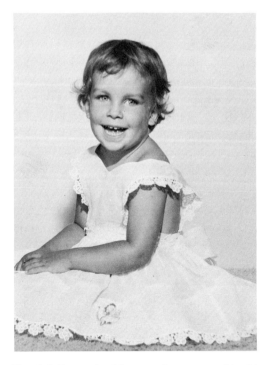

Fig. 6-4. Proper dentition contributes to good health and appearance.

sils may require special care or removal should they prove obstructive of normal speech and breathing functions.

Skin changes also are noted in this period. The light, delicate, and supersensitive skin of infancy gives way to a tougher "hide" of childhood.

Neural and muscular changes

In infancy a high percentage of body weight is fat, bone, and the organs of the body. The amount of muscle tissue is small, and it constitutes a relatively small proportion of the body weight. During the toddler and preschool period there is an ever-increasing percentage of muscle tissue and body weight devoted to muscles. The soft baby fat of infancy gives way to the appearance of muscles and adult conformation. The protruding abdomen of infancy becomes the trim and frequently slender form of childhood.

Maturation of the nervous system permits greater coordination and organization of the child's behavior. Microscopic inspection of the nervous system would reveal that nerve fibers, once only partially differentiated, now have become separated and insulated from each other by the myelin sheath. Myelinization is the term given to the process of development of the protective shields around nerve fibers. This maturational change permits greater specificity of functioning within the nervous system. The brain as well undergoes great evolutionary changes during this period. By age 2 years the brain has grown to nearly three times its birth weight, to a weight of approximately 1,000 gm. This is roughly 75% of its size at maturity. Brain size and weight, perhaps more than any other feature, are most nearly complete by the end of the toddler and preschool period. By the date of school entry the brain will be fully 90% of the adult size and weight.

Sensory and motor development

By the advent of the toddler and preschool years, *sensory* functioning is highly developed. Except for some of the fine points in discrimination, which may be affected by the final maturation of the nervous system through completion of myelinization, the apparatus is complete. It is possible that there is a continuing growth of tactile sensitivity, but further changes in sensory functioning will be of a learned rather than a maturational type. Our major emphasis in this section will be on developmental changes produced by maturation of the skeletal and muscular systems. These systems in conjunction with the sensory apparatus interact to form the behavioral refinements that are a vital part of growing up.

Motor development of the child will have progressed by age 2 years through a series of stages in the evolution of his locomotion. He will have been able to sit, crawl, creep, stand, and walk with support before he actually embarks on independent walking, which becomes well developed in the toddler stage. None of these events is possible if there has not been sufficient maturation in the child. Training may be used to refine already-present responses, but it cannot be used to accelerate the maturational processes. Unusually early walking can occur only if there has been sufficient maturation of the involved muscular and neural structures to make this possible.

By the time the child is 3 years old he shows a wide variety of motor responses. No longer is he forced to toddle uncertainly in moving from place to place. He is now able to run. He can move quickly, avoid objects, move easily up or down stairs, and jump, both down from objects and up onto low ones. In other motor activities he can successfully pedal a tricycle, throw objects with some degree of accuracy, and maintain his balance even on uneven ground or where other hazards are present.

By age 4 the preschooler is able to extend his jumping behavior, skip, and play games requiring gross motor coordination. Even when 5 years old, he will not be able to play the popular game of hopscotch that many children engage in during the early school years. Coordinated motor activities such as batting a ball and catching swiftly moving objects still elude all but the very skilled child.

In finer movements such as the use of hands and fingers, the toddler and preschooler goes through a rapidly evolving set of skills in which he is able to manipulate objects, stack blocks in building a "house," and show increasing skill with a pencil. Only able to produce a wobbly straight line at age 2, by age 3 he is able to copy a circle, by age 4 he may be able to add body features to a crude picture of a man, and by the time he is 5 years old he may be able to produce a square. Most children by age 5 can draw recognizable pictures of a series of objects: a man, a car, a house, and other familiar objects.

LANGUAGE DEVELOPMENT

The rudiments of speech are present by the end of the infancy period. The child uses a few simple words, which at first are labels for persons, objects, or acts but which soon may stand for entire sentences. For example, the word *doll,* depending in part upon the inflection, may mean "This is my doll," "Give me my doll," "Where is my doll? I want it," or "I dropped my doll; please pick it up for me."

By 18 to 24 months most children are beginning to combine words as in "Want Mama" or "Where ball?" Words are omitted from what an adult considers a complete sentence, but the meaning is clear. Most noteworthy is the regularity of word orders from the very beginning of these combinations. The child does not confuse order but puts subject, predicate, and object in their proper sequence when he uses them.

Vocabulary usually grows rapidly between the ages of 2 and 2½ years. By 2½ the child is able to communicate his needs quite well to adults, and by the time he reaches the end of the preschool period he will probably have nearly 10 times as many words available to him as he did at age 2. Most children use complete sentences by the age of 4 and can convey feelings as well as meaning by appropriate use of inflections and intonations. Articulation has become clearer and more precise in most children. Exceptions occur if the child stutters or has other speech handicaps or if parents encourage baby talk or reinforce immature communication.

Whereas extensive variations exist on a cultural basis as to the numbers and types of words children use, studies indicate that children today are more nearly uniform in language development and show higher levels of performance in language skills during the late preschool period than was true in earlier genera-

tions. One possible explanation that has been advanced is that working class children are not as disadvantaged when compared with children from other families as they were generations earlier. With adequate incomes, better educa-

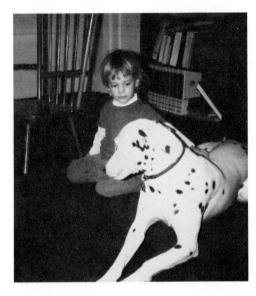

Fig. 6-5. Communication can take many forms.

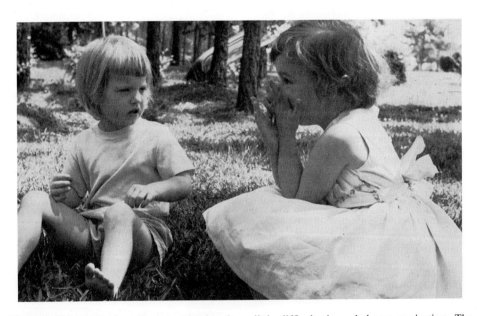

Fig. 6-6. Communication. Two preschoolers have little difficulty in verbal communication. The social response of a need for privacy is conveyed by the cupped hands. (From Heckel, R. V., and Jordan, R. M.: Psychology; the nurse and the patient, ed. 2, St. Louis, 1967, The C. V. Mosby Co.)

tional facilities, and the presence of many forms of mass media of communication—radios, television, audiovisual training aids in schools—differences appear to be on the decline. Differences continue to exist between social classes in the level and ease of acquisition of language skills, but they do not reflect the profound differences once noted. Similarly the sex differences in language skills once strongly emphasized by researchers no longer seem so pronounced. This may reflect a breakdown in the separation of training for boys and girls that was prevalent in earlier generations. Our culture no longer views the woman as weak, helpless, and incapable of education. Instead, females today receive highly similar education and may strive for occupational goals that are identical with those of males. As a result differences once thought to be inherited now appear to be merely a result of differing emphases in training.

As was indicated briefly in the section on infancy, Piaget describes the period from 2 years to maturity as the period in which intelligence develops from the beginnings of organized symbolic behavior (language) to the ability to use hypothetical reasoning, or, in other words, from concrete representation to the increasingly abstract. This, of course, is reflected in the language of the child. As his intellectual capacities emerge, he is able to recognize and describe classes of objects, deal with them on an abstract level, and form new and meaningful relationships between objects and events.

Problems in language development

A number of problem areas exist in language development. Among these are problems arising from stuttering, inadequate training, cultural limitations, and sensory or intellectual deficits that impede learning. Each may act to prevent the child from acquiring necessary learning experiences at appropriate periods during his development.

Speech problems such as stuttering are quite common and should be expected during the early phases of language development. Early speech is marked by many a false start, halting attempt, and inadequate production of words. This begins with the use of meaningful speech

and may continue for a number of years. Some experts believe that anxious and concerned parents who feel the child should be more proficient in his speech development may reinforce his concern about his speech and thus prolong the difficulties by conveying their anxieties to the child. Other theorists see stuttering as an expression of deep-seated concern and difficulty within the child. Both theories obviously cannot deal with many of the known factors about stuttering.

Whereas it is well established that emotional difficulties can bring on and prolong stuttering behavior, it has been observed that stuttering is far more pronounced in boys than in girls. Does this mean that boys are more disturbed than girls? Probably not, but it may reflect something about the relative ease with which boys and girls can acquire language skills. Similarly it may reflect the fact that girls, lacking physical strength, rely more upon verbal behavior. As a result they develop language skills earlier and perfect them to a higher degree than boys. We are confronted with a series of possible explanations with only partial research evidence to support any of them.

In spite of the fact that many children will at some stage of their development show blocking, stammering, or stuttering in their speech, the great majority will overcome this without professional help. By the time the child enters school in most cases he will have perfected language skills to the degree that stuttering is no longer observable.

The problems arising from inadequate training and cultural limitations are less obvious. In general they result in lower levels of language skills, lower measured intelligence, and an overall pattern of limitations in communication, which may build an ever-widening gulf between the child and his social environment. Much of the early learning of speech seems to be on the basis of a constant repetition of sounds provided by parental figures and imitated by the young child. If contact with parents is limited or the types of language patterns provided is inadequate, the child will show a language deficit quite early in his development.

Sensory defects or intellectual limitations similarly will operate to limit the child's first-hand experience with language. In the case of intellectual limitations, he will be unable to perform the basic steps in the acquisition of language. He will be unable to class words or objects sufficiently to ensure their retention. If he has difficulties in sensory areas that limit his ability to hear or to see, his chances for acquiring understanding of specific objects and their relationships are greatly limited. The blind child who hears the word *sky* will have a great deal of difficulty in conceptualizing this since it is not included in his personal experience. Although others may use many words to describe "sky" to him, he will never be able to comprehend this concept as fully as can the young child who is able to see. Deafness provides such a language block that, unless the child has had a great deal of training, he may be totally unable to speak.

Problems abound in the development of speech. They cut across all cultures and all ages of individuals. Although compensating mechanisms are available, any sensory deficit or intellectual deficit may prevent the full acquisition of language skills.

PSYCHOSOCIAL DEVELOPMENT

During infancy few demands are placed on the child for conforming to any specific social patterns. To be sure, the parents prefer that the child be happy and comfortable so that he will not cry and yet have a fairly regular schedule. He should sleep long enough that other members of the family may get adequate rest. For these behaviors he is rewarded with a great deal of affection and attention, while other needs are fully met. Parents do not expect a great deal in return for the services they provide for the child. Most do not exact strict conformity to a series of social rules or behavior patterns. Even where parents do make such demands, the young child is not sufficiently mature to respond adequately to them.

It is during the second year that the first major social demands are made of the child. Up to this time parents accept in a matter-of-fact way the problems of keeping the baby clean and dry by frequent diaper changes. In the second year various social demands are placed on the child, limiting his mobility to designated areas, exercising some control during self-feeding, and

controlling his agitation when some of his desires are blocked or frustrated. For example, light fixtures and electric outlets are not play toys. The knobs on a television set must not be touched. Bedtime is at a certain hour. Lipstick belongs to mother, not to baby.

Most parents will begin the rudiments of toilet training during the second year. Unfortunately toilet training is often an area of stress between parents and children. Frequently mothers will expect children to be trained far earlier than is possible, as indicated in our knowledge of the age at which muscular control can be gained. Parental concern and hostility with regard to toilet training may lead to intense conflicts, anxiety, frustration, and aggression. Many parents fail to realize that the concern and difficulty they are causing in the child have an effect that is the exact opposite of what they are trying to convey. In times of stress even adults have been known to lose bladder and bowel control. The child under stress, who has only minimal control over his sphincters, is much more likely to have accidents and difficulties when emotionally upset. In cases where parents are punitive, the accident, which is now more likely to occur, causes further retaliation. What frequently results is disaster. The child, disturbed over his inability to please his parents, will generalize his emotional difficulties to a series of other situations. He may think of himself as bad or evil because he is unable to please them. He may develop resentment and aggression toward parents because of their unwillingness to help or understand him, and this may result in even further disturbances in interpersonal relationships. The child may anticipate that other adults and other persons will react to him in a punitive or rejecting way because of his training difficulties.

Anthropologists and psychologists have reported many differences in toilet-training practices found within our own culture and in comparisons with other cultures of the world. In our culture Sears, Maccoby, and Levin (1957) found that lower class mothers tend to be more punitive and restrictive in toilet training as compared with middle class mothers. It was thought that middle class mothers had more exposure to popular trends in child rearing and thus developed more permissive attitudes. These results were in essential agreement with work done earlier by Davis and Havighurst (1946). Other societies show a range of behaviors from the very punitive to the extremely permissive. Psychoanalytical writers and some psychologists have made much of the subject of toilet training in attempting to explain the emergence and development of personality. Examples of this theoretical approach can be studied in Whiting and Child (1953). (For positive suggestions on teaching mothers about toilet training see Chapter 9.)

Identification

Much of the process of socialization occurs through identification. In identification the child takes on the behaviors, characteristics, and ways of responding observed in other persons in his environment.

It leads the child to think, feel, and behave as though the characteristics of another person belong to him. Usually in the young child this person is a parent whose behavior is imitated by the child as if it were his own. This can be seen in play with dolls when the children act as mother and father and serve a miniature tea party. Tones of voice, gestures, and other behaviors may similarly be incorporated. At this age adult standards are accepted without question, and the child engages in a whole series of role-playing behavior in which both positive and negative aspects of the parent are reflected.

Children tend to take on certain characteristics of both parents, regardless of sex. During the early years, particularly in the toddler and preschool period, the primary source of identification is with the mother. This could lead to later problems for the male child. However, the mother can do much to limit any complete identification with her on the part of her son. The father can be the model for his children, although his contact with them is necessarily limited by his being out of the home during much of the waking period.

Most theorists are generally agreed that the basis for identification is a search on the part of the child for security and a movement away from anxiety. If the child identifies with the parent, he feels as if he had acquired his parent's

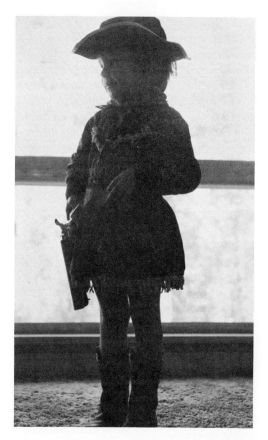

Fig. 6-7. Identification. Our young hero or heroine learns to identify with cowboys or cowgirls seen on television.

strength and adequacy as well. Also he is likely to be rewarded by overt demonstrations of love, attention, and other positively reinforcing behaviors. Even in the absence of positive reinforcement, the child may learn that by behaving in a particular manner he will avoid being punished or negatively reinforced.

Other mechanisms are operating in identification as well. The child recognizes parents as having a high degree of control over the environment; they may move freely within it and may engage in social behavior and interactions that the child wishes to emulate. By identifying with the parent the child realistically hopes to reach some of the same goals after a time.

Problems in identification

Unfortunately not all homes offer adequate models for identification. In many families one or the other parent is punitive, rejecting, or possessed of a series of undesirable behavior patterns. What can this do to the child? Let us consider the case of a male child whose father has a number of undesirable characteristics. Perhaps he rejects the child and shows him no love. Under these circumstances it will be extremely difficult for the child to identify with the father and take on his traits. Perhaps as a result of this unfavorable experience with the most important male figure in his life, he identifies more closely with the mother. In this process of identification he may take on a number of feminine characteristics that may put him in conflict with the culture in which he lives. In spite of this further dilemma he may find his cultural role less traumatic than that of identifying with a rejecting, negativistic person. If a child is rejected by the opposite-sexed parent, he may grow up to be well identified with his sexual role but unable to interact satisfactorily with members of the opposite sex. He may anticipate the kind of rebuff or rejection he received as a child.

This is not to imply that all children whose families include inadequate figures with which to identify will grow up to have disturbances in interpersonal relationships. This is far from the case. Quite frequently other persons in the environment may take on major parental roles that the parents themselves are unable to fulfill. Grandparents, other relatives, or members of the neighborhood community may serve as positive sources of identification for the child. These persons, labeled transitional figures (Heckel, 1964), serve as a stable link for the child in the total process of identification. Lacking satisfactory role models within his family, the child may utilize transitional figures in his process of emotional development. Although this is more characteristic at later stages of development, young children can and do seek support, even during the toddler and preschool years.

In other instances even young children may realize that unfavorable conditions in their own home may not be characteristic of all other situations; they may not generalize their "home" problems to others. In most normal families problems are far less intense. Most parents, although not perfect, have many characteristics

with which children readily identify. As a result they are generally viewed as warm and receptive, providing the child with a desirable role model.

Oedipal period

The oedipal period, or oedipal phase as it is sometimes called, is a process in which the child has a strong desire for love and affection from the opposite-sexed parent. It has some of the characteristics of identification in that the child is viewed (at least by psychoanalytical writers) as identifying with an adult role in the need to interact in a love relationship with the mother or father. Under these conditions the boy is a rival with the father for the mother's affections, and the girl is a rival with the mother for the father's affections. Freud and his followers placed many sexual overtones on this interaction, although this view is not held by all present-day theorists. Most now recognize the strong need for attachment and love between parent and child but minimize the sexual aspect.

The oedipal complex may exist to a very strong degree in some families and be much weaker in others. It is a normal process but is not now considered by most theorists as always necessary to the successful maturation of the child.

Problems growing out of the oedipal situation are not unlike the difficulties in identification. It the child has many unfulfilled oedipal needs, the chances of emotional disturbance at later periods of development are much greater. Heckel (1963), in a study of young girls who had lost their fathers before or during the first two years of life, found them to have serious adjustive difficulties, precocious sexual interests, and disturbed interpersonal relationships. It was thought that these were not due to the loss of the father alone. In each instance the mother was passive, dependent, and unable to provide some of the strength and support that might have been supplied by the missing father.

In other words, the personality of the remaining parent is extremely important.

Development of social standards

By the onset of the preschool period, following the infant and toddler phases, most children have already developed a strong sense of right and wrong. Each of the earlier experiences with the parents will have had a part in the developing of the child's value system, his conscience, and his ideals. The experiences in which he has been rewarded, has been punished, or has encountered a series of "no's" as well as those things for which he has been given permission begin to be sorted, classified, and understood as the young child develops his powers of conceptualization. If his training and experience have been erratic and inconsistent, it is easy to understand how his conscience may develop with loopholes, blind spots, or other deficits. Much of conscience is developed by the need to please parents and a fear of their disapproval. Should the child think about violating one of the parents' principles, his immediate reaction might be to feel anxiety. When he violates one of their principles, he feels guilt. As indicated earlier, if the training has been inconsistent, he may or may not experience the appropriate reaction when he has broken some standard. During this period the chief transmitters of right and wrong for the child with regard to the culture and to the family patterns of behavior are his parents. They will set the stage for what the child believes and what he will follow as his standards as well as what he will disregard as being unimportant or unnecessary.

We are all familiar with the problems that arise when the parents set one standard of behavior for the child but practice a different one themselves. These inconsistencies also cause the child to reflect irregularities in the development of his own social standards. Unless the parent provides an adequate role model for the child in adhering to behaviors that the parent desires for the child, the possibility is that these behaviors will be rejected by the child also. Children learn primarily from examples set by parents whose behavior they internalize rather than by precept.

The acquiring of conscience and ideals is a long process and combines formalized teaching, the observation of parental value systems, shaping by the parent, and the positive aspects of wishing to please parents and receive their rewards. These mechanisms in combination will result in the end product we see as the social

standards of the child. Signs of the development of social standards appear early in the developmental sequence. With maturity the values acquired in childhood generalize to a wide variety of situations. The character developed in this earliest formative period will have a great part in shaping the behaviors of the mature adult.

Interests

In the second and third year of life the child is interested in his own body. Toilet training tends to focus an interest on genitals: differences between sexes, differences between adults' and children's bodies, and interest in excreta. (See p. 16 for detailed discussion.) The toddler discovers he has legs that can carry him away from and to his mother. He loves to explore his environment and touch, handle, and taste everything that he can get into his hands. The work of Berlyne (1960) is a major source of information on curiosity. To run around pushing or pulling a toy delights the toddler. Then he finds he can assist in undressing. He wants to be independent, to feed himself. The toddler likes to have his own possessions: his chair, his spoon, his bed, his blanket, his towel, etc. This helps to give him a feeling of esteem and of belonging that adds to his security. The more secure he is, the more he turns attention to other objects. He enjoys climbing into his

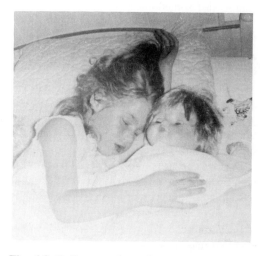

Fig. 6-8. Dolls are real people to 5-year-olds. Note the protective arm around the doll.

stroller and being taken on a walk. Although a cuddly toy or a teddy bear is nice to hold as he goes to sleep, the toddler likes to play with materials with which he can do something. The 2-year-old does not play with others yet but may play well side by side with a like-aged child. This is called parallel play. He enjoys books that have a familiar picture in them: shoes, coat, umbrella. He likes recognizing familiar objects and turning the page himself. Mother Goose rhymes are popular for their rhyme as well as for the words. Pictures of animals are enjoyable. Color in pictures makes them more interesting.

Later the growing child likes picture books of transportation as airplanes, cars, trains. By 3 and 4 years he likes stories with repetition and reiteration like "The Gingerbread Man" and "The Little Red Hen." Listening to children's songs and stories on a record player is popular. Some children's stories lend themselves to acting out, such as "The Three Little Pigs" or "Goldilocks and the Three Bears." By 5 years the child is ready for a short story with a plot, such as "Little Black Sambo."

When the child is familiar with his own body and immediate surroundings and has attained a certain amount of self-reliance, he turns his attention to objects outside himself. Four years of age is the peak of questions: What makes the clock go "tick-tock"? Where do babies come from? The child does not want a lengthy explanation, just something brief and to the point; otherwise his interest is lost. If a child says, "What makes the bridges stay up?" an acceptable answer might be, "Bridges are carefully built so cars can cross them."

As the child progresses in the preschool period he enjoys a trip to the library for a book, visiting a farm, going to the zoo, looking at a fire engine, etc. As indicated, children become interested in the world around them. The greater their own security and independence, the greater their quest and interest in the world around them. This period is what Erickson calls the stage of initiative.

In the preschool period pets are of interest. Children may lavish affection on them. That a dog, for example, has to have water and food makes him almost a human object.

Certain play materials that are popular with preschool children are conducive to learning to share, participate, and take turns. These include a small wagon, blocks, doll dishes and doll, slide, and jungle gym. More than one child can play with these. Although these is still a lot of solitary or individual play, shifting groups of two or three children may stay together a short time. True, the children need supervision to see that they use acceptable techniques to attain their desires and to not hurt other children.

By the end of the preschool period children will be able to interact in a fairly cooperative manner. Social development is further refined in middle childhood.

Most interactions will be planned by others or arranged informally with immediate neighbors. Boundaries set up for this group may be limited to the yards or homes of neighbors on either side. Although as adults we may view this as quite restrictive, the child sees the yard, the sidewalk, or the neighbor's house as filled with a host of new objects that hold fascination for him. Generally a child can find hours of entertainment in his own yard, watching butterflies or bugs in summer, snowflakes in winter, or even drops of rain falling on a window when he is confined inside.

Sex differences in interests

Masculine and feminine behaviors are in many ways culturally developed and not so strongly biologically prescribed as has previously been believed. The evidence of discrimination against women in opportunities for independent living, jobs, salaries, and legal status has long been there for all to see but has recently been brought into the open by the women's liberation movement. The stereotypes of male and female characteristics are rapidly changing, and much of what follows may soon be in large part outdated.

During the toddler and preschool years parents may begin to see results of their shaping of interests in both boys and girls. In a paper describing ongoing research at the University of California, Berkeley, Dr. Jeanne Block reported (1975) a negative effect of sex role emphasis in the behavior of nursery school girls. No differences can be found between the sexes at age 3 in solving problems when barriers must be overcome. But by age 4 there is a noticeable change in the girls; they are no longer so active, give up sooner, and are more likely to ask for help than boys. Many girls have already learned that such dependency is expected of them. By age 5 children are keenly aware of sex-appropriate interests and behavior. Now boys may take an interest in playing ball with the father, whereas the girls' play may center on activities considered to be feminine. The girl may play mother, nursing and caring for a doll, or she may play the role of housewife, cooking, sewing, cleaning, etc.

Some crossover will be permitted. Girls may play some games and activities usually restricted to boys, whereas boys may still be permitted to play house with girls their age or help mother take care of the house. As the boy nears the end of the preschool period there will be much stronger pressures on him to adopt more masculine interests and activities. Feminine interests in boys beyond this preschool period will lead to rejection if they are held during the school years. Although girls may not be censured for having an interest in boys' activities, they may not be well accepted by other girls.

If we wish to see more women enter the sciences and professions or become leaders in politics and in business, basic changes must be made in the way girls have too often been brought up. They must be encouraged to be independent and self-assertive rather than to be submissive and as a result to have to obtain what they want by indirection and subterfuge. Recently this does seem to be happening, but many parents are still imbued with the notions of former generations and the change will not be easy.

Social interactions

As we have indicated, the social interactions of the child will be largely governed by the actions of the parents. When parents encourage external associations, the child will develop rapidly during this period—from an egocentric being, interested only in his own personal needs, to a socially interacting, responding child. Although he will use in his interactions a series of defensive behaviors such as with-

drawal, denial, and repression or perhaps more aggressive reactions, his basic orientation will be social in nature.

Some of the mechanisms we identified in discussion of the child's problems will be used when difficulties occur in his interpersonal relationships. Frustrated by unsatisfactory interactions, the child may temporarily regress in his behavior, he may engage in aggressive verbalization in the form of quarreling, or he may seek to place the blame on other persons, other situations, or even on inanimate objects. The child thus has at his disposal a whole series of reaction patterns with which to meet problem situations when they occur with other persons. Although many of these reactions work quite well in dealing with other children, they may be much less effective in meeting interpersonal problems with parents. Parents will see these present in each of their children at some time. In the hospital setting, also, children who are

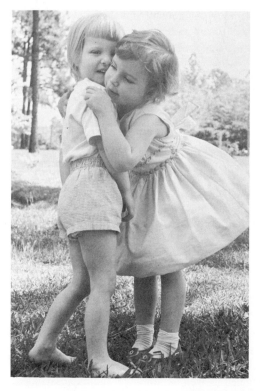

Fig. 6-9. Social interaction. Probably in imitation of adult behavior, the hug is used by preschoolers in greeting one another.

frustrated, anxious, or fearful may show the same behaviors we have already mentioned: withdrawal, denial, repression, projection, regression, etc.

Families differ widely in what they will permit the child to use as defensive reactions. Some parents will reward and approve of the child who is quiet and withdrawn, and he uses this as his major defense. Other families will demand a compliance or acquiescence, either behaviorally or in verbal form, from the child. In other instances the family may tolerate aggressive responses from the child when interpersonal difficulties occur. Regardless of the pattern of response utilized, much of his behavior will be directed toward solving the problems of interacting with others and socializing the frustrations that occur as a result. Living cooperatively with other persons is at best a difficult problem. It is only when the child learns suitable methods of dealing with his feelings and the feelings he arouses in other persons that he can successfully maneuver in his home environment. Quite frequently many of the problems of social interaction are eased and relieved by the child's entering a nursery school where he may have an opportunity to interact under supervision with other children his own age.

Contribution of nursery schools

Nursery schools supplement the home experience but in no way replace it. They are typically open only in the morning until lunchtime. Usually children are 3 years old before being admitted.

Attendance at school can release the mother from the child's care to do various errands or to help meet her other responsibilities.

Nursery school aids the child's development in several ways. Being away from the mother for a short time increases emotional independence and growth. The child learns that satisfaction can be obtained from adults outside the family. In general self-reliance is promoted in every aspect of development. Studies indicate that a higher level of social interaction is attained as well as initiative and expressiveness. There is exposure to literature, art, and music, although on a very elementary level. Social science experiences are usually provided, such as

a visit to a farm. Types of play equipment in nursery schools such as a sandbox, slide, or jungle gym may not be able to be provided in the home or even a large area outdoors for play.

Nursery schools help the child towards a readiness for the experience of school at the typical age of 6 years. Early learning of the fact that persons other than the parents are capable of exercising control over the child's behavior is of great importance. Until the child learns that others can assert such control, he will be in a state of conflict with other persons. If learning this lesson is delayed until the first year of school, changing the child's guidance is of benefit to parents and to individuals who will encounter the child in later periods of life.

Problems of the toddler and preschool child

Toddler and preschool children face a number of adjustive problems in relating to other children and to their own families. Some of the most prevalent problems are the appearance of aggressive behavior, tantrums, fears, jealousy, and dependency. Each may operate to limit the child's effectiveness in social situations, and each may require discipline or control by the parents.

Aggression

Research on behavior has revealed that aggression is a natural consequence of frustration. A large part of the process of socialization for children is devoted to the curbing and control of aggressive impulses. Even with the pressure of social controls, children continue to express aggressive tendencies. They may do this for a number of reasons. In some families aggression is condoned and even reinforced. Some children learn very early in life that they must be aggressive to receive attention and other forms of reward. In other instances environments are so frustrating that they result in the expression of overt aggression even though the consequences for such expression may be unpleasant.

Socialization operates to curb aggressive impulses in several ways. Some parents provide a positive role model for the child to follow in which aggressive impulses are curbed or channeled into more socially acceptable areas. In other instances the child is made to feel guilty for expressing aggression. He may also develop anxiety about the expression of aggression, and this may force him to avoid situations in which feelings of aggression might be experienced. Pressure of parents to conform is often quite intense. Mothers and fathers frequently admonish children by saying, "My little boy (girl) would not do something like that," or "If you do a thing like that, something bad will happen."

As a result of such admonitions most children learn quickly to channel their aggressive impulses into more subtle mechanisms of expression. Quite frequently they conform in the presence of parents—only to displace aggression onto toys, other children, or household objects. Many a family pet has been the long-suffering victim of a child whose parents completely inhibit all his aggressive responses.

Temper tantrums

Temper tantrums appear early in the developmental sequence. They occur most frequently when the child first meets frustrations from parents and the environment. During infancy frustrations are relatively few. As the child enters the toddler and preschool phase, he is confronted by many new circumstances and situations, all of which pose special problems for him. He is expected to conform and change his behavior in many ways. Restrictions are placed on his expressions of aggression, his desire to range freely is restricted, he may be punished when he violates some of the "no's" that parents set, and he may be punished when he violates the rights of other persons. All this is very trying to the child, who has been used to having all of his needs met during the earlier periods of development. As a result he may rage against persons and situations that he feels are restricting him.

Most children at one time or another show temper tantrums and rages. Why do some children give these up quite quickly and others persist with this form of aggression in some form even into adulthood? Let us consider a case in point. Johnny, age 3, an only child, had grown up in the home of quite permissive parents.

They seldom frustrated any of his needs except where harm might come to him. On a shopping trip with his mother he was attracted by a large stuffed toy in the supermarket. His mother was not particularly interested in buying this for him and tried to force him to leave. Johnny resisted and flew into a rage, throwing himself onto the floor, kicking his heels, and slapping his hands on the floor. The embarrassed mother, concerned by what other persons might think, took the stuffed toy to the checkout counter and bought it for the child.

What really happened in this situation? The child showed aggression and rage at being thwarted. The mother, anxious to avoid a scene, gave in to the child and bought him the desired object. This very act by the mother reinforced the possibility that in future situations the child would again show temper tantrums. In effect she had rewarded the undesired behavior. We know from learning theory that when a response is rewarded the possibility of its occurring again is greatly increased. Thus the mother had laid the groundwork for a series of problems with the child in the future. When temper tantrums and other forms of aggression are even occasionally rewarded, the chances of their reappearing are good.

Conversely, if the parents or other authority figures in the child's life do not reinforce temper tantrums, if negative behaviors are not rewarded, they will drop out because they serve no useful purpose. Proper control of this behavior may be gained by ignoring it. Psychologists have found that even punishment may reinforce such behavior if the temper tantrum is thrown to gain attention. Punishment represents an undesirable form of attention but is still attention.

Fears

With the acquisition of language and a broadened environment the child encounters many new hazards and obstacles that have a potential for inducing fear. It is not possible to predict for any one child what will be feared and what will be tolerated. Many times a child's early learning experiences may attach negative attitudes or fear to things that are neutral for other individuals. Typical fears during this period are fears about dreams, fear of the dark, fears of separation, and fears related to ambiguous or poorly understood situations.

When fears are on a pathological level the child is afraid of a whole series of events and situations and overreacts to them. Simple fear responses such as withdrawal, dependency, clinging, and other fear reactions can usually be removed by educative processes. The child who fears a dog may respond more positively to the animal when it is petted by the parent or a friend of the child. In other instances minor fears may often help the child learn new and effective ways of dealing with situations that he cannot control or master. He may develop skills in social interaction to avoid being left alone; he may even learn to ride a bicycle to avoid walking past a yard that contains a large, noisy dog. Other examples abound in developmental histories. Children do many things because they are afraid of appearing silly, stupid, or unsophisticated. Fear will often provide motivation for behavioral change when other methods fail.

Jealousy

Jealousy is an emotion that is most often experienced in families in which there is more than one child. Although jealousy can also develop because of having to share one or the other parent, this appears to be less of a problem than is the case with siblings. Jealousy is typically aroused when another child enters the family and commands a great deal of attention from both parents. During the early stages of infancy the parents must give a great deal of time to the care of the infant. The older child, once the center of attention, now feels that he has been replaced and is no longer wanted or loved. It is natural that much of his aggression would be directed toward the intruder. In some cases the aggression felt is so strong that it results in the older child's hitting, pinching, or otherwise abusing the new infant.

Although it is not possible to remove all jealousy, parents can do a great deal to relieve the intensity of these feelings. It is quite normal, if we have been operating on one level of behavior and are then forced to play a lesser role, for us to feel frustrated or angry and, if our place has been taken by another, to be jealous of the person who replaced us. Recognizing such

"loss" in the eyes of the child, the parents may draw him into the care and development of the new infant. By helping with the infant, planning activities for him, and sharing in family decisions, the child can gain a feeling of participation and belonging to the family group. The extension of privileges to him may also, in part, compensate for his difficulties. To be sure, as the younger child grows older he may look with jealousy on the older child's privileges, but this can be handled by rewarding and recognizing abilities on each level.

When jealousy is present but not overt, it often takes the form of regressive behavior on the part of the child. In the case of Ken the arrival of a baby brother resulted in his regressing to a more infantile stage of behavior. He begged for a bottle, began wetting his pants, and showed other signs of behaving as a small child. The parents, recognizing the symptoms as jealousy of the new child, made a special effort to have him feel that he was an important part of the family and in part responsible for the care of the new child. They also sought means of rewarding him for acting his age. The result was a disappearance of the symptoms and a development of a positive attitude toward the new child.

Dependency

Dependency is a normal characteristic at certain stages of development in the child. In his early life he is completely dependent upon parents for meeting all his needs. As he matures, the child will seek to maintain a strong dependency relationship because of the security, protection, and comfort it provides. However, he will also be torn to move away from the family constellation because of the positive rewards offered for social interaction with others. Parents typically reinforce more dependency in young girls than in young boys. Codes of behavior for girls are stricter, and maintaining them is somewhat more difficult. As a result parents ordinarily do not release girls' dependency attachments as readily as those for boys.

In the preschool period there is some pressure on the child to give up many of his dependency relationships. When he expresses dependency, either on parents or on the teacher in nursery school, he may be seen as being a baby or different from others. As a result he may be teased or scolded, which negatively reinforces the undesired behavior.

Dependency is often used as a substitute for aggression as a means of dealing with frustrating situations. Children may also adopt a pattern of dependency because this is the role model provided them by the parents. In other instances dependency is utilized as a reward by parents to motivate the child for a series of tasks. Dependency is present in all people to some degree. The amount of dependency the child will show will be a direct reflection of the pattern of rewards offered by the parents. When they reinforce nondependent social behaviors, the tendency for the child to cling will be low. If, on the other hand, they restrict activities and increase fears of external contacts, or if the child has a high need for nurturing, the chances are excellent for his maintaining a high level of dependency, not only in childhood but also in later periods of development.

Falsehoods

Sometimes the preschool child, especially at the ages of 4 and 5 years, is accused of "lying." The young child actually confuses fact and fantasy many times. The child should not be accused of lying but should be helped to differentiate between fact and fantasy. "You mean you are pretending this?" an adult might inquire when the child makes a comment that is obviously wrong. After all, the child is read stories, so why should he not make up a story? Adults are paid money to write stories; the better the story, the more money they receive. If the child is imaginative, he should be given a chance to tell a make-believe story to an audience.

Truthfulness in older children is aided, first of all, by a wholesome relationship with parents. Seeing that the child receives adequate attention and affection will eliminate undesirable attention-getting devices. For example, the child might tell the parent he did something that he did not do but for which he would receive attention. Severe punishment for any misdeed is to be avoided; then the child will not fear severe consequences if he tells the truth. Truthfulness is promoted by example and by positive reinforcement for telling the truth. Also, if the child thinks he will not be believed even when he tells the truth, training in truthfulness is almost impossible. The habit of objectively discussing a troublesome situation will help to avoid untruthfulness. In addition, realistic expectations of children at different ages will prevent frustration, enhance self-esteem, and increase the probability of the child's telling the truth.

REFERENCES

Baumrend, D.: Current patterns of parental authority, Dev. Psychol. Monogr. **4**(Part 2):1, 1971.

Becker, W. C.: Consequences of different kinds of parental discipline. in Hoffman, M. L., and Hoffman, L. L., editors: Review of child development research, vol. 1, New York, 1964, Russell Sage Foundation.

Berlyne, D. E.: Conflict, curiosity and approval, New York, 1960, McGraw-Hill Book Co.

Biller, H. B.: Father, child and sex role, Lexington, Mass., 1971, D. C. Heath & Co.

Bronfenbrenner, U.: Two worlds of childhood: U.S. and U.S.S.R., New York, 1970, Russell Sage Foundation.

Davis, A., and Havighurst, R. Y.: Social class and color differences in child rearing, Am. Sociol. Rev. **11**:698, 1946.

Dielman, T. E., et al.: A check on the structure of parental reports of child rearing practices, Child Dev. **42**:483, 1971.

Dwyer, J., et al.: Feeding the pre-school child, Postgrad. Med. **47**:264, March, 1970.

Escalona, S.: Understanding hostility in children, Chicago, 1954, Science Research Associates, Inc.

Goda, S.: Speech development in children, Am. J. Nurs. **69**:276, February, 1969.

Heckel, R. L.: Shifting patterns of affection; transitional figures, Ment. Hyg. **48**:451, July, 1964.

Heckel, R. L.: The effects of fatherlessness on the preadolescent female, Ment. Hyg. **47**:69, January, 1963.

Hurlock, E.: Developmental psychology, New York, 1975, McGraw-Hill Book Co.

LaRue, M.: Head start in a Tennessee county, Am. J. Nurs. **70**:114, January, 1970.

Lichtenberg, P., and Norton, D.: Cognitive and mental development in the first five years of Life: A review of recent research, Bethesda, Md., 1970, National Institute of Mental Health.

McCandless, B.: Children: Behavior and development, New York, 1967, Holt, Rinehart & Winston, Inc.

Miles, M. S.: Body integrity fears in a toddler, Nurs. Clin. North Am. **4**:39, March, 1969.

Mussen, P., Conger, J., and Kagan, J.: Child development and personality, ed. 2, New York, 1974, Harper & Row, Publishers.

Pre-school child malnutrition, primary deterrent to human progress, Pub. No. 1282, Washington, D.C., 1966, National Academy of Sciences–National Research Council.

Read, K.: The nursery school, ed. 3, Philadelphia, 1960, W. B. Saunders Co.

Rosenham, D.: Prosocial behavior of children. In The young child: Review of research, vol. 2, Washington, D.C., 1972, National Association for Education of Young Children.

Sears, R. R., Maccoby, E. E., and Levin, H.: Patterns of child-rearing, Evanston, Ill., 1957, Row, Peterson & Co.

Spelke, E., et al.: Father interaction and separation protest, Dev. Psychol. **9:**83, 1973.

Spock, B.: Raising children in a difficult time: A philosophy of parental leadership, New York, 1974, W. W. Norton & Co., Inc.

Sutton-Smith, B.: Child psychology, New York, 1973, Appleton-Century-Crofts.

Tizard, B., et al.: Environmental effects on language development, Child Dev. **43:**337, 1972.

Vaughan, V. C., III: Growth and development. In Vaughan, V., III, and McKay, R. J., editors: Nelsons textbook of pediatrics, ed. 10, Philadelphia, 1975, W. B. Saunders Co.

Watson, R.: Psychology of the child, ed. 3, New York, 1973, John Wiley & Sons, Inc.

Whiting, Y. W., and Child, I. L.: Child training and personality, New Haven, 1953, Yale University Press.

7
MIDDLE CHILDHOOD

This chapter covers the period from 6 to 13 years of age, with minor variations because of earlier onset of adolescence. Descriptive titles for this age span abound. It is known as middle childhood, the preadolescent phase, or the school years. Whatever the title, it is a critical period of development during which the child for the first time is brought into full and continuing contact with others outside the home. As a part of this moving away from the family the child will develop more fully his social and sexual roles; he will acquire academic training while learning to read and write and to communicate in other ways. Perhaps most important will be his testing in the world at large of the value systems established during earlier years.

In this first testing of value systems and their impact on other persons, children are frequently faced with some of their most difficult conflicts and anxieties. They may find that their own value system varies from that of other children of their age; they may hear teachers expressing concepts and ideas that are unacceptable in their own home; they may learn that they themselves do not "fit in" and may be unable to find means whereby they can belong, thus discovering that their intellectual skills may be inadequate to meet the demands of the new situation. To cope with the many new stresses of the outside world children during this period quite often develop extensive defensive behaviors and mechanisms that serve to reduce anxiety and allow the individual to live more comfortably with himself.

In the course of this chapter we will look more closely at these events as well as observe the physical development that takes place during this period.

PHYSICAL DEVELOPMENT

From infancy the child's growth has been extremely rapid. By age 6, the beginning of this period, boys weigh about 48 pounds (22 kg.) and girls about 47 pounds (20 kg.). Boys and girls are about equal in height, standing about 3 feet 10 inches (approximately 117 cm.). During this period growth is a slow but steady increase. In height the child will grow approximately 5% per year and in weight about 10% per year. By the time he is 12 years of age he will weigh some 84 pounds (38 kg.) and be about 59 inches tall (150 cm.). There is a sex differential in such values because for some girls the growth spurt may have already begun, and girls will on the average exceed boys in both height and weight. The difference amounts to an average of 3 pounds in weight and 1 inch in height. The growth chart for this period of development (Table 7-1) shows the evolution of weight changes in boys and girls. Note that at 10½ years girls pull even with boys and that at 11 years they first take the lead in height and weight. This female advantage continues until 14½ years of age, or well into the adolescent period.

Skeletal changes

By age 6 many of the proportions of the child have taken on a character that will be maintained into adulthood. Bones lengthen and become harder, and ossification centers are present in nearly every instance. With the passage of additional time bone contours may change slightly. During the adolescent period the union of the epiphysis and the diaphysis takes place. Since making an x-ray study of the entire body of young persons is not practical, a great deal of reliance has been placed on x-ray films of changes in the hand and wrist as an index of skeletal maturation. Through use of this and similar techniques it is possible to gauge the developmental progress of any child over a period of time.

Table 7-1. Height and weight tables for children in middle childhood*

	Percentiles (boys)				Percentiles (girls)		
	10	**50**	**90**		**10**	**50**	**90**
6 years				*6 years*			
Weight in pounds	40.9	48.3	56.4	Weight in pounds	39.6	46.5	54.2
Weight in kilograms	18.55	21.91	25.58	Weight in kilograms	17.96	19.96	24.58
Height in inches	43.8	46.3	48.6	Height in inches	43.5	45.6	48.1
Height in centimeters	111.2	117.5	123.5	Height in centimeters	110.5	115.9	122.3
6½ years				*6½ years*			
Weight in pounds	43.4	51.2	60.4	Weight in pounds	42.2	49.4	57.7
Weight in kilograms	19.69	23.22	27.4	Weight in kilograms	19.14	22.41	26.17
Height in inches	44.9	47.6	50.0	Height in inches	44.8	46.9	49.4
Height in centimeters	114.1	120.8	127.0	Height in centimeters	113.7	119.1	125.6
7 years				*7 years*			
Weight in pounds	45.8	54.1	64.4	Weight in pounds	44.5	52.2	61.2
Weight in kilograms	20.77	24.54	29.21	Weight in kilograms	20.19	23.68	27.76
Height in inches	46.0	48.9	51.4	Height in inches	46.0	48.1	50.7
Height in centimeters	116.9	124.1	130.5	Height in centimeters	116.8	122.3	128.9
7½ years				*7½ years*			
Weight in pounds	48.5	57.1	68.7	Weight in pounds	46.6	55.2	65.6
Weight in kilograms	22.0	25.9	31.16	Weight in kilograms	21.14	25.04	29.76
Height in inches	47.2	50.0	52.7	Height in inches	47.0	49.3	51.9
Height in centimeters	120.0	127.1	133.9	Height in centimeters	119.5	125.2	131.8
8 years				*8 years*			
Weight in pounds	51.2	60.1	73.0	Weight in pounds	48.6	58.1	69.9
Weight in kilograms	23.22	27.26	33.11	Weight in kilograms	22.04	26.35	31.71
Height in inches	48.5	51.2	54.0	Height in inches	48.1	50.4	53.0
Height in centimeters	123.1	130.0	137.3	Height in centimeters	122.1	128.0	134.6
8½ years				*8½ years*			
Weight in pounds	53.8	63.1	77.0	Weight in pounds	50.6	61.0	74.5
Weight in kilograms	24.4	28.62	34.93	Weight in kilograms	22.95	27.67	33.79
Height in inches	49.5	52.3	55.1	Height in inches	49.0	51.4	54.1
Height in centimeters	125.7	132.8	140.0	Height in centimeters	124.6	130.5	137.5
9 years				*9 years*			
Weight in pounds	56.3	66.0	81.0	Weight in pounds	52.6	63.8	79.1
Weight in kilograms	25.54	29.94	36.74	Weight in kilograms	23.86	28.94	35.88
Height in inches	50.5	53.3	56.1	Height in inches	50.0	52.3	55.3
Height in centimeters	128.3	135.5	142.6	Height in centimeters	127.0	132.9	140.4
9½ years				*9½ years*			
Weight in pounds	58.7	69.0	85.5	Weight in pounds	54.9	67.1	84.4
Weight in kilograms	26.63	31.3	38.78	Weight in kilograms	24.9	30.44	38.28
Height in inches	51.4	54.3	57.1	Height in inches	50.9	53.5	56.4
Height in centimeters	130.6	137.9	145.1	Height in centimeters	129.4	135.8	143.2

*Modified from measurements guide by Howard V. Meredith, Iowa Child Welfare Research Station, The State University of Iowa; from Vaughan, V. C., III: Growth and development. In Vaughan, V. C., III, and McKay, R. J., editors: Nelson's textbook of pediatrics, ed. 10, Philadelphia, 1975, W. B. Saunders Co., p. 42.

Table 7-1. Height and weight tables for children in middle childhood—cont'd

	Percentiles (boys)				Percentiles (girls)		
	10	**50**	**90**		**10**	**50**	**90**
10 years				*10 years*			
Weight in pounds	61.1	71.9	89.9	Weight in pounds	57.1	70.3	89.7
Weight in kilograms	27.71	32.61	40.78	Weight in kilograms	25.9	31.89	40.69
Height in inches	52.3	55.2	58.1	Height in inches	51.8	54.6	57.5
Height in centimeters	132.8	140.3	147.5	Height in centimeters	131.7	138.6	146.0
10½ years				*10½ years*			
Weight in pounds	63.7	74.8	94.6	Weight in pounds	59.9	74.6	95.1
Weight in kilograms	28.89	33.93	42.91	Weight in kilograms	27.17	33.79	43.14
Height in inches	53.2	56.0	58.9	Height in inches	52.9	55.8	58.9
Height in centimeters	135.1	142.3	149.7	Height in centimeters	134.4	141.7	149.7
11 years				*11 years*			
Weight in pounds	66.3	77.6	99.3	Weight in pounds	62.6	78.8	100.4
Weight in kilograms	30.07	35.2	45.04	Weight in kilograms	28.4	35.74	45.54
Height in inches	54.0	56.8	59.8	Height in inches	53.9	57.0	60.4
Height in centimeters	137.3	144.2	151.8	Height in centimeters	137.0	144.7	153.4
11½ years				*11½ years*			
Weight in pounds	69.2	81.0	104.5	Weight in pounds	66.1	83.2	106.0
Weight in kilograms	31.39	36.74	47.4	Weight in kilograms	29.98	37.74	48.08
Height in inches	55.0	57.8	60.9	Height in inches	55.0	58.3	61.8
Height in centimeters	139.8	146.9	154.8	Height in centimeters	139.8	148.1	157.0
12 years				*12 years*			
Weight in pounds	72.0	84.4	109.6	Weight in pounds	69.5	87.6	111.5
Weight in kilograms	32.66	38.28	49.71	Weight in kilograms	31.52	39.74	50.58
Height in inches	56.1	58.9	62.2	Height in inches	56.1	59.8	63.2
Height in centimeters	142.4	149.6	157.9	Height in centimeters	142.6	151.9	160.6

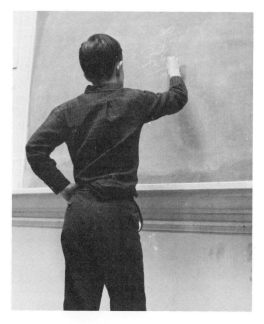

Fig. 7-1. The child in elementary school. By the time the child reaches elementary school age, or middle childhood, his body has begun to take on the long, lean appearance that is proportionately much like that of the adult.

Neuromuscular changes

Accompanying the skeletal development are those changes that occur in the muscles of the body. There are sex differences in the proportion and distribution of fat and muscle tissue in boys and girls, but for each sex there is a much greater percentage increase in muscle tissue during this time than in former years. It has been reliably reported by a number of investigators that during the elementary school period both boys and girls double their strength and physical capacities, although girls consistently do less well than boys in activities requiring physical strength.

In matters of coordination the differences are less pronounced. Girls frequently excel in tasks that require hand-eye coordination and attention to details. Conversely, boys show a greater degree of organization and coordination in tasks requiring interaction of a number of muscles and gross movement.

Play activities during this period reflect the child's growing awareness of and use of muscles and motor skills. During the childhood years both boys and girls learn to ride bicycles, skate, play ball, write, and draw with increasing skill.

Dentition

Not only is the period of these school years important in the social realm, but it also represents the "breakthrough" of permanent teeth. It is a time, too, when children are likely to lose some of their visible teeth. From the age of 6 to 12 years the process is one of replacing the deciduous teeth with the permanent ones. Quite often parents develop undue concern about the positioning of newly erupting teeth. In most instances, however, the proper aligning takes place naturally and easily. In the sixth year the first molars appear, followed shortly thereafter by the upper front or central incisors. Others erupt during successive years with appearance of the last, the third molars (or wisdom teeth), occurring by late adolescence.

Physique and personality

It does not require much personal experience in dealing with other persons to realize that there is a strong relationship between physique and personality. This is most obvious in cases in which the individual suffers from some deficit or handicap such as deafness, blindness, speech defect, chronic medical disorder, crippling disorder, or abnormal glandular condition. Such conditions limit the individual's social contacts and prevent his playing a normal social role in his age group.

More subtle but more encompassing in their scope are the general effects of physical development and physique on personality as seen in normal children.

Psychiatrists, psychologists, and others have long been interested in the possible relationship between personality and body type. Extensive study of thousands of subjects has brought forth a number of different classifications, the most popular of which has been the one labeling persons with short, fat builds as *endomorphs;* long, thin persons as *ectomorphs;* and muscular, athletic persons as *mesomorphs.* Since very few people fit exactly into any one of these categories, additions to this classification system have been made. These have included breaking the body down into three separate areas and providing a rating scale based on the degree to which any one of the characteristics is present. This information has been correlated with personality characteristics of individuals in the hope of finding some definitive relationship between characteristics of personality and body type.

Some general relationships have been established, but the results are still inconclusive, partly because of the tremendous effect of culture upon physique. Our culture, for example, is one in which many of us are slightly overweight. This is less prominent in children than in adults but is still important enough to affect the body conformation of many children. Similarly in some more deprived cultures everyone is "skinny" because adequate supplies of foodstuffs are not available.

Although evidence concerning body types and personality may be still inconclusive, many other factors relating to physique are now definite and well established. These are a result of the general response of persons within our culture to certain physical characteristics and of the physical limitations placed on a child by his height, weight, and build. The short, fat boy with poor motor coordination will rarely be rewarded by his playmates for being the "best" in sports. As a result of negative reinforcement in the sports area, he may turn to other activities and interests. A well-coordinated boy or girl, on the other hand, will be in demand for athletic activities and as a result receive much reinforcement for efforts in this direction. He or she will frequently be first chosen among the children for "choose-up" games and will naturally move into leadership roles as a result. Many a child will play some special or specific role for his group in order to receive its attention and approval. The fat boy may become the "jolly, fat boy" because this is what others seem to expect of him and it is the simplest way for him to remain a part of the group and receive its benefits.

In one study on delinquency Glueck and Glueck (1950) included 1,000 boys, 500 delinquent and 500 not delinquent, and found that the delinquent group contained three times as many boys who were mesomorphic or athletic in build than the nondelinquent group. Conversely the tall, thin ectomorphic type was found 10 times as often in the nondelinquent group. Other researchers have generally supported this finding. Interpreting these results is somewhat difficult. One likely hypothesis is that the athletically built young person is more likely to take part in social situations than other individuals, and thus he has a greater potential for coming into conflict with some of the rules and regulations of society. The tall, thin, ectomorphic individual is much more often found to be withdrawn, introverted, or thoughtful. Many of his activities center on the home or in areas that are not group centered. As a result his chances of coming into conflict with society are considerably lower.

Although these relationships seem indicative of definite trends, a question is frequently raised as to the possibility that children who appear to be of one build between 6 and 12 years of age may change their body type during adolescence or at maturity. To put it in more popular terminology, "Can the 97-pound weakling become the well-muscled, athletic adult?" Although there is some slight shifting caused by the action of hormones, in general the type of build that

an individual will have in later life is reasonably well established in childhood. A loss of baby fat and a broadening of shoulders can be expected in boys, but the developmental lines are present early and remain fairly consistent. Training and exercise can do much to capitalize on inherent characteristics but gross changes are only rarely encountered. Nutrition specialists say that overeating in childhood with resulting overweight causes structural changes that make it much harder for the adult to keep his weight within normal limits.

PSYCHOSOCIAL DEVELOPMENT
Sex role and sex typing

By the time the child reaches school, forces have been at work for many years, shaping his personality characteristics along well-defined lines. These will not always follow the usually expected patterns, but there are "normal" guidelines or stereotypes set forth in our culture. For example, boys are expected to be athletic, outgoing, strong, assertive, and aggressive. Girls are expected to be neat, meticulous, and social; they too are to be athletic—but only to a limited degree and in special areas of interest. Not only do parents shape the behavior of children in these particular directions but movies, television, books, and schoolteachers also work further toward the adoption of these general behavior patterns. The patterns are sufficiently well defined so that even in the first grade those boys who do not conform to the expected roles are termed sissies and girls who fail to conform to their norm are labeled tomboys. By the age of 10 or 12 years, behaviors are so well defined that most children can clearly label both feminine and masculine stereotypes with little hesitation.

Children's ability to label and distinguish appropriate behaviors for boys and girls results in their reinforcing individuals who conform to expected patterns and punishing or rejecting individuals who fail to do so. For the child who is initially unable to conform the result is that he must face an increasingly difficult job if he is to meet the demands of his social group adequately. Quite frequently this results in the individual's renouncing his social group and becoming an isolate. This is true for both boys and

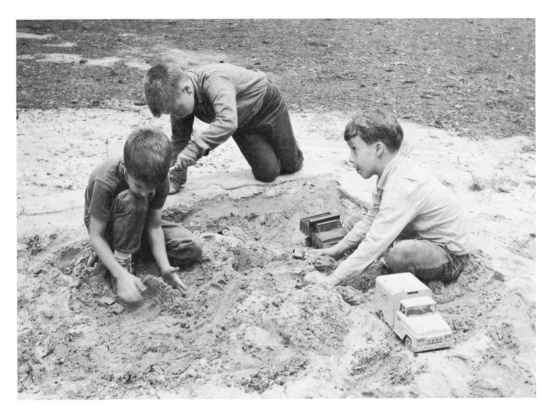

Fig. 7-2. Play. Imaginative play is still popular, although games tend to be somewhat different for boys and girls. Sex typing of behavior becomes prominent.

girls who have difficulties in living up to group expectancies. One of the difficulties these days is that mores are changing so rapidly that adults as well as children are having difficulty in keeping up with them.

Class factors

Expected roles differ somewhat depending upon the social class background of the child. This is in part due to differences in child-rearing practices and to the different standards for later behavior when the child has become an adult. In studies contrasting lower class families and those from middle class settings, there has been some definitive indication that children in the lower class environment are able to identify specific role behavior much earlier than is the case in middle class families. Boys in the lower class families tend to choose exclusively masculine interests at a point where, in middle class families, these are less well defined.

Several factors are important in this differen-

tiation, which is noticed all through life. Middle class men as compared with men of lower class groups show many more interests that are usually considered feminine or neutral at the time they enter college. Things frequently identified as being feminine are interests in art, music, and literature. Often it is not that persons having such interests fail to possess others as well. In many cases these are simply the reflection of a broad, inclusive range of interests rather than a lack of identification with an appropriate role. Frequently they merely reflect the level of interest found in the child's home and family. In middle class homes there is provided a constant exposure to a wide range of special-interest materials. In the lower class family, in contrast, enriching materials such as art, music, and literature are found less frequently. The child grows up in his home atmosphere, identifying closely with the role of the father or mother. When the parent has a limited range of interests the child will reflect a similarly limited pattern.

Thus many aspects of life are affected: value systems, recreational activities, future goals, aspirations, dreams—all will be shaped by social class. As the child matures the social class influence will be provided by others outside the immediate family. Some churches are essentially upper class, whereas others follow more traditional or lower class patterns. These will be influential in asserting further the values of the particular social class to which the individual belongs. Club memberships, too, will be drawn along such lines. Schools attended will be determined by the neighborhood in which one lives; thus the chance of further shaping to a class pattern will be present during the school years. Values only partially imparted during childhood will become more and more fixed as the child passes through the school age. The pressure for the bussing of children out of their neighborhoods to achieve racial and social class integration is motivated largely by the desire to minimize the factors just outlined.

Peer group relationships

Relationships with the peer group are the most important variable in social interaction for the child in the school years. Mussen, Conger, and Kagan (1974) indicate that the chief values to be gained in peer relationships by the child are modifications of his behavior to be acceptable to his peers, opportunities to develop patterns of interaction with age mates, methods of dealing with dominance and hostility, techniques for relating to persons in positions of leadership and authority, the development of personal leadership skills, and opportunities to work through or to share various social problems. Important among the values is the therapeutic opportunity to share common problems in dealing with adults. All these factors interact with the learning experiences of the child to provide him with a more realistic and workable concept of himself and his own behavior.

No child will adapt perfectly to all the many requirements of him by his peer group. Perhaps the values of the peer group are so different that he will be forced to give up the potential rewards of interacting with others and continue to abide by the rules and regulations set forth by his own family. This may force him to be an outsider or an isolate but lessen the possibility of severe conflict within the home setting. The great majority of children are quite eager to interact meaningfully with others in the group. They show a high degree of motivation to be liked and accepted by classmates. Failing to gain this acceptance, they are frequently motivated to make appropriate changes in behavior in order to change their status. As a rule it is only when their attempts at interaction have been consistently unrewarded that children adopt a completely negative pattern and withdraw entirely from the group. Fortunately most children's behavior is readily shaped. When an understanding of the group rules is established, the individual is usually able to modify his behavior and become a part of the young society.

When children attempt to become a part of a group, they may first resort to behavior patterns learned in the home. If this fails, their next course of action is to imitate the behaviors of those individuals they perceive to be in leadership roles or at least those warranting high degrees of acceptance. Quite frequently this results in the individual's being incorporated into the group. In other instances, if the particular behaviors are leadership behaviors, he may first have to fight the present leader in order to play a more important role. This is quite characteristic of the behavior of young boys. With young girls the interaction is less likely to result in physical violence, yet there is much maneuvering and seeking for an appropriate basis for social interaction.

The gang

Groups in early childhood are only poorly organized. Youngsters may interact and play together for short periods of time without forming lasting attachments. By the time children reach the school years relationships become more formalized and show the characteristics of a gang. At first gangs are only lightly structured with a changing membership—one that cuts across all social classes. By the age of 10 or 11 years boys in gangs may take up special interests such as football, baseball, or other sports activities. This tends to form more solidly the relatively flexible lines of gang membership seen earlier. Thus persons who are unskilled

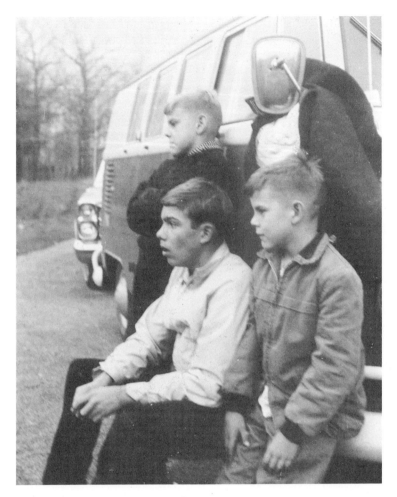

Fig. 7-3. The gang. In this period the gang begins to emerge. Social interaction is important and shared on a close, intimate basis. These boys watching a game share a pessimistic view of the action.

physically may be forced into a minor role within the gang or dropped entirely. Girls' gangs are less formalized throughout the middle childhood years unless they turn into such adult-supported groups as the Brownies, Girl Scouts, or Camp Fire Girls organizations.

It is characteristic of older gangs in the middle childhood years to be either all boys or all girls. The informal grouping at age 6 or 7 years may be highly mixed, but after these first few years shaping is carried on by schools, parents, and other interest groups to separate the activities for boys and girls. This separation continues until the emergence of dating behavior and adolescence.

Social status

In the beginning school years status among children depends less on economic, ethnic, and racial factors than is true at later periods of development. Initially popularity and group status are based on such characteristics as leadership, participation, and positive and friendly attitudes toward others. There is some sex differentiation observed, the boys being rewarded with social acceptance for behaving in "masculine" ways, whereas girls receive highest acceptance when they play "feminine" roles in which friendliness and acquiescence are considered far more important than aggressiveness.

Psychologists interested in studying group

status have long made use of sociometric techniques. One sociometric technique involves asking group members to indicate the persons they would (1) most like or (2) least like to interact with under a specified set of circumstances. In a study by Heckel (1952), subjects were asked to name the three persons they would most like to room with and the three persons they would least like to room with while in college. Similarly sociometric data can be collected on a variety of circumstances: whom the individual would most or least like to play with, go camping with, etc. Such data, when accumulated, can be used to construct a sociogram—a device for indicating the degree of acceptance, rejection, or avoidance shown within a group of subjects. The most typical pattern found for the average child in grade school indicates mild acceptance and few rejections. In any group there are individuals who stand out and are widely chosen or widely rejected because of their behavior. Still another unit, appearing to have little impact on the total social process, is the isolate—the child who is neither chosen nor rejected by other children.

As we have indicated, there is little class or caste pattern clearly discernible in the early school years. However, by the time the individual has reached the age of 10, 11, or 12 years all these factors seem to play a role in acceptance or rejection. Reinforcement for acceptance and rejection may come from several sources. Not infrequently children in grade school will be echoing sentiments of their parents who, because of prejudicial attitudes, may insist they not interact or play with certain children.

Many children will fail to attain acceptance by the peer group because their own values may not coincide with those of many other members. For example, the child who has been reared in another section of the country or under extreme deprivation may fail to understand or be unable to cope with the value systems of children whose backgrounds are much different from his own. Also as children grow older the child who is different in the sense of being physically unattractive, poorly dressed, or lacking in social graces will be rejected because these values are important to older children.

Status in the middle childhood years undergoes striking change. It moves from a classless and colorless attitude based almost entirely on acceptance and nonaggressive attitudes to a highly structured system involving social and behavioral bases for acceptance. In the later years the values of the child's family will be more fully understood and be more solidly the basis for many of his acceptances or rejections. If he rejects the values of his own family, he may well turn to his peer group for establishing a new set of values in the hope of gaining increased social status.

It should be quite obvious by now that when we speak of social status and acceptance we are speaking, at least in part, of friendship. Children tend to choose their friends to fill a wide variety of social interaction roles. During the early school years there is a tendency on the part of children to choose for their friends persons from their own sex. Although this segregation is not complete during the first school years, many forces act to keep the two sexes apart. Girls are encouraged to engage in activities that are quite different from the competitive, aggressive activities encouraged in young boys.

Children themselves tend to support parental attitudes by making fun of the boy or girl who shows undue interest in members of the opposite sex. It is only toward the end of the middle school years that interactions and friendships between the sexes are encouraged. Most often these occur under very specific and well-governed situations. Children in the fifth and sixth grades may, for example, take ballroom dancing where they are required to interact in a formal social situation with members of the opposite sex. In other situations such as birthday parties, church groups, and school functions, there is a gradual breakdown of sex segregation as the children approach adolescence. Even though boys or girls might wish to choose a member of the opposite sex as a friend during the childhood years, they probably would be discouraged in this by parents, teachers, and other children. In spite of these many prohibitions, conversations with young boys and girls reveal that they are quite conscious of and attracted to members of the opposite sex. Initial attempts at interaction often fail because boys attempt to respond to young girls much as they would to male playmates, and girls expect from boys treatment similar to that accorded them by other girls. As a result both groups often observe most comfortably from a distance until socialization is sufficiently complete that a common basis for interaction is established, like that which develops from the more or less formal social settings already mentioned.

Family relationships

A great burden is placed upon the stability of the family relationship when the child first ventures away from home to enter school. It is then that all the instabilities, the insecurities, the defects in training and education are brought into sharp focus. The child who has grown up with insecurity and uncertainty may have been able to derive sufficient support from constantly being with the mother prior to entering school. After this entry, however, he can no longer be reassured by seeing his mother. Instead, he is at the mercy of his concern and anxiety. It is this type of child who may develop school phobia and refuse to attend school. Similarly the child who has been overprotected and prevented from engaging in the necessary process of socialization may be unable to meet the demands on a level of maturity sufficient to let him function well in a school setting. The child who has been idolized by parents to the extent that he expects the world to revolve about him also encounters difficulties upon school entrance. These represent only a few of the typical problems that children present to the first-grade teacher. Each has its own particular dynamics, and each may be dealt with in the school setting with some degree of success. Most children do encounter some adjustive difficulties initially. These tend to dissipate once the ground rules and regulations for school life have been established.

The problems facing the child who meets initial adjustive difficulties do not end there. Because of the establishment of a certain set, he may continue to respond in ways that will make him unacceptable or unpopular with other children. Unless both the child and the parent are able to alter their attitude and behavior, the adjustive difficulties may continue throughout school.

Most serious of the adjustive difficulties that face the child are those that stem directly from problems within the family. The incidence of adjustive difficulties in school among children from homes where parents have been divorced or separated, where there is marital discord, or where neglect or rejection of the children is present is much higher than that observed for any other causal factors. Poverty, for example, is far less important in producing negative behaviors in school than are the factors relating to parental adjustment. When adjustive difficulties exist for the parent, an inevitable result seems to be some neglect or rejection of the child. Acceptance and warmth on the part of the parent may be able to overcome many of the "negative" environmental factors that may surround the child. Children can tolerate inadequate clothing more readily than neglect and hunger more readily than rejection. Young children are nearly as versatile as adults in dealing with problems relating to rejection, neglect, and lack of love. They may show aggression, withdrawal, or even psychosomatic symptoms. It is not unusual to see psychosomatic elements in the form of rheumatoid arthritis, a variety of skin disorders, ulcerative colitis, asthma, and even tachycardia listed among the symptoms of disturbed children. In attempting to track down the psychological basis for the behaviors exhibited, psychologists and psychiatrists have found that in nearly every instance there have been instabilities, insecurity, and inconsistency in the parents' behavior toward the child. Although predisposing factors related to the specific psychosomatic illness were present, emotional events were often the principal precipitating factors in specific attacks of the illnesses.

Family control

The degree of control exercised by any family has many dimensions. Part of family control is and has been related to the social class background of the parents. We are able to find great differences between upper class, middle class, and lower class families with regard to both the exercise of and the type of controls utilized. With considerable differences in systems for controlling behavior it is likely that symptoms will be found to vary from one social class to another when studies are made of symptomatic behavior in children.

Lower class homes characteristically have a dominant, authoritarian structure in which parents use punishment or the threat of punishment to control much of the child's behavior. They permit him little latitude in his activities and grant him little freedom of choice. Children who grow up in this atmosphere—and who do not openly rebel against it—generally are characterized by being shy, somewhat withdrawn, self-conscious, and acquiescent in the presence of adults. As would be anticipated, their greatest problems in adjusting to other persons come from difficulty in self-direction due to feeling insecure and inferior to other children who have had greater degrees of freedom in their experience.

A feature more commonly seen in middle class training is the overly permissive parent who grants the child a much greater latitude in expressing himself, making his own decisions, and having fewer of his requests or demands frustrated. Quite commonly children in this category are in great need of structure. This is reflected in behavior of the acting-out variety in which children show antagonism, rebellion, or irresponsibility and frequently are disobedient to authority figures. Whereas in social groups they show outgoing, ascendant behavior, they often present adjustive difficulties because limits have not been established on their social behavior.

This is not to imply that differences are strictly drawn along class lines. A high percentage of lower class families are permissive and a high number of persons in middle class families are of the authoritarian type. On the average the middle class family is more permissive and the lower class family is more authoritarian. These general behavior patterns are accompanied by other behaviors relating to the display of affection, child care, and attitudes toward children—in which mothers of middle class background are much more able to display affection and mete out far less punishment than the mothers from lower class background. These factors have been described quite effectively in a book by Sears, Maccoby, and Levin (1957). With these apparent social class differences in regard to the proper method of child care, it is easy to understand why communication difficulties may exist between children of differing class backgrounds. Through similar experiences a basis for interaction and communication is laid. When divergence exists in child-rearing practices, it can be anticipated that these will show up even more dramatically in the communication problems that children face when they are placed in a new situation. These different child-rearing practices also color a great many other factors in life. Children growing up in an authoritarian home may have a much lower regard and affection for parents than those found in children who grow up under more permissive circumstances. Attitudes of acceptance and respect toward parents may be far greater among middle class families than in lower class families, where a higher degree of ambivalence and rejection may be directed toward parental figures. This is partly because of treatment of the child and partly because parents from lower class families rarely represent the cultural ideal of an appropriate role model for the child. It is difficult for a child coming from a lower class family to speak proudly or boast about a father who engages in any occupation that is the basis for low status, ridicule, or humor. Middle class occupations rarely, if ever, evoke similar responses.

Siblings

Before moving away from discussion of the family constellation, it should be noted that a considerable influence upon the child's behavior will be exerted by the presence or absence of brothers or sisters. Many research studies have been conducted on the effects of having older brothers or sisters as well as on the type of discipline and its impact in only-child and in multiple-membered families. Not only must the child who has siblings learn to deal effectively with parents but he must also learn to deal with special problems that arise as a result of having brothers or sisters. This type of problem affects a considerable number of persons in the United States. Well over 80% of families have more than one child. Thus the child at some time has to determine his new role in the family, the degree and type of responsibility he will be permitted to express, and how he will deal with the addition of other children who are younger than himself.

Some of the factors that have been researched indicate that the oldest child in the family is often characterized by the ability to take responsibility, to demonstrate a more serious, conscientious approach, and to show less aggression than younger siblings. It has also been determined that the youngest child in the family frequently enjoys the most permissive atmosphere, being able to express aggression more openly and with less personal threat than any other child.

Adjustment outside the family has generally been viewed as being less difficult for the child with siblings than for one who grows up as an only child. Of necessity the former will have worked through a number of problems in dealing with the feelings and the behavior of other persons before he enters school. His process of socialization will generally be more complete than that of a child without siblings. Although these represent only a few salient points concerning the presence or absence of siblings in the life of the child, they do indicate that these are of some importance in understanding the total dynamics of any child the nurse will encounter in the hospital or in the home.

EMOTIONAL DEVELOPMENT

Of the many problems that face the child during the school years, most dominant are those relating to fear and anxiety. Up to the onset of school life the child has been fairly well cared for and protected in his limited social environment by the activities of mother, father, grandparents, and older brothers and sisters. Now he is expected to turn outward away from the family, and meet the challenge of the external world. Most prominently this is found in the school settings. The child does this, realizing full well that he has very limited equipment for dealing with his environment and the people in it. His acceptance and his survival may depend on his ability to adapt to a whole series of new circumstances and situations, which he may only partially understand and which may attract but at the same time repel him. He must learn to please three groups, which may sometimes be at odds with one another—his teachers, his parents, and his friends. Somehow during this period he must work out a system that balances the many forces acting on him in such a way as to meet his own needs as well as please and satisfy other persons. How well and how effectively he is able to do this will depend in part on his early training and experience. If he has been raised to be sensitive and aware of the feelings and needs of others, he may do a much more effective job in working out a satisfactory balance. If he has been raised in a home that did not make him so aware and sensitive, he may encounter the constant frustration of failing in social situations.

In any case these continuous encounters with new situations often arouse a great deal of anxiety and fear in him. The source of the anxiety may have many forms. If he has developed a strong conscience, he may be made to feel guilty because of demands placed on him by his peer group. Frequently the members engage in activities that are neither approved nor condoned by parents or teachers, such as sexual exploration, masturbation, aggression, and other less accepted behavioral patterns. He must decide whether to stay a part of the group and engage in these behaviors or to withdraw to a peripheral position and remain in the good graces of his family.

For most children the situation is never completely resolved. They engage in furtive and tentative exploratory behaviors that do arouse in them feelings of guilt—but not of sufficient strength to deter their behavior completely. It is only for the child who grows up in an atmosphere of permissive control that these problems will be minimized. It is necessary that limits and parameters be established for each child within which he can operate comfortably. These should not be so severe as to strangle emotional development.

With regard to fears the world of the young child is literally jammed to capacity with situations that are capable of producing intense fear responses. Because of his size and personal inadequacy, animals, older persons, natural forces, or separation from parents may all produce highly realistic and specific fears. Quite often a lack of experience on the part of the child may expand these circumstances far out of proportion. He may through imagination develop an entirely unrealistic picture about the need for care and caution or learn to be afraid of certain of life's hazards. As the child becomes more mature through the middle childhood years, he develops more ways of coping with fears and anxiety. Education itself is an important factor in lessening many of the fears that are of an unrealistic nature. Common among the unrealistic fears are fears of ghosts, mythical creatures, distant events, animals, etc. Mussen et al. (1974) point out that in many instances these unrealistic fears persist not because the child really believes in danger from these sources but because they are substitutes for fear responses that might more appropriately have been directed at the parents. A child may be fearful of lions and the harm they might do him to a quite unrealistic degree when in reality the fear is one displaced from the father, who is threatening to him, and onto a safer object—the lion.

Other fears and anxieties are developed by the role that the child is forced to play or because of the personal characteristics that he may bring into the schoolage environment. If he is a member of a minority religious or racial group, he may have already encountered situations that are the basis for both fear and anxiety. If he has not to this point had such experiences, often parents will warn him to be on the lookout or be aware of the possibility of rejection or hostility directed toward him because of these factors. A number of observers have noted that, whereas children of kindergarten or first grade age may have already developed verbal prejudices, which are expressed openly, they often do not have accompanying behavior to reinforce the statement. Thus it has been noted in some schools where problems of integration have occurred that some white children who expressed negative attitudes toward blacks would still in their schoolground activities engage freely and easily in play with them. An appropriate linking of the words and their own behaviors had not been developed. This, of course, suggests that prejudicial attitudes largely reflect parental attitudes, and it is only after a considerable period of indoctrination that prejudicial attitudes and

behavior become linked together. It has been noted that modification of prejudicial attitudes is much more readily achieved in the younger children through educational procedures and controlled social interaction. Such modification has been shown in some southern cities where white students in formerly segregated classes have elected black students to class offices. This is an emergent problem from the early school years. It will not see its most exaggerated form until the adolescent and college years.

Adjustment to school

We have indicated that the transition from the safety and protection of the home to the school environment is one of the most difficult transitional periods in the life of the child. Demands placed on children in the first grade are often unique in the child's experience. Even those who have had nursery school or kindergarten background are rarely prepared for the organization, regimentation, and demands for achievement that will be set for them in the first grade. The majority of children, especially those who have older brothers and sisters, look forward to the opportunity to learn the skills of reading, writing, and arithmetic. Even play activities among preschool children often center on the school. This doubtless serves a useful purpose in introducing the child to some of the demands that will be placed upon him. If the acquiring of knowledge in the school setting were a short-term and easy process, problems for both the child and teacher would be greatly lessened. Many children, after entering school, are quite disappointed that they cannot learn to read and write in a matter of days or hours. Repetition, drill, and practice—so necessary in the acquisition of basic skills—represent demands for discipline and attention that require the harnessing of energies that prior to the children's school entry were allowed to range free or were only lightly controlled.

Educators have long been concerned about educational policy that says that at 6 years of age each child is automatically ready to begin school. The experience of educators, physicians, psychiatrists, psychologists, and nurses has made them keenly aware that there are great differences among 6-year-olds in both intellectual and emotional development. Many children are emotionally mature enough to face school at age 5, whereas others may not be able to make the transition until they are 7 or 8 years of age. The emotional strains placed on the child in separating for a large part of any day from parents can be especially traumatic for the shy, insecure child who feels uncomfortable even when parents are by his side. Whereas most children at 6 years of age will be able to make the emotional transition with only a little foot dragging or reluctance, an added year's maturity for the less secure child may make the difference between ultimate school success and failure.

Part of the child's readiness for entering school is in reality the mother's readiness to accept this new stage of development in her child. Quite frequently a mother reacts to having all her children in school as a sign that they are now nearly grown and that she is approaching middle age. Not infrequently mothers will unconsciously cling to the youngest child and attempt to delay his maturing. Many cases have been reported in which mothers verbally tell their children to go to school but also cling to them emotionally and make it difficult or impossible for them to attend.

For satisfactory schoolwork in the middle childhood years the child should be as nearly free from emotional stress as possible. The learning that is to take place during these formative years will be the most important learning that has taken place since his acquisition of speech. Bad attitudes toward school, poor learning habits, and a faulty acquisition of the fundamentals of reading, writing, and problem solving, if these are inadequately learned or are distorted by emotional problems, may forever undermine the child's ability to handle academic situations and learning tasks satisfactorily. A large part of learning will require his use of interpersonal skills in communicating with the teacher and with other students. He must not only be able to express himself in raising questions or supplying answers but he must also be sensitive to the questions, answers, and interactions that other persons have. Each of these will contribute to his total knowledge of subject matter, of himself, and of other per-

sons. He must be able to conceptualize, organize, and express a whole new world of intellectual skills and concepts.

Transition from home to school is not always a difficult process. Educators have long realized the possible complications of the situation and as a result have tried to provide first grade teachers with training and skills that allow them to cope more adequately with potential problems of the young child. During preschool years the primary figure in the life of the child is the mother, and first grade teachers are almost invariably women. Educators are careful to select teachers who have sensitivity, warmth, and ability to deal with the many problems of children. It is not simply a matter of the teacher's guiding their development of skills in learning to read, to write, to draw, and to engage in problem-solving behavior. Many of her activities will center around recognizing the personal needs of the child and seeing that social behaviors are developed or modified and are shaped to agree with the general needs of the class and of the child in interaction with the class members. The teacher in effect is a mother substitute, performing for a portion of the day many of the activities formerly carried on by mothers. The nurse or parent who visits a school lunchroom will be interested by the actions of the "school mother," first checking that children have clean hands, then observing their manners during the meal, and seeing that they "eat their vegetables," clean their plate, drink their milk, and return the plate or tray to the kitchen. These are not isolated activities. Similar behaviors on the part of the teacher take place in the classroom. She must see that children do not become so nervous, excited, or upset that they lose bowel or bladder control—not an infrequent happening in the school setting. In some cases children are too shy to raise their hands to be excused to use the bathroom. The teacher must therefore be attentive to the nervous squirmings or twitchings that may warn of impending disaster.

Like the parent the teacher also sets limits and imposes rules on the behavior of the child. Mussen et al. indicate that in general teachers' values are of the middle class variety and that they reward such behaviors as cooperation, friendliness, neatness, and obedience while punishing disobedience, lying, cheating, and stealing. Aggressiveness except under controlled conditions is also frowned upon. There is some variation in permissiveness as applied to boys and girls, although this is held almost exclusively to the playground setting.

Considering the value systems that the teachers attempt to provide for the children and the values they themselves hold, it is easy to understand why children from different cultures, lower class backgrounds, or groups whose social values are at variance with those of the teacher are quite frequently rejected or unrewarded in their contacts with school.

Not all teacher-child relationships follow ideal patterns. Some children may lack the social attributes needed for satisfactorily relating to teachers. Others may possess intellectual deficits or unusually high abilities that upset normal classroom routine. Also, teachers may possess personality attributes and prejudices that prevent them from understanding or handling behavior that differs from the norm they have been led to expect.

Most often both teacher and child will react to each other on the basis of past experiences with other adults and other children. The child who has come from a warm, responsive home will in most instances generalize such feelings toward his teacher. The stage is thus set for a positive school relationship. Conversely, children coming from homes in which they are rejected, mistreated, or unloved will anticipate similar treatment from teachers and other persons outside the home. Quite frequently their behavior will reflect negative attitudes toward social interactions with adults. If, however, the teacher is perceptive and recognizes the basis for the child's behavior, she may be able to provide him with a new learning situation in which at least one adult responds to him without rejection or hostility. This leads in turn to a change in the child's set to respond, and new learning has taken place.

Children prefer school situations with structure and limits. This does not mean that they prefer a teacher who is only a disciplinarian. They seem to prefer teachers with characteristics they would desire in a warm, loving parent.

Jersild studied the characteristics of teachers who were liked or disliked most in school settings and found that children wanted teachers who were kind, cheerful, fair, impartial, attractive, helpful, democratic, and enthusiastic, to mention a few of the most desired characteristics (Jersild, Telford, and Saurey, 1975).

These characteristics follow through all years of education. Most of us have had experiences with instructors who were domineering or hostile in their responses to students. Almost invariably they have been less effective than teachers who were supportive and encouraging of student efforts. The result of these bipolar teacher attitudes is seen in teacher-centered as opposed to group-centered activity. In teacher-centered activity the teacher makes all the decisions about the necessary ingredients of the teaching situation; in the group-centered approach a different kind of consideration is given to the individual needs, feelings, and expectations of the children. This is not to imply that the children determine what they will learn and at what point, but their needs and views are considered in forming the approach to the material to be covered.

From numerous studies on the type of leadership provided by a teacher there has been an indication that it is possible for students to be highly productive under a strict and authoritarian teacher. Yet pupils working under such a system express far less personal satisfaction with what they have done and about the school setting. In school settings where there is a more democratic atmosphere, production and learning can be high also, and pupil satisfaction is much higher than in authoritarian settings.

What does this mean for the child in school? Quite simply it has been demonstrated on many occasions that the individual working in a situation in which he feels personally satisfied and accepted shows more consistent performance and higher levels of motivation than are possible in any other structure. As a result children who are able to work in a motivating environment achieve consistently more effective learning and better social adjustment than would be possible in any other situation. Of course, the child who enters school from a home in which a high level of self-esteem has been fostered by loving but firm parents has a great advantage regardless of the situation he encounters in school.

LEARNING PATTERNS IN THE MIDDLE CHILDHOOD YEARS

In this section we will present some of the characteristics of the schoolage child: his patterns of thinking, how he learns, how he communicates, and what he has achieved to this point in his development. In addition, the relationship between educational achievement and physical condition of the child is discussed.

Thinking and learning

One of the most striking advances in the development of the child that emerges during the middle childhood years is his growing ability to engage in logical thinking. During his earlier life, particularly from 2 to 7 years of age, his thinking is frequently prelogical or precausal. In prelogical or precausal thinking the child's explanations of events may attribute them to something in a sort of pure fantasy, things as the child would like them to be, or quasi-explanations, which in reality are not explanations. For example, one child in describing why we have months of the year said that we "have March so that children can fly kites." In answer to the question, "Why do we have night?" the child replied, "So that we can sleep." Prelogical or precausal answers reflect a lack of social experience and a lack of ability to develop cause-and-effect relationships.

During the years from 7 to 11 in normal children, there is an emergence of logical patterns of thought. At about this time the child becomes able to establish cause-and-effect relationships between events. He also learns to seek and find alternative explanations for events around him if his first attempts at explanation proves inadequate for solving his problem. No longer will he commit such basic errors as attributing of life to inanimate objects: "Is a boat alive?" "Yes, a boat is alive because it moves." This explanation by a young child is representative of the type of error called animism, which is rarely made by children after age 7 or 8.

There are many other aspects to thinking that are taken up in detail in other works, particularly the studies reported by Jean Piaget. He has been foremost among researchers on the thinking processes in children. An excellent summary of his work is provided by Flavell (1963). Other researchers have followed the lead provided by Piaget and have found great differences in the rate of attainment of concepts and thinking in children based on what appear to be purely cultural grounds. Individuals who have limited interaction with others—limited social experience—almost invariably retain prelogical and precausal thinking far beyond the point found in individuals who live in enriched environments. In some instances lack of enrichment is the result of an emotional characteristic in which the child is disturbed or withdrawn in his interactions with others.

Learning has many characteristics in common with thinking. Initially in childhood the learning process is one of association, positive teaching or direction, imitation, and trial and error. The child acquires knowledge of individual objects and events but is unable to respond to all classes of objects. By the middle childhood years, however, the ability to discriminate between classes of objects is well established. Learning during this period follows the classic pattern, taking place when a response made by the child leads to reduction in an operating need or drive. In humans motivation is far more complex than in animals. As a result we work for a great many goals and are highly motivated to achieve varying types or degrees of these. With many motives operating the opportunities for reinforcing different behaviors are quite great. Thus the child is being constantly reinforced during every waking moment.

Communication

Thinking and learning are of little use to the child unless he is able to communicate his experiences to others effectively. At age 6 he is quite able to communicate. His vocabulary is large, usually in excess of 2,500 words. Although at this initial stage he is unable to communicate many complex ideas or use many of the words that adults use readily, by the time he is 12 or 13 years old his vocabulary will be three times as large as it was at 6 years.

Much of the communication, particularly with other children, is in the form of imaginative play or in trying on new social roles. It has been estimated that on any given day children of school age will engage in 3 to 5 hours of active play. During this developmental phase much of their play requires verbal interaction. Wide varieties of concepts, words, and expressions are used. There is an emergence of slang expressions, nicknames, and in some instances "made-up" words or vocabulary.

In addition to peer interaction, television plays a large part in the language development of today's child. Many "children's programs" are developed with adult concepts and vocabulary, making them pleasant to persons of all ages. The child is thus exposed to a greater range of learning than might ordinarily be achieved simply through playing with other young children or talking to parents, who may continue to speak to him as if he were still a small child.

The child in his early school years is equipped with a sizable vocabulary, the beginnings of logical thinking, and other characteristics that are of importance: his muscular coordination is sufficient to permit him to draw recognizable animals and human figures; he is able by age 7 to draw a diamond; he is able to repeat five digits with ease before he is 8 years old; his ability to follow complex directions is highly developed; and he can perform simple arithmetic operations. By the time he reaches preadolescence he will be able to use and define a great many words; he will have acquired a great deal of specific knowledge about places, persons, and events; and his motor coordination will be equal to that of some slower adults.

Physical status and school

The achievement of many educational goals will be reached only if the child has progressed satisfactorily in his physical development. There are many variations in rates of development, and there are many health conditions that can impede the normal development of the child during the middle childhood years. Eliminating the very obvious conditions such as mental deficiency we find that children with other forms of handicap also suffer in relation to normal children in the development of satisfactory educational progress. Problems such as hearing loss, blindness, motor impairment, or emotional disturbance as well as some glandular conditions and chronic medical disorders all operate to limit the child's stamina, motivation, and ability to benefit from normal class procedures. As a result most studies of children with handicaps have demonstrated that they do not do well in school when compared with more normal children. In some instances certain types of defects are related to cultural deprivation. Children who are handicapped by conditions such as bad tonsils, defective teeth, or visual defects that are correctable may be showing effects of an environment that cannot compensate for or correct minor but handicapping defects. Dietary deficiencies may be reflected only in the child's appearing slightly underweight and yet may operate to keep the child at a low energy level and thus unable to function competitively in a school situation with other children from better environments. Today many schools have programs of providing both medical care and dietary supplements for individuals who cannot afford minimal personal care. Such programs can aid but never completely overcome the handicaps that may stem from this particular type of situation.

SUMMARY

Middle childhood is a period of steady but slower growth in height and weight. Permanent teeth begin to erupt at 6 years and, except for the second and third year molars, are complete by 12 years. In the last part of this period some girls may show secondary sex characteristics. Menstruation may have begun. There is a great deal of individual variation in this.

When the child enters school at 6 years, his world expands and enlarges. His ability to cope with it depends somewhat on his readiness to begin school, whether he has accomplished previous developmental tasks. According to Erickson, infancy is a period when trust is learned; in the toddler and preschool years the child continues through stages of autonomy and then initiative and is now ready at the beginning of middle childhood to enter the stage of industry.

In this period, he needs to feel accomplishment from intellectual learnings in school and from extracurricular activities out of school. To be able to read and write opens a new world to the child. Skill in games or activities as skating, bicycle riding, jumping rope, and/or playing tennis should each bring a sense of achievement. If these skills are not learned in this period, an adolescent may feel self-conscious in learning them later. As some activities are popular throughout life, lack of skill in a given recreational activity may limit recreational enjoyment in adulthood. Academic and recreational skills aid a child in developing a wholesome self-concept.

Social behavior, which had its beginning in responsiveness to people, then in learning to share and take turns in the preschool period, is further modified in middle childhood by contact with peers, teachers, and other authority figures outside the immediate family. The child gains experience in group participation from belonging to a given class in school, having a camping experience, and in participation with his peers or particular "gang" in recreational activities. In many ways members of a peer group tend to discipline one another. Group approval is desired; therefore the behavior of an individual member may be modified.

Social concepts and values change as the child participates in community affairs such as delivering papers, paper drives, going to church, and belonging to such organizations as the Y.M.C.A. and scouts. In addition, vacation trips broaden the growing child's horizon. Discussions of local and national elections as well as hearing newscasts on television all help to make him more aware of the world in which he lives. Concepts of playing fair and loyalties are derived in good measure from participation in school activities and in any activity with his peer group, both in school and after school.

A conscience is further developed in this period. This is particularly influenced by the adult supervision he receives. Positive reinforcement is essential. When a child does misbehave, the parent should explain to the child why his action is wrong so the child can better evaluate his own behavior in the future. A child who has a poorly developed superego is more likely to exhibit irresponsible social behavior and may later become delinquent.

The attitudes of authority figures such as teachers, parents, and others influence the child's self-esteem and behavior. Whether adults around him are permissive, authoritarian, or democratic has an effect on how he handles hostility and aggression, whether he feels rebellious or cooperative. Parents can promote his initiative and self-direction or repress it.

Communication skills are increased with the ability to read and write. A marked increase in vocabulary enables the child to participate better in social groups. Through the early middle childhood especially the child tries out new roles in imaginative play. With better communication skills it is easier for an adult to talk over problems with him, and the child can better express his feelings and beliefs. Songs, stories, poetry, word games, and signals that scouts use are all forms of communication.

Family background influences a child's progress in school. Middle class families are apt to show more interest in educational achievement than those from a low socioeconomic level. The child is usually exposed to more intellectual activity in a middle class or well-to-do family.

Also the disadvantaged child is apt to have less language development and cognitive skills. He may have feelings of inadequacy that influence his academic achievement.

Children who need help should be identified early for special counseling: a child with learning difficulties, a child with health problems, or a child who tends to stay by himself. With help, these children may be able to achieve and succeed.

According to Freud, this is a period of latency. As mentioned, each child tends to play with children of his own sex. On the other hand, this is a period when each child further learns his or her sex role. The child is fortunate who comes from a family in which both the mother and father are present. When a father is present he serves as a role model for his son and influences him toward masculinity. If the father is absent a boy may experience difficulties in proportion to the length of the absence. Girls in a father-absent home may be more shy and have difficulties in relationships with males.

REFERENCES

Anderson, R. E.: Where's Dad? Paternal deprivation and delinquency, Arch. Gen. Psychiatr. **18:**641, 1968.

Baumund, D.: Current patterns of parental authority, Dev. Psychol. Monogr. 4(part 2):1, 1971.

Biller, H. B.: Father, child, and sex roles, Lexington, Mass., 1971, D. C. Heath and Co.

Birth, H. G., and Gassory, G.: Disadvantaged children: Health, nutrition, and school failure, New York, 1970, Grune & Stratten, Inc.

Breckenridge, M., and Vincent, E. W.: Child development: Physical and psychological growth through adolescence, ed. 5, Philadelphia, 1965, W. B. Saunders Co.

Campbell, J. D.: Peer relations in childhood. in Hoffman, M. L., and Hoffman, L. W., editors: Review of child development and research. vol. 1, New York, 1964, Russell Sage Foundation.

Cervantes, L. F.: Family background, primary relationships, and the high school dropout, J. Marriage Family **5:**218, 1965.

Coopersmith, S.: The antecedents of self-esteem, San Francisco, 1967, W. H. Freeman and Co., Publishers.

Dielman, T. E., et al.: A check on the structure of parental reports of child rearing practices, Child Dev. **42:**893, 1971.

Flavell, J. H.: Developmental psychology of Jean Piaget, Princeton, N.J., 1963, D. Van Nostrand Co., Inc.

Gardner, R., and Mariarty, A.: Personality development at preadolescence, Seattle, 1968, University of Washington Press.

Glueck, S. and Glueck, E.: Unraveling juvenile delinquency, Cambridge, Mass., 1950, Harvard University Press.

Harris, S., and Braun, J. R.: Self-esteem and racial preference in black children, Proc. Ann. Convent. Am. Psychol. Assoc. **6:**259, 1971.

Heckel, R. L.: The effects of fatherlessness on preadolescent female, Ment. Hyg. **48:**451, July, 1964.

Heckel, R. L.: The prediction of social success or failure in the college situation, Furman studies, Spring, 1952.

Hetherington, E. M.: Effects of father absence of personality development in adolescent daughters, Dev. Psychol. **7:**327, 1972.

Hurlock, E. Developmental psychology, New York, 1975, McGraw-Hill Book Co.

Jersild, A. T.: Characteristics of teachers who are "liked best" and "disliked most," J. Exp. Educ. **9:**139, 1940.

Jersild, A., Telford, C., and Saurey, Y.: Child psychology, ed. 7, Englewood Cliffs, N.J., 1975, Prentice-Hall, Inc.

Kagan, J.: Personality development, New York, 1971, Harcourt Brace Jovanovich, Inc.

Kandel, D. B., and Lesser, G. S.: Parental and peer influences on educational plans of adolescents, Am. Sociol. Rev. **34:**213, 1969.

Leverthal, T., and Sills, M.: Self-image in school phobia, Am. J. Orthopsychiatry **34:**685, 1964.

Mitchell, D., and Wilson, W.: Relationship of father-absence to masculinity and popularity of delinquent boys, Psychol. Rep. **20:**1173, 1967.

Mussen, P. A., Conger, J., and Kagan, J.: Child development and personality, Ed. 4, New York, 1974, Harper & Row, Publishers.

Sears, R. R., Maccoby, E. E., and Levin, H.: Patterns of child-rearing, Evanston, Ill., 1957, Row, Peterson, & Co.

Stone, L., and Church, J.: Childhood and adolescence, ed. 2, New York, 1968, Random House, Inc.

Watson, E. H., and Lowrey, G. H.: Growth and development of children, ed. 5, Chicago, 1967, Year Book Medical Publishers, Inc.

8
ADOLESCENCE

DEFINING ADOLESCENCE

Adolescence is often called a period of storm and stress, of anxiety and turmoil. Virtually everything changes for the young person. His body is developing new proportions, and he is subject to new and different physiological urges, especially sexual. He looks and is expected to behave like an adult, but he feels insecure and threatened by the very independence he craves. He must establish new relationships with his peers, especially those of the opposite sex, and he is expected to decide on and prepare for a vocation and for adult responsibilities including marriage. He is no longer a child.

According to Blos (1975), adolescence is the second period of individuation; the first is completed in the third year of life when the child first realizes that he is a separate individual. The adolescent must shed family dependencies so that he may become a member of the adult world. His capacity for logical thinking has increased so that it may function on a verbal, symbolic, hypothetical level without concrete support. This may lead in the beginning to worry about what is real and what is not and is perhaps central to concern over establishing an identity as described by Erikson (1963).

Identity realization is a lifelong process, beginning in infancy and developing throughout childhood. However, adolescence is the critical stage in which all the changes just mentioned plus the increased capacity for logical thinking converge to bring to the young person the realization that he is an individual, different from all others, with a special configuration of traits. Normally he is increasingly accepted by himself, by his peers, and by society at large as a person in his own right. Self-acceptance, often so difficult for adolescents, is primary, a necessity for the acceptance of others. In this rapidly changing society, as one young woman expressed it, it is extremely difficult to know from day to day where one stands. Adults are often little help because they cannot keep up with the changes themselves, probably not as well as the adolescents. With increasing age often comes resistance to change and a desire to do things as one has always done them. This increasing rigidity aggravates the difficulty the older generation may have in adapting to young people's acceptance of or even enthusiasm for change.

It has been said that the very term *adolescence* is an invention of modern western society, that primitive societies encountered less difficulty in the transition from childhood to adulthood. To be sure, primitive societies prescribed rigid transitional rites for both boys and girls at puberty (Muensterberger, 1975). These are difficult for the adolescent, but when certain practices are the unchangeable reality for all one accepts them as best one can without open revolt. When there is freedom and opportunity to decide for oneself, things become difficult even if desirable. In the relatively free Athenian society of 2,400 years ago Socrates was condemned to death for his "impious" ideas and for "corrupting" youth by getting them to think for themselves in disagreement with authority.

Elders have always complained about young people, but never has there been a more difficult period than now, when young people have been released from restraint and are expected to behave rationally and in accord with their parents' ideas although there are few or no regulations and guidelines to which they must conform. No longer are there chaperones at parties and dances; young people may go out in the family car and do as they please. History has shown that for adults as well as young people the release of restraints has promoted rebellion, revolution, and marked turmoil. Many examples can be seen in history: the first few centuries preceding the fall of Rome, the Renaissance in western Europe; the effects of the freeing of the serfs in 1861 in Russia. The old saying, "Give them an inch and they'll take a mile," contains a great deal of truth.

These periods of unrest as a rule seem to precede an advance in civilization, a change for the better, increased freedom and self-determination for the people. However, ultraconservative forces that resist change are pitted against those who wish to change too fast and too radically with resulting turmoil and unrest. The world seems to be going through such a period now. This makes it difficult for us all, but especially for the young.

• • •

Throughout the childhood years parents usually have maintained constant control and supervision over the social, intellectual, and emotional development of each child. All activities have been carried out with some degree of supervision by teachers, parents, nurses, counselors, or other responsible persons acting for the parents. The only exceptions to this are cases in which the home is of marginal quality and children are rejected, neglected, or unwanted. In some few cases overpermissive parents may be willing to permit younger children to engage in unsupervised activities.

With the approach of adolescence there is a movement away from the home on the part of all young persons. As the child seeks to emancipate himself from his family, there is often resulting stress and conflict. Parents only grudgingly recognize the adolescent's need to identify himself as a distinct and different person in contrast with his childhood role as an appendage of a family. In most cases they reluctantly permit his "leaving the nest."

As if this were not enough to produce problems for the adolescent, he must also face a changed response from the culture. Other persons in the community who once regarded some of his behavior as cute, clever, or charming may regard that same behavior at this later stage as inappropriate, immature, or undesirable. Even though his age may be little more than that of a child, demands will be placed on him to react

with reserve, dignity, and adult logic. This is exceedingly difficult when the inclinations on the part of the young person are to behave as he had only a year or two earlier. Least fortunate in this regard is the boy or girl who matures early and who chronologically is quite young but physiologically appears several years older.

With increased demands for training and education in any culture there is a consequent delay in the age at which marriage can take place. This poses one of the major problems to the adolescent in advanced cultures. Although the young person is fully capable of reproduction, wants his independence, and in some instances is sufficiently mature to handle adult responsibility, he is likely to be forced by reason of our highly technological society to delay close, long-term relationships until the completion of his education. Although once it was possible to acquire full-time employment offering a good future at age 16 to 18 years, today it is virtually impossible for the individual who has less than a high school education to develop a secure and meaningful future. High school graduates of today also must consider the possibility of spending additional years in training or collegiate education to find adequate employment. Not only is the adolescent expected to delay any formation of long-term relationships with members of the opposite sex, but he must commit himself at an earlier and earlier date to follow a particular educational plan or career. Many years ago high school was simply high school, with a curriculum that was very general and often of the college preparatory type. Today there are many subspecialties available to the high school student. He may take a technical course, a vocational course, a college preparatory course, an accelerated course, or perhaps a major in agriculture. Although it is possible that he may change his mind and his vocation at some later period in his training, this is done only with difficulty. Preparation for work has begun earlier and earlier in the educational process so that today there is some consideration of occupational categories and career choices even in the eighth grade. Such decisions require an earlier maturity for the adolescent of today. Yet conversely we extend his years of dependence on the family for supplying his educational and financial needs, sometimes well into adulthood. This has the opposite effect of delaying maturity. Consider the case of a physician, who must complete 4 years of college, 4 years of medical school, a year of internship, and then a residency in the specialty of his choice that may last from 3 to 5 years. During all these years he may be in part dependent upon his family for survival. Quite often he will be between 32 and 34 years old by the time he is first ready to be independent of the many persons who have supported him during his period of education. Although such a case is the exception, there are many occupations that now require long periods of training. Consider the preparation for nursing, which during its early years was commonly carried out in a relatively short time. Today many programs award a bachelor's degree in nursing, whereas others offer advanced degrees in special areas such as nursing education. It is possible for the nurse today to spend 7, 8, or even more years after high school to become fully trained to serve as an instructor in a school of nursing. Although technically an extended training period does not force the person to remain adolescent for all these years, his financial limitations and his lack of independence may keep him from acquiring full status as an adult.

PHYSICAL GROWTH

The major physiological changes of adolescence are the occurrence of a first menstrual period, or menarche, in girls and the emergence of secondary sex characteristics in boys, particularly the appearance of pigmented pubic hairs. These mark puberty and the onset of adolescence and occur primarily between 11 and 15 years of age. In some cases there is a precocious arrival of puberty, and some girls as young as 9 years begin menstruation. In other instances glandular underfunctioning may delay the appearance of puberty until as late as the seventeenth or eighteenth year. In such cases it is often necessary for a physician to administer hormones to aid in bringing about the changes involved.

These physiological changes are produced in part through the action of gonadotropic hormones, which are secreted by the anterior pituitary gland. The pituitary (or master) gland controls hormonal balance within the body. Secretion of gonadotropic hormones produces a stimulation of sex glands within the body, with the resultant production of sex hormones and the development of sperm and ova in males and females. The action of the sex hormones is to produce secondary sex characteristics and to promote growth of bone and muscle, which have a major part in the accelerated growth during adolescence.

Accelerated growth

Table 8-1 indicates that there is a rapid acceleration of growth during the adolescent period. Although there is some variation as to the time at which this takes place, for boys it generally begins at approximately 13 years of age and lasts until 15, with age 14 being the year of maximum growth. In girls the growth spurt begins at about age 11 and lasts until 13 or 14 years. In general the twelfth year is considered the period of maximum growth in girls. During this time the increase in height and weight is greater than for any other given period of time in the child's life.

Although growth continues in succeeding years, the growth rate in girls after 13 years of age is much slower than during the period of acceleration, whereas boys show a decrease after age 15 in their rate of growth.

Girls show significant changes in body conformation. There is a beginning of the accumulation of fat in the shoulders, breasts, hips, and thighs as the result of hormonal action. The onset of menarche signals that final growth will be attained within the succeeding 3 to 5 years. Weight changes during this period may continue, and it is not unusual for a girl to gain an excessive amount of weight during the early adolescent period—weight that may stay with her until maturity.

In boys adolescent acceleration in growth is evident in the increase in length of legs, which gives many adolescents a gangling, high-hipped appearance. Boys with normal development during this time show a widening of shoulders and an increase in size of pectoral and latissimus muscles, which produce an athletic or masculine appearance. Boys usually do not show

Table 8-1. Height and weight tables for adolescent boys and girls*

	Percentiles (boys)				Percentiles (girls)		
	10	50	90		10	50	90
12½ years				*12½ years*			
Weight in pounds	74.6	88.7	116.4	Weight in pounds	74.7	93.4	118.0
Weight in kilograms	33.84	40.23	52.8	Weight in kilograms	33.88	42.37	53.52
Height in inches	56.9	60.0	63.6	Height in inches	57.4	60.7	64.0
Height in centimeters	114.5	152.3	161.6	Height in centimeters	145.9	154.3	162.7
13 years				*13 years*			
Weight in pounds	77.1	93.0	123.2	Weight in pounds	79.9	99.1	124.5
Weight in kilograms	34.97	42.18	55.88	Weight in kilograms	36.24	44.95	56.47
Height in inches	57.7	61.0	64.1	Height in inches	58.7	61.8	64.9
Height in centimeters	146.6	155.0	165.3	Height in centimeters	149.1	157.1	164.8
13½ years				*13½ years*			
Weight in pounds	82.2	100.3	130.1	Weight in pounds	85.5	103.7	128.9
Weight in kilograms	37.29	45.5	59.01	Weight in kilograms	38.78	47.04	58.47
Height in inches	58.8	62.6	66.5	Height in inches	59.5	62.4	65.3
Height in centimeters	149.4	158.9	168.9	Height in centimeters	151.1	158.4	165.9
14 years				*14 years*			
Weight in pounds	87.2	107.6	136.9	Weight in pounds	91.0	108.4	133.3
Weight in kilograms	39.55	48.81	62.1	Weight in kilograms	41.28	49.17	60.46
Height in inches	59.9	64.0	67.9	Height in inches	60.2	62.8	65.7
Height in centimeters	152.1	162.7	172.4	Height in centimeters	153.0	159.6	167.0
14½ years				*14½ years*			
Weight in pounds	93.3	113.9	142.4	Weight in pounds	94.2	111.0	135.7
Weight in kilograms	42.32	51.66	64.59	Weight in kilograms	42.73	50.35	61.55
Height in inches	61.0	65.1	68.7	Height in inches	60.7	63.1	66.0
Height in centimeters	155.0	165.3	174.6	Height in centimeters	154.1	160.4	167.6
15 years				*15 years*			
Weight in pounds	99.4	120.1	147.8	Weight in pounds	97.4	113.5	138.1
Weight in kilograms	45.09	54.48	67.04	Weight in kilograms	44.18	51.48	62.64
Height in inches	62.1	66.1	69.6	Height in inches	61.1	63.4	66.2
Height in centimeters	157.8	167.8	176.7	Height in centimeters	155.2	161.1	168.1
15½ years				*15½ years*			
Weight in pounds	105.2	124.9	152.6	Weight in pounds	99.2	115.3	139.6
Weight in kilograms	47.72	56.65	69.22	Weight in kilograms	45.0	52.3	63.32
Height in inches	63.1	66.8	70.2	Height in inches	61.3	63.7	66.4
Height in centimeters	160.3	169.7	178.2	Height in centimeters	155.7	161.7	168.6
16 years				*16 years*			
Weight in pounds	111.0	129.7	157.3	Weight in pounds	100.9	117.0	141.1
Weight in kilograms	50.35	58.83	71.35	Weight in kilograms	45.77	53.07	64.0
Height in inches	64.1	67.8	70.7	Height in inches	61.5	63.9	66.5
Height in centimeters	162.8	171.6	179.7	Height in centimeters	156.1	162.2	169.0

*Modified from measurements guide by Howard V. Meredith, Iowa Child Welfare Research Station, The State University of Iowa; from Vaughan, V. C., III: Growth and development. In Vaughan, V. C., III, and McKay, R. J., editors: Nelson's textbook of pediatrics, ed. 10, Philadelphia, 1975, W. B. Saunders Co., p. 42.

Continued.

Table 8-1. Height and weight tables for adolescent boys and girls—cont'd

	Percentiles (boys)				Percentiles (girls)		
	10	**50**	**90**		**10**	**50**	**90**
16½ years				*16½ years*			
Weight in pounds	114.3	133.0	161.0	Weight in pounds	101.9	118.1	142.2
Weight in kilograms	51.85	60.33	73.03	Weight in kilograms	46.22	53.57	64.5
Height in inches	64.6	68.0	71.1	Height in inches	61.5	63.9	66.6
Height in centimeters	164.2	172.7	180.7	Height in centimeters	156.2	162.4	169.2
17 years				*17 years*			
Weight in pounds	117.5	136.2	164.6	Weight in pounds	102.8	119.1	143.3
Weight in kilograms	53.3	61.78	74.66	Weight in kilograms	46.63	54.02	65.0
Height in inches	65.2	68.4	71.5	Height in inches	61.5	64.0	66.7
Height in centimeters	156.2	173.7	181.6	Height in centimeters	156.3	162.5	169.4
17½ years				*17½ years*			
Weight in pounds	118.8	137.6	166.8	Weight in pounds	103.2	119.5	143.9
Weight in kilograms	53.89	62.41	75.66	Weight in kilograms	46.81	54.2	65.27
Height in inches	65.3	68.5	71.6	Height in inches	61.5	64.0	66.7
Height in centimeters	165.9	174.1	182.0	Height in centimeters	156.3	162.5	169.4
18 years				*18 years*			
Weight in pounds	120.0	139.0	169.0	Weight in pounds	103.5	119.9	144.5
Weight in kilograms	54.43	63.05	76.66	Weight in kilograms	46.95	54.39	65.54
Height in inches	65.5	68.7	71.8	Height in inches	61.5	64.0	66.7
Height in centimeters	166.3	174.5	182.4	Height in centimeters	156.3	162.5	169.4

the accumulation of fat that gives girls a rounded, "feminine" appearance.

Boys normally exhibit changes in the larynx and vocal cords caused by androgenic hormonal secretions. Since the vocal structures are undergoing change, voice quality may fluctuate between the levels of childhood and those common to maturity. This is responsible for some of the unusual "croaking" sounds that adolescent boys are noted for.

There are other general changes that take place in both boys and girls. Though changes in facial characteristics the soft, round baby features gradually disppear. The forehead becomes higher and wider. Lips, formerly thin and childlike, become full, and the mouth also takes on width and added dimension. The chin, which is quite frequently receding in childhood, begins to show more prominence. Overall bodily proportions change. The head, which was so dominant in infancy and childhood, now accounts for a much smaller proportion of the total body size. Arms, legs, and trunk tend to show much

more rapid acceleration in growth during adolescence than the face and head. Head size, for example, is 90% complete by age 10, but other proportions of the body are not nearly so complete at that time. During succeeding years growth is concentrated in other areas.

These are far from the only changes that take place during the development of the adolescent. Almost all parts of the body undergo growth and elaboration during the adolescent period. Internal organs of the body take on added size. There is a change in the skeletal structure of the body with accelerated calcification of bones, which once showed a high level of cartilage and fibrous tissue that caused them to be pliable, soft, and spongy. Cartilage undergoes calcification, and the total bone structure becomes denser and more rugged. Although this has been a continuous process throughout childhood, during the adolescent growth spurt the change becomes more rapid. In girls much of this ossification process has become complete by 17 years of age; in boys this may occur by 18 or 19

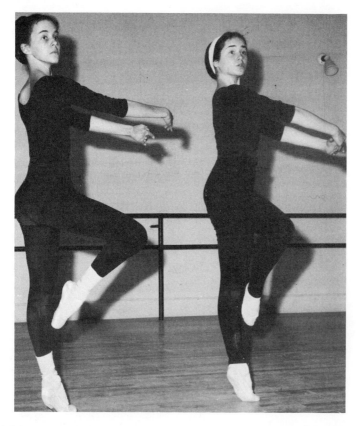

Fig. 8-1. Adolescence. The general impression that girls or boys lack coordination during the adolescent period can be quickly dispelled by watching the actions of young ballerinas such as the sisters pictured here. In many cases they can attain a level of perfection in executing difficult maneuvers that would not be possible later in their lives.

years of age. In some instances there is a continuation of growth and development of bony structure until the age of 20 or 21 years. Changes that occur during early adulthood are chiefly of the thickening type rather than elongation.

These skeletal changes are accompanied by changes in the percentage of muscle tissue in the body of the young person. In the young child less than 20% of the body weight is devoted to muscle tissue. However, by the age of 16 years, when much of the growth acceleration has been completed, as much as 44% of the body weight is in the form of muscle tissue. As muscle tissue accumulates, the child becomes much more able to demonstrate strength, coordination, and agility than was possible when his muscles were less prominent and less able to

provide the strength and support necessary for many of the vigorous activities characteristic of adolescence. Both girls and boys show great increases in speed, coordination, and strength during the adolescent period. This acceleration in girls continues until they reach the age of 14 or 15 years, when it stabilizes. In boys the coordinated activities show an increase until a later period, up to 17 or 18 years. Whereas boys generally show an overall superiority in speed and strength, the results are not quite what they seem. For example, a woman of today may do as well as many men of an earlier period of time. In a recent Olympic contest many of the women who competed in running, broad jumping, and hurdling events performed at levels exceeding those of earlier male Olympic champions. Thus, although men may still

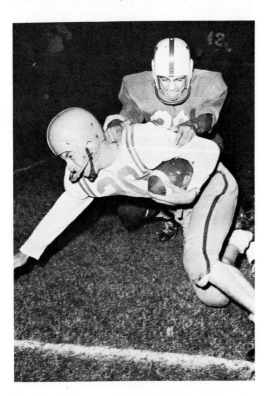

Fig. 8-2. Adolescence. Boys during late adolescence clearly show the physical vigor and power that sets them apart from females of the same age. These high school football players reflect a type of gross strength and coordination that would be of little use in activities shown in the preceding ballet illustration. (Courtesy Bryant English.)

maintain a slight edge, there is a gradual lessening of the sharp differences once noted between men and women in certain coordinated activities. There are many things that may account for this, such as improved nutritional standards and a lowering of the former barriers to female participation in a wide variety of physical sports.

Reproductive organs

The appearance of secondary sex characteristics and the dramatic change that takes place in the reproductive system of the adolescent have already been discussed. In boys the growth of reproductive organs is considerable. Outwardly there is a change in the size of the penis, the testes, and the scrotum. Pubic hair appears, and the ability to ejaculate is characteristically pres-

ent within a year after the appearance of pubic hair. In the succeeding 2-year period there is a development of axillary and facial hair in the male. Internally there are various changes and secretions that will affect other organs of the body such as the larynx.

In girls there are a number of early signs that precede the onset of menstruation or menarche. Chief among these are the increase in the diameter of the areola and the beginning growth of breast tissue. The areola and the papilla, or nipple, form the breast bud. As development continues the nipple increases in size and projects outward, while breast tissue continues to multiply. During this same period of growth the uterus loses its infantile quality, taking on added size and a new position more suitable for childbearing.

Variation in ages of onset of puberty and menarche

Many of the growth and development charts prepared in the United States during the 1920's and 1930's are inadequate for today's use. There has been a steady increase in average height and weight for both boys and girls in this country as well as in many other sections of the world. Recent studies made in Japan reveal that facilities that were adequate in grade schools before World War II and immediately afterward are too small today. Along with this noted increase in height and weight has been an earlier onset of puberty and menarche. Although the figures do not reveal striking changes, they do present a consistent picture of earlier development and greater growth rate.

Explanations for this appear to be largely based on nutritional factors. No doubt increased health facilities, better sources and supplies of vitamins, adequate medication, and, perhaps more important, better preventive methods have removed many of the diseases and dietary conditions that might impede the growth rate. Other studies of areas in which there is extreme deprivation of food or inadequate medical care reveal that the onset of puberty and menarche is frequently delayed by these conditions. Although no evidence is forthcoming to support the contention that children from tropical countries mature earlier than others, evidence does indicate that in some of the colder climates there appears to be a later development of puberty and menarche. Explanations for these findings are not necessarily outside the realm of the diet-deprivation hypothesis.

PSYCHOLOGICAL AND SOCIAL BEHAVIORAL CHANGE

The changes that accompany adolescence produce changes in the way the young person views himself and in the way other persons view him, his behavior, and his role in society. How an individual views himself is referred to as his self-concept. This is a complex combination of the way in which the individual sees himself in relation to the world around him. His view is rarely an objective one. It is a view based on the way other persons have reacted to him in the past; it is colored by his goals and ideals and also by private thoughts, feelings, and attitudes that may be unknown to other persons around him. The self-concept is in part formed by each individual in comparing what he considers his characteristics with the characteristics he perceives in other persons. In some instances the adolescent may seek perfection from himself and view himself as far less adequate than other persons around him. In other instances parents may force an unrealistic self-concept on the individual, who may feel that under no circumstances will he ever fail and that everyone will treat him with the regard and concern his parents have shown. Mussen, Conger, and Kagan (1974) indicate that some of the basic characteristics that individuals use in assessing their own self-concept are (1) behavioral evaluations relating to good or bad behavior, (2) being intelligent as opposed to lacking skills, and (3) being well developed or handsome as opposed to having an inadequate or undesirable physical structure or body image.

Because the adolescent has had little experience either with his new body image or with the many social opportunities that are now available to him, he may reflect more critically upon himself or his behavior and look for behavioral standards set by others—either those in his peer group or persons slightly older than himself. Frequently parents are unable to supply the support and information so necessary for adjustment and reassurance during this period. Although the adolescent faces the new social situations with limited experience, he may be forced to draw on his experience, inadequate as it may be, when judging himself in relation to the world around him. Children growing up in families that make them feel unwanted or inadequate find these feelings intensified during the adolescent period.

Severe problems faced by adolescents relate to the onset of the adolescent period itself and particularly the secondary sex characteristics that go along with it. Boys and girls who are later in maturing than their peers frequently suffer humiliation, embarrassment, and extreme personal concern regarding their delay. Reassurance by family physicians rarely outweighs the fact that they observe in their peers the appearance of characteristics that they themselves do not possess. In addition they observe the increased acceptance that the larger, more developed males and females receive from other group members. Although the relationship between physical development and leadership qualities is not always high, it appears to be a strong factor during the early adolescent period.

Let us now look a little more closely at certain variations in the self-image: the ideal self and the real self. The ideal self is a combination of idealized attitudes, characteristics, and behaviors. These are gained basically through internalization of parents' standards but often find expression through adulation of adolescent heroes such as movie stars, football players, or outstanding members of the community. The ideal self may be patterned after the important characteristics the adolescent perceives in these persons. Quite often what he sees is not the total person but only a few dominant features such as success, wealth, fame, or physical attractiveness. Building these characteristics into what he or she might like to be, the adolescent may envision an ideal self that is completely unrealistic and out of reach. When the teenager is able to see these ideal levels in a realistic fashion, when he sees them as desirable characteristics or things that might be attained after years of struggle and hard work, the conflicts arising from the ideal self are not severe. Unfortunately many teenagers see these as goals that they

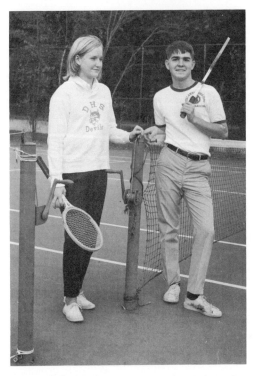

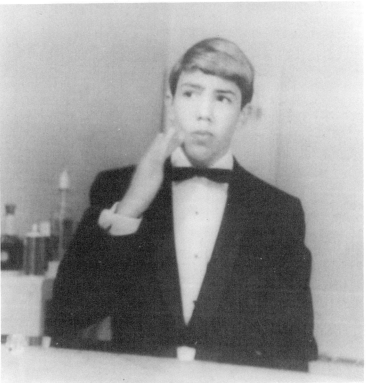

Fig. 8-3. The body image in adolescence reaches a high level of maturity in form and grace for both boys and girls.

should have now. The slender, small-breasted girl feels that she should have the overdeveloped figure of a Hollywood starlet while she is still 14 years of age. Boys commonly wish to be athletic heroes even though in adolescence they do not have the height, weight, or motor coordination necessary to achieve their goals. Nearly all teenagers establish ideals. Sometimes these ideal persons are socially deviant or delinquent. When such an ideal has been set for the individual, he may be reflecting the antisocial values of his subculture or he may be reflecting serious adjustive problems in which he individually feels the necessity to rebel and fight against society.

For most persons the ideal self does not pose insurmountable problems. To be sure, there may be daydreams and fantasies in which desired characteristics are attained. Quite often these daydreams and fantasies, where not carried to excess, lead to constructive planning in which the adolescent works toward the development of his personal characteristics and behavior in the model provided for him by those he admires. Nurses, physicians, and teachers frequently are taken as ideal models. As a result a great responsibility is placed on any person functioning in the service setting. Adolescents, influenced by their behavior and approach to life, will frequently mold much of their own behavior in a similar pattern.

Let us turn our attention to the real self. This real self is an elusive combination of the individual's self-image, his ideal self, the self that he reveals to others around him, and the self seen by persons who might objectively observe and measure his behavior. A parallel may be drawn between the view of the individual's personality and the view of a cube. Certain aspects are visible from certain angles of the cube: The closer or more rigid is the position of viewers, the less of the total cube, or of the individual himself, can be seen. The objective observer stands at some distance to view the personality or cube as a whole.

Striving for maturity

Striving toward maturity comes from two sources. Society demands of the adolescent that he acquire the appropriate behavior to adjust in adult society. The adolescent himself, as he develops physical maturity, seeks to attain the rewards of society that are a part of adulthood. Adulthood has many positive benefits for the adolescent. Not only may he acquire more status and recognition from other persons by behaving and functioning as an adult, but other rewards also are open to him. As an adult, he may marry, engage in approved sexual activity, raise a family, and work in an occupation that returns adequate financial rewards—all of which may act to enhance his status in the community. As an adolescent or a child none of these things was available to him. Nearly all forms of sexual behavior are disapproved, early marriage is restricted, employment opportunities are unavailable, and status for the very young is almost nonexistent. In effect the adolescent is forced, often against his desire, to become completely dependent upon his family or other members of society. Independence is a hard-won and much-sought-after freedom for the adolescent.

Before he is granted the recognition of being considered an adult he is expected to have attained emotional maturity and stability, demonstrated the ability to handle stress, assumed a series of increasingly responsible roles, and become able to look beyond his own immediate needs in recognizing the rights, privileges, and feelings of other persons around him.

With these difficult and demanding characteristics it is easy to see that few persons we regard as adults have mastered these behaviors. No adolescent can possibly have attained all this no matter how sophisticated and self-confident he may appear on the surface. Development of the self-esteem he must achieve if he is to be a happy and successful adult is hindered by excessive expectations too early. Life beyond adolescence is still a period of growth and development in which persons usually continue to improve their understanding and increase their ability to meet social demands effectively.

In our culture, perhaps more than in others, there is a recognition of the rights of the individual. These rights include a freedom of choice in his pattern of life as to education, employment, choice of a mate, where he will live, and what he will do with his spare time. However, he can fulfill these goals in a mature way only if it is not done at the expense of other persons. Parents and others close to the young person have a great deal to do with his attainment of the self-respect and self-confidence necessary. This may be called self-love in the sense in which it is used in the biblical admonition, "Love thy neighbor as thyself." Without positive feelings for oneself, it is impossible to love and respect others.

Adolescent sexual behavior

Adolescent sexual behavior differs in different societies and is motivated and shaped by the social and psychological environment as well as by physiological development. Increased glandular activity and physical development bring about significant changes and increase the possibility that sexual responses may occur. Also, as the adolescent becomes more a part of the adult world, he comes in contact with more and more of the sexual aspects of the adult social environment. These take many forms. Books, magazines, movies, television, advertising, and a large part of the verbal and social interaction among adults are concerned with love and sex.

The adolescent, with his increased access to extracurricular activities and to relationships outside the home and school with peers of both sexes, may spend a large part of his time in satisfying his curiosity. His interest may take many forms. In addition to the vicarious sources, many adolescents engage in erotic and autoerotic sexual behavior. Autoerotic behavior, in which the individual uses masturbation in one of its many forms to reach sexual gratification, is more commonly found in boys than in girls. Studies have consistently shown that by late adolescence more than 90% of males will have achieved orgasm through masturbation. Girls report somewhat less than half the incidence of masturbatory activity attributed to boys.

As the adolescent boy and girl approach marriage and adulthood, the incidence of orgasms, sexual experiences, and sexual knowledge increases significantly. In the past greater cultural permissiveness has resulted in a much greater increase for boys than for girls. A variety of factors accounts for this. The possibility of the girl's becoming pregnant is probably the most important. The accessibility of the sexual apparatus to the male for manipulation also may have its effect. Not only has our society been more permissive with regard to sexual attitudes in boys but it permits wider degrees of freedom in social mobility for boys. Girls rarely have been permitted to move about freely in the community unless parents were aware of where they were going, whom they were going with, and at what time they would return. Although boys frequently have some limitations of a similar type, parents have been less concerned with their activities. The possibility of loss of status, reputation, and acceptance because of sexual acting out is less in boys and has been almost universal for girls. Indeed, precocious sexual activity for boys is sometimes seen as a status symbol among other adolescent boys, and there are indications recently that this may be becoming true for girls also in certain sections of society.

There has been during the twentieth century a marked change in the frequency of premarital intercourse for girls (Mussen, Conger, and Kagan, 1974, p. 573). This began in the grandmother's generation. According to the original Kinsey report, only 2% of girls born before 1900 had had premarital intercourse by the age of 16 and 8% before the age of 20. This percentage gradually increased, but there has been a recent acceleration to 30% by age 16 and 57% by age 19. The corresponding figures for boys, 44% and 72%, respectively, reflect a very small change from the figures for the preceding generation.

It must be reemphasized that the changing mores in regard to sex stereotypes are already influencing behavior. Girls are demanding their share of athletic support and opportunity. Clothing for the two sexes is becoming similar. Options are increasing for both sexes.

Block's study (1975) defines the stereotype as expecting boys to be active, competitive, assertive, and energetic; girls are expected to be considerate, empathetic, loving, and tolerant. A combination of these qualities, called androgyny, seems to result in a more flexible adult in both sexes with higher self-esteem. In adolescence, however, the aggressive, competitive boy and the more conventionally "feminine" girl may be more popular. The development of androgynous characteristics is highly related to child-rearing practices and is more likely to characterize middle class families. Young people entering college are likely to exhibit more flexible patterns than those not seeking a college education.

Parents and sex

Researchers have found that one of the most significant factors regarding stability and maturity with regard to sexual behavior is under the direct influence of the immediate family of the young person (Bernard, 1961). They have shown that in families where sex education is provided by the parents the incidence of sexual problems and difficulty is greatly diminished. When parents are unwilling or unable to provide training, knowledge, and information for the child with regard to the facts of sexual behavior, he must turn to others. A primary information source is found in other persons of his own age group. This is an unreliable and often ill-informed source of information. In other instances older brothers or sisters, neighbors, or other persons in the community may supply some of this knowledge. Frequently this, too, is of an undesirable quality. There has been a movement toward having such information offered through the school systems, but some parental groups have violently opposed the idea. Some church groups have provided information, but occasionally well-intentioned but ill-informed and embarrassed lay persons conducting such meetings have increased anxieties and problems rather than diminished them. Outside the family this role in instruction is most often played by physicians and nurses. Through the years there has been a recognition that medically oriented and trained individuals have access to considerable information regarding not only the sexual apparatus but some of the psychological and sociological implications of sexual behavior. Under ideal circumstances this information giving should be handled by a combination of sources—the parents and a professional person in medicine or a medically related area who has had special training in supplying sex information.

The reasons why parents refuse to supply sexual information to their children as their questions develop and emerge are many. The child whose general questions have met with matter-of-fact answers is frequently aroused to excessive curiosity when he suddenly encounters an area in which he gets no answers and may be given reproof by parents. Frequently parents are embarrassed, humiliated, or upset when questions arise in the sexual area. Yet the supplying of this information is vital to the healthy, normal development of the child and adolescent. There are countless cases of young girls whose mothers had failed to inform them of even such basic occurrences as the onset of menstruation and who suffered enormously because they were unaware of the physiological facts of life. Even more prevalent are cases in which young women have approached marriage almost totally ignorant of sex and the reproductive process. Not infrequently young girls have been encountered who believed that kissing was the manner in which pregnancy occurred. Guilt is often reinforced in boys by inculcating feelings of worthlessness and sin in them when they engage in normal, nearly universal practices such as masturbation. Fortunately, parental guilt regarding sex and sexual matters has been decreasing in recent years. During the Victorian period and the early part of this century, attitudes with regard to sex were rigid and prohibitionistic. Today's educational system has opened many doors, and there is a more open attitude toward discussing sex. The result has not been promiscuity for adolescents. Instead, it has led to closer and more meaningful relationships between parents and children and a decrease in anxiety about sexual matters in young persons.

Social interaction in adolescence

During the formative years of infancy and childhood there is little concern about the interaction between boys and girls. During preschool years play groups generally are mixed, and activities are centered on play experiences suitable for both boys and girls. During the early school years boys gradually become more interested in active athletics, whereas most girls until recently have participated in less vigorous games. Although it was never universally the case and has become increasingly less prevalent, by the age of 9 or 10 boys and girls have been likely to play largely with members of their own sex and often have been embarrassed to associate with the other sex.

This pattern undergoes a dramatic change with the onset of adolescence. Not only does the peer group encourage and expect interaction with members of the opposite sex but parents as well often become concerned if sons or daughters fail to develop along expected patterns. Parents also expect interactions with the opposite sex to be well controlled, uninvolved, and conducted with a great deal of social judgment. The age at which such interactions are expected and the freedom allowed vary a great deal with social class and ethnic groups. In general, as stated at the beginning of this chapter, excessive parental expectations regarding adolescent responsibility and general behavior have accounted for much of the uncertainty and turmoil characterizing many in this age group.

Burdened with these many and complex factors, it is little wonder that the average adolescent has difficulty establishing satisfactory interaction with members of the opposite sex. Not only has there been a period of indoctrination in which there was little or no interaction but there has been in most instances a series of prohibitions or ''dont's'' set forth by parents on proper social interaction. Boys generally receive fewer of these ''don'ts'' than girls, but each is informed concerning his proper role. With adolescence that role changes. The adolescent is required to draw on his past experiences to make appropriate responses to members of the opposite sex. A large part of the anxiety about interaction will come from what he has observed in his role models—the parents. For children who grow up in a home where parents are on generally friendly terms, have few arguments, and are able to externalize love and guidance to their children, the role models are positive and the children frequently will adjust well to the demands of adolescence. Conversely, when there has been much stress and strife in the home relationship with quarrels, rejection, unhappiness, and in some cases divorce, both boys and girls will approach heterosexual relationships with anxiety, fear, and extreme doubt as to the possibility of ever working out satisfactory relationships.

Negative attitudes formed in childhood are not insurmountable. Suitable counseling and guidance can reshape attitudes and lessen anxiety. If the counselor or therapist is skillful in handling young people, he will find this age group particularly amenable to change. They are old enough to think logically and to consider new ideas but not yet rigidly set in ways and beliefs. According to Heckel (1964), a neighbor or other adult friend may help the young person with his emancipation problem. He serves as older friend and counselor, often to great advantage.

For those who are able to break through the many barriers that exist in forming heterosexual relationships, a considerable period of time is spent in learning the social interaction skills necessary to relate effectively to others. Conversations and discussions of boys and girls during this period are concerned with standard setting regarding dates, social behavior, marriage, sexual relations, and various stratagems for interacting with individuals perceived as desired companions. Part of the reason for the extensive time spent by adolescents on these topics is the fact that for each area of our country and each subcultural grouping there are variations of behavior that may be considered unacceptable or ''square'' in others. Much of this information cannot be obtained from books. Written sources frequently attempt to cover a broad spectrum of recommended behaviors but can only rarely be related to a specific instance in a particular area. Young persons are forced to learn the norms for behavior in their own particular group from trial and error or discussion.

Failing to learn the appropriate behavioral standards and patterns may lead to rejection for the young person. This is one of the most painful and difficult experiences to be faced during the adolescent period. Some years ago Taylor (1938) studied the reactions of high school boys and girls to determine what they considered desirable in persons of the opposite sex. Her findings, although obtained more than 30 years ago, are applicable today. Young persons still are concerned about the same features or character-

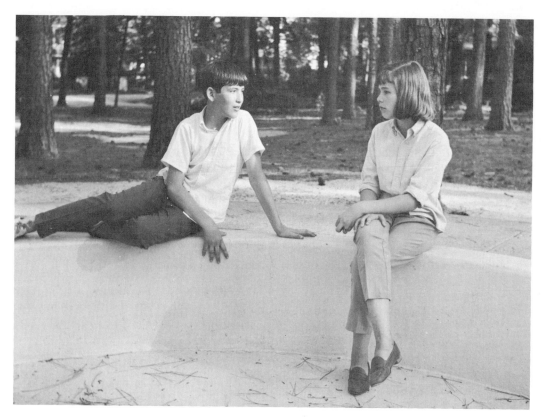

Fig. 8-4. Dating behavior. Dating and social interaction with the opposite sex play an important role in the learning process for the adolescent. Here are seen the first and very tentative interactions between two young teenagers.

istics of opposite-sexed peers. Boys indicated that the following were the most desired characteristics in girls in order of rank: attractive personality; looks; being considerate, a good conversationalist and good listener, feminine, skilled in a variety of activities, and intelligent; a sense of humor, commanding respect, and not using excessive makeup. In a similar manner high school girls expected a boy to have an attractive personality; get along with all types of people (including parents); have good physique; be a good conversationalist, a good listener, intelligent, and not conceited; have a sense of humor, and be neat and clean in appearance, courteous, and a good dancer.

In spite of fads and fashions that may occur at any one period of time, these same characteristics are still important. Sloppy attire may occasionally be in fashion for both boys and girls, but it represents merely a transient change

and may be found to occur in only a relatively small percentage of young persons. What would you as a nurse see as desirable characteristics in members of the opposite sex? In retrospect, would you say that your views have changed since high school in this regard? Chances are that in ranking the foregoing characteristics you too would place them in about the order shown. Several years ago an informal spot check of college students revealed that approximately the same order held true for that group as well.

These same traits are the ones sought by young persons in choosing a mate. When these characteristics are present in a potential mate, the focus on premarital sexual concerns is considerably reduced. This is, of course, a delicate balance. The adolescent is motivated toward finding sexual gratification. He is also seeking to do this in an acceptable way and develops considerable guilt and concern regarding sexual matters. When two young persons have a wide range of interests and activities in common, it is easier to lower anxiety and concern and to decrease the frequency of sexual relationships, which may lead to further concern, anxiety, and guilt. Mutual interests do not in and of themselves remove the possibility of sexual acting out but do prevent a young boy and girl from having "nothing else to do." Few adolescents engage in sexual activity with complete abandon and conviction; most have reservations, guilt, and doubt. If they abstain, they may fear a loss of love or a loss of status among peers, or they may feel that sexual activity is a way of proving that they are grownup. Young persons with a wide range of interests and capabilities are less likely to fall victim to such arguments.

Development of adolescent value systems

Where do value systems come from in the adolescent? What factors in his early experience or training serve to provide the values of judgmental skills that will help tell him whether his behavior is correct or incorrect? Even with such knowledge, why do some young persons fail to follow these guidelines and embark on other patterns of behavior, which may be considered less desirable or even harmful? Changes in value systems result from phenomena already discussed, such as the movement toward independence, the increased reliance on other persons in the same age group, the identification with persons outside the family, and the results of teaching and training from within various institutions of the country—schools, churches, and formalized training settings such as the Y.M.C.A. and social clubs. Each of these institutions as well as the family prescribes certain practices and behaviors for young persons. Membership in organizations requires conformity to their accepted behaviors or at least the overt appearance of conformity.

As long as the value systems proposed by others appear to be functional and to work for the individual, there is probably only a moderate degree of deviation from those standards—deviation due to curiosity, inquisitiveness, or desire for exploration. However, if the adolescent finds that the teaching and training he has received render him unable to meet the demands of the social group of which he is a member or if it leaves him with the majority of his problems unsolved, he will undoubtedly seek to explore other value systems and other forms of judgment.

In spite of the amount of sifting and sorting that goes on in adolescent value systems and moral judgments, adolescents are most likely to maintain something close to the values set forth by their parents. Children tend to select the same churches, frequently go to the same schools or colleges, vote for the same political candidates, and show the same general patterns for handling anxiety as do their parents. This is no mere coincidence. Parents and other groups are intolerant of individuals who do not follow their dictates or prescribed patterns of behavior as part of the identification process, and to avoid conflict and anxiety children during the early years adopt the general system put forth by their parents. In most instances they find that this behavior solves many of the problem situations in which they find themselves.

With some parents conformity is induced by developing a feeling of guilt or concern in the child. When he does not follow the prescribed patterns of behavior indicated by the parent or by institutions of which he is a member, he develops extreme feelings of guilt—of having done wrong. The ability to recognize a difference between one's own behavior and that prescribed or desired by other persons is the beginning of the formation of a conscience. Conscience may be defined as conformity to one's own standard of right conduct. Guilt feelings arise when these standards are violated.

By the onset of adolescence these value systems are relatively complete. Most of the early training has been thoroughly incorporated into the value system of the young person. If you will recall how frequently the child has been confronted with "No, no, mustn't," "That is bad," or "You shouldn't do that," you will have some idea of how long the process of indoctrination has been going on. It has in effect been working from earliest infancy until the present. It will not diminish during the adolescent years.

At this time, however, there may be many other sources of stimulation that will put forth additional goals or values. As these other forces do occur, they inevitably will modify to some degree the early training of the child. If his early value system were perfect and met all his needs completely, there undoubtedly would be little change. Unfortunately, this is not the case. Sometimes inner urges such as sexual desire will be so great that the individual will find himself in conflict with his early value systems. In other situations things that worked quite well at age 5 or 6 no longer are adequate to meet the demands of the social situation or of the peer group in which the young person finds himself. He must then either modify his value system or withdraw to a safe position. Since the lure of the peer group is considerable, chances are there will be some modification of his value system to fit more comfortably with those of his friends. Rarely will movement toward the peer group completely upset the former value system. If the original system was totally inadequate or if the persons providing that system of values were rejecting of or disliked by the young person, changes will be greater or in some cases extreme.

Changes also may be dramatic and sweeping when an individual is able or is forced to move from one social class to another or from one section of the country to another. In these instances he may find that his early concepts are inadequate or inappropriate for the new situation. Conflicts of great magnitude frequently lead to severe emotional disorders requiring professional help, or the individual may find himself isolated from all other persons in his new peer group. For most adolescents the process is one of adjusting and focusing values. It is during this period that the constant adjustment of personal values may also act to shape some of the opinions about desired careers or vocations.

Selecting a vocation

As cultures become more complex, the matter of career selection becomes increasingly important. Even today career choice poses few problems in the more primitive cultures where there are only limited occupational opportunities. Some of the island cultures in the western hemisphere offer few alternatives for young boys to choose. They may follow the sea on fishing boats for traders, engage in a marginal agricultural economy, seek jobs as household servants on American islands, or work in some of the small shops on their home island. Girls have even less opportunity. They may marry and raise a family, work on the small farms, or long for the day when they can escape the confines of their island and go to Europe or the United States under one of the quota systems or as domestic workers. This occupation often permits them to enter other countries under special visa arrangements.

In our country the problem is a large one. Every year sees the period during which young persons must make some career commitment appear earlier and earlier. Once vocational guidance and help was provided after completion of high school; today it is found in almost every large high school in the country. Many junior high schools also offer career planning and guidance. Today many guidance counselors talk about introducing help in vocational choice and career planning even in the grade school.

Why this increased emphasis? Because of the highly technological demands of our society, many types of work require a specialized level and type of intelligence and ability. The early recognition of these qualities permits a fuller development of stages that are preliminary to entering these careers. If children have physical handicaps or limited intellectual abilities, early planning may lead them into careers as productive, useful citizens, whereas excessive delay may prevent their ever acquiring the skills needed to function effectively in society.

These factors have in the past been especially important in the lives of boys. They have been expected to prepare themselves to support not only themselves but also wives and families; this remains true in many families and at many levels of society. However, today many women prepare themselves for gainful employment not only to supplement the family income in these inflationary times but also for personal fulfillment. Of course some women assume full support responsibilities for themselves or in a one-parent family. Women today are seeking broader horizons and in many cases do not anticipate gladly a career limited to homemaking.

With the population explosion and resulting motivation to have smaller families the incentive to achieve a satisfactory career outside or in addition to the home is further strengthened.

Adequate vocational guidance in career selection has many positive benefits to both boys and girls. In addition to providing for the future by making the young person financially self-sufficient, there are many rewards from appropriate career choice. For example, an early choice of career may shorten the length of time that the young person must spend in a relationship of dependency on family or other groups underwriting his education. By developing career choices early the young person is able to demonstrate a number of positive, goal-oriented characteristics that promote development into maturity. These allow him to advance toward independence from the family along mature and socially desirable lines. Other persons his own age will recognize and reward him for his development in these areas. The young person who has committed himself to some educative program receives additional rewards from adults who recognize his abilities.

The actual choice of a career is a complex and fascinating process. In many instances the individual will attempt to follow in his father or mother's footsteps and become a part of the same business or profession. In other instances the reaction patterns are negative toward parental figures and the young person seeks a career other than that held by one or the other parent. In still other instances personal needs or drives may cause a young person to follow some specific career. Nursing, social work, psychology, and medicine have special appeal for persons who desire or who need to work with other persons in a helping capacity. Those whose needs are to dominate others or to lead may seek careers in the military service, in law, in politics, or in certain types of business. Any career choice involves a combination of these and many other factors. Not only must the individual have the necessary talents to follow a specific career but he must also have information about the characteristics required for success, and he must have some knowledge of the career itself. Many persons growing up in remote sections of our own country are uninformed or unaware of many potential job areas. Boys growing up in the poverty-stricken Appalachian region in these recent years may see few vocational choices open to them. Girls from the same area may see little future except marriage to an occasionally employed husband and a life of hard work. With increasing emphasis on education and training many persons who now feel doomed to lives with bleak or uncertain futures may be equipped to become productive, useful workers in careers that were unknown to their parents.

Family influence

The family exerts many pressures on career choice for the young person. Among them may be a wish to have him follow in his father's or mother's footsteps or to enter a career that the parent may have desired for himself but had no opportunity to achieve.

Social factors

This introduces the social class factor into vocational choice. Children who grow up in lower class families may be forced by limited education, inadequate training, or limited personal ability to seek employment in the same general areas of unskilled or semiskilled occupations that their parents have. When they are able to "break through" socioeconomic barriers and obtain a better education or training beyond that generally available to the members of their culture, they may become upwardly mobile and reach a higher status occupation than did their parents. Many parents are ambitious for their children to have a better chance than they enjoyed and will sacrifice a great deal to bring it about. If this happens, however, young people must sever many of the ties that were a part of their previous status. The very act of their breaking away from the former culture may lead to rejection by other members of this group. Former friends may classify them as being "high-hat" or "stuck-up." At least there will be ambivalence created for the person of lower class status if he attempts to alter that status.

The middle class value system quite consistently encourages its members to strive for white-collar occupations, which often require training beyond the high school years—in technical schools, junior colleges, business schools, and universities. Blue-collar or laboring occupations are viewed as undesirable, and considerable pressure is exerted on children from middle class families to choose occupations that have high status.

Upper class groups are probably unique in that almost invariably they will be given extensive education beyond high school. Even those children who are not able to qualify for education in a university will be sent to fashionable finishing schools where they will acquire the social veneer necessary for them to function effectively in their class. Since upper class status is often determined by the inheritance of wealth, it is handed down from generation to generation unless family fortunes change. Permissible occupations for members of the upper class have been limited, although it has been possible for women in that group to take up a number of service occupations, which may give the appearance of fulfilling a social obligation. Since this class is small and exclusive, its impact on our total culture is small, at least in terms of person-to-person relationships.

Group membership

Of much greater concern are the factors relating to membership in religious and racial minority groups. In many instances mere membership in these groups forces the individual into a low status role in nearly every community. In many parts of this country, for example, only rarely have blacks been able to occupy middle class occupational roles, even though their education may equip them for much higher positions. Outside of teaching and governmental service, well-educated blacks in the South have entered law, gone north, or been forced to accept positions beneath their general level of ability. This situation has changed a great deal in recent years. More and more blacks are being hired in clerical positions and other white-collar, middle class occupations. Some are rising to the top.

Most minority groups within our country face a series of restrictions that may operate to lessen the chances of their children's receiving training and education that will let them rise above their family's class status. Even when they overcome the handicaps of inadequate schools, overcrowded classrooms, and limited opportunity, private colleges may restrict their enrollment to the number of students for which they have facilities. Public school systems in recent years have removed barriers, and students are more frequently admitted to schools of their choice.

In some cases parents' ambitions for their children are unrealistic and out of line with their potential. Some children are forced to strive for goals beyond their capacities simply because parents wish their children to enter a profession or to achieve a higher status than they themselves held.

Careers for women

One final problem in vocational choice cuts across all groups. This problem is the competition between a career and motherhood for young girls in our society. There has always been a reluctance to accord homemaking and motherhood real status. As a result, nearly every girl in high school feels she must follow a career. Many psychologists today advise that young women prepare themselves for three careers. They believe that the most effective women today are those who have had several years' work experience based on training during adolescence and early adulthood prior to marriage. This would represent their first career unless they decide not to marry or, if married, not to have children. If such decisions are made and adhered to, the woman has a better choice of a wide variety of careers and an excellent opportunity to advance as far as her capabilities permit. More and more women are reaching positions of high influence and power in the community and the nation. Of course, some succeed in reaching high status even when they have family responsibilities as well.

A second career would be fulfilling the duties and responsibilities of motherhood and raising a family. Too often, little emphasis, planning, and training are provided for this. Many women feel that children involve completely giving up their careers. Successful planning is a highly individual matter. Some women are most successful and happiest as mothers when they combine another career and motherhood. By delegating routine duties to others they can carry out both roles. The result is a higher level of satisfaction for both mother and child than would be possible if the mother were forced to play the single role. The skills necessary to function in this double role are more demanding and more difficult than those necessary for success in a career outside the home. A recent study (Curtis, 1976) in which women combining motherhood and a career were interviewed revealed one thing nearly all had in common. They were overworked and tired; also, many were lonely. Even supposedly liberal fathers did not really share responsibility for home and children, especially where details were involved, such as appointments for doctors or music lessons.

The third stage of development in career life for women would take place after their children are grown and the intervening years of family responsibility are past. Women may become depressed and develop a sense of uselessness. It is at this time that careers given up at the time of marriage may take on added importance. In the field of nursing, particularly, women whose families are grown may return to active nursing duties after several months of refresher courses. Here their professional skills combined with those learned through their experiences in motherhood can provide some of the best nursing available.

PROBLEMS OF PARENTS

The role of the parents during the adolescent years of their children is anything but smooth. The unpredictability of the adolescent creates an atmosphere of uncertainty filled with potential for conflict. It is difficult for the parent to remember that the adolescent needs encouragement, not condemnation. Parents are too frequently ready to demand and control when their child is developing independence, but at the same time they expect him to act responsibly as an adult.

The young person would like more independence and less responsibility; his parents want the opposite. Gradual assumption of both responsibility and independence is the goal, but most parents have had no training in how to assist gracefully with this process. They should know when to let go and when to hold on; they should realize their valuable role in helping the adolescent understand what is happening to him and how to cope with it. Yet many parents are more an obstacle than a help; they seem to have forgotten or repressed their own difficulties at this crucial period and often increase their child's turmoil, uncertainty, and guilt by their lack of understanding. Adolescents are usually trying to grow up and act as adults but are not yet entirely ready, and when they find themselves criticized at every turn hostility and counterproductive acting out may occur. On the other hand, the adult who does understand—who can communicate with his child, hold his confidence, and listen to what he has to say—can be of enormous help to the adolescent through this trying period of change.

Occasionally parents attempt to live vicariously through their children. When this occurs parents often push too early for involvement in occupations, dating, or peer group involvement, or conversely they do not permit sufficient socialization. Fathers particularly are protective of their daughters and resent the young man who takes his little girl away from home.

Yet the approval, understanding, and affection of the father are of great importance to the young girl, who learns through him how to accept herself as a woman and how to adjust successfully to men. The conflict between mother and daughter, which is likely to peak in early adolescence, may be aggravated by the mother's unconscious envy of her daughter as she progresses through this period in the bloom of youth that the mother feels she has lost. An immature mother is equally upset by her son, for whom no woman is good enough. The rigid demanding father who has forgotten his own adolescence may expect adult responsibility and serious purpose too early. Anthony (1975, p. 493) summarizes as follows:

If an adult remembers how much of himself has gone into the making of the adolescent, he will be able to sympathize and empathize to an extent that should make for a partnership based on mutual respect and affection. The matter was well summed up by BenHaMelikVehaNazir Hasdai in 1230 A.D., "Your son at five is your master, at ten your slave, at fifteen your double, and after that your friend or foe, depending on how you bring him up."

YOUTH IN THE PRESENT ERA

As already indicated, one of the main tasks of adolescence, central to the task of becoming an adult, is the establishment of a firm sense of identity, a definition of oneself as a person (Erikson, 1963). If the relationship between parents and adolescent is positive, the process is greatly facilitated, and the young person passes through this critical period with a minimum of conflict and disturbance.

Because of lack of instruction and training, many parents with the best of intentions are not equipped to help their child through this difficult period of his life. Also, parents' own personality problems may handicap them. As a result serious trouble may and frequently does develop.

The idealism of youth, their concern with moral values and standards, is to be encouraged and applauded but is not sufficiently appreciated by adults. "Rap sessions," often extending far into the night, occur among college students and in other places where young people congregate. The most involved moral and philisophical questions are discussed, probably more intensely than they ever will be again. This is not only because young people are idealistic but also because they are struggling to understand their own burgeoning impulses of aggression, sex, etc. They wish to improve society not only to bring it closer into line with the standards they have been taught in their childhood but also to assuage feelings of concern and guilt about their own impulses that they do not understand, have not been brought up to accept, and need to rationalize.

Conflict with society

The present era is difficult for everyone because of the rapid change and technological advance and because of the uncovering of dishonesty and double dealing in high places. The display of chicanery, violence, intergroup hatred, and demagoguery on the television screen in one's own living room intensifies the conflict between ideals and reality. If in addition the parents are viewed as hypocrites who preach one set of values and act according to another, the adolescent, trying to develop his own standards, may become utterly confused.

Many young people not only in the United States but in many countries around the world have become disillusioned with society. The more intelligent and sensitive the adolescent is, the more likely he is to realize the discrepancies between rhetoric and behavior. Parents and counselors must be wise indeed to be able to counter the cynicism that is likely to result. Stage, screen, media, and literature do little to help but too often emphasize negative aspects of behavior and life in general. Optimism about human nature is in short supply.

The idealism of the young is apparent, nevertheless, in their striving for an open society, for more communication among people of varying ages and ethnic groups, for more understanding and love of one's fellowman. It is their disillusionment with the behavior of those in high places, whom they had been taught to emulate and admire, that is in part responsible for the so-called alienation of youth in modern society. Since the word *alienation* comes from the Latin word meaning "other," this condition can be considered as stepping to a "different drummer," to quote Thoreau.

To be expected is the alienation of young and old who suffer from discrimination and deprivation because of race, color, religion, or other difference from the dominant majority. Their poverty, poor education, and lack of resources to share in the luxuries and advantages they see around them are seen as resulting from this discrimination. Quite rightly they resent it, and many, especially when young, act out against it in hostile, even antisocial, behavior. Again it is the sensitive, intelligent youths who are the most angry. The more information they have about advantages others enjoy but they lack, the more alienated they become. Worst of all they may come to accept in part the majority's characterization of them as inferior, with resulting impairment of their self-concept as worthwhile, important human beings. To counter this, encouragement of pride in one's race, culture, sex, or other distinctive background is of great importance. One hopeful sign recently is that cultivation of such pride in

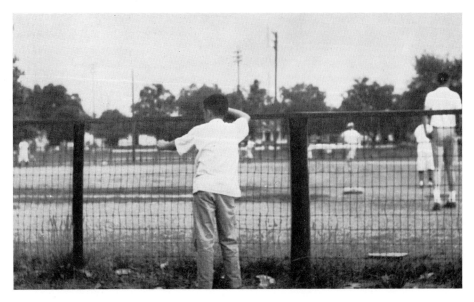

Fig. 8-5. A crisis. Not all crisis interventions occur in situations of conflict. The isolate excluded from participation with other children may be more in need of help than the child who acts out his feelings against society. (From Heckel, R. V., and Jordan, R. M.: Psychology; the nurse and the patient, ed. 2, St. Louis, 1967, The C. V. Mosby Co.)

various groups is occurring. Perhaps we are beginning to learn that conformity to majority customs and ideas is not necessarily a virtue.

Today rebellion among youth is not restricted to the poor and deprived but may and does involve young people from middle and upper class environments. If it is moderate and nonviolent, this disenchantment with life as it is may signal a change for the better when young people reach adulthood and enter positions of prominence in the society. No one can be proud of many things that have been happening—dishonesty in high places, attempted imposition of our standards on others in parts of the world with different cultures, intolerance of disagreement, unconscionable invasions of privacy by bugging and wiretapping. The list could be extended.

In response to their disenchantment, young people react in various ways. Some drop out, leaving college or a job. The communes and hippie groups such as those in the Haight-Ashbury area are examples. These young people are often idealistic and wish to get away from a society that they consider devoted to material gain without consideration for the feelings and well-being of others. They emphasize openness, love, caring, and autonomy or independence. They want their gratifications now, not in some ill-defined distant future.

The difficulty has been that these young people have not usually been autonomous but have had to obtain food and other necessities in some way—from families, part-time menial jobs, or stealing and other antisocial behavior. Probably for this reason more than others, most of the hippie communities did not last. Their successors are more conservative; young people are moving back to the country in increasing numbers, where they live off the land, grow their own food, and become independent as did their ancestors who homesteaded or moved west. The relative scarcity of available land is, of course, a problem.

Another group to be considered is the relatively large number of young men who left the country or went underground rather than fight in what they considered an immoral war in Vietnam. This took courage; many who refused the draft are still expatriates. The country has probably lost some highly intelligent young men, potential leaders, in addition to some who were merely taking advantage of the situation to avoid unpleasant duty.

Other young people, disillusioned with society, have become activists in order to change things of which they disapprove. A majority try to accomplish this by accepted methods; they helped in the 1968 presidential campaign of Eugene McCarthy; when slightly older they participated as interns in government or even ran for Congress and were elected in the 1974 freshman group. They are showing themselves to be more outspoken and active than newly elected congressmen have been in the past. The going is rough, but most of them are continuing the fight and have been reelected.

Radical dissenters, on the other hand, believe that revolutionary changes are necessary to reform this "corrupt" society and are ready to use violence if necessary to bring about change. They assert that the end justifies the means. They reject traditional values and consider themselves a counterculture. Many do not realize that being against a culture merely for the sake of being against it without offering any feasible alternative accomplishes little. To dress in sloppy clothes or refuse to keep clean merely because one's parents or society in general disapproves is showing as much dependency as if one behaves conventionally merely because authority says so. No personal values are involved in either case.

Juvenile delinquency

After this general description of modern adolescents and slightly older youth, a discussion of specific consequences is in order. Emotional problems develop in difficult situations, especially when parents and other persons in authority do not help the young person in his attempts to understand our rapidly changing mores.

Emotional problems may induce depression, withdrawal, or even suicide, which statistics show to be increasing rapidly among people 15 to 30 years of age. These people, unless suicide attempts succeed, often become patients in hospitals or clinics. The nurse with understanding and empathy may be of inestimable value in helping the young person face life again.

When problem behavior of the adolescent is directed outward instead of inward, when he acts out his conflicts, he is likely to come in contact with officials of the law and be termed a delinquent. He does not even need to go outside the home to get in serious trouble, for his parents may take him to court as "incorrigible," "unmanageable," or "out of control." Our standards of conduct for children are more stringent than for adults, who could not be arrested for incorrigibility unless it involved aggravated assault or other criminal behavior. Children can also be brought into court for skipping school or running away from home. These status offenses, not criminal for adults, are supposed to protect the child against himself. Recently there have been legal complaints against these discriminations on the grounds that the child is not permitted due process that would be granted an adult.

In general the rate of delinquency has been increasing at a greater rate than the adolescent population since 1948. In the past boys have been more likely to act out and be brought to court than the more passive girls by a ratio of four or five to one. Their offenses were likely to be aggressive ones involving burglary, larceny, car theft, and malicious mischief; girls were arrested more frequently for incorrigibility, running away, or illicit sexual behavior. (Boys are rarely arrested on similar sex charges.) The ratio of boys to girls is now rapidly changing, with delinquency among girls having increased faster than among boys every year since 1965. Also, girls are now more likely to engage in aggressive offenses similar to those committed by boys.

Compulsory schooling, intended to provide everyone with the opportunity for education, can backfire for the small percentage (but large numbers) of children who do not adjust to school. Approximately 2%, mostly adolescents, drop out of school each year; this can number more than 1,000 a year in a single county. Many more stay but profit little or not at all.

If it is determined that a child is mentally retarded, he may be given special education, although such opportunities are not available in all areas. But, if he has reading problems such as dyslexia or emotional problems, rarely is anything done to help him. He is usually pushed ahead because of his age, regardless of his achievement; he may reach the ninth grade, for example, with first grade reading ability. Then, if he has any sensitivity and courage, he leaves an impossible situation with his self-concept often irreparably damaged. Usually he cannot get a job and may hang around on street corners with the road to delinquency wide open for him. Yet special educators and counselors know well how to remedy many of these problems. Even by purely economic standards this is "penny wise and pound foolish." By humanitarian standards it is tragic.

The relationship of delinquency to emotional problems has long been recognized. The first child guidance clinic in connection with a juvenile court was established in Chicago in 1909 by a psychiatrist, William Healy. This was followed by others, notably the Wayne County Psychopathic Clinic at the juvenile court in Detroit in 1916 (Ives, 1974). In 1912 the first psychological study of institutionalized delinquent girls was initiated at the State Home for Girls in Trenton, New Jersey (Otis, 1960). These were attempts to treat delinquent behavior by psychological methods and are still very much in use today in clinics all over the country.

The nurse, whether she be called a psychiatric, pediatric, or school nurse, is likely to come into contact with the potentially delinquent child, probably before he has been arrested. Therefore she can have a positive influence on the child's behavior in the early stages of his deviance. Training in understanding the child in trouble is of utmost importance to the nurse. In fact, many adolescents in difficulty will confide that they first began to notice they were "different" as soon as they entered school at the age of 5 or 6 years. Here is a great opportunity for the school nurse to gain at a very early age the confidence of the child who is unpopular, a loner, or frightened.

Delinquency is reported to be more prevalent among youths of lower socioeconomic status. Environmental influences may promote delinquent behavior, especially in the urban ghetto or where unemployment is high and young people have little constructive activity during their prolonged leisure. When asked if he could not find companions who did not steal, one 10-year-old boy answered after considerable thought, "I think there's one red-headed boy who lives on the corner two blocks away who does not steal." What can be expected in such circumstances? Boys clubs, scout troups, the Big Brother movement, the Y.M.C.A. and Y.W.C.A., and neighborhood centers may help, but where delinquency is the accepted tradition the boy or girl who does not participate may not be accepted by his peers.

Nevertheless, the proportion of delinquency in deprived areas is undoubtedly exaggerated in the statistics because ghetto youth are more likely to be arrested for minor offenses than middle class youths, who would be taken home to their parents or remanded to them by the court. The incidence of delinquency in suburban affluent neighborhoods is increasing. Affluence does not necessarily bring happy family relationships, and the single most predictive indicator of adolescent delinquency is a poor relationship with parents (Mussen, Conger, and Kagan, 1974, p. 636). Children with a good relationship rarely become delinquent. Also, parents whose social or professional obligations keep them out of the home much of the day and who have little time left to know and understand their children often do not provide sufficient guidance, supervision, or an adequate role model for young people. Adolescents need a stable family unit and parents who are accessible as much as younger children do.

Society has not been successful in treating delinquency, which continues to increase. Punishment or incarceration in so-called correctional institutions usually makes matters worse, embittering the young person and exposing him to more sophisticated deviants who often complete his indoctrination into a life of crime. There may be rare exceptions where the young delinquent comes under the influence of a truly understanding, sensitive, superior counselor, who might be the nurse. But as a rule even good psychiatric or psychological treatment, social casework, or foster home placement offers only temporary remissions before the child goes back into the environment that caused the trouble in the first place. In fact, as a reward

Table 8-2. Drugs commonly used by adolescents on a nonprescriptive basis (this is not intended to be complete but does include commonly utilized drugs)

Drug group	Common name, trade name	Habituating or addictive	Extent of usage
Psychotogenics			
Cannabis sativa	Marijuana (grass, pot, hemp, hash)	No	Extensive in urban areas, especially in late adolescence
Lophophora williamsii	Mescaline, peyote	No	Rare except in border areas and West coast
Psilocybe mexicana	Psilocybin	No	Rare
Ergot derivatives	Lysergic acid (LSD)	No	Widely used, but only rarely on a continuing basis
Stimulants			
Sympathomimetics	Amphetamines (Benzedrine, etc.)	Yes	Widely used among students, especially during exam periods
Analeptics	Pentylenetetrazol	No	Rare
Nicotinics	Nicotine (cigarettes)	Yes	Extensively used, most often initially in imitation of adults
Xanthines	Caffeine (coffee, tea, etc.)	Yes	Culturally approved, widely used
Sedatives, hypnotics			
Barbiturates	Phenobarbital	Yes	Extensive usage, although less popular with advent of tranquilizers and wider usage of marijuana
Bromides	Potassium bromide	No	Rare in adolescents, more common in adulthood
Alcohol	Various beverage forms	Yes	Widespread as a major form of expression of "adult" status in adolescents, especially by high school age
Anesthetics, analgesics			
General anesthetics	Ether, nitrous oxide, chloroform	No	Occasionally used in small amounts to produce high or novel experience; quite dangerous, misuse often causing death
Local anesthetics	Cocaine	Yes	Widely distributed, but only occasionally found in adolescent usage, mainly in late teens
Analgesics	Opium (heroin, morphine)	Yes	A major source of drug abuse in all areas of United States
	Demerol	Yes	Rare in adolescents, common in adult addiction
Psychoactive drugs*			
Phenothiazines	All marketed under various trade names and readily available on prescription basis	Occasionally, especially Librium, Miltown	Often taken for relief of anxiety in imitation of adults
Rauwolfia compounds			Only rarely used today
MAO (monoamine oxidase) inhibitors			Used in imitation of adults, often taken from their supplies to produce a lift

*Many psychoactive drugs are used to offset the effects of other drugs, to reduce hangover, to offset depression after use of marijuana, etc.

for good behavior he is usually sent back home. It is as if medicine cured a person of tuberculosis and then he was sent back into an environment where the disease was rampant.

The drug problem

One situation that has aggravated the tendency toward increased delinquency is the current excessive use of psychoactive drugs. Whereas previously this was largely an adult problem, now such substances are readily available to adolescents and even to children. No social class, race, or religious group is immune. Various drugs commonly used by adolescents are given in Table 8-2.

Causes of the upsurge in drug use are many and involved. One explanation is that our society is increasingly a drug culture. According to television advertisements, drugs are a cure for almost anything; just take a pill and your trouble will vanish. The prescribed use of tranquilizers and "pep pills" (amphetamines) is widespread and far in excess of what patients really need. When young people see television messages and notice that their parents take a pill for almost any slight discomfort or worry, they are more inclined to do likewise, although the drugs they use are usually different from those their parents approve.

Young people do not at first realize the danger of some of the drugs they are encouraged by peers or pushers to use until they have become psychologically dependent or physiologically addicted; by then it is often too late to stop. Parents become extremely emotional and confused about the entire drug problem. They become very upset over the use of marijuana, for example, which the older generation made illegal as long ago as the 1930's. Yet so far as research to date shows, marijuana is not so dangerous to the user or to the community as alcohol or nicotine, both of which may be legally used to excess. Marijuana is confused with the much more dangerous narcotics and is even legally called a narcotic although this is not scientifically true. All this confusion aggravates the problem and gives young people an opportunity to point out the hypocrisy and even falsehood of adult reactions.

Now the National Institute of Alcohol and Alcoholism reports that 9 million Americans are alcoholics and that only about one tenth of these are receiving treatment. The drinking of alcohol was forbidden in the United States two generations ago with very bad results in the rise of crime, bootlegging, and deaths or psychosis from toxic alcohols consumed when nothing else was available. Evidently we learned little or nothing from this "noble experiment" in our handling of the new addictions.

Another unfortunate outcome of adult preoccupation with drugs is the administration of tranquilizers, amphetamines, and other drugs to hyperactive children in school. Often this is done without adequate examination to determine whether the child is minimally brain damaged, has a physical problem requiring medication, or is emotionally troubled and in need of understanding and counseling instead. In these instances a compassionate professional

nurse may be of inestimable value in seeing to it that no drugs are administered without careful medical screening.

The transition from a prescribed pill to an illegal one is easy, and deeper causes are often hidden. In Vietnam, where drugs were readily available, many young men became accustomed to using marijuana and harder drugs to escape from the hardships they were enduring, and they brought back their habits with them. Our increased contact with Asian and other sources of illicit drugs caused importation to escalate, thus increasing ease of access to potential users in the United States.

Simple curiosity may occasionally start the adolescent on the use of drugs since young people like to experiment and "try everything once." It may be at first a rebellion against adult constraints. However, when it persists to the point of dependence or addiction, it usually reflects deep distress, unhappiness, and emotional conflict. As S. Rado says, psychological investigation of drug addiction "begins with the recognition of the fact that not the toxic agent but the impulse to use it makes the addict" (Wieder and Kaplan, 1975, p. 348). Again it must be stressed that where there is communication and a positive, mutually trusting relationship between generations drug abuse is much less likely. When one intelligent former heroin addict was asked how parents could behave differently so that young people would not become addicted he replied, "Well, ma'am, it would help if they'd talk with us, not at us."

Marijuana

The large majority of adolescents who have experimented with illicit drugs have used marijuana. It has been reported that by 1972 at least 24 million persons in this country had used the drug and that 51% of college students report having tried it (Mussen, Conger, and Kagan, 1974, p. 624). For most of these it is experimental only and does not lead to psychological dependence. It is not addictive. In normal dosage its physical effects are not remarkable: an increase in pulse rate, some alteration of blood pressure, and a minimal loss in muscle strength and steadiness. It promotes relaxation and enjoyment in emotionally stable people who are among friends. As one young user said, "When I'm depressed and hate the world, if I sit in a circle with my friends and smoke pot, I feel happy, forget my troubles, and love everybody."

Low doses of alcohol and marijuana seem to have similar effects (Wieder and Kaplan, 1975). Historically, when alcohol has been proscribed by religious law, marijuana or hashish replaces it. Younger adolescents, moreover, seem to prefer marijuana, which is not so diffuse and overwhelming to them as alcohol. Certainly it has not in this country proved as dangerous to public safety as alcohol.

Use of marijuana does not lead to the use of stronger drugs except that, since it is illegal, it introduces the user to pushers and underworld characters. Once known to these people, the young person can more easily be influenced to experiment further. Were marijuana to be decriminalized, this hazard would be minimized.

In larger amounts or if cannabis, the effective chemical, is isolated and given in concentrated doses, this substance can produce effects similar to those of hallucinogenic drugs. In unstable individuals excessive anxiety, suspiciousness, or even paranoid ideation may result. Similar behavior can result from alcohol intoxication.

Other psychotogenics

The psychotogenic drugs are so named because they produce psychotic symptoms, including hallucinations, delusions, grandiosity, euphoria, and feelings of unreality. Best known are LSD trips. Mescaline, peyote, and psilocybin are less frequently used.

Toxic psychotic effects may also be produced by the sniffing of various chemical substances such as glue, gasoline, and cleaning fluid. These may produce permanent brain damage and are therefore extremely dangerous.

LSD trips may lead to experiences of a sense of timelessness, vivid panoramic visual hallucinations, and the illusion that superior and lasting insights are emerging. Changes in body image lead to subjective experiences of fusion or union with others (Idem, p. 352). It may be the drug of choice for those who cannot break their shell of isolation without pharmacologic help. On the other hand, it may also produce enhanced feelings of isolation, depersonalization, and panic. It may lead to an acute psychosis.

Barbiturates, tranquilizers, and amphetamines

Barbiturates, tranquilizers, and amphetamines are often prescribed and are overused by adults as well as by adolescents. The young person may find these pills in the family medicine chest, and such an experience may go far to convince him that drugs are all right to take.

In the United States the barbiturates, prescribed as sleeping pills, account for more than 3,000 deaths a year from overdose (Mussen, Conger & Kagan, 1974). They are addictive and after a period of brief relaxation act as a depressant. Continued usage results in intellectual impairment.

The amphetamines (speed), while not physiologically addictive, are extremely dangerous physically. Sophisticated drug users leave them alone, for they know that "speed kills." They are nevertheless used by too many young people as an energizer and may be alternated with the depressing barbiturates in a vicious cycle. Amphetamines, Methedrine, and cocaine diminish awareness of fatigue; increase feelings of assertiveness, self-esteem, and restlessness; and decrease judgment and accuracy. If amphetamines are taken in combination with alcohol, as has been done even by college students preparing for examinations, the fatal potential is increased.

Anesthetics and analgesics: opiates and cocaine

Until recently the most dangerous of drugs, the opiates and cocaine, were largely confined to the most depressed sections of society. But now heroin, originally synthesized to help patients withdraw from morphine, has become widely used by middle class young people as well. It has been known as the "drug of despair." As do the other opiates and the synthetic methadone, it produces a state of quiet lethargy following a brief euphoria. The user is no longer involved with external reality, withdraws, and can shut out his pain while having fantasies of wish fulfillment and self-sufficiency.

Tolerance develops quickly, and the dosage must be continually increased. This leads to addiction with the urgent need to obtain the drug whatever the cost and the ever greater possibility of overdosage and death. Persons under its influence are not likely to commit acts of violence, but they may steal or push drugs on others to obtain money for this extremely expensive habit. Young girls, some in their early teens, may resort to prostitution to obtain the means to buy the drug. Criminal sanctions are stringent for mere possession of the drug, to say nothing of pushing it or stealing to obtain the money. The adolescent who uses heroin has placed himself in a situation dangerous to his health, his freedom, and eventually his life. Once he is addicted, withdrawal is difficult and probably will involve submission to one of the long-term residential treatment programs. These are arduous, and many young addicts cannot tolerate them, leave the program, and continue on their self-destructive course.

The prospect for controlling drug use is not encouraging. The peak year was 1969, after which the number of drug abusers abated. But the latest information is that the number is rising again. All of us who work with people can help to dissuade those who are tempted to use drugs or who have already started. Educational programs for parents and children that involve physicians, nurses, psychologists, social workers, teachers, and others will help. Most help of all is communication among peers, between parents and children, and between teachers and students with mutual respect for each other and a lack of patronizing lecturing. Persons who have had drug problems themselves and have conquered the habit are of inestimable value in working with those trying to break away. They can enforce strict discipline and give advice and caring warmth without causing resentment and negative reactions on the part of those they try to help. Of course the ex-addict himself must be a caring person if his interaction is to be effective.

Available help

To want to change patterns of behavior and achieve an acceptable self-direction in his life, the adolescent must have the desire to change his behavior. Communities vary in the help they can provide. Of course, the psychiatrist or psychologist in private practice can provide individual counseling and therapy. There are often community mental health centers in which there is a team, usually composed of a psychiatrist or psychologist, a social worker, and often a psychiatric nurse. There the adolescent may have individual or group therapy or both. In group therapy, problems are worked out in

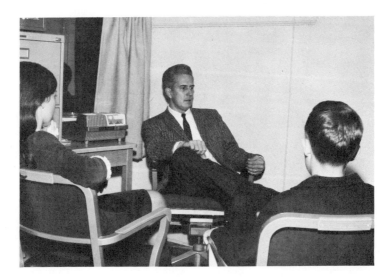

Fig. 8-6. Group psychotherapy with adolescents. Treatment of the problems of young children may involve active play, especially when the child is too young to express his feelings verbally.

conjunction with others. Information is fed back to each individual from other persons, showing him or telling him how his behaviors affect others in the group. Only rarely is it possible to develop the full degree of understanding and insight into the rights, privileges, and feelings of others that can be attained in group psychotherapy.

Sometimes help can be secured from the outpatient services of a psychiatric hospital. In addition, there are crisis intervention centers that care for situational problems for no longer than a 6-week period. They help the individual to be able to function normally again in society.

SUMMARY

Emphasis upon the teenage period is a relatively recent development, although conflict between generations and complaints of older persons about youthful behavior go back thou-

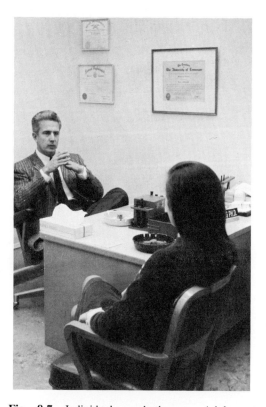

Fig. 8-7. Individual psychotherapy. Adolescent counseling usually involves a face-to-face relationship in which problems are discussed and verbally shared.

sands of years. Now there is recognition that the years following puberty constitute a period of stress for most young people. Major physiological changes take place; there is a rapid acceleration of growth, and the body image changes; the capacity for logical thinking increases and develops; and new instinctual urges, especially the sexual, burgeon. Psychologically the adolescent seeks to emancipate himself from his family and become independent. His interests move away from the home; the opinions of outsiders, especially peers, become important.

While all this is going on the understanding, trust, and tolerance of the parents is of great importance but often in short supply. Parents realistically expect the young person to be able to accept more responsibility but at the same time may surround him with restrictions, deny reasonable privileges, and resent his striving for independence. In contrast to earlier days the adolescent often must remain financially dependent well into adulthood while he completes a college education or, if he leaves school early, while he hunts for scarce jobs. Unemployment among young people, especially in minority groups in the cities or for those with less than a high school education, is extremely high.

Most young people pass through this difficult period successfully and eventually become fairly well adjusted as adults. It is essential that every young person develop a sense of his own identity, know who he is as a separate and different individual. This process is greatly facilitated when communication between generations remains open, where there is loving concern, tolerance, trust, and understanding. With the rapid changes in mores that characterize the present era, many older people themselves find it difficult to adjust and thus are of comparatively little help to their children, who are also confused and uncertain.

In evaluating the situation it is important to realize that young people today are perhaps more idealistic than their predecessors. They value honesty and openness in interpersonal relations; they do not have so many inhibitions; they believe in allowing the individual to develop his own standards without too much interference from authority, whether parental, societal, or religious. If this trend continues, there may be a real advance in civilization when this generation assumes positions of power. Nevertheless it makes it more difficult for youth today to tolerate the dishonesty, misuse of power, and self-seeking that have been uncovered in high places.

Therefore too large a minority have become alienated. This may be understood in part as a reaction against the unfairness of society on the part of those subject to discrimination or deprivation. But many of the disenchanted have not been deprived but have rejected the contemporary American value system with its emphasis on materialism, its involvement in wars all over the world, and its denial of social justice to special groups. These young people want to change the system, often by conventional means, sometimes by "dropping out." A minority, usually those whose relationships with parents and other authorities have been troubled, have despaired of bringing about change without violence and revolution. This group, while comparatively small, receives more than its share of publicity.

This situation may be in part responsible for the increasing incidence of juvenile delinquency. Also unemployment, deprivation, failures in school, and decreased respect for authority are important causation factors. Paradoxically, increased freedom for minorities and women's liberation may also play a part. The rate of delinquency among girls has risen much faster than among boys although it has not yet reached the same level. All of our efforts at treating delinquency, whether by punishment or psychological or social methods, have so far proved ineffectual. It must be stressed again that satisfactory parent-child relations and mutual trust (beginning in infancy) seem to provide the best preventative.

The increasing use of psychoactive drugs among youth is a highly disturbing problem for which no adequate solution has been found. The drugs used range from the relatively innocuous such as caffeine and aspirin through the medium range such as marijuana to the highly dangerous sedatives, depressants, and narcotics. Some of these are used to escape from pain and distress, to overcome feelings of unworthiness by bringing dreams of omnipotence and creative excellence, to overcome feelings of isolation and alienation with a sense of fusion and merging with others, or to find meaningful personal experiences or unusual sensory delights in an otherwise bleak existence. The pattern of drug use is not random; different drugs are used to satisfy different needs. A better understanding of the relationships between personality problems and choice of drug might facilitate a solution to this serious problem. Continuing education of all those involved with young people, including physicians and nurses, is imperative.

REFERENCES

Ambron, S. R.: Child development, Corte Madera, Calif., 1975, Rinehart Press.

Anthony, E. J.: Two contrasting types of adolescent depression and their treatment. In Esman, A. H., editor: The psychology of adolescence: Essential readings, New York, 1975, International Universities Press.

Bernard, J. S.: In Duvall, E. M., and Duvall, S. M., editors: Sex ways in fact and faith, New York, 1961, Association Press.

Block, J. H.: Reconceptualizing some psychological constructs in view of recent research on sex roles. Unpublished paper presented at District of Columbia Psychological Association meeting, December, 1975.

Blos, P.: In Esman, A. H., editor: The psychology of adolescence: Essential readings, New York, 1975, International Universities Press.

Curtis, J.: Working mothers, Reviewed in Washington Post, January 15, 1976.

Developmental psychology today, Del Mar, Calif., 1971, Communications Research Machines, Inc.

Douvan, E.: Commitment and social contract in adolescence, Psychiatry **37:**22, February, 1974.

Erikson, E. H.: Youth, change, and challenge, New York, 1963, Basic Books, Inc.

Gesell, A., Ilg, F. L., and Ames, L. B.: Youth, the years ten to sixteen, New York, 1956, Harper & Row, Publishers.

Gimpel, H.: Group work with adolescent girls, Nurs. Outlook **16:**47, April, 1968.

Gordon, J. E.: Personality and behavior, New York, 1963, The Macmillan Co.

Heald, F., editor: Adolescent nutrition and growth, New York, 1969, Meredith Corp.

Heckel, R. V.: Shifting patterns of affections; transitional figures, Ment. Hyg. **48:**451, July, 1964.

Hurlock, E. Developmental psychology, ed. 4, New York, 1975, McGraw-Hill Book Co.

Inhelder, B., and Piaget, J.: The growth of logical thinking from childhood to adolescence, New York, 1959, Basic Books, Inc.

Ives, M.: History of public service in psychology. Unpublished paper presented at American Psychological Association convention, September, 1974.

Jersild, A. T.: The psychology of adolescence, New York, 1963, Macmillan, Inc.

Kinsey, A. C., Pomeroy, W. B., and Martin, C. E.: Sexual behavior in the human male, Philadelphia, 1948, W. B. Saunders Co.

Kinsey, A. C., Pomeroy, W. B., Martin, C. E., and Gebhard, P. H.: Sexual behavior in the human female, Philadelphia, 1953, W. B. Saunders Co.

McCandless, B. R.: Children and adolescents, New York, 1961, Holt, Rinehart & Winston, Inc.

McCary, J. L.: Human sexuality, ed. 2, New York, 1973, Van Nostrand Reinhold Co.

Miller, E.: Adolescence; on the road to womanhood, Nurs. Outlook **8:**505, September, 1960.

Muensterberger, W.: The adolescent in society. In Esman, A. H., editor: The psychology of adolescence: Essential readings, New York, 1975, International Universities Press.

Mussen, P. H., Conger, J. J., and Kagan, J.: Child development and personality, ed. 4, New York, 1974, Harper & Row, Publishers.

Otis, M.: Psychological studies at the state home for girls, 1912-1914. In David, H. P., editor: The welfare reporter: Fifty years of psychological studies in the New Jersey State Department of Institutions and Agencies, Trenton, N.J., 1960, New Jersey State Department of Institutions & Agencies.

Rakinovitch, R.: Psychology of adolescence, Pediatr. Clin. North Am. **7:**65, 1960.

Rosenthal, M. S., and Rothner, I.: Drugs, parents, and children, New York, 1973, The New American Library, Inc.

Schonfield, W.: Body image in adolescence? A psychiatric concept for the pediatrician, Pediatrics **31:**845, 1963.

Smith, B. S.: Child psychology, New York, 1973, Appleton-Century-Crofts.

Spindler, E. D.: Better diets for teen-agers, Nurs. Outlook **12:**32, February, 1964.

Stare, F.: Good nutrition from food, not pills, Am. J. Nurs. **65:**86, February, 1964.

Stearns, G.: Nutritional health of infants, children, and adolescents, Proceedings of National Food and Nutrition Institute (agricultural handbook No. 56), Washington, D.C., 1952, U.S. Department of Agriculture.

Strang, R.: The adolescent views himself, New York, 1957, McGraw-Hill Book Co.

Taylor, K. W.: Do adolescents need parents? New York, 1938, Appleton-Century-Crofts.

Weider, H., and Kaplan, E. H.: Drug use in adolescence: Psychodynamic meaning and pharmacogenic effect. In Esman, A. H., editor: The psychology of adolescence: Essential readings, New York, 1975, International Universities Press.

9

PROMOTION OF HEALTH

Because of the ever increasing emphasis on promotion of health, this chapter is devoted to this subject. The nurse may see the child at home, in a well child conference, in a special clinic, at school, at camp, or in a physician's office. When the nurse cares for the ill child in the hospital the nursing care plan for the child should include guidance toward optimum health as well as help with the problem that brought him to the hospital.

In the following pages, first an introduction is given to health assessment and promotion. This includes a guide sheet for general information about the child's family, their health, and the child's previous health history. Also included are suggestions for establishing the climate for health assessment, suggested observations of environmental conditions to note during a home visit, and interpersonal relationships for which to watch. These factors help in the understanding of the child so the nurse can give the best service to the child.

Specific health assessment guides and suggestions for pertinent health guidance at different age levels are given in each section of this chapter: infancy, toddler and preschool period, middle childhood, and adolescence.

To give optimum health guidance the nurse needs to know as much as possible about the child and his environment as well as available health services and resources in the community. Because of her knowledge of health, the school nurse may be used as a resource person for teachers who have the responsibility for health instruction.

Guides for information and assessment

Fig. 9-1 is a guide for general information about the child and his parents. It could be used in a setting outside the hospital. It is important to know whether the child is living with one or both parents, whether he has siblings, the educational background of his parents, the language spoken in the home, and the health of parents and siblings. Before deciding what health guidance may be necessary, not only is general information about the family necessary but also the health history and general health status of the child. Through observation in a well child conference or elsewhere, some understanding of the parent-child relationship can be deduced. If a home visit is made, the environmental conditions in which the child lives can be noted.

A suggested guide for physical assessment of children of different age levels is included in each section of this chapter (Figs. 9-2, 9-13, 9-19, and 9-20). With the guide is also a suggested form to use in obtaining information about the child's general development, hygiene, and interests, together with a list of pertinent health topics for guidance of children of varying developmental levels.

A physical examination guide is used most often in a well child conference as one way of knowing whether a child is growing and developing as expected. Another reason for its use is to see whether there is any abnormality that needs medical attention. If so, the nurse refers the child to a physician.

Even when a physical examination is not actually performed in a home visit, the nurse can learn to observe closely, to listen carefully, and to watch for any indication that suggests deviation from good health and expected growth and development.

Role of the nurse in establishing climate for health assessment

The appearance of the nurse, her posture, and her facial expression all have meaning to the child's mother or caretaker. Since one assumes

160

GENERAL INFORMATION

Name of child _____ Birthdate _____ Sex _____ Address _____

Parent	Age	Race	Nationality	Occupation	Education in years	Religion	Living in home?

Siblings

Names	Age	Grade in school	Health status (good, poor)

Other members of household

Name	Age	Relationship

Who usually takes care of the child? _____

Health history of family:

Hypertension, diabetes, heart disease, cancer, health problems of parent and/or children

Health history of the child:

Mother's prenatal care: None _____ Private doctor _____ Public health clinic _____

Other _____

Length of pregnancy _____

Prenatal complications: None _____ Toxemia _____ High blood pressure _____

Hemorrhage _____ Other _____

Length of labor _____

Delivery by: Physician _____ Midwife _____ Other _____

Place: Home _____ Hospital _____ Other _____

Type: Spontaneous _____ Other _____

Weight at birth _____ Length _____

Health at birth: Good _____ Breathing difficulty _____ Blood transfusion _____

Convulsions _____ Jaundice _____ Other _____

Illnesses of this child _____

Immunizations and ages at which given _____

_____

Fig. 9-1. Assessment form.

that the nurse likes people, the opportunity to see and talk to the family members should bring pleasure to her. A cheerful nurse dressed in a well-fitting uniform with her hair neatly done and a healthy glow to her skin is apt to convey a feeling of strength and well-being. The smile, the posture, and the manner of the nurse in speaking or gesturing can convey interest in the patient and gladness in seeing her. Throughout her contact with the family, the nurse must remember that her facial expression and her tone of voice can communicate acceptance or rejection; it can communicate her interest just as much as anything she says.

The relationship between the mother and the nurse influences the child; if the mother accepts the nurse, the child is more apt to do so.

Much of the communication to a young child is of a nonverbal type. Because the infant distinguishes between strange and familiar people by 6 months of age, the nurse might let the mother hold the infant while she examines him; however, smiling at the infant and talking to him helps him to get used to other faces and people than his mother and to associate pleasure with it. A great deal relative to the child's development, health, and interpersonal relationships can be observed without handling the infant and young child. It takes a baby or young child time to get used to the newcomer: the nurse. If the nurse offers a rattle or toy to the infant, the latter may smile and/or vocalize.

To gain the cooperation of infants and young children, a gentle voice, touch, and manner are helpful. Sudden, abrupt movements are to be avoided. Further familiarity with an object helps dispel fear. Even an infant can finger the stethoscope or otoscope. Watching the light in the otoscope go on and off is of interest to most children regardless of their age. The nurse might take a young child's doll and pretend to examine the ears and listen to the chest.

For a nurse to pat the doll or teddy bear of the toddler or preschool child denotes her affection for the child. The teddy bear or doll is very real to the child: a live person. To misuse the child's favorite toy or toss it aside roughly is viewed by the child as a direct hurt to him.

To further gain the preschool child's and older child's cooperation the nurse can use a more direct approach. She can introduce herself and

explain what she is going to do. She can make friends with him before doing the examination. It might be helpful to learn the child's interests and general hygiene as indicated on the health assessment guide for his age level. Even with a toddler or older infant, getting information from the mother about general hygiene and care gives time for the young child to get used to the presence of the nurse.

Of course, the school-age child and adolescent can give the nurse much of the information himself, but he too needs time to learn to trust a new person in order to communicate well. Giving information about school, a pet, and recreational activities may help the older child to see that the nurse is interested in him. This helps in establishing rapport. The schoolchild may view the nurse with real interest. The nurse should explain who she is and why she is present.

The fact that the preadolescent and adolescent are interested in their bodies and want to be "all right" is helpful to the nurse in explaining the physical examination and in giving health guidance.

The adolescent may feel he can talk more freely to the nurse in the latter's office than he can at home where there are others present. The adolescent can accept more responsibility for his own health than the younger child can. If a feeling of trust exists, the adolescent girl may be more willing to attend family planning clinics. It is important for the adolescent to feel the nurse is his or her nonjudgmental friend.

Home visit

On a home visit the nurse has the opportunity to see the physical characteristics of the child's environment, the mother-child relationship, and the health of the particular child whom she came to see. She has the opportunity to inquire about the health of the other members of the family. Of course, basic information about the family may have already been obtained when the child was in the clinic or on a previous home visit.

Physical environment: cleanliness, safety, neatness

These factors can be judged by the locale of the home, its appearance, the home furnishings, and the outside yard if there is one. Before she enters the home the nurse can observe factors in the environment such as housing, sewage disposal, and water supply. If any of these is judged to be unsafe, she can refer these matters to the sanitarian in the local health agency. The nurse can also see if there are screens on the windows to protect the family from flies and mosquitoes.

If there is a yard, is it safe for the children or are there glass and debris that could be harmful? If there is no yard, where do the children play? Perhaps there is a nearby park.

Inside the home the nurse can look for signs of rodent infestation. If there is a toddler or crawling infant, the nurse should particularly look at the living room and kitchen for potential hazards to the child. The small child or infant puts everything in his mouth. It is necessary for insecticides, bleaches, cleaning agents, medicines, and the like to have covers fastened securely and to be placed on a shelf out of reach.

The general appearance of the mother or both parents and children gives some idea of cleanliness and neatness. Clothes may be faded and old but clean and neat.

The furnishings of the house may be sparse but adequately clean. On the other hand, they may be the reverse, with a pile of soiled clothes in the corner. Whether there is a separate bed for the child and whether there is a refrigerator are pertinent facts to know. Are there any play materials for the child? If so, are the child's possessions placed in a separate drawer or box? Is there a hook within the child's reach for his towel and his coat or outdoor clothing? Is there a small chair for the child? In other words, is the home planned with the child's needs in mind or just the parent's? Of course, lack of funds may be the reason for no separate bed or play materials. If necessary, a referral to family and child welfare services can be made.

Mother-child relationship

Spontaneous warmth and friendliness of the child toward the nurse when she enters the home is a good omen because in order to have positive feelings toward others the child has to have experienced affection himself. Congenial laughter shows a certain amount of relaxation, a lack of tenseness.

Does the child talk to the mother or approach her? Is clinging behavior seen, or does the child perhaps simply stand near her? Does the child stand near the mother when a stranger comes into the home? In turn, what does the mother say about the child or to the child, and what does she do in the nurse's presence? Does the mother show any kind of affection to the small toddler such as patting him or lifting him into her lap? What tone of voice does she use in speaking to the child? Does she participate in her child's play? Does she spontaneously tell the nurse some of his activities and accomplishments? It is significant if the nurse has found the child playing outside the home and the screen door of the house locked. Does the mother not want to be disturbed by the children? Inside the house, was the child in a separate room with the door shut or was he with his mother?

Children need to feel a warmth of affection, a sense of belonging, a chance at achievement, and recognition. These psychological needs are met differently at varying ages. Does the home environment of this particular child provide for the psychological needs of the child?

Crossness and irritability to the children might be due to ill health of the mother, financial worries, or fatigue. Although the nurse may have come to visit the home because of a child's presence there, she should see if there is any way the mother herself needs help. To the degree that the mother's needs are met, the child's are more likely to be met. Possibly referral to an appropriate agency for financial assistance is indicated; if the family lives in the country, the suggestion that foods costs might be reduced if the family were to grow a vegetable garden may be helpful. If the mother feels fatigued, perhaps the nurse and the mother can discuss the organization of the mother's day so that she will have adequate rest. It would probably not be effective for the nurse to say, "Get 8 hours of sleep at night and you'll feel better." The mother may think, "Oh, if I only could!"

The mother needs recreation also, preferably with her husband. If just once a week she can get away from the children and home and do something that gives her pleasure, it helps her mental hygiene. One interest outside the family is helpful, such as membership in a club or church group. On the other hand, going to a neighbor's house to chat awhile provides some recreation.

After one contact with the family it is wrong for the nurse to assume that she really understands family relationships. What she sees and interprets is a first impression. Several contacts with the family might change her first impression.

Summary

There is an increasing emphasis on the importance of teaching health promotion. To do this best it is helpful to have information about the parents, siblings, and other members of the family group. In addition, a health history of the child is important. Fig. 9-1 is a suggested guide for obtaining this information. A physical assessment of the child's present health and a knowledge of his development, interests, and general hygiene help give a basis for needed health guidance. An understanding of the home environment (perhaps from a home visit and/or an understanding of family relationships) aids the nurse in her plan for teaching. Good communication and rapport between the nurse and her clients is particularly vital if teaching is to be effective. Health guidance varies according to the interest of the mother and/or child, their level of understanding, and the age of the child. Suggested health topics for guidance are given as part of the health assessment forms. A detailed discussion of health promotion and guidance at different stages of growth (infancy, toddler and preschool period, middle childhood, and adolescence) is given in each of the following sections of this chapter.

PROMOTION OF HEALTH IN INFANCY (28 DAYS TO 1 YEAR)
Health problems

Health problems of infants under 1 year of age, in terms of mortality, are shown on Table 9-1. After certain causes of mortality in early infancy, congenital anomalies rank second, symptoms of ill-defined diseases third, influenza and pneumonia fourth, and then accidents. In studying Table 9-1 one may see that the particular problem causing the greatest number of deaths is congenital anomalies; with

Table 9-1. Deaths under 1 year and infant mortality rates in United States, 1973*

Cause of death†	Number	Rate‡
Certain causes of mortality in early infancy (760-769.2, 769.4-772, 774-778)	30,391	968.8
Asphyxia of newborn, unspecified (776.9)	5,380	171.5
Immaturity, unqualified (777)	5,369	171.2
Hyaline membrane disease (776.1)	4.467	142.4
Respiratory distress syndrome (776.2)	4,091	130.4
Birth injury without mention of cause (772)	1,852	59.0
Condition of placenta (770)	1,318	42.0
Congenital anomalies (740-759)	8,953	285.4
Symptoms and ill-defined conditions (780-796)	4,208	134.1
Influenza and pneumonia (470-474, 480-486)	3,562	113.5
Influenza (470-474)	52	1.7
Pneumonia (480-486)	3,510	111.9
Accidents (E800-E949)	1,691	53.9
Inhalation or ingestion of food or other object causing obstruction or suffocation (E911, E912)	485	15.5
Accidental mechanical suffocation (E913)	336	10.7
Septicemia (038)	805	25.7
Diarrheal diseases (009)	648	20.7
Meningitis (320)	492	15.7
Hernia and intestinal obstruction (550-553, 560)	477	15.2

*Modified from Summary Report Final Mortality Statistics, Rockville, Md., 1973, Public Health Service, U.S. Department of Health, Education, and Welfare (Table 10).
†According to International classification of diseases, eighth revision, 1965.
‡Per 100,000 live births in specified group.

asphyxia, unqualified immaturity, hyaline membrane disease, respiratory disease syndrome, and pneumonia next in consecutive order. Since asphyxia, immaturity, and hyaline membrane disease are usually associated with the neonate, the problems of congenital anomalies and pneumonia loom very large during the later infancy period. Accidents accounted for well over 1,000 deaths.

Congenital malformations need early identification and treatment, whereas accidents may possibly be prevented through anticipatory teaching. When the infant is ill, as with respiratory infections, he needs prompt medical attention. People who have colds or respiratory conditions should not handle the infant. The infant under 1 year of age has little resistance to infections.

Factors that relate to the role of the nurse in promoting the general health of the infant are discussed on the following pages.

Assessment of health

The nurse assesses the health of the infant to see if he is growing and developing normally, to see if there are unusual findings that should be referred to a physician, and to better see what guidance she may need to give the parents to further promote the infant's health. A suggested guide is given in Fig. 9-2.

The well infant has a clear skin, bright eyes, and an interested expression. He cries very little. He has a good appetite and sleeps with his mouth closed. His bowel movements are of normal color, number, and consistency. (For description of stools, see p. 406.) The infant gains steadily in height, weight, and ability to do things. In assessing his health a physical examination should be done, development should be noted, and information about general hygiene and care should be obtained. Appendix A provides milestones in development and suggested guidance at various months. Familiarity with norms of development is essential for the nurse. Norms are important in judging wide deviations. Motor, social, language, and adaptive behavior are all evaluated in judging the infant's developmental level. Mental development of the infant is judged by his general developmental abilities in social, motor, language, and adaptive behavior.

In a physical examination measurements are taken of the height, weight, and circumference of the head, chest and abdomen. (See Figs. 6-3 and 6-4 for percentile charts for measurements of weight, length, and head circumference.) Infants whose measurements are below the tenth percentile or above the ninetieth percentile are unusual.

In general the circumference of the head is the largest part of the body at birth, but by 6 months the circumferences of the head, chest, and abdomen are about the same. By 1 year of age the circumference of the chest is larger than that of the head. In successive examinations it is important to note if the infant is growing taller and heavier or remains the same. Also, is the head enlarging or are the measurements the same? On the other hand, if the head circumference grows more than 2 cm. in 1 month, it should be reported. This may indicate developing hydrocephalus (excessive amount of cerebrospinal fluid in the head). The infant may have microcephalus (a small brain that is arrested in development). If measurements have remained the same, in addition it should be noted whether the head is symmetrical or if it has an odd shape. Is the head brachycephalic and has it a flat occiput as seen in children with Down's syndrome? The most frequent cause of craniosynostosis (premature closing of the sutures) is premature closing of the sagittal suture that results in a long, boat-shaped head, a condition that does not allow the brain room to expand. This as well as hydrocephalus can be corrected so that brain damage does not result.

Still focusing on the head, the character of the fontanels should be noted. The posterior fontanel usually closes by 2 months and the anterior between 12 and 18 months. If open, are they depressed, bulging, full? The amount a fontanel is open should be noted (1 by 2 cm., etc.). A bulging fontanel is usually indicative of increased intracranial pressure.

Other observations of the head include the condition of the scalp, the hair, and any swellings in any area of the head such as caput succedaneum. The amount of hair an infant has varies. Some have a lot; others have little. If hair is present except at the back of the head, the infant may have been left on his back for long periods of time and worn off his hair.

The facial expression and responsiveness are noted as well as whether the face is symmetrical on both sides. This is best observed while the infant is smiling, laughing, or crying.

The skin of the infant should be observed for tissue turgor, rashes, bruises, moles, swellings, or discoloration. Dryness of the skin and mucous membranes should be noted. Rashes should be described by location, whether macular or papular, whether infected, etc.

Text continued on p. 172.

SECTION 1: PHYSICAL EXAMINATION

Directions: Fill in blanks with appropriate information.

MEASUREMENTS

Height _____ Weight _____ Respirations _____ Blood pressure _____

Circumference: Head _____ Chest _____ Abdomen _____

SKIN

Color _____ Tissue turgor _____ Bruises _____ Rash _____

Moles _____ Other _____

SENSORY DEVELOPMENT
Eyes

General observations: Color _____

Expression: Dull _____ Bright _____

Inflammation: Eyes _____ Eyelids _____

Discharge: Right _____ Left _____

Dried secretions on eyelids: Right _____ Left _____

Pupils react equally to light: Right _____ Left _____

Focus on object _____ Follow moving object _____

Strabismus (Observe position of light reflected in cornea; should be in center of each pupil.):

   Right _____ Left _____

Ears
(Use otoscope as necessary.)

Normal configuration and position _____ Other _____

External ear normal _____ Cysts, malformations _____

Pain: Right _____ Left _____

Canal: Clean _____ Wax _____ Foreign body _____ Discharge _____

   Other _____

Tympanic membrane color (normally gray) _____ Handle of malleus visualized _____

Concave eardrum _____ Cone of light reflex (from otoscope) fans out externally _____

Hearing (Shake bell or rattle behind child, first on one side, then the other.): Right _____ Left _____

Nose

Nostrils patent (Close one nostril with finger and observe breathing through other nostril.):

   Right _____ Left _____

Dried secretions _____ Discharge (describe): Right _____ Left _____

Fig. 9-2. Guide for health assessment of infant.

SECTION 1: PHYSICAL EXAMINATION—cont'd

Mouth and throat

(Use tongue depressor and flashlight as necessary.)

Lips: Moist _____ Dry _____ Cracked _____

Mouth breathing _____ History of snoring when asleep _____

Condition of gums _____ Buccal membrane _____

Teeth: Number _____ Condition _____

Pharynx clearly visible _____ Exudate on tonsils _____

Tonsils: Inflamed _____ Obstructing view of pharynx _____

Soft and hard palate intact _____

HEAD

Shape: Symmetrical _____ Other _____

Scalp: Smooth _____ Dry _____ Scaly _____ Sores _____ Swelling _____

Protrusion _____

Hair: Texture (fine, coarse) _____ Dandruff _____

Fontanels: Posterior: Closed _____ Open _____ Anterior: Closed _____

Open _____ Characteristics if open: Normal _____ Full _____ Bulging _____

Depressed _____

Control of head: Raises head when prone _____ Lags when sitting up _____ Holds erect

and steady _____

Face: Alert expression _____ Other _____

Symmetrical (note when infant is crying or laughing) _____ Rash _____

NECK

Supple (full range of motion) _____ Symmetrical _____

Lymph nodes palpable _____ Cervical _____ Posterior cervical _____

LUNGS

(Use stethoscope as necessary.)

Expand symmetrically _____ Contour of chest _____

Quality of respirations: Wheezing _____ Grunting _____ Quiet _____

Retractions _____ Rales _____

Abdominal respiration _____ Other _____

HEART

Quality of heart sounds _____ Rate _____ Intensity _____ Rhythm _____

Murmur _____ Unusual sounds _____

Fig. 9-2, cont'd. Guide for health assessment of infant.

Continued.

SECTION 1: PHYSICAL EXAMINATION—cont'd

ABDOMEN

Soft _____ Anything unusual (hard, distended) _____

Contour: Symmetrical _____ Protuberant _____

Protrusions or swelling _____

Masses _____ Bowel sounds heard with stethoscope _____

Umbilicus: Clean _____ Healed _____ Protuding _____ Other _____

Anything unusual about liver _____ Spleen _____ Kidneys _____

EXTREMITIES
Arms and hands

Flex easily at elbows, wrists, finger joints _____

Edema _____ Color _____ Nodules _____ Rash _____

Temperature (unusual warmth or coolness) _____

Other _____

Nail beds: Color _____ Circulation (Apply pressure to see if color returns

   quickly.) _____

Feet

Flex easily _____ Extend _____ Abduct _____ Adduct _____

Position normal _____ Other (equinovarus) _____

Legs

Equal in length _____ Edema _____ Color _____ Rash _____

Nodules _____ Unusual warmth or coldness _____

Other _____

Hips

Test for dislocated hip (see p. 342).

BACK

Shoulders even _____ Vertebrae straight _____

Anything unusual (moles, tuft of hair, protrusion) _____

GENITALIA
Female

Labia symmetrical _____ Clean _____ Inflamed _____

Discharge (describe) _____

Presence of clitoris _____ Vaginal orifice _____ Urinary meatus _____

Fig. 9-2, cont'd. Guide for health assessment of infant.

SECTION 1: PHYSICAL EXAMINATION—cont'd

Male

Penis with urethral opening at end _____ If not, describe _____

Testes in scrotum: Right _____ Left _____

Circumcised _____ Foreskin easily retracted _____ Clean _____

ANUS

Patent _____ Fissures _____ Normal configuration _____

NEUROMUSCULAR DEVELOPMENT
Reflexes

Moro reflex* (extension of trunk, extension of limbs followed by flexion and adduction) _____

Stepping reflexes (Support infant around trunk and place soles of feet on flat surface; normal infant

takes alternating steps.) _____

Rooting reflex (Stimulate side of cheek and infant turns his mouth and face to stimulus.) _____

Grasping reflex† (palmar and plantar) (Place fingers on palm of hand or foot; infant grasps ex-

aminer's fingers.): Right palmar _____ Left palmar _____ Right plantar _____

Left plantar _____

Incurvation reflex‡ (Run finger down paravertebral area first on one side of spine, then on other;

causes incurvation of spine toward stimulated side.) _____

Sucking reflex (Stroke lips.) _____

Tonic neck reflex§ (With infant supine, turn head sharply to one side. Arm and leg on side to which

jaw is turned extend; leg and arm on opposite side flex.) _____

Pupillary response to light _____

Blinks at dazzling light _____ Equality of pupils _____

Babinski sign‖ (Stroke along lateral margins of foot from heel forward to base of great toe. Infant

normally hyperextends toes. This is a positive response.): Right _____ Left _____

Biceps reflex: Right _____ Left _____ Triceps reflex: Right _____ Left _____

Brachioradialis reflex: Right _____ Left _____

Motor system

Muscle tone: Good _____ Flaccid _____ Hypotonic _____ Spastic _____

---

* Response disappears by age 6 months; absence prior to 8 weeks indicates neurological defects.
† Response lessens by age 3 to 4 months.
‡ Response disappears by age 4 weeks.
§ Response disappears by age 3 to 4 months.
‖ Positive sign is normal in first 12 to 18 months of life and abnormal after age 18 months.

Fig. 9-2, cont'd. Guide for health assessment of infant.

Continued.

SECTION 2: GENERAL DEVELOPMENT

GROSS MOTOR DEVELOPMENT
Postural development
Head: Lag in sitting posture _____ Holds erect and steady _____

Sits alone _____ Stands _____

Locomotion: Crawls _____ Walks with one hand held _____ Walks alone _____

Use of hands
Palmar grasp _____

Reaches for objects: Both hands _____ One hand _____

Transfers objects from one hand to other _____

Uses index finger and thumb _____

Builds tower of two blocks _____

SOCIAL DEVELOPMENT
Smiles: In response to adult smile _____ Spontaneously _____

Plays with fingers _____

Laughs _____

Vocalizes: Responsively (to adult) _____ Spontaneously _____ Expressively _____

   Jargon _____

Words: One word _____ Single words _____ Sentences (two or more words put to-

   gether) _____

Complies with suggestion such as "Give it to me." _____

Points (when desires distant object) _____

Waves hand _____ Plays peekaboo _____ Pat-a-cake _____

Cooperates in dressing _____

EMOTIONAL DEVELOPMENT
Cries: When? _____ Seldom _____ Frequently _____ What does mother do when

   infant cries? _____

Usually happy _____ Irritable _____ Responsive _____ Hyperactive _____

   Lethargic _____

Behavior with others than family _____

Anything special that pleases infant _____ Anything that upsets infant _____

Fig. 9-2, cont'd. Guide for health assessment of infant.

SECTION 2: GENERAL DEVELOPMENT—cont'd

RELATIONSHIP WITH OTHERS
Relationship with father
Does he share in care of infant? _____ If so, how? _____ Time spent playing with infant _____

Relationship with mother
Attention of mother to infant's needs _____ (as observed)

Response of infant to mother _____

Method of mother comforting infant _____

Does mother sing to infant? _____ Rock infant? _____

How much time does mother play with infant? _____

Siblings if observed
Behavior toward infant _____

Infant's response _____

SECTION 3: GENERAL CARE

GENERAL CARE
Bathing
Sink _____ Tub _____ Other _____ Time of day _____

Sleeping
Own crib _____

Time of nap: A.M. _____ P.M. _____

Length of nap: A.M. _____ P.M. _____

Bedtime _____ Time awake in A.M. _____

Elimination
Stools: Number per day _____ Describe (amount, color, consistency) _____

Urination: Number of diapers wet in 24 hours _____

Clothing
What articles or clothing are usually put on infant? _____

Diapers: How washed _____ Times rinsed _____

PLAY AND SOCIALIZATION
Taken outdoors in stroller _____ How long? _____ Where? _____

With what does infant play? _____

Adults who play with infant _____ When? _____ How? _____

Siblings play with infant _____

Fig. 9-2, cont'd. Guide for health assessment of infant.

Continued.

SECTION 3: GENERAL CARE—cont'd

NUTRITION

Describe feeding in 24-hour period: Milk or formula _____ Solid food _____ Water _____

Fruit juice _____

HEALTH TOPICS FOR GUIDANCE

Nutrition
Bathing
Clothing
Play
Emotional needs: affection, sensory stimulation, relief from tension
Care of infant when he cries
Immunizations
Prevention of accidents
Recreation and health of parents
Relation of siblings to infant

Fig. 9-2, cont'd. Guide for health assessment of infant.

The sensory organs to be examined include the eyes, ears, nose, and mouth.

The eyes are examined for inflammation of the eye or eyelid, any discharge from either one, whether pupils react equally to light, whether the infant can focus or follow a moving object, and whether there is any sign of strabismus (cross-eye); anything unusual or abnormal should be reported to a physician.

The examination of the ears includes noting whether the external ears are of normal configuration or have cysts or malformations, whether there is any discharge from the ear canal, the appearance of the canal and tympanic membrane when seen by an otoscope, and whether the infant can hear. In looking at the tympanic membrane of the ear canal the nurse should pull the auricle of the ear back and down to straighten it in the infant and young child. (In the older child the auricle of the ear is pulled back and up.) Normally the color of the tympanic membrane is gray. Certain landmarks should be visualized, such as the handle of the malleus. The eardrum should normally be concave. Light in the ear from the otoscope should fan out externally. Hearing of the infant can be tested by shaking a bell or rattle behind the infant first on one side, then the other to see if he makes a response. An infant 4 or 5 months of age usually turns his head in the direction of the sound.

The nose is examined for patency of nostrils and any sign of dried secretions or discharge. A tongue depressor and flashlight are needed to see the buccal membrane of the mouth, whether the soft and hard palate are intact, and whether the tonsils are so large that they obstruct the view of the pharynx. Inflammation or exudate on tonsils should be noted. Any white exudate should be noted as it may signify the presence of thrush.

The suppleness of neck can be tested by placing one hand behind the infant's head and pressing the head forward and down. Symmetry of both sides of the neck should be noted and the muscle on each side felt for the possible presence of a mass. Congenital torticollis is sometimes associated with a difficult delivery. If it is present, a mass is felt in the sternocleidomastoid muscle. The head is tilted toward the affected side while the chin is turned toward the opposite shoulder. There may be asymmetry of the face with this condition.

The neck is palpated for cervical nodes. Normally they cannot be felt.

Before auscultation of the lungs the nurse

should note the contour of the chest to see if both sides expand symmetrically and whether respirations are abdominal. Abdominal respiration is frequent and normal in the newborn. Quiet respirations are normal but, if there is grunting, wheezing, or retractions, this may signify respiratory distress. Are there any swellings or markings on the chest? In auscultating the chest the sounds of inspiration and expiration should be evaluated in several different areas of the chest. Palpation and percussion of the chest should be included in the examination. Vesicular breath sounds are the normal breath sounds heard on inspiration and expiration. They are high pitched during inspiration and low pitched during expiration. Variations from this are abnormal.

The rate of the apical heartbeat can be counted. One must remember that both the respiration and pulse of the infant increase when the infant cries or is active. The rate is lower when he is quiet or sleeping. The quality, rate, intensity, and rhythm of the heartbeat are especially noted. Any abnormal murmurs or sounds should be reported. The particular areas to be examined include the aortic area (second right intercostal space near the sternum), the pulmonic area (second left intercostal space), the left third and fourth intercostal spaces along the sternum, and the apical area (fifth intercostal space).

The nurse auscultates for normalacy of heart sounds. The first heart sound (S_1) is the loudest of the sounds. It is the systolic part of the cardiac cycle produced by closure of the mitral and tricuspid valves. It is best heard at the apex. The closure of the semilunar valves (aortic and pulmonic) is the diastolic part of the cardiac cycle. The second heart sound (S_2) is evaluated at the second left intercostal space near the sternum. The second sound is normally split and varies with respiration. The S_1 and S_2 sounds of the heart are the most important. Frequently in children a third heart sound (S_3) is heard at the apex. Other heart sounds are abnormal.

The abdomen is gently palpated for the presence of organomegaly or masses. Normally the liver is palpable 2 to 3 cm. below the right costal margin during infancy, but this is not true after 1 year of age. The tip of the spleen may normally be felt below the left costal margin at all ages. The kidneys are normally not palpable.

Extremities are examined to see if all joints flex easily and can be adducted and abducted. Any edema, pain, swelling, nodules, or unusual warmth or coldness is noted. Likewise a difference of color in opposite extremities is noticed. An infant's feet are often in a varus position, but if the examiner can straighten them easily there is no cause for worry. The young infant may appear bowlegged because the muscles on the outside of his leg are more developed than on the inside of his leg. The tibia is straight. Legs are compared to see if they are of equal length. Hips can be tested for congenital dislocation as described in Chapter 13.

The back of the infant is inspected to see if the shoulders are even and the vertebrae straight. A swelling, tuft of hair, or dimple at the base of the spine should be noted. A dimple is very common and does not signify a pathologic condition unless a discharge or swelling occurs. A discharge could mean that there is a communication between the skin and spinal cord or a superficial infection. In most cases it is not until adulthood that the discharge or swelling occurs. Prompt medical and surgical treatment is advised.

The genitalia of girls are inspected to see if there is a clitoris, a vaginal orifice, and a urinary meatus. Whether the labia are symmetrical is noted as well as whether there is any inflammation or discharge. The genitalia of boys are inspected to see if there is a urethral opening at the end of the penis, if both testicles are in the scrotum, and if the infant has been circumcised. There is a minimal degree of phimosis until 8 months, when the foreskin can be easily retracted. In bathing male infants, forceable retraction should be avoided. The foreskin is retracted gently as far as it will go.

The anus is inspected to see if there are any fissures in the mucous membrane of the anus and if the anus is patent.

In the neurological examination the reflexes are tested and the tone of the muscles is noted. If a muscle is flaccid, hypotonic, or spastic, a referral is made to a physician. The following reflexes are tested as in adulthood: pupillary

biceps, triceps, brachioradialis, and patellar reflexes. The Babinski reflex should be negative
after about 18 months of age but positive in
infancy. Other infantile reflexes include the incurvation, Moro, tonic neck, stepping, sucking,
and rooting reflexes. By 6 months of age these
reflexes normally have disappeared. (These reflexes were described in Chapter 4 and are
briefly explained on the assessment guide.)

The infant health assessment guide in Fig.
9-2 has three parts: physical assessment, general development, and general care (hygiene, play
and socialization, and nutrition). A summary of
possible topics for health guidance is given.
These topics are discussed at length in the following pages under guidance toward health.

Guidance toward health
Emotional needs

The infant needs to be mothered, to have relief from tension, and to have sensory stimulation. The latter is also a social and intellectual
need. Mothering means cuddling, rocking, and
gently caressing the infant. It includes seeing
that the infant's needs are met promptly. Prolonged periods of crying should be avoided. If
the infant is hungry, he needs to be fed. If cold
or uncomfortable, he needs warmth and comfort. The infant is not a miniature adult and
cannot wait. As the infant grows older, he
needs play materials and someone to play with
him. Providing him with auditory and visual
stimulation is part of showing real affection.
When the infant is fed, the mother can hold the
infant and become further acquainted with him.
Bath time provides another opportunity to caress, talk, and play with the infant. Through the
process of associating pleasantness and comfort with the mother the infant grows to love the
mother and/or others who share his care. As the
infant grows older, he is awake for longer
periods of time in the late afternoon and evening so that the father and older siblings have a
chance to touch, talk, and play with him.

The infant needs to see a warmth of facial
expressions and happy smiling faces as well as
to feel comfort and closeness through tactile
sensation. (The distressing effects of maternal
deprivation were discussed in Chapter 1.) Loud
quarreling voices are upsetting to the infant.

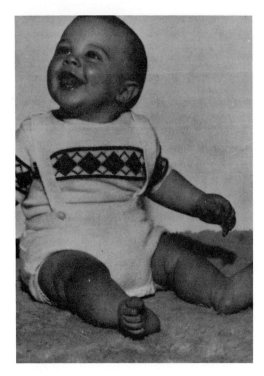

Fig. 9-3. A healthy baby is a happy baby.

By 5 months of age he reacts to an angry facial expression.

To best promote the infant's mental hygiene
the mental hygiene of those around him must
also be good. To care for an infant is work, and
there are times when any mother may feel hostility. Ambivalent feelings are normal; however, if the mother receives sufficient rest, has
recreational diversions, and has her own emotional needs met, she can better provide for the
infant's needs for warmth and affection. If the
nurse will discuss with the mother the latter's
need of rest and recreation, she indirectly helps
the infant.

In home visits and in child health conferences
the nurse has an excellent opportunity to observe the mother-child relationship. It is the interaction between the two that is important. She
should notice whether the mother tries to meet
the infant's needs and her consistency in so doing. If the infant cries or tries to wiggle out of
her lap, what does the mother say or do? If the
mother feeds the infant, does she poke the bottle into the infant's mouth and then gaze around

the room, or does she focus her attention on the infant?

Sensory stimulation is not only an emotional need but is also an intellectual and social one. Play and exercise of the infant are discussed later in this chapter on p. 180.

Social needs

The infant needs to have an enlarging circle of acquaintances. Besides his immediate family, he should become accustomed to seeing relatives and friends of the family. When they come into the home they should not be allowed to disturb the infant if he is sleeping, but, if the infant is awake, they can look at him and speak to him. The infant who is 6 months old knows the difference between a familiar person and a stranger. Safe on his mother's lap, he may look at a stranger with interest. Further familiarity helps him to be more friendly. When the older infant is ready for closer contact with a stranger, he offers her a toy, puts out his hand, or crawls toward her. The infant, not the adult, should make the move for closer acquaintance. Friends of the older siblings should be instructed in this also. It is advisable for the office nurse and public health nurse to let the infant make the first move toward friendship. Many times it is better if the nurse permits the mother to undress her infant or hold him for the doctor instead of doing this herself. Taking the infant from the mother frequently puts the infant on the defensive.

In the infancy period it is desirable for the emerging toddler to associate pleasure and satisfaction with other people so that he can gain a sense of trust. In order to enjoy people he does need contact with them. If no provision is made for this, by the time the infant is 1 year of age he may be unduly shy in front of others.

The infant can be left with a relative or neighbor for an hour or two when the mother goes grocery shopping, has her hair done, or goes out with her husband. This encourages emotional self-reliance.

General hygiene

Infancy is the all-important time for positive attitudes to be formed toward bathing, eating, and sleeping. If these routines are unpleasant,

the child may develop negative behavior toward bedtime, mealtime, and bath time and become increasingly resistant to them. It is easier to educate than to reeducate, and every effort should be made by the adult to see that these routines are enjoyable during infancy.

Bathing. The mother should plan to give the infant a bath when she is not rushed or feeling tense. The convenient time may be after older siblings have gone to school, after the infant's noon meal, or before the infant's bedtime. The time does not matter, but how the bath is given does matter. During the first few months of the infant's life, the mother needs to be careful that the infant is held firmly so that he does not feel insecure in the tub. The feel of the warm water should be soothing to him. Smiling and talking to the infant help him to relax. Quick, abrupt movements should be avoided. (For bath procedure in a tub see p. 74.) As the infant gets older, he likes to move around in the tub or possibly to finger a rubber bath toy or hit the water with his hand. After his bath the mother might well place the infant on a large bed to exercise. She may use this time to play with him, talk with him, and caress him.

Sleeping. When the infant is put in his crib to sleep, conditions should be comfortable. Clothing should fit him. If pajamas have feet in them, they should be long enough. Infants grow very quickly! The mattress should be firm. The room should be darkened and should be at a comfortable temperature. If the adult is comfortable in the room, then probably the infant is also. Blankets are often kicked off by older infants; after the infant falls asleep the blanket can be gently rearranged over him. Ordinary household noises can continue when the infant is sleeping, but a blaring radio or television is disturbing.

During the neonatal period the infant may sleep 22 out of the 24 hours, but he awakens at intervals of 3 to 4 hours because he is hungry, is uncomfortable, or needs attention. His pattern of sleep changes with age. By 3 months of age he should be sleeping for 6 hours without waking at night, and gradually he stays awake for longer periods in the daytime. By 6 months of age he usually has a nap in the morning and one in the afternoon. At night he sleeps for about 12 hours. The infant develops a certain rhythm of sleeping if placed in his crib at the same hours each day.

Eating. Eating behavior in infancy is directed toward the maintenance of nutritional requirements for growth and development and the introduction of a variety of food flavors. Conditions relative to eating should enable the infant to learn to recognize food and feeding as a source of enjoyment and love.

Nutritional needs. The infant's formula or breast milk will be his major source of nutrients in the early months of infancy. As in the neonatal period, the formula composition is calculated on the basis of protein, calorie, and fluid needs, which are determined by the infant's body weight. The infant normally doubles his birth weight by 5 months of age and triples it by 1 year; thus the formula composition must be constantly adjusted to maintain the rate of growth.

Since the volume of formula gradually increases as more milk is needed to meet the protein requirement, the amount of water used to dilute the formula will gradually decrease. If evaporated milk is used, only an equal volume of water may be needed to dilute it by the time the infant is 6 to 8 months of age. If a commercially prepared formula (Similac, Enfamil) is used, the dilution is usually one can of formula concentrate to one can of water. The prepared formulas are also available with added iron. For example, one can of concentrated Similac with iron formula per day will supply an infant the minimal daily requirements of essential vitamins and iron that he needs for normal growth and development. If whole milk is used, no extra water is needed. Whole milk should not be given until after 12 months of age because of the poor digestability due to the large curd size. The infant can be given sterile water from a bottle or cup between feedings.

As the infant grows, his stomach capacity increases, and he is able to take a larger amount of formula at each feeding. By the second or third month the infant will take 4 to 6 ounces at a time and will probably not require a feeding in the middle of the night. By 6 or 7 months the infant usually takes four 8-ounce feedings a day.

When the nurse makes a home visit or talks

to the mother in the clinic, she should question her regarding feeding practices. The nurse should be able to determine whether the formula is adequate by comparing the mother's report of the formula composition, total volume, number of feedings, and amount taken at each feeding to the infant's requirements for protein, calories, and fluid. If the infant is not growing satisfactorily, the formula may be at fault and adjustments will have to be made. If the formula is adequate, intestinal malabsorption, a metabolic defect, or another disease condition may be the cause of the infant's failure to thrive. In any case the nurse's findings should be reported to the physician.

The infant may be receiving too much formula and gaining too much weight. A fat, flabby infant is not necessarily a healthy one, and the mother should realize that overfeeding may be just as harmful as underfeeding.

Supplements to formula. Breast milk and formula adequately meet the infant's need for protein, calories, and fluid, but both lack certain specific vitamins and minerals to meet the infant's requirements for optimum growth.

ASCORBIC ACID. Ascorbic acid is required for collagen, bone, and tooth formation. Without sufficient ascorbic acid the infant may develop scurvy. To avoid this the infant should receive 35 mg. of ascorbic acid a day.

Ascorbic acid is an extremely labile vitamin; it is readily destroyed by heat and exposure to oxygen. The pasteurization and sterilization processes reduce the amount of ascorbic acid in cow's milk. Breast milk contains some ascorbic acid, but the amount is dependent on the mother's diet. To ensure an adequacy of ascorbic acid for the infant some form of supplementation is usually begun in the first 2 to 4 weeks of life.

Orange juice should not be offered until 8 months of age because of hyperallergenic qualities. Tomato juice is also a source of ascorbic acid, but since it contains only half the amount of ascorbic acid as orange juice, twice as much would have to be given. Small infants will usually not take this much tomato juice so it should not be offered until the infant is about 2 months of age. It may be given in a bottle, a cup, or a spoon.

The physician may prescribe synthetic ascorbic acid in tablet form if he suspects the infant may be allergic to citrus fruits. One 50 mg. tablet crushed and dissolved in cool water is the usual daily prescription.

VITAMIN D. Vitamin D is essential for the utilization of calcium and phosphorus in the formation of teeth and bones. A deficiency of vitamin D results in rickets.

As with ascorbic acid, the amount of vitamin D in breast milk depends on the mother's diet, but it is generally inadequate to meet the infant's requirement of 400 I.U. per day. Most cow's milk is fortified with 400 I.U. of vitamin D per quart, but small babies do not drink a quart of milk in a day; therefore, additional supplementation is necessary.

Vitamin D can be supplied as liquid preparation or as cod-liver oil. Some vitamin D preparations also contain vitamin A and ascorbic acid. The kind to be used will be determined by the physician. The nurse's role is to emphasize and teach the mother accurate measurement of the prescribed amount. A large dose of vitamin D is toxic and can result in overcalcification with subsequent bone deformation.

Some commercially prepared formulas have been supplemented with vitamin D. This makes additional supplements theoretically unnecessary; however, if the infant habitually does not take all the formula, the vitamin D intake may be inadequate.

IRON. Most full-term infants whose mothers were adequately nourished during pregnancy will be born with a body store of approximately 300 mg. of iron. As the infant grows and his blood volume expands, this store of iron will be used for the synthesis of hemoglobin and myoglobin. The store will eventually be depleted unless it is replenished by dietary intake. Since both cow's milk and breast milk are deficient in iron, the baby will need supplements from other foods. Iron-enriched cereal is generally recommended.

Introduction of cereals. The question of when to begin cereals is still the subject of controversy. Since the full-term infant does have a store of iron that should last 3 to 6 months, some physicians believe that cereals need not be introduced until that time. There is also evidence that the infant's absorption and utilization of iron are not efficient before 6 months of age, although newer research suggests this might not be the case with respect to iron-enriched cereals.

Others recognize that spoon feeding cereal to the infant requires learning a new eating technique, and time is needed for both the infant and the mother to adjust to it. It is generally the case in practice to introduce cereals at an early age so that by the time the infant actually does have a physiological need for iron he will be taking cereal well.

Commercially prepared infant cereals are tolerated by most young infants. Rice and barley are generally introduced first because they tend to be the least allergenic. Mixed cereals should be avoided until it has been established that the infant has no sensitivity to any of the individual grains included in the mixture.

The mother should begin by diluting a teaspoon of cereal with some of the infant's formula. The mother can expect the infant to take no more than this the first few times. The amount and consistency will be increased until the infant of 6 or 7 months of age is taking 4 to 5 tablespoons of cereal a day.

The cereal should be offered on a small spoon. Its consistency should be thin enough so that the infant partly sucks it off the spoon. In general it is best to offer the cereal before the formula when he is hungry and ready to eat. If given the bottle first, he may not accept the cereal. The same is true later when pureed fruits and vegetables are offered.

The mother should be prepared for difficulties she is likely to encounter. She can expect more cereal to end up on her, on the infant's bib, and on the floor than in the infant's stomach during the first few feeding sessions. If the mother thinks the infant must eat cereal only for nutrition's sake, she may be tempted to avoid the mess by punching a large hole in a nipple and feeding the cereal in a bottle. The nurse should assure the mother that the infant will learn to eat cereal from a spoon if she is patient and that this aspect of feeding is an important step in the development of desirable eating behavior.

Addition of other solid foods. The same general principles used in the introduction of cereals will be applied in the introduction of other solid foods. The nurse will want to remind the mother that new foods should be introduced one at a time, beginning with a small amount, which will be increased gradually as the infant's appetite requires.

A single new food should be tried for 5 to 7 days in succession before introducing another. This allows the infant time to become thoroughly acquainted with each new flavor. It is also economical if the mother is using commercially prepared baby food, since opened jars should not be kept in the refrigerator longer than 3 days. If the infant eats the same food 3 days in a row, he should finish the jar in that time.

When an infant spits out a new food, it is more often a sign that he has not yet adjusted to its flavor or texture than an indication of his outright dislike of it. The mother should handle these situations in a matter-of-fact manner. If the mother thinks the spitting is cute and she laughs and cuddles him, the infant will think he is being rewarded for spitting and he will continue it with each new food he tries. On the other hand, if the mother is punitive about the mess he makes, the infant will not learn to associate eating new foods as a pleasurable experience. Neither should the mother make an unpleasant face when feeding the infant a food she herself dislikes.

Opinions differ regarding the sequence in which new foods should be offered. Since all the infant's nutritional needs can be met by breast milk or formula and proper vitamin supplementation until at least 3 months of age, the decision about which foods to begin first is more often based on individual preference and the infant's willingness to accept them. Most infants will accept pureed fruits and vegetables at 2 to 3 months of age; pureed meats can be given at about 4 months. An example of a suggested schedule of when to introduce solid foods is given in Table 9-2.

Commercial baby foods are the most convenient, but for economical reasons the mother may want to use fruits and vegetables eaten by the rest of the family. Ripe bananas may be mashed and given to the infant raw, but all other fresh fruits and vegetables must be cooked, pureed, and strained. Sugar and seasoning should not be added. If canned fruits and vegetables are used, they should be rinsed in water to remove excess syrup and salt before they are pureed. It is important that the infant learn to accept a variety of fruits and vegetables. They will be a major source of vitamin A, vitamin C, and iron in later life.

Plain meats such as pureed beef, chicken, pork, veal, lamb, and liver can be introduced once the infant has adjusted to fruits and vegetables. The chief nutritional contribution of meats is protein, B vitamins, and iron. Meat

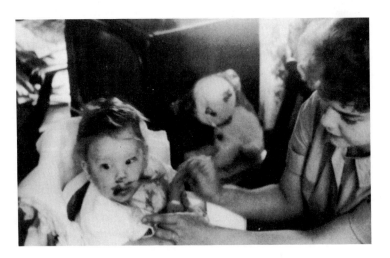

Fig. 9-4. For an infant, enjoyment of eating is important, not neatness.

Table 9-2. Introduction of solid foods*

3 weeks
   Rice cereal: begin with 1 tablespoon of cereal and 1
      tablespoon of formula (feed cereal with a baby spoon);
      increase quantity of cereal as baby needs it; feed it
      twice a day.
6 weeks
   Barley, wheat, oats, etc.: 2 tablespoons twice a day
   Fruit (apricots, applesauce, peaches, etc.): ¼ to ½ jar
      twice a day
2 months
   Vegetables (squash, carrots, beets, etc.): ¼ to ½ jar
      twice a day (Do not give spinach.)
   Fruits: ¼ to ½ jar twice a day
   Cereals: 2 to 4 tablespoons twice a day
   Juices: 2 to 4 ounces twice a day (Do not give orange
      juice.)
3 to 4 months
   Vegetables, dinners, meats, cereals, fruits: three solid
      food meals per day
6 to 8 months
   Eggs, dinners (meats and vegetables), table food
      (mashed), junior baby foods, orange juice
8 months
   Begin teaching baby to feed self with spoon. Teach baby
      to drink out of glass.
15 to 18 months
   Discontinue bottle feedings.

*From Instructions for the care of your new baby, Baton
Rouge, La., 1977, Louisiana State University Pediatric
Department, Earl K. Long Memorial Hospital.
NOTE: When starting a new food, give it by itself for 5 to
7 days before beginning another food. If a rash, diarrhea,
spitting up, or vomiting occurs discontinue that specific
food and begin another one.

and noodle or meat and vegetable combinations
should be avoided in infancy. They usually contain more starch than meat and tend to confuse
the small infant who is just learning to discriminate between food flavors.

Once the infant has become familiar with
fruits, vegetables, and meats, a daily food pattern should be established. This helps to introduce the infant to social and cultural eating customs and lays the foundations for routine eating
behavior that is desirable in later life.

Table foods. By 6 or 7 months of age most
infants are ready to learn to chew. It is believed
that if the transition from pureed to coarser textured foods is postponed too far beyond this
time, future feeding problems may occur.

Commercial junior foods are convenient, but
it may be more economical for the mother to
feed the infant table foods. It is unwise, however, to suggest table foods without first determining what the family typically eats. The
nurse might want to take a family diet history so
that the physician can see which foods from the
family table are appropriate for the infant. The
mother will need some counseling in meal
planning and food preparation if the history reveals that diet improvements are necessary.

Coarsely chopped cooked vegetables,
mashed, baked, or boiled potatoes, and peeled,
raw, ripe fruits are suitable table foods for the
6-month-old infant. By 7 or 8 months of age
finely ground, boneless, fat-free meat can replace the pureed varieties. The mother may occasionally give the infant cottage cheese or
pudding as a milk supplement. When teeth
begin to erupt, dry toast, crackers, or zwieback
help the infant to learn to chew and feed himself.

The yolk of a hard-cooked egg may be introduced when the infant is 6 months old, but,
because of the possibility of allergy, egg whites
should be withheld until the infant is 9 to 12
months of age. By the time the infant is 1 year
old he should be able to eat a wide variety of
plain table foods without having to depend on
special baby foods to any great extent.

Weaning. Breast-fed babies are usually
weaned between 6 and 9 months of age or when
tooth eruption occurs. If the mother's milk is
diminishing or if she contracts a serious illness
that would interfere with lactation, the infant
may be weaned before the age of 6 months. If
the infant is weaned early, the transition should
be from breast to bottle. Young infants derive
pleasure from sucking that should not be denied. If the infant is weaned after 6 months of
age, it is probably easier to go directly from the
breast to a cup; however, this is largely an individual decision that is left to the physician and
the mother.

When the formula-fed infant begins to want
to hold his own bottle (around 8 months of age)
it is a good time to teach him to hold a cup. To
be easy to grasp the cup should be small
(possibly the size of a fruit juice glass) so that
the infant can put his two hands around it. If
he is used to sipping water or orange juice from

a cup, he may accept milk from a cup more easily.

Cup feeding should be introduced gradually. The infant should not be forced to abandon the bottle until he is well acquainted with the cup-feeding technique. The two methods will overlap for a while, but by the time the infant is 12 to 18 months of age the bottle should be discarded since drinking from it becomes a habit. The longer the child clings to the bottle, the harder it is for him to relinquish it.

Clothing. The infant's clothing should be in accord with the environmental temperature, the activity of the infant, and the stage of development. For example, a dress would be in the way of a 10-month-old girl in the crawling stage. Overalls or pants would be much more practical. In hot weather a cotton sunsuit is more comfortable than a shirt and pants. Clothing for infants should be washable and easy to put on and take off. Sweaters and shirts that open like coats are less likely to make the infant feel restrained when he is being dressed.

In selecting clothing the mother should avoid garments of wool that would be used next to the skin. The infant's skin is delicate and easily irritated; cotton is probably best. Buttons on the clothing should be small and sewed on tightly so the infant cannot take them off and swallow them. Garments with drawstrings or lace around the neck are hazardous and should be avoided. Lace can irritate the delicate skin. If waterproof pants are used, they should be loose and made to allow for ventilation. Otherwise, moisture under the pants may cause a diaper rash, besides making the infant unduly warm.

During the early months of life the infant sleeps a great deal and needs mostly diapers, shirts, jackets, and blankets. Infants grow quickly, and it is a mistake to buy much during the first few months of their life. Later, when they are taken for outings in a carriage, stroller, or car, suitable outdoor clothing should be of a type that enables the mother to dress the infant with a minimum of pulling arms and restraining motions. Shoes are not needed until the infant is walking; then they are used to protect his feet from splinters, glass, and other dangers. The shoes should conform to the outline of the foot: broad at the toes and narrow at the heel. The shoes should be a thumb's width longer than the foot and ¼ inch wider at the toes. If the infant begins to wear shoes before 1 year of age, he may need a pair almost monthly because of his rapid growth. Between the first and second year the infant needs a new pair of shoes every 2 or 3 months. New socks have to be bought just as frequently unless they are stretch socks.

Play and exercise. At first being carried, rocked, bathed, and held constitutes a certain amount of exercise and stimulation for the infant. In his second and third month he needs attractive objects at which to look—perhaps tied to his crib. By 4 months of age he grasps an object with both hands and carries it to his mouth so that toys should be given him to handle. For safety's sake they need to be durable and washable with no sharp edges or small detachable parts that the infant could swallow. A toy that is attractive and makes a noise when handled adds to enjoyment. When the infant is old enough to begin to crawl, pots and pans that fit inside each other are a delight to him, as is taking off the fitted covers of pans and putting them on again. Playing peekaboo when the infant is 9 or 10 months of age is fun.

During bath time the mother can talk to, caress, and play with the infant. Bath time means play time to the infant, especially when he can sit up in the tub. An infant enjoys trying to catch the floating toys in the tub and slapping the water with his hand.

When the infant discovers he can make various sounds with his voice, he spends time just vocalizing as an amusement. By 4 months the infant tries to respond vocally when an adult talks to him. Vocalization sometimes takes place when the infant is pleased about some activity or has a sense of well-being. He feels well and wishes to be sociable.

By 7 months of age the average infant can sit up alone, and this gives a different viewpoint of his surroundings. He can see more. His buggy, crib, or chair should be moved to different parts of the room so that he can see different objects. This *is* entertainment for him. Sometimes placing him on a screened-in porch provides amusement.

Before the infant is able to crawl he should be placed in a playpen or on a blanket on the floor

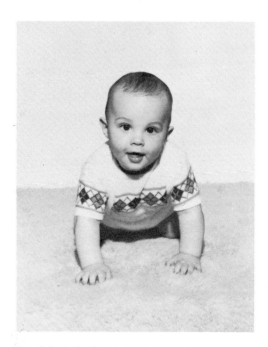

Fig. 9-5. A healthy baby is an active, alert baby.

so that he can kick his legs, stretch, and turn over without any fear of falling. He needs to feel freedom. When he is old enough to crawl, this is a fascinating activity indeed, but it is essential that the home be safe for him. There should be no pins, bobby pins, or other small objects on the floor that the infant could swallow, and breakable items should be kept from his reach. Unused light sockets should be covered. Screens must be so well fastened that they cannot be pushed out. If low tables have round corners rather than sharp square corners, bumps and bruises are avoided.

In general the infant enjoys play of a sensory type—something that provides auditory, visual, and tactile pleasure. In the second half of the first year of life his play is more outgoing. He seeks contact with people and finds objects to touch, taste, and feel. Through play he learns about his immediate environment. In the first 6 months he learns more about himself. He surveys his hands, finds his voice, learns he can

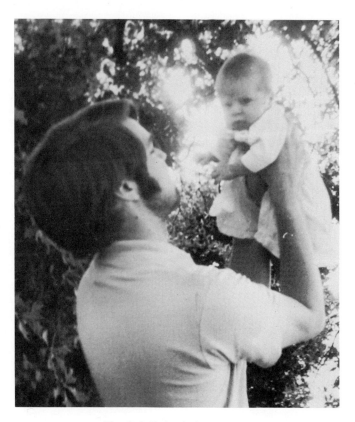

Fig. 9-6. Father is important, too.

turn over, and later examines and plays with his feet. He becomes familiar with people's faces as they bend over him or hold him close to them. During the second 6 months, when he sits up, then crawls, and then pulls himself to a standing position, his perception of people and his environment changes.

In summary, the infant younger than 1 year has his need for sensory stimulation met through social contacts with people, handling of objects, exploration of himself, and finally sensory exploration of his immediate environment.

Fresh air and sunshine. The infant needs to have morning and afternoon outings in pleasant weather. In summer he should remain inside during the hottest part of the day. This time varies in different localities. The infant's skin is tender, and he blisters easily when he is exposed to sunlight. Moreover, his surface area is large in comparison to his weight; therefore he becomes dehydrated faster than an adult when playing outdoors. The infant's physician may make definite suggestions about the length of time the infant is to be outside. Exposure to extremes of temperature or windy days is not conducive to promotion of health.

Prevention of accidents

Aspiration and/or inhalation of foreign objects is the most common type of accident in infancy. Of what significance is this for the nurse? First, feeding technique should be considered. The infant should be held for feedings. The practice of propping a bottle is unsafe. After the infant is fed he should be placed on his abdomen or propped on his right side. If he does regurgitate any of the feeding, there is considerably less danger of his apirating any of it if he is on his abdomen or side.

Second, when the infant is old enough to purposefully grasp any object, he is likely to put it in his mouth. Articles small enough to swallow (coins, buttons, safety pins, bobby pins) should be kept out of his reach. When the infant is old enough to crawl and enjoy playing with pots and pans in the kitchen cupboard, such household articles as cleaning agents, drain cleaners, bleaches, kerosene, or insecticides should have covers that fit tightly and should be placed on a shelf out of reach of the infant. The

same is true for all medicines; however, the toddler is more likely to explore these articles than the creeping infant.

Toys should be sturdy enough so that, if the infant bites on them (and he will), they will not break and perhaps injure his mouth. It is better to have the eyes of a stuffed teddy bear embroidered on the bear than for them to become loose and have the infant possibly swallow or aspirate them. Toys should not have small pieces that the infant could swallow or aspirate.

The infant should have a safe area in which to crawl. Toward the end of the first year he begins to use his thumb and forefinger to pick up tiny objects such as common pins from the floor. Guards should be placed around fireplaces and open gas heaters. Stairways should be protected. If there is a wading or swimming pool outside, the infant must be closely watched to prevent his falling into the water and possibly drowning.

In addition to aspiration or inhalation of an object, other accidents that can easily occur should be avoided. An infant should not be left alone in a house or in an automobile. When riding in a car, the infant should be fastened into his car seat and the driver of the car should closely observe good driving rules.

If the infant is placed in a high chair, he should be supervised and not left alone. Not only is there danger of his falling but also the infant may get tangled with the straps on it. Crib sides should be up at all times when the infant is in his crib. If the infant is placed on a couch or large bed, precautions should be taken to prevent his falling. He must not be left alone.

The nurse has an opportunity to teach prevention of accidents in the hospital, clinic, doctor's office, child health conference, or infant's home. There are many ways to do this, depending on the particular situation in which the nurse is working. Examples include giving direct verbal instructions, using posters and literature, and praising the mother who demonstrates safety habits in the care of her infant.

Medical supervision

The infant requires closer medical supervision during his first year of life than he will need at any other period. The infant's mother

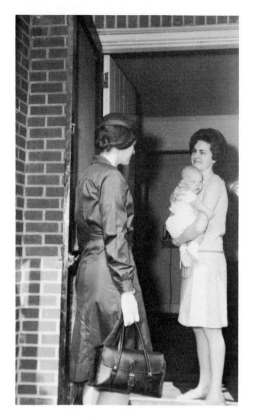

Fig. 9-7. Public health nurse makes an instructive visit.

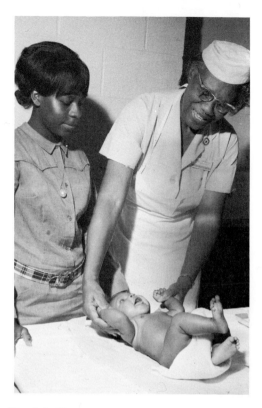

Fig. 9-8. The public health nurse shows the mother how to hold the infant for physician's examination in a child health conference. The diaper is unpinned on one side, and the infant's arms are held in a relaxed position, but out of the physician's way.

may take him to a private physician or to a child health conference, which is usually under the auspices of the county health department. From his medical supervision the mother learns whether the infant is growing and developing normally. In addition, she receives directions about his nutrition and general care; finally, the infant needs protection from communicable diseases for which there are specific immunizations or vaccinations. Of course, if the infant shows signs of any illness or abnormality when seen in a well child clinic, he is referred to a physician for treatment.

Child health conference. On the infant's admission to a child health conference, the nurse takes a history from the mother, including significant factors relative to the infant's birth, developmental record, feeding behavior, nutrition, stools, and any problems the mother has or believe she has relative to the infant. Another nurse then weighs the infant, takes his temper-ature, and measures the length of his body and the circumference of his head. In doing this the nurse has the opportunity to notice anything unusual and can attach a note about it on the chart or call the physician's attention to it when he examines the infant. After the physician examines the infant, immunizations are given by the nurse in accord with the physician's recommendations and the policies of the county health department. At this time the nurse should make sure the mother understands suggestions the physician has given her.

An ideal time for group education of mothers about child care is when they are waiting to have the physician see their infants. A short talk by a nurse on some phase of the infant's health may be helpful to them, or possibly a demonstration of types of food for the infant's diet.

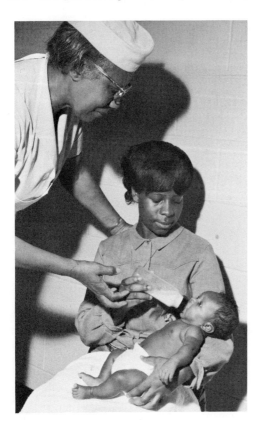

Fig. 9-9. The public health nurse in a child health conference is teaching the mother the correct technique to use in bottle-feeding an infant: The neck of the bottle is filled with milk, and the upper part of the infant's body is elevated while he is taking the formula.

Table 9-3. Revised schedule for active immunization and tuberculin testing of normal infants and children in the United States*

2 mo.	DTP†	TOPV‡
4 mo.	DTP	TOPV
6 mo.	DTP	§
12 mo.	Tuberculin test‖	
15 mo.	MMR¶	
18 mo.	DTP	TOPV
4 to 6 yr.	DTP	TOPV
14 to 16 yr.	Td # and thereafter every 10 years	

*Approved by the Committee on Infectious Diseases, American Academy of Pediatrics, 1977.
†DTP = diphtheria and tetanus toxoids combined with pertussis vaccine.
‡TOPV = trivalent oral poliovirus vaccine. This recommendation is suitable for breast-fed as well as bottle-fed infants.
§Optional TOPV in endemic areas.
‖Frequency of repeated tuberculin tests depends on risk of exposure of the child and on the prevalence of tuberculosis in the population group. The initial test should be at the time of or preceding the measles immunization.
¶MMR = Measles-mumps-rubella combined vaccine.
#Td = combined tetanus and diphtheria toxoids (adult type) for those more than 6 years of age in contrast to diphtheria and tetanus (DT), which contains a larger amount of diphtheria antigen. *Tetanus toxoid at time of injury:* For clean, minor wounds, no booster dose is needed by a fully immunized child unless more than 10 years have elapsed since the last dose. For contaminated wounds a booster dose should be given if more than 5 years have elapsed since the last dose.
Storage of vaccines: Because biologics are of varying stability, the manufacturers' recommendations for optimal storage conditions (e.g., temperature, light) should be carefully followed. Failure to observe these precautions may significantly reduce the potency and effectiveness of the vaccines.

Individual teaching can be done whenever an opportunity presents itself.

Medical protection from infection

Prophylaxis against specific diseases. There are certain diseases from which the infant may be protected: diphtheria, pertussis, tetanus, rubeola, rubella, and poliomyelitis. (See Tables 9-3 and 9-4 for the recommended immunization procedures.) Immunization against rubella is advised for girls approaching puberty; indeed, sometimes it is given before the child enters school. If a pregnant woman contracts rubella during pregnancy, especially in the first trimester, the baby may be born with certain defects, particularly of the heart, the eyes, and the brain.

In explanation of the recommendation for tetanus toxoid, it should be pointed out that children frequently have cuts, accidents, or burns and that, if the child has not had tetanus toxoid, he will have to be given tetanus antitoxin. If antitoxin from horse serum is used, there may be severe reactions.

The public health nurse has an opportunity in prenatal and postpartum classes as well as in her home visits and in child health conferences to teach the mother about immunizations. The hospital nurse has an opportunity to teach about immunizations before the new infant is discharged and/or when an infant is hospitalized. The nurse in the pediatrician's office should

Table 9-4. Primary immunization for children not immunized in infancy*

Age 1 to 5 yr.

First visit	DTP, TOPV, tuberculin test
1 mo. later	Measles, rubella, mumps
2 mo. later	DTP, TOPV
4 mo. later	DTP, TOPV
6 to 12 mo. later or preschool	DTP, TOPV
Age 14 to 16 yr.	Td—continue every 10 yr.

Age 6 yr. and older

First visit	Td, TOPV, tuberculin test
1 mo. later	Measles, rubella, mumps
2 mo. later	Td, TOPV
6 to 12 mo. later	Td, TOPV
Age 14 to 16 yr.	Td—continue every 10 years

NOTE: Physicians may choose to alter the sequence of these schedules if specific infections are prevalent at the time. For example, measles vaccine might be given on the first visit if an epidemic is underway in the community.
*Approved by the Committee on Infectious Diseases, American Academy of Pediatrics, October, 1973.

check patients' records to make sure immunizations have been given and should remind mothers to bring infants or children back for booster injections. Immunizations are important not only as one factor in keeping the child well but also in avoiding the severe complications of some diseases. Myocarditis is a serious complication of diphtheria. Paralysis may follow poliomyelitis. Pneumonia may follow pertussis if vomitus is aspirated. Encephalopathy may be a complication of both pertussis and rubeola (red measles).

Administration of immunizations and vaccinations

Caution. An acute febrile illness is reason to defer immunization until the subsequent visit or until the infection is properly controlled. Minor infections not associated with febrile reactions, such as the common cold, are not contraindications.

Routine influenza immunization is not currently recommended for normal infants and children because the vaccines vary in effectiveness and produce unacceptably high numbers of local and systemic reactions. Also, influenza virus infections cause low morbidity and mortality. Children with chronic, high-mortality rate illnesses such as chronic bron-

chopulmonary disease, metabolic disease, glomerulonephritis, nephrosis, neurologic disorders, and rheumatic heart disease should receive influenza vaccine. The influenza vaccine should not be given to anyone who has a history of an allergy to egg or chicken since this vaccine contains egg protein that could produce a severe allergic reaction.

A patient without a history of previous immunization who has a large contaminated wound should receive tetanus immune globulin (human) intramuscularly. Also the immune globulin may be used to infiltrate around the wound when it appears grossly contaminated. If tetanus immune globulin (human) is not available, equine or bovine tetanus antitoxin can be used after appropriate eye and/or skin testing for sensitivity is carried out. If desensitization is necessary, any satisfactory approved method of desensitization is carried out with the physician in attendance. Never inject a serum or perform a skin test unless a syringe containing 1 ml. of a 1:1,000 solution of epinephrine is within immediate reach because of the dangers of anaphylactic shock.

If the wound is minor and clean, active immunization may be begun without administration of tetanus immune globulin.

Techniques of administration. The nurse in a child health conference or in a doctor's private office usually administers immunizations. If the child associates any discomfort and pain with the nurse, he is likely to cry not only when he next sees her but also when he sees anyone else in a nurse's uniform. The skill with which the injection is given will influence the child's discomfort. After the injection has been given the nurse should pat and speak to the infant and perhaps offer the older infant or child a toy with which to play so that he can associate something pleasant with the nurse. The deltoid or the rectus femoris muscle or the vastus lateralis muscle of the thigh can be used for giving immunizations. Because of the danger of hitting the sciatic nerve, the use of the gluteal muscles should be avoided in infants or young children.

The serums used for prophylaxis of specific communicable diseases should be kept refrigerated. When transported from the health department to a child health conference, they should be in containers surrounded by ice. Care should also be taken to see that the solutions are not outdated.

Reactions to immunizations. Mild temperature elevations are the most common reactions. The occurrence of a severe reaction consisting of high fever (over 103° F. or 39.5° C.), somnolence, or convulsions is cause for caution in subsequent injections. Most physicians suggest that acetaminophen (Tylenol) or aspirin be given to the infant immediately when the infant returns to his home after immunization so that he will not be uncomfortable and fretful. Local reactions to the injection such as swelling, pain, and redness may be relieved by applying cold compresses to the affected area. The physician should be consulted if the infant continues to be ill after 24 to 48 hours.

Tuberculin test. The subject of tuberculin tests is included here because of the importance of early case findings so that treatment can be begun. Unfortunately tuberculin tests are not routinely done in either doctors' offices or child health conferences.

The intracutaneous test of Mantoux is the most frequent method of determining the sensitivity of a child to tuberculosis. Another test that is being used for survey purposes is the tine test.

MANTOUX TEST. The Mantoux test is usually done on the inner surface of the forearm. The selected dilution of tuberculin, usually 0.1 ml. of purified protein derivative (intermediate strength), is injected in the anterior surface of the forearm between the layers of the skin. A tuberculin syringe and a No. 26- or No. 27-gauge needle with a short bevel is used. The reading of the test is made 48 to 72 hours after the injection. Erythema alone is not significant. It is the presence and extent of the induration around the site that is important. The diameter of the induration should be measured in millimeters. Induration larger than 10 mm. is considered positive. Smaller ones may be due to various other factors, and the child should be retested. Purified protein derivative comes in three concentrations (first, intermediate, and second strengths). First strength purified protein derivative is the most dilute.

TINE TEST. The tine test equipment consists of a stainless steel disk with four tines or prongs attached to a plastic handle. The tines have been dipped into a solution of old tuberculin. The set is easy to store and is disposable. It eliminates the need to store bottles of tuberculin.

POSITIVE REACTIONS. If the tests are strongly positive for tuberculosis, the child either has tuberculosis or has had an initial infection from which he has recovered. The child is evaluated in regard to the status of his tuberculosis, whether active or inactive. Infants and children under 6 years of age and adolescents who have positive tuberculosis tests are usually placed on isoniazid for periods of not less than 1 year. It is to be remembered that the complications of tuberculous meningitis and acute miliary tuberculosis in the first 2 years of life account for the high mortality rate in childhood tuberculosis.

Frequently grandparents are sources of tuberculosis infection for children. Their coughs have gone unnoticed. It is imperative that a search be made of all contacts of the child until the desired information is gained. The public health nurse should be involved in this search. Until the person who has tuberculosis is found and treated, others will be exposed to the condition.

Avoidance of contact with the person who has active tuberculosis is the only positive means of not getting the disease. Milk for infants and children should come from tuberculosis-free cattle. All milk should be pasteurized, but if raw milk is used, it should be boiled before consumption by infants and children.

BCG. BCG (bacillus of Calmette-Guérin) is a vaccine that produces a partial immunity to tuberculosis. The duration of immunity is unknown. After it is given the purified protein derivative reaction of the person, if previously negative, turns positive. The use of BCG vaccine is limited to those having frequent contact with tuberculosis patients or to very young or elderly patients who are located in areas where there is tuberculosis. For example, a newborn infant could be administered BCG vaccine before being discharged to be cared for by the mother if the mother has a recent history of arrested pulmonary tuberculosis.

Prevention of nutritional deficiency diseases

Prevention of nutritional diseases again emphasizes the role of the nurse in teaching infant nutrition to mothers (or parents). The public health nurse can reinforce the guidance of the physician, whether it be in the hospital, child health conference, outpatient department, or home.

If an infant is given an adequate diet, the chances of development of nutritional disturbances will be minimal. The most common nutritional disturbances are iron deficiency anemia and malnutrition. Knowledge of these conditions is part of the nurse's background in fundamentals of nutrition; therefore only a few implications for the child's care are given here.

Iron deficiency anemia. The most common form of anemia in children under the age of 2 years develops when the child is not fed enough iron-rich foods such as iron-fortified cereal, egg yolk, and meat. Solid foods rich in iron should be offered before the formula when the infant is fed to offer the greatest available sources of iron. An infant needs a maximum of 32 ounces of formula per day at any age. If the infant is taking all the solid foods he should, then he is generally unable to take a quart of milk in a 24-hour period.

Iron deficiency anemia is characterized by red blood cells that are smaller than normal and very deficient in hemoglobin content. (See Appendix B for normal blood values at different ages.) This type of anemia can be referred to as hypochromic microcytic anemia. It occurs most frequently between 8 months and 2 years of age. The usual history obtained from the mother is that the child drinks at least 2 quarts of milk per day and refuses most other foods. The child is usually pale, listless, irritable, anorexic, and obstinate in his refusal of solid foods.

Treatment consists of addition of 100 mg. of elemental iron per day to the diet by giving an oral iron preparations. Two to three months is the average length of time it takes to restore the blood values to normal. If the anemia is severe enough to produce heart failure or if the child has a severe infection, it may be necessary to effect a more rapid correction by whole blood or packed red blood cell transfusion. Parenteral iron preparations are available but are used infrequently in children. The oral iron therapy usually produces a rapid improvement in the mental and physical condition of the child, and at the same time it increases the child's appetite for foods other than milk so that he gradually receives a more nutritionally balanced diet.

The role of the nurse is, first, to see that a well infant is under medical supervision so that the mother will receive guidance about the infant's nutrition and, second, to supplement this guidance as necessary relative to techniques in feeding so that the mother will carry out the physician's directions.

When the public health nurse sees the mother at child health conferences, she should be careful each time to ask what the infant is being fed. In home visits the nurse should look at the infant and notice his color, activity, brightness of the eyes, and texture of the skin as well as his general growth. If the nurse notices pallor, listlessness, irritability, possibly fat that is flabby, or other indications suggestive of iron deficiency, she should urge the mother to take the infant for a medical evaluation.

If the nurse sees the infant in the hospital, the administration of oral iron preparation ordered is her responsibility. If in the outpatient department, she is responsible for giving the mother directions in administering the iron preparation. The medicinal iron should be given to the infant between meals since milk and milk products contain phosphorus and cereals have a considerable amount of phytates, which form insoluble salts with iron.

When the infant is receiving treatment for iron deficiency anemia (either in the hospital or in the outpatient department), the nurse is in a splendid position to do teaching about general hygiene of the infant and/or to refer the infant to a public health nurse so the family can receive guidance on nutrition and general hygiene as necessary.

Scurvy. Scurvy is a disease caused by a deficiency of vitamin C. It can be specifically avoided by adequate intake of citrus fruits (such as orange juice or tomato juice) or vitamin supplement.

The mother of the infant with scurvy may notice that the infant cries when she diapers him or holds him. Pain is due to changes in the long bones of the child. Swelling and sometimes subperiosteal hemorrhages are present. The infant may lie motionless on his back with legs semi-flexed (a frog-leg position). The term *pseudoparalysis* has been used in relation to this. Scurvy may be further evidenced by hemorrhages in the gums, mucous membranes, and skin and also by blood in the stool and urine.

When he is admitted to the hospital, the nurse should handle the infant very gently and as little as possible. This is the one type of infant that the nurse should *not* pick up to feed or cuddle—until he has less pain. When an infant is better, he will begin to move around by himself. At that point the nurse can pick up the infant. Administration of ascorbic acid either parenterally or orally or both will correct the deficiency. Other than handling the infant carefully, the nurse's chief role is in giving the infant prescribed ascorbic acid orally. In addition to ascorbic acid, orange juice or tomato juice is given.

During the infant's hospitalization the nurse has a chance to teach the mother nutrition and feeding habits of infants. What the physician is going to tell the mother or what the nurse will say should not be left until the day the infant is discharged. Sometimes it is desirable for the nurse to have the mother repeat what the doctor has advised to see if the mother has really understood the directions. The nurse should also inquire about the medical supervision of siblings (if there are any) and their nutritional habits.

Rickets. An infant or child with rickets may display one or more of the following characteristics:

1. Craniotabes (softening of the occiput)
2. Enlarged epiphyses of wrists and ankles
3. Delayed closure of the anterior fontanel
4. Caput quadratum (square or box-like appearance of the head)
5. Dental defects (cavities and defects of the enamel)
6. Rachitic rosary or beading of ribs at the costochondral junction
7. Pigeon breast deformity of the chest
8. Harrison's groove (depression under the border of the chest)
9. Defects of the spinal column (scoliosis, kyphosis, lordosis)
10. Deformity of the pelvis (rachitic)
11. Genu valgum or genu varum (knock-knees or bowlegs)
12. Retarded growth and development

The treatment of rickets consists primarily of the administration of vitamin D. The daily administration of 1,500 to 5,000 I.U. (6 to 20 drops of a preparation containing 10,000 units per gm.) will produce healing demonstrable on roentgenograms within 2 to 4 weeks. The large dose should be continued until the healing process has well begun; thereafter a maintenance dose of 400 I.U. daily is adequate. Bone deformities such as knock-knees or bowlegs may require corrective appliances during the healing stages.

Nursing care. When this child is admitted to the hospital, an important aspect of the care provided by the nurse is to see that he receives vitamin D as ordered by the doctor and to carefully supervise his mealtime. (See p. 202 for a discussion of eating habits.) Other responsibilities of the nurse are to take precautions against the child's falling since his bones fracture easily and to try to prevent respiratory infections to which the rachitic child is very susceptible. He should be placed in a room where there are no children with infections.

Teaching the mother (or parents) about nutrition is again important, just as with the mother of the infant with scurvy. If the diet of one child in the family is inadequate, it is possible that the whole family's diet is inadequate and unbalanced. The local public health nurse is frequently able to counsel and advise the family regarding dietary measures if necessary.

Infantile tetany. Tetany due to a deficiency of vitamin D is an occasional accompaniment of rickets. It is now rare because of the widespread prophylactic use of vitamin D. It occurs most frequently between the ages of 4 months and 3 years; rarely it is observed before 3 months of age. The serum calcium level falls below 7 to 7.5 mg. per 100 ml., which produces muscular irritability.

Tetany, regardless of cause, is characterized by twitching or convulsion, carpopedal spasm, and laryngospasm. In carpopedal spasm the hands are abducted, the wrist being flexed and the thumb drawn across the palm of the hand. The foot is drawn inward and downward. In laryngospasm there is a high-pitched inspiratory cry. Carpopedal spasm can be obtained by placing a constricting or blood pressure cuff around the upper arm very tightly (Trousseau's sign). If the facial nerve is percussed in front of the auditory meatus, there is a contraction of the facial muscles on that side (Chvostek's sign).

Active treatment is designed to raise the serum calcium above the tetany level. The level may be obtained by administration of 4 to 6 gm. of calcium chloride or lactate in milk or 5 to 10 ml. of a 10% solution of calcium gluconate intravenously if oral medication is impractical. Calcium gluconate should not be given subcutaneously or intramuscularly because of the dangers of local necrosis.

Malnutrition. Malnutrition occurs when an inadequate intake of calories is continued for a prolonged period of time. The deficit may also be a lack of proteins, amino acids, or minerals. When the body does not receive the proper nutritive requirements it is forced to draw upon its own tissues for maintenance. Malnutrition may arise because of an insufficient food supply, ignorance of food requirements, or poverty or in association with a disease in which prolonged vomiting, diarrhea, abnormality of absorption, or prolonged intravenous feeding occurs. The incidence of malnutrition is decreasing in the United States since the implementation of government-sponsored food stamp programs.

Marasmus. The clinical signs and symptoms accompanying marasmus may be insidious and may reach an advanced state before its seriousness is appreciated. The picture of advanced marasmus is quite characteristic (Figs. 9-10 and 9-11). The skin hangs in folds, especially in the extremities and buttocks, due to atrophy of the subcutaneous fat. In young infants the sucking pads in the cheeks are the last fat depots to be used up, apparently because the fat there is more saturated and less readily mobilized. The bones and joints become prominent and the hands clawlike. The abdomen is scaphoid or distended. Physical activity is diminished, temperature is subnormal, and bradycardia may result. The infant's general appearance is that of a toothless old man.

As starvation progresses, resistance to infection is lowered, deficiency of one or more vitamins may occur, and low serum iron and

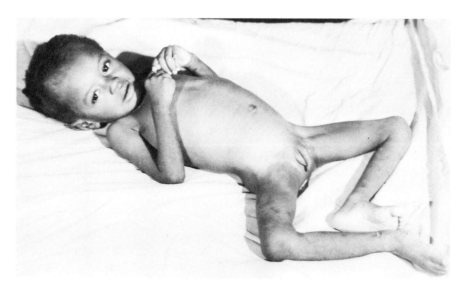

Fig. 9-10. Malnutrition in patient 10 months of age. Subcutaneous fat has disappeared. Note the child's apathy and misery and healed impetiginous lesions on the legs.

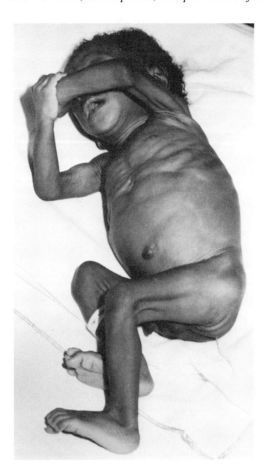

Fig. 9-11. Malnutrition and emotional deprivation in a 9-month-old child. Note "clasping" position of hands over child's head.

protein levels may result. As activity and peripheral circulation decrease, bed sores may develop.

In the management of marasmus the possible causes must be kept in mind. Parenteral feeding may be necessary if the condition is caused by gastrointestinal disease. The usual types of formulas are satisfactory for oral feedings but should be introduced cautiously; the child's ability to handle food is limited by the poor condition of the digestive tract. Many infants may require as much as 200 calories per kilogram of actual body weight before recovery begins. Recovery may be slow at first, but when it occurs it is usually complete. Sometimes, if the condition has been serious and of long duration, there is some impairment of stature as well as intelligence and behavioral development.

Nursing care is directed toward providing abundant emotional security and attention in the form of cuddling, holding, rocking, and feeding. Care of the skin is most important to prevent bed sores. The mother needs instructions and supervision in child care while the child is in the hospital. In addition, the hospital social worker may be helpful in aiding the mother to satisfy her own emotional needs. On discharge the mother should be referred to community social service agencies to help her obtain food for the child. Contact should be made with the public health nurse to help continue the instructions and supervision of the mother in care of the child.

Kwashiorkor. Kwashiorkor is a severe form of protein malnutrition. It is seen most commonly among children in underdeveloped countries when breast feeding is discontinued and the infant is placed on a diet of insufficient protein quality. It is rare in the United States and occurs most frequently between 18 months and

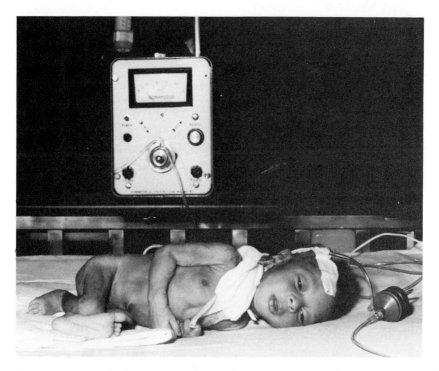

Fig. 9-12. Malnourished child receiving hyperalimentation. Note indwelling silicone rubber catheter that has been threaded into superior vena cava, Sigmamotor infusion pump, and Millipore bacterial filter.

5 years of age. Pathologic findings include atrophy of smooth and cardiac muscle, fatty infiltration and fibrosis of the liver, and atrophy of the mucous membrane of the gut. Symptoms include edema, retarded growth, alterations in skin and hair pigmentation, vitamin deficiencies, muscle weakness, and a mental state of apathy and irritability. A mortality rate of 20% to 30% occurs even with expert management. Treatment and prevention of kwashiorkor require the inclusion of adequate amounts of high-quality protein, vitamins, and minerals in the diet. Nursing care is essentially the same as in marasmus.

Summary

Infancy constitutes a period of rapid growth. The infant needs close medical supervision first of all to see that he is growing and developing as expected. The earlier any defect or abnormality is cited and treated, the better. In addition, the mother or parents may need guidance about the infant's nutrition and feeding habits, immunizations, and prevention of accidents. Also, physical, social, and emotional needs of the infant may need interpretation to the mother. For example, cuddling and playing with the infant do not spoil him. He needs to be given attention and to have sensory stimulation. The nurse should be careful not to try to give too much information at any one time. She should instead give it in accord with the previous knowledge of the mother, the immediate need of the mother, and her interest and her ability to understand. Complimenting the mother when she functions in a capable manner may stimulate the desire for further learning.

PROMOTION OF HEALTH IN THE TODDLER AND PRESCHOOL PERIOD
Health problems

Accidents are the leading cause of death in children 1 to 4 years old. As shown in Table 9-5, congenital anomalies, influenza and pneumonia, malignant neoplasms, homicide,

Table 9-5. Deaths and death rates
for children 1 to 4 years old, both sexes*

Rank	Cause of death†	Number	Rate‡
	All causes	11,548	84.5
1	Accidents (E800-E949)	4,300	31.5
2	Congenital anomalies (740-759)	1,331	9.7
3	Influenza and pneumonia (470-474, 480-486)	1,043	7.6
4	Malignant neoplasms, including neoplasms of lymphatic and hematopoietic tissues (140-209)	1,027	7.5
5	Homicide (E960-E978)	258	1.9
6	Meningitis (320)	254	1.9
7	Diseases of heart (390-398, 402, 404, 410-429)	237	1.7
8	Enteritis and other diarrheal diseases (008, 009)	186	1.4
9	Acute bronchitis and bronchiolitis (446)	141	1.0
10	Meningococcal infections (036)	138	1.0

*Modified from Facts of life and death, Rockville, Md., 1974, Public Health Service, U.S. Department of Health, Education, and Welfare (Table 28).
†According to International classification of diseases, eighth revision, 1965.
‡Per 100,000 population in age group.

and meningitis rank next in order. Education of parents in prevention of accidents to toddlers and young children should reduce the accident mortality. Periodical health examination to detect any abnormalities plus prompt medical attention when the child is ill are imperative in any attempt to reduce the other health problems. Good general health will help the child's resistance if he has an infection in this period.

Role of the nurse

The nurse's contacts with a child of this age do not differ much from her contacts with the infant except that in some instances the child health conference is limited to children under 2 years of age. True, there is a preschool roundup of children who will be entering the first grade in the fall. At this roundup health assessments can be done. The child can receive the immunizations and vaccinations recommended by the state health department.

Another contact of the public health nurse is in nursery schools, kindergartens, or day nurseries. Sometimes the nurse is invited to talk to mothers' clubs or groups about the health problems and care of preschool children.

The factors that the nurse needs to know in promoting the health of the toddler and preschool child are discussed in the following pages: assessing the child's health, eating and sleeping habits, toilet training, play and exercise, sex education, discipline, accident prevention, and medical supervision.

Assessment of health

A suggested guide for assessment of health of children in this age group is shown in Fig. 9-13. Also included is a summary of data to be obtained regarding development and care as well as suggested topics for health guidance.

An explanation of physical assessment of the infant was given on p. 165. In the physical assessment of the toddler and preschool child, only the differences in growth and development from those of infancy will be discussed. For example, the average child can understand simple directions, walks alone at 15 months, talks in short sentences at' 2 years, and has erupted his temporary set of teeth by 2½ years. His anterior fontanel closes by 18 months of age. It is possible to give preschool children an audiometric examination, a Snellen vision test, and a detailed neurological examination. Infantile reflexes have disappeared. The head circumference is 90% of its adult size by 6 years of age.

The 12 cranial nerves can be assessed as outlined on the assessment guide. Assessment of cerebellar function helps to appraise motor coordination. By 3 years of age this can be tested by having the child walk several steps heel to toe, touch his nose with his index finger when his eyes are closed, run in place, twist both hands as though screwing a light bulb, stand on one foot briefly, and pat his knee with the palm of his hand and then the back of his hand. A child from 1 to 3 years of age will normally be expected to have difficulty in performing these tasks.

The motor system can be tested through inspection of muscles for size, tone, and strength

Text continued on p. 201.

SECTION 1: PHYSICAL EXAMINATION

Directions: Fill in blanks with appropriate information.

MEASUREMENTS

Height _____ Weight _____ Respirations _____ Blood pressure _____

Circumference: Head _____ Chest _____

SKIN

Color _____ Tissue turgor _____ Bruises _____ Moles _____

Swelling _____ Rash (describe) _____

Other _____

SENSORY DEVELOPMENT
Eyes

General observations: Color _____ Expression: Dull _____ Bright _____

Inflammation: Eyes _____ Eyelids _____

Discharge: Right _____ Left _____

Dried secretions on eyelids: Right _____ Left _____

Pupils react equally to light: Right _____ Left _____

Strabismus (Observe position of light reflected in cornea; should be in center of each pupil. For older

child, 3 to 5 years, cover one eye at a time and have child fixate on distant object straight ahead.

Note if uncovered eye moves in either direction.): Left _____ Right _____

Visual acuity: Test with Snellen chart after 3 years of age.

Ears

(Use otoscope as necessary.)

Normal configuration and position _____ Other _____

External ear normal _____ Cysts, malformations _____

Pain: Right _____ Left _____

Canal: Clean _____ Wax _____ Discharge _____ Lesions _____

Foreign body _____ Other _____

Tympanic membrane color (normally gray) _____ Handle of malleus visualized _____

Concave eardrum _____ Cone of light reflex (from otoscope) fans out externally _____

Hearing (For small child: Shake bell or rattle behind child, first on one side, then the other. For older

child, 3 to 5 years, audiometer may be used.): Right _____ Left _____

Nose

Nostrils patent (Close one nostril with finger and observe breathing through other nostril.): Right _____

Left _____

Dried secretions _____ Discharge (describe): Right _____ Left _____

Continued.

Fig. 9-13. Guide for health assessment of toddler and preschool child.

SECTION 1: PHYSICAL EXAMINATION—cont'd

Mouth and throat

(Use tongue depressor and flashlight as necessary.)

Lips: Moist _____ Dry _____ Cracked _____

Mouth breathing _____ History of snoring when asleep _____

Condition of gums _____ Buccal membrane _____

Teeth: Number _____ Condition _____

Pharynx clearly visible _____ Exudate on tonsils _____

Tonsils: Inflamed _____ Obstructing view of pharynx _____

Soft and hard palate intact _____

HEAD

Shape: Symmetrical _____ Unusual (describe) _____

Scalp: Smooth _____ Dry _____ Scaly _____ Nodules _____

Other _____

Hair: Texture (fine, coarse) _____ Dandruff _____ Nits _____ Pediculi _____

Other _____

Fontanels: Posterior: Closed _____ Open _____ Anterior: Closed _____ Open _____

Characteristics if open: Normal _____ Full _____ Bulging _____ Depressed _____

Face: Symmetrical _____ Expression: Dull _____ Alert _____ Interested _____

Rash _____ Anything unusual _____

NECK

Supple (full range of motion) _____ Symmetrical _____

Lymph nodes palpable _____

Thyroid, thymus, trachea in midline _____

LUNGS

Expand symmetrically _____ Contour symmetrical _____

Barrel shape _____ Abdominal respirations _____

Breathes quietly _____ Grunting respirations _____

Wheezing _____ Other abdominal sounds _____

Rales _____ Wheezing _____ Retractions _____

HEART

Quality of heart sounds _____ Rate _____ Rhythm _____ Intensity _____

Murmur _____ Unusual sounds _____

Fig. 9-13, cont'd. Guide for health assessment of toddler and preschool child.

SECTION 1: PHYSICAL EXAMINATION—cont'd

ABDOMEN

Contour: Symmetrical _____ Protuberant _____ Distended _____ Hard _____

Other _____

Respiratory movements of abdomen (not usually seen after third year) _____

Scars _____ Protrusions _____ Other _____

Masses (Palpate abdominal organs gently.) _____

Umbilicus: Clean _____ Protruding _____ Discharge _____ Other _____

Bowel sounds (Listen with stethoscope.) _____

EXTREMITIES
All joints

Full range of motion _____ If not, explain _____

_____

Arms and hands

Edema _____ Color _____ Nodules _____ Rash _____

Unusual warmth or coolness _____ Other _____

Nail beds: Color _____ Circulation (Apply pressure to see if color returns quickly.) _____

Clubbing of fingers _____

Legs

Edema _____ Color _____ Unusual warmth or coolness _____

Nodules _____ Rash _____ Other _____

Equal in length _____

Hips

Test for dislocated hip (see p. 342).

BACK

Scapulae equal _____ Vertebrae straight _____ Moles _____

Protrusions _____ Swelling _____ Other _____

Iliac crests even _____

GENITALIA
Female

Labia symmetrical _____ Clean _____ Inflammation _____

Discharge (describe) _____

Presence of clitoris _____ Vaginal orifice _____ Urinary meatus _____

Fig. 9-13, cont'd. Guide for health assessment of toddler and preschool child.

Continued.

SECTION 1: PHYSICAL EXAMINATION—cont'd

Male

Penis with urethral opening at end _____ If not, describe _____

Testes in scrotum: Right _____ Left _____

Circumcised _____ If not, foreskin easily retracted _____ Clean _____

ANUS

Patent _____ Fissures _____ Anything unusual _____

NEUROMUSCULAR DEVELOPMENT

First olfactory cranial nerve

Identification of familiar odors (oranges, peanut butter, etc.) _____

Second (optic) cranial nerve

Visual acuity: Snellen Test _____

Peripheral vision (Have child focus on object such as examiner's nose; move finger through all hemi-

spheres; ask child when he can first see the finger.): Nasal side (should be 60 degrees) _____

Temporal side (should be 100 degrees) _____ Vertical (should be 130 degrees) _____

Third (oculomotor), fourth (trochlear), and fifth (abducent) cranial nerves

Unequal movement of pupils (Have child follow examiner's finger moving through all quadrants.):

Right _____ Left _____

Pupillary light reflex in corresponding spots on pupils: Yes _____ No _____

Nystagmus _____

Sixth (trigeminal) cranial nerve

Motor division: Symmetry of strength of muscles of jaw (Try to pull tongue blade away as child bites

hard on it.) _____

Sensory division (Touch forehead, cheeks, and jaw with point of pin.): Sensation present _____

Sensation absent _____

Symmetry of response: Right _____ Left _____

Corneal reflex (Touch cornea with wisp of cotton.) _____

Seventh (facial) cranial nerve

Motor division: Symmetry _____ (Have child wrinkle forehead, smile, and raise eyebrows.):

have child close eyes while examiner tries to open them by pushing upward on eyebrows): Equality

of strength _____

Sensory division (Have child put out tongue and put sugar then salt on anterior sides of it.): Iden-

tifies: Salt _____ Sugar _____

Fig. 9-13, cont'd. Guide for health assessment of toddler and preschool child.

SECTION 1: PHYSICAL EXAMINATION—cont'd

Eighth (acoustic) cranial nerve

For small child, shake bell or rattle behind child, first on one side, then the other. For older child, use

audiometric test. _____

Ninth (glossopharyngeal) and tenth (vagus) cranial nerves

Hoarseness of voice _____ Ability to swallow _____ Gag reflex _____

Eleventh (accessory) cranial nerve

Strength and symmetry of sternocleidomastoid muscle (Turn child's head against opposing pressure

on one side, then the other.): Right _____ Left _____

Strength and symmetry of trapezius muscle (ability to lift shoulders simultaneously against opposing

pressure): Right _____ Left _____

Twelfth (hypoglossal) cranial nerve

Have child press tongue against each cheek: Right _____ Left _____ Symmetry _____

Cerebral function

For young child, use development test. For older child, use psychometric examinations. Note general

behavior and levels of consciousness.

Cerebellar functions

Touches nose with index finger with eyes closed (Repeat once or twice; note consistent past pointing.)

_____

Pats knee with palm of hand, then with back of hand (Repeat several times.) _____

Twists both hands as if screwing a light bulb (Child should copy twisting motion demonstrated by

examiner.) _____

Stands straight with feet together and eyes open _____ With eyes closed _____

Walks heel to toe several steps _____

Stands on one foot (age 4 years) _____

Runs in place _____

Motor system

Muscle size: Normal _____ Hypertrophy _____ Atrophy _____

Muscle tone: Good _____ Flaccid _____ Spasticity _____ Hypotonia _____

Symmetry (Measure muscles in calf of leg and compare with similar muscles of other leg.) _____

Muscle strength (Have child push against resistance from the examiner.) _____

Symmetry of resistance in arms (Have child extend arms out straight: try to push them apart.) _____

(Try to push them together.) _____

Fig. 9-13, cont'd. Guide for health assessment of toddler and preschool child.

Continued.

SECTION 1: PHYSICAL EXAMINATION—cont'd

Motor system—cont'd

Other groups of muscles tested same way _____

Abdominal muscles (ability to do several sit-ups) _____

Abnormal muscle movements: Twitching _____ Tics _____ Tremors _____ Chorei-

form movements _____ Jerking involuntary movements _____

Sensory system: primary sensation

Superficial tactile sensation (Test symmetrical areas of body with wisp of cotton. Have child close

his eyes and point to spot he felt sensation.) _____

Superficial pain (Test symmetrical parts of body with sharp and blunt ends of pin. Have child close

his eyes and tell whether pin is sharp or blunt.) _____

Temperature (Fill one test tube with hot and one with cold water; have child close his eyes and touch

him with alternate tubes.) _____

Vibration (Use large tuning fork. Ask child to tell when vibration stops. Places tested for vibration

include sternum, elbows, knees, toes, iliac crests.) _____

Cortical and discriminatory sensation

Two-point discrimination (Ask child to close eyes and tell if one or two points are pressing on skin.

Test several areas.) _____

Point localization (Have child close his eyes and ask him to point to spot where object touched him.

Use wisp of cotton, test tube, or pin.) _____

Extinction phenomena (Test of parietal lobe in child older than 6 years. Touch child simultaneously

in two homologous parts; ask where he was touched; he should feel two places.) _____

_____

Reflexes*

Plantar grasp reflex† _____ Biceps reflex _____ Triceps reflex _____

Brachioradialis reflex _____ Achilles tendon reflex _____ Patellar reflex _____

Globular reflex (Tap bridge of nose and eyes will close; check for symmetry.) _____

Blink reflex (Shine light suddenly in eyes.) _____

Babinski reflex‡ _____

*The following infant reflexes should have disappeared by age 6 months: Moro reflex, tonic neck reflex, rooting reflex, stepping reflex.
†Absence indicates possible spinal cord lesion.
‡Should be negative after age 18 months.

Fig. 9-13, cont'd. Guide for health assessment of toddler and preschool child.

SECTION 2: GENERAL DEVELOPMENT

GROSS MOTOR DEVELOPMENT
Postural development

Creeps _____ Stands with one hand held _____ Stands alone _____ Walks with

one hand held _____ Walks alone _____ Runs _____ Climbs _____ Stands on

one foot momentarily (3 years) _____ Hops on one foot _____ Skips (5 years) _____

Use of hands

Picks up cube and places it in cup (1 year) _____

Builds tower of blocks (number) _____

Draws with pencil: Circular scribble (2 years) _____ Man (4 years) _____ Triangle from

copy (5 years) _____

LANGUAGE DEVELOPMENT

Single words (number) _____ Sentences (2 years) _____

Follows simple commands _____ Knows full name _____ Age _____ Sex _____

Counts pennies (number—should be 10 at age 5 years) _____

Names four colors (5 years) _____

SOCIAL DEVELOPMENT

Plays simple ball games (1 year) _____ Says "bye-bye" _____

Indicates some needs by pointing _____

Feeds self _____ Manipulates spoon well _____

Helps to undress (2 years) _____ Dress _____

Helps to put things away _____

Washes hands _____

Play: Parallel play _____ Beginning to share and participate (social interaction) _____

Asks questions _____ Role playing _____

EMOTIONAL DEVELOPMENT

Usually happy _____ Irritable _____ Usually quiet _____ Active _____

Hyperactive _____ Listless _____ Lethargic _____

Activity child especially likes or causes of happiness _____

Activities that especially upset child _____

Time spent away from mother _____ Behavior when away from mother _____

Attachments to particular adults _____ Behavior when strangers are present _____

Attachment to inanimate objects for security _____

Continued.

Fig. 9-13, cont'd. Guide for health assessment of toddler and preschool child.

SECTION 3: GENERAL CARE

SLEEPING

Has own bed _____ Sleeps with another child _____ Time of nap _____ Length of

nap _____ Bedtime _____ Time awake in A.M. _____ Sleeps quietly _____

Restless _____ Nightmares _____

NUTRITION

Does child still take milk by bottle? _____

Describe food eaten in last 24 hours: Breakfast _____ Lunch _____ Dinner _____

   Snacks _____

ELIMINATION

How frequently does child void? _____

Number of stools per day _____ Describe (amount, color, consistency) _____

Dry in daytime _____ Nighttime _____

Goes to toilet by self _____ Manages clothing by self _____

CLOTHING

Clean _____ Serviceable _____ Adequate _____

DENTAL CARE

Brushes teeth _____

Visits dentist periodically _____

PLAY

Play materials child especially likes _____

Is there a place for him to store his toys? _____

Plays outdoors _____ If so, where? _____

Plays alone _____ Plays with other children _____

Enrolled in nursery school _____ Day nursery _____

Enjoys presence of other child or children _____

DISCIPLINE

Is child usually cooperative? _____

Reaction of mother if child is uncooperative _____

PROBLEMS

What problems does mother see in care of child? _____

_____

_____

Fig. 9-13, cont'd. Guide for health assessment of toddler and preschool child.

SECTION 3: GENERAL CARE—cont'd

PARENT-CHILD RELATIONSHIP

Behavior of child when mother is present (as observed) _____

Behavior of mother with child (as observed) _____

Time mother spends in play with child (describe) _____ _____

Time father spends in play with child (describe) _____

Time father spends in caring for child (describe) _____

Does mother enjoy child? _____ Does father? _____

Does either parent punish child? _____ If so, how? _____

_____

Why? _____

Recreation of mother and father away from child _____

SIGNIFICANT OTHERS

Other adults who spend time with child _____

What do they do with child? _____

How does child react with them? _____

HEALTH TOPICS FOR GUIDANCE

Nutrition
Play materials and play
Sleep and naps
Elimination
Immunization
Prevention of accidents
Self-help with clothing
Dental care
Health of parents
Self-reliance
Limitation of behavior

Fig. 9-13, cont'd. Guide for health assessment of toddler and preschool child.

as noted in the assessment guide. Twitching, tremors, and jerky or involuntary movements, if present, should be noted.

The sensory system is assessed by testing tactile sensation and reactions to superficial pain, temperature, and vibration as described on the assessment guide.

The well toddler or preschool child is active and has a clear skin, bright eyes, an animated expression, good posture, and endurance. He increases steadily in height and weight. His appetite is good and he sleeps well. He has a pleasant disposition. A cross, irritable child is not a well child.

As mentioned previously as part of the assessment, information about the child's development and general care is obtained as well as a physical examination. Based on information gained, health guidance can be given. Detailed discussion of health factors for children of this age is given in the section entitled "Guidance toward health."

Behavior characteristics

For a detailed description of this period of childhood see Chapter 6. For convenience of the reader, a brief review of a few behavior characteristics and patterns will be given.

The typical toddler walks or runs with his feet rather far apart and is still a little unsteady in his balance. He falls easily. He is a busy person, poking his finger into everything he can. Anything he can pick up and put in his mouth, he will. Adults must be careful not to leave within his reach small objects that he can swallow or any medicines or poisonous substances such as insecticides. The toddler is discovering himself as a person. There is much he can do by himself: ambulating with no help, feeding himself, playing with objects, helping to undress, etc. He can speak in short sentences by 2 years and thus may easily communicate. Erickson has described this as the stage of autonomy. The toddler wants to be independent and becomes negative and upset when crossed. To let him do as much as possible for himself is helpful. He is rigid and ritualistic only because this offers him security, that is, to have routines (eating, bathing, going to bed) done the same way each time. Separation from familiar people and/or a familiar environment (for example, hospitalization or absence of his mother for a period of days) is anxiety provoking. No matter how independent he is, when strangers come into the home he is apt to run quickly to his mother and stay by her.

The 3-year-old is more mature and more flexible. He wishes to please adults. His increased vocabulary aids his ability to relate to others. He often asks "Why?" not for information but to get the other person to talk to him more so he, in turn, can say more. His play is largely individualistic, but a beginning of sharing is seen. The 3-year-old enjoys using a tricycle. He takes responsibility to go to the bathroom himself and thus keeps dry in the day time. At 3 to 4 years he keeps a dry bed at night.

The 4-year-old is an aggressive person. He may defy authority. He is curious and asks questions about the world around him. Walking, climbing, eating, and bathing are routine matters now. He explores the environment around him. Trips to a zoo or farm or a walk in the woods takes on new meaning; this is a stage of initiative and curiosity. Although he shares, he still is not capable socially of organized group play. He plays by himself more than with others. He can skip and draw a man with head and legs.

The 5-year-old child is a more stable, calm person than the 4-year-old child. There is little, if any, infantile articulation. He enjoys being near his mother and is proud of his father. He can count 10 objects correctly. He prefers companionship to solitary play.

Guidance toward health
General hygiene

Eating. Nutritional needs and psychological factors that influence eating continue to play a role in growth and development in the toddler and preschool years. Goals for nutrition should include recognition and acceptance of a variety of foods and an increased ability for self-feeding. It is important to emphasize that regular meal schedules and good food habits established in the toddler and preschool periods will have a lifetime impact.

Nutritional needs. After a year of rapid gains in height and weight during infancy, the child's growth rate begins to slow down gradually, so it can be expected that the energy needed for growth will also decrease. Energy requirements for the toddler are 100 calories per kilogram per day. Although this calorie requirement is a slightly higher allowance than during the later months of infancy, it is lower in relation to body weight from ages 1 to 3 than in the first year of life. The energy requirements for the toddler per pound of weight are the lowest they will ever be during childhood. Changes in body composition that accompany growth and development make it extremely important that these calories be provided by high-quality foods.

The child is no longer dependent on others to carry him about; he is beginning to stand by himself and walk. This indicates that the skeletal muscles, especially those of the back, buttocks, and thighs, should begin to increase in size. Normally the increase in muscle mass accounts for about one half of the total weight the child will gain in the toddler years. To allow for this growth the toddler should have at least 2 gm. per kilogram of good-quality protein per day. Such foods as milk, meat, fish, eggs, cheese, peanut butter, or dried peas and beans need to be included in the child's diet each day. Without sufficient protein the child's muscles will be weak and his posture will be poor.

The long bones, although not growing as rapidly in length, are mineralizing and being strengthened to stand the stress of walking and carrying weight. They need good supplies of calcium, phosphorus, and vitamin D. These nutrients are also important for the deciduous teeth that are beginning to erupt. Two cups of milk plus the milk the child eats as cheese, on cereal, or as ice cream and pudding is sufficient to meet the recommended dietary allowance of 800 mg. of calcium a day.

The reduced energy needs of the toddler relative to his body weight can cause a decrease in appetite—the term *physiologic anorexia* is sometimes applied. Consequently the mother might complain that the child does not seem to be eating as well as he did in infancy, that he plays with his food and does not finish all that is on his plate.

One possible reason may be that the mother is giving the child too much food. It is often difficult for the mother to visualize how much food is appropriate, especially in view of the change in appetite. A way to help her understand the child's nutritional needs is in terms of her own requirements. If the mother herself is eating a good diet, she should be consuming about 2,000 calories and 46 gm. of protein a day. The toddler needs approximately half of these amounts.

Another rule of thumb for the 2-, 3-, and 4-year-old is to offer 1 level tablespoon of each different food for each year of age. For example, an appropriate dinner menu for a 2-year-old might be 2 tablespoons of boneless, lean, cut meat, 2 tablespoons of mashed potatoes, 2 tablespoons of raw or cooked vegetables, ½ slice of bread, ½ serving of dessert, and ½ to ¾ cup milk.

Some mothers have trouble getting their young children to accept vegetables. Nutrition surveys reflect this in that the diets of toddlers and preschool children tend to be frequently deficient in vitamins A and C. It is always easier if the vegetables are not overcooked, not too hot, and not allowed to get cold and soggy. Plain, raw, crisp vegetables are usually favored over creamed cooked ones. The child may have trouble with tough or stringy parts. It is less difficult for the toddler to eat vegetables if the stalks of such varieties as broccoli and asparagus are cut into small pieces and the strings are removed from celery before they are given to the child.

Sometimes mothers who are having feeding problems with their toddlers tend to think that as long as the child drinks his milk his nutrition will be all right. As a result the child is drinking more than a quart of milk a day and eating few other foods. Over a period of weeks or months on such a diet it is not unusual for the child to require treatment for iron deficiency anemia. To prevent such situations the nurse must help the mother understand the change in appetite that will occur when her child reaches the toddler years and emphasize the need for including a variety of foods from the Basic Four food groups in the diet each day. In the preschool years the same variety of foods should be offered but in slightly larger quantities. The child from 4 to 6 years of age needs 1,800 calories and 30 gm. of protein each day.

Physiological factors. A 24-hour recall and food history should be taken routinely to determine what the child is being offered and how much he usually eats. If food variety and portion sizes are appropriate but the mother still complains that the child does not eat well, the nurse should consider physiological factors that influence the appetite.

Illness itself may be a reason for a poor appetite. The child with an elevated temperature does not eat as much as he usually does; in fact, if a child is listless or cross and does not wish to eat, his temperature should be taken. A low hemoglobin level may also produce a relative anorexia.

Exercise and activity, especially in the outdoor air, will stimulate the appetite; conversely fatigue will decrease it. The child may be too tired to eat. The toddler and preschool child need a nap after lunch. The child 4 to 5 years old might not sleep, but a rest on his bed for an hour is relaxing.

Snacks. The interval between meals is important. The toddler and preschool child have a small stomach capacity. Small mid-meal snacks of nutritious foods such as cheese sticks, ice cream, and pieces of fruit contribute to the child's nutrition and are fun to eat, but constant nibbling throughout the day should be avoided. This prohibits proper emptying of the stomach. The result is that the child will not be hungry at mealtimes.

A common practice of mothers of 1- to 2-year-olds is giving them apple or grape juice in a baby bottle between meals. Mothers sometimes think that, because they come from fruits, these juices make good snacks, and the baby bottle prevents having to clean up spills. The practice should be discouraged for two reasons. First, the child is old enough to begin to take liquids from a cup. Second, apple and grape juice have a high sugar content. Constant sucking from a bottle is associated with a high incidence of dental caries among toddlers and preschool children.

Another popular snack for young children is sugar-coated breakfast cereals. While these cereals are usually enriched with some B vitamins and iron, the high sugar content negates the benefits of added nutrients. *Plain* whole grain and enriched cereals are more appropriate occasional finger snacks.

Psychological factors. The following factors can help the child to enjoy mealtime:

1. Food that is easy to handle. "Finger foods" such as carrot sticks, lettuce, hard-boiled eggs, bananas, apple slices, orange slices, and hot dogs are popular with children. Other vegetables and meat should be cut in small pieces.

2. Simple and attractive foods. A child of this age is alert and interested in his environment; he is anxious to examine and learn new things. Eating can be a delightful experience. Since he is no longer eating strained or pureed foods, the toddler can begin to recognize the variety of textures, colors, and flavors of differ-

ent foods. However, most children are not gourmets; they do not like highly spiced or strongly flavored foods. Combination dishes should be served with discretion. If the child is given a complicated casserole, chances are he will separate all the parts before eating it or he will not eat it at all. This is because the child likes to know exactly what is on his plate.

Curiosity can be used as a motivation for introducing new foods. As in infancy, this should be done gradually—one at a time. The child should not be bribed to try something new, nor should he be scolded if he does not like it. He can always give it another try at a later time.

3. Small portions. The child may make no attempt to eat a large serving. A glass of milk or fruit juice needs to be small in size. It is easier to give seconds than it is to coax a child to eat a large serving.

4. Company with meals. It is more fun to have other children at the table or to be with other people at mealtime than it is to be alone. True, preschool children and toddlers cannot eat and talk at the same time, but the presence of others keeps the child from feeling lonesome, and helps him learn to associate mealtime and eating as enjoyable social experiences.

5. Example of others. Since children like to imitate their elders, they will want to sample foods that others eat. Conversely, if adults indicate their dislike for certain foods, the child will too. Adults should be aware of how sensitive the child is to their own reactions towards food. The child should be allowed to make up his own mind regarding likes and dislikes.

6. Social behavior of adults. Cheerfulness, serenity, and matter-of-factness (rather than coaxing, bribing, or threatening) are more conducive to the child's eating what is in front of him. If the adults say "please" and "thank you," the child in time learns these expressions in relation to their proper use and will use them also.

7. Physical conditions of eating. Cheery surroundings, a well-ventilated room, and comfortable eating conditions all add to the possibility of the child's eating more than he might otherwise. The chair in which he sits should be of the right height so that the child

will not be placed in an awkward position at the table and have to reach way up for his food. The toddler might be placed in a high chair at the table where he can see other members of the family and the food they eat. A plastic bib placed on the toddler like an apron will protect his clothing since he is a messy eater. The rug or floor might be protected by a newspaper under the child's chair so that the mother can relax and help the child enjoy mealtime. Suitable eating utensils are important also. While he is between 1 and 3 years of age the young child needs a straight-sided spoon and a dish with sides on it since he does not have control of his fine muscles as an older child does. Between 1 and 2 years of age he is able to manage a small cup with straight sides. Soup can be put in a cup for the child to drink. A 3-year-old child can learn to use a fork—preferably a salad fork since it is wider and the food stays on it better. The 3-year-old child can eat from a plate rather than a bowl. Lettuce can be added as a "finger food" or it can be placed between bread in a sandwich. It is difficult for a child to eat lettuce with a fork or spoon.

8. Readiness for mealtime. No child likes to stop playing immediately and be called to supper. The mother should give him a warning that it will soon be mealtime so that he may finish the activity in which he is engaged. She should see that his hands are washed and that he is toileted; then he is ready to come to the table. The routine of washing hands prior to mealtime helps to get his mind set toward another activity.

9. Conditioned eating behavior. Many psychologists believe that the meanings people attach to food in early childhood condition their eating behavior for life. In our society certain foods carry social connotations that the child readily learns. For example, sweets such as cookies, candy, and cake are often considered "treats"; dessert is sometimes a "reward" for finishing a meal. Some parents use sweets to placate the child when they cannot give him the attention he requires or demands.

We do not know for sure what ill consequences for the future these practices have. Some believe that one cause of obesity may be that people have learned to turn to food treats as a means of self-gratification when things go wrong. A "sweet tooth" has a known association with dental caries, and some have suggested that it may play a role in the onset of diabetes and atherosclerosis.

This does not mean that we must divorce food of its social meanings, but food should not be used as a reward, nor withholding it as a punishment. The nurse can help parents appreciate the problem by emphasizing that young children will learn to enjoy all kinds of food if they are given the chance and that high-sugar, empty-calorie foods are not the way to show children that they are loved.

Rest and sleep. Both rest and sleep relieve muscle fatigue and help to maintain stability of the nervous system. The amount a child needs varies a little with each child just as it does with individual adults. If the child has had enough sleep, he awakens in a happy mood and wants to get up. If he is cross and listless, he has not had enough sleep. In general children have both a morning and an afternoon nap up to 18 months or 2 years; however, some children discontinue their morning nap by 1 year of age. Others may continue a morning nap but not sleep in the afternoon.

The total sleep at night remains somewhat constant, but the nap shortens as the child gets older. When the child is 5 years old and attends kindergarten, he needs a period of rest after lunch even if he does not sleep. Rest slows down the metabolism. The 1-year-old child needs from 12 to 17 hours of sleep, the 2- and 3-year-old need from 10 to 16 hours, and the 5-year-old, 9 to 14 hours.

During the toddler and preschool period the aims in sleeping habits are a willingness to go to bed, independence, and ability to fall asleep quickly. In accomplishing these aims there are several factors to be considered: the physical condition of the child, psychological aspects, and the physical environment.

Physical condition of the child. Hunger, fatigue, daytime nap, elimination, and digestion all influence the child's ability to sleep. The child who has had an afternoon nap of 2 hours probably is not ready to go to bed at 7:00 or 7:30. Bedtime and naptime need to be suited to the individual child and to the family. If a father does not come until late, he needs to see his children then. Their schedule should be so arranged that they will be awake for at least a short time when he is home.

If a child has an early dinner at 5:00 but is put to bed at 7:30, he needs a nourishing snack before starting to bed. A sandwich, a glass of milk, fruit, or a bowl of cereal can answer this purpose. Discomfort from indigestion will not allow the child to relax. A quiet period of play is more conducive to the child's ability to fall asleep readily than is a strenuous active romp. His elimination needs should receive attention before he gets into bed since a desire to void or defecate also influences sleep.

Psychological aspects. Emotional upsets, scoldings, overexcitement, punishment, and unpleasant associations with bed and bedtime interfere with the child's willingness to go to bed and his ability to fall asleep quickly. If he is accustomed to being rocked or to using a particular blanket and he then cannot be rocked or the blanket is not available, the child becomes upset and it may be some time before he goes to sleep.

Before the toddler is taken to bed the mother or mother-substitute should help him to pick up his toys and put them away. This helps to emphasize that playtime is finished and it is time for something else. A 4- or 5-year-old child may, in addition to this, need warning that it is *almost* time for bed. This lets him have time to complete whatever he may be doing with blocks or some particular toy.

The routine of going to bed should be socialized. It should be a pleasant contact for both parent and child—a time when they talk with each other and become further acquainted. After he has had a warm (not hot) bath and is in comfortable night clothing, he may wish to tell mother or father about the events of the day that were important to him. Sometimes parent and child plan the next day together. When the mother works, bedtime and an evening chat become very important. On the other hand, the father may like to use this time to get to know his little son or daughter better. Any unpleasant happening in the day should be straightened out by evening. The child should never be threatened with punishment the fol-

lowing day. All should be calm and well when the child is ready to fall asleep.

Sometimes it is comforting to the child to sleep with a particular stuffed animal or doll—one that is sort of soft and cuddly.

It is well to accustom the child to sleeping in the dark, but, if the child is visiting relatives, the possession of a small flashlight ready for his use in the night if necessary helps to give him confidence.

Physical environment. The number of children or of children and adults in a bed, the bed itself, the adequacy of coverings on the bed, the comfort and adequacy of night clothing, and the ventilation all influence the sleep of the child. If possible, the child should have a bed of his own. A warm, lightweight blanket is usually more comfortable to the child than a heavy blanket, which is not necessarily warm. The bed or crib should be large enough for the child and should have a firm mattress.

Because the toddler often kicks off his blankets before falling asleep, pajamas with feet in them are usually convenient to use in the winter. When the child is asleep, the blanket can be rearranged. Pajamas or nightgown should fit. If the garment is too tight, it constricts the child's movements and limits his ability to relax; if too large, it fails to serve its purpose. Pajamas are most serviceable when made so that the bottom part buttons onto the top. Then, when the 2-year-old child wets his diaper at night, the mother can change the diaper and adjust the clothing with a minimum of disturbance to the child.

The room should be well ventilated, and extremes of temperature should be avoided. If the room temperature is comfortable to the adult, it is probably comfortable to the child.

Suggested routine at bedtime. The routine at bedtime may include the following: having some quiet activity before bedtime, being warned that bedtime comes soon, putting away toys and games, observing a regular hour of bedtime, associating pleasantness with bedtime (a socialized routine), having a warm bath, attending to toilet needs, using comfortable night clothing and bed clothing in a well-ventilated room, and finally saying goodnight. The attitude of the adult should be matter-of-fact throughout the routine. The adult *expects* the child to go to bed.

Naps. Again, the hour for the naps should be consistent. Removing play clothing and putting on night clothing suggest sleep. The room should be darkened. The child should be comfortable. The child may like to hold one particular toy. It is neither necessary nor wise for the mother to remain at the bedside until he falls asleep. This furthers the child's dependency. If a day then comes when mother cannot stay with the child, he will lie and fuss and have trouble going to sleep. Ordinary household noises should continue, but an effort should be made to avoid loud or unusual noises.

Coming into the child's room promptly when he wakens and attending to him promptly helps to avoid giving the child a feeling of lonesomeness.

Toilet training. Toilet training is a subject that often evokes much discussion. Mothers are anxious to do right, and toilet training is often made too great an issue. Toilet training takes a long time. It includes the child's learning his responsibility for getting to the toilet on time, managing his clothes by himself, flushing the toilet, and washing his hands. Even at 5 years the child may need reminding about handwashing after going to the toilet. Toilet training could be considered a part of the physical and motor development since control of sphincter muscles is essential, but keeping dry is also the acceptable social behavior. Infants soil themselves, but a big boy or girl does not. It is quite possible that, even if parents did nothing about toilet training and the child was one of several children, he might stop wetting himself in order to be like the older children. He does not want to be a baby.

In infancy, if the child's diaper is changed when wet, gradually the infant learns the comfort of a dry diaper and fusses or voices discontent when he is wet. Accustoming the infant to a feeling of dryness is the first step in toilet training. Next, when the child is old enough to understand the use of the commode, when he can walk, and when he has a bowel movement at the same time each day, the mother can place him on a toilet chair a few minutes before he has a defecation. A child's toilet chair has some advantages over a toilet seat placed on an adult toilet: the child does not have to be picked up and lifted onto it, and there is no possibility of his falling from it. If the child is at all resistant, the mother should abandon her efforts until a later time. If the child is interested in using the toilet chair, a definite word or phrase such as "defecation" or "bowel movement" should be taught the child. The mother's manner should be gentle and matter-of-fact. Impatience and punishment are likely to lead to resentment in the child. If the child has a defecation, he should be praised. No issue should be made of failures, and certainly the child should not be left on the chair more than 5 minutes at the most.

It is difficult to state an age at which to begin, but probably the mother is wasting her time to begin when the child is younger than 24 months since he is interested in so many other activities. He has little motivation except approval from mother until he becomes conscious that other people in the household use the bathroom and shows some desire to conform to their behavior.

In planning to help the child control urination the mother could keep a chart and see how frequently the child wets himself. Until the child is dry for 2 hour intervals, it is not advisable to begin training. In general small children void as soon as they wake up. So when the mother decides to begin training the child, she can place him on the toilet as soon as he wakes up in the morning, immediately after his nap, and then according to her charted observations of the child's frequency. Comments regarding the importance of the mother's attitude, teaching the child a suitable vocabulary, and equipment to use are the same here as for training in defecation. Sometimes a mother will find that if she seats a child on the toilet after breakfast, the child has a bowel movement and voids at the same time. In general a child does have a defecation after a meal, so it is good to establish the habit of his going to the toilet at that time, but no coercion should be used.

Usually a 2-year-old child will stay dry in the daytime if the mother or mother-substitute takes the responsibility of getting him to the toilet on time; therefore training panties might be used.

Coercion should be avoided. At 2 years of age the child still wets the bed at night so diapers should still be put on him at bedtime.

If the child is going out to play in the snow and has a heavy snowsuit to put on, then perhaps it is safer to put diapers on the 2-year-old child. By 3 years of age the child assumes responsibility for going to the toilet himself, but the child is usually 4 years of age before he keeps a dry bed at night.

In helping him to keep a dry bed at night the parent should take the child to the toilet the last thing before he goes to bed; then, depending on the child's rhythm of urination, he might be taken again at the time the parents go to bed. The child should sleep in a junior bed rather than a crib so that he can get out of bed himself in the morning to go to the bathroom. His sleeping clothing should be such that he can manage them without any adult help. The practice of limiting fluids before the child goes to bed is questionable. The child may feel thirsty, which can keep him awake at night, or he may feel rebellious and resentful at fluids' being withheld. Furthermore, limiting fluids may have an undesirable effect on the kidneys.

During the toilet-training stage children usually show a curiosity about their genitalia. Little girls may wonder if something is wrong with them because they do not have a penis. The little girl may wish to stand up as her brother does to void. It is a good thing to let children of opposite sexes see each other at this stage of development so that they know there is a difference. Words such as rectum, buttocks, and penis should be added to the vocabulary of children in the toilet-training stage since they are interested in that part of the body.

New experiences such as moving or going on a trip are not favorable times to begin training; if the training has been begun, accidents will occur at such times.

Play and exercise

Toddler. The toddler needs provision for space in which to run and play outdoors as well as inside. A screened-in porch is helpful or a yard with a fence around it. A back yard without a fence is probably safer than a front yard since the toddler could so easily run out into the street. Inside there should be a particular place for his toys so that he knows where they are. An open shelf is useful. The toddler needs a chance to practice using his legs. His balance is not good even at 2 years of age. He runs with his feet wide apart. He squats frequently instead of sitting down or leaning down. Walking and running are new gleeful experiences to him.

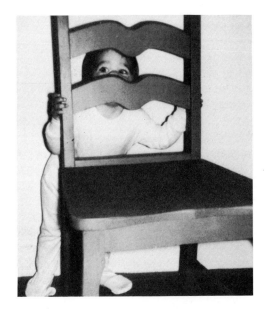

Fig. 9-14. This toddler enjoys playing peekaboo.

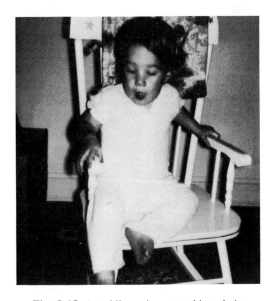

Fig. 9-15. A toddler enjoys a rocking chair.

Often he resents being carried. The toddler discovers he is a person separate from his mother, although the 2-year-old still clings to her in front of strangers.

If there is no yard in which to play, the mother might take him to a nearby park. Toys that can be pushed or pulled are popular, as are nests of boxes. Putting pegs in a wooden peg board is equally popular by 18 months of age.

Bath time can be a playtime. Cars, large blocks, cloth books, a low swing, and a large box to climb into provide entertainment for the toddler.

Play of the toddler not only aids him in motor development but also helps his sensory development, because he knows an object is smooth or rough only by feeling it. The toddler who learns to play by himself contentedly is learning emotional independence. An adult does not have to be with him each moment. Play objects stimulate his curiosity and intellect. Children under 3 years of age do not usually play with other children, but they are aware of what another child is doing and may do the same thing. This is called parallel play. A child from a large family is likely to play together with another child sooner than the only one in a family.

Preschool child. Provision needs to be made for indoor and outdoor play for the child of 3 to 5 years. Since big muscles are developed sooner than small muscles, the child at this age needs more large than small material. Outdoors, such toys as tricycles, swings, jungle gyms, slides, and wagons are popular and allow for big muscle movement and exercise. Play materials with which more than one child can play aid social development since they can be shared. Children talk when they share materials, so the use of language as a social function is stimulated instead of just use of language to express needs.

Creative materials—a sandbox, an easel, or large drawing paper to use with crayons or in finger painting—lend themselves to self-expression by children. Doll equipment (doll, doll clothes, doll carriage), housekeeping materials, and large trucks encourage dramatic play. Many uses can be made of both large and small blocks.

Preschool children's play is characterized by

love of activity for activity's sake alone and also by a great deal of imitation and imagination. Children engage in play rather than play games. It is predominantly a toy age. The child plays more alone than with others. He may at times play blocks, for example, with one other child; then a third child may join, and the first one may leave. It is a shifting group.

In addition to providing space for play, play materials, and supervision, as was suggested for the toddler, provision for companionship of

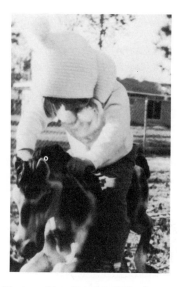

Fig. 9-16. A rocking horse is lots of fun for a 2½-year-old.

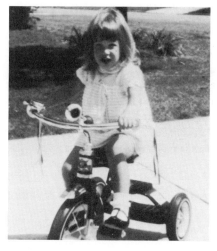

Fig. 9-17. Tricycles are popular with 3- and 4-year-old children.

the children, if even for a short time each day, is necessary. Children do not learn how to get along with other children except by being with them. The child who is not used to being with others has a difficult time when he starts school. His attention may be focused on adjustment problems instead of school work.

Adults need to supervise play and to instruct a child as to the use or possibilities of materials. An adult should also see that materials are safe and that children do not intentionally hurt each other. To have a policy that children should keep their hands off other children is advisable.

In summary, the children need a definite time to play, a place to play, companionship, play materials, and supervision. In good weather the child should be outdoors for a period in the morning and in the afternoon.

Discipline

The term *discipline* is often misused. Many people imply that the meaning of discipline is the use of stern measures with a threat of punishment. This is erroneous. Disciplining a child means teaching the child the acceptable ways of behavior. The child is not born knowing what is right and what is wrong. As an infant, he soon learns that he can put a toy in his mouth and bite on it, but he cannot do this to soap and be happy about it!

A toddler's mother often complains, "He gets into everything!" Is this really wrong? The infant old enough to crawl and the toddler old enough to walk or "trot" around love to explore their environment. They want to feel, touch, taste, and look at everything. If there were no curiosity, no research would be done and world progress would be at a standstill. On the other hand, accidents should be avoided (p. 212).

The home must be arranged so that it is not necessary to say "no, no" to the child constantly. He needs to be provided with suitable play materials and a space indoors and outdoors where he can play and run without a lot of taboos. If no suitable activity is provided, he may get into trouble as well as injure himself with various objects.

Commands should be kept at a minimum.

Instead of saying, "Pick up your toys," the parent might say, "It's time to pick up your toys." Adults do not care to be commanded, and neither do children. Treat the child with courtesy and let him know he is loved. This eliminates the need for attention-getting behavior on the part of the child. Give choices when possible. Does it matter if the child wears a blue sweater instead of a yellow one? Does the child wish to play with his blocks or does he prefer his big truck? These choices do not matter to the adult, but they give the child a sense of importance. The adult should maintain a sense of humor while with the child and laugh with him, not at him. Wholesome companionship is helpful to the preschool child. It is nice for the child to have contact with another person who is around his size.

Avoid setting too high a standard of behavior for the toddler and preschool child. The toddler does not know how to take turns with a toy and could not comprehend this if told. The 4-year-old child is beginning to have concepts of taking turns and sharing equipment.

At the end of the day children usually do not behave as well as in the morning. Fatigue influences their behavior. If children are fussing with each, a change of activity or giving the children some food—ice cream, fruit, or a glass of milk—sometimes helps.

Between the ages of 18 months and 3 years a child is often called negativistic because of conflicts between parents and child. This is due to the struggle of the small child to assert himself as a person. He is not a baby. He wishes to do things for himself. The child of 2 years of age should be allowed as much independence as possible. Conflicts, whenever possible, should be avoided—perhaps by techniques suggested in the foregoing paragraphs.

Punishment should come only as a natural result of doing wrong. If a given child persists in throwing blocks when parents have instructed him to build with them, then the blocks might be taken away until the child says that he knows how to use them. The parent should encourage the child to control his own behavior. If a given child is repeatedly annoying and hitting another one, the child who is misbehaving should be removed from the situation (told to sit

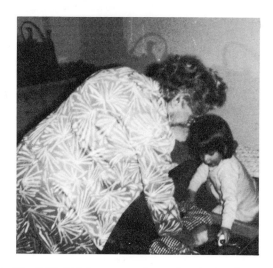

Fig. 9-18. Helping to unpack grandmother's suitcase provides an interest for this 20-month-old girl.

in his room or in a certain chair) *until he says he is ready to join the others*. The child must understand, of course, the reason for his isolation or punishment.

The phrase *naughty child* or *bad child* should not be used. It is the behavior, not the child, that is bad. The adult likes the child but not his behavior. If the adult says to the toddler, "bad child," the child will feel that the adult has rejected him. Rejection has devastating influences.

Spankings are a *splendid* outlet for the emotions of harassed parents! There is no relation between a spanking and a wrongdoing. A spanking humiliates the child, and, if it is a repeated punishment, it soon grows ineffective. It also teaches the child that older and bigger people can strike little ones. This can help make the child a bully when he is larger.

In summary, the major factors in teaching discipline are (1) adequate attention and recognition of the child, (2) the behavior pattern that the adult gives to the child, (3) provision of suitable recreation, and (4) reasonable expectations of the child's behavior.

Sex education

Since sex education is so much a part of general care of the child and may constitute a problem if not handled correctly in the formative years of the child's life, it would be well to discuss it briefly. (For other information and details of sex education refer to pp. 16, 20, 229, and 240. A bibliography on sex education is included at the end of Chapter 2.)

Sex education and sex information are not the same thing. The age of 4 is the child's peak of asking questions, not about himself but about phenomena around him. Running and walking are no longer a novelty to him as they were at 2 years. Managing utensils when eating is more or less mechanical, and he can partially dress himself. So he turns his attention to things he sees around him. "Where do babies come from?" is a common question at this age. A simple but truthful answer given in a matter-of-fact way guards against misinformation. The manner of the adult in answering shows the child whether there is something wrong with such a question or whether that can be discussed just as any other question can.

Too much information should not be given but rather an amount and type in accord with his interest and capacity for understanding. "A baby grows inside the mother" is a good start for more information. This may be enough, or the child may ask, "How does the baby get out?" "It comes through a special passage called the birth canal." An expectant mother may wish to further explain that she will go the hospital when the baby is ready to come out so that a doctor will help. Afterward she will rest in the hospital because she is tired from carrying the baby.

The child may forget information given and ask the same questions later, but as discussed in Chapter 2, the child's interest in different aspects of sex varies at different developmental levels. In the preschool period he is particularly interested in the origin of the new baby and a description of the new baby. (The baby sleeps a lot, takes milk from bottle and breast, and has to be carried since he cannot walk for some time. The new baby cannot talk. He makes sounds and cries when he wants something.)

However, as stated previously, sex information and education are not synonymous terms. Sex education begins in infancy with the mother's acceptance of the sex of the baby. It continues with the parents' attitudes toward the body of the baby when touching and handling him during his bath, when changing his diapers, and while dressing or undressing him.

Toilet training furthers sex education. The child learns the names of sex organs and some of the body processes of excretion as well as an attitude toward body functions.

The toddler and preschool child sees differences between the bodies of little boys and girls (if there are siblings) and between children and adults. It is almost inevitable that he learn these things incidentally since small children go into the bathroom together, undress in the same room, and see parents bathing or dressing. Words should be added to the child's vocabulary such as nipple, breast, penis, umbilicus, urinate, and defecate or bowel movement.

Protective attitudes and courtesy of the father toward the mother are seen by the child as well as behavior of grandparents to each other and to the child's parents. He may observe the function of mothering in animal life, such as the mother cat feeding her kittens.

If parents play with him and administer to his needs, he associates fun and comfort with this in addition to deriving a certain understanding of functions of parents toward children.

To reiterate: sex education begins at birth. Its real importance in the child's early years lies in the attitudes that are formed toward sex. Specific information may be forgotten. This can be given again later. If wrong attitudes toward sex and toward the body are learned in this period, it is very hard to reeducate the child toward a different viewpoint.

Accident prevention

In the 1- to 4-year age group the three chief causes of death from accidents are automobiles, fires, and drownings. The incidence of accidents in the home is high, but not all of these are fatal. Poisonings are frequent in this age group. The deaths from automobiles largely occur when the child is a pedestrian, not when he is a passenger in a car. The child may be playing in the street or driveway.

In the toddler and preschool period the parents should protect the child from accidents and also begin his safety education. The street is not a good place to play. Parents should obey signal lights and tell children that green is "go" and

red means "stop." In crossing a street with his parents the child should have the example of parents' looking both ways before crossing.

Some deaths from fire in this age group might be prevented if parents made sure there were two entrances or exits to the home or apartment where they live so that they would not be trapped. Guards should be in front of open gas heaters or fireplaces to reduce the hazard of clothing catching fire. Children should not be left alone where there is a lighted stove. If coal-burning stoves are used, ventilation should be good. Matches should be in metal containers. Electrical devices should be checked periodically. Cloths that have cleaning oil on them should be destroyed as soon as possible. Handles of cooking utensils should be turned so that a small child cannot reach up and pull down the hot contents of a pan over him.

Drownings might be prevented if the child were carefully supervised when he went near a swimming pool, pond, or creek. Also, the child should never be left in the bathtub alone.

Some accidents do not result in death but in crippling conditions. As more accidents occur in the home than anywhere else, every effort should be made to have it a safe place. The home should be in good repair. Loose boards on porch steps should be fixed. Stairs should be kept free of objects. Screens should be kept in windows so that children cannot fall out if a window is open. Also, window screens should be so well fastened that they do not fall if the child pushes against them. If venitian blinds are used at windows, the loops should be cut open to eliminate the danger that a child might accidentally hang himself. If refrigerators are discarded, doors should be removed so that children will not be trapped inside. Toys should be checked for safety to make sure that they have no splinters or sharp edges or any small parts that a child might swallow. Guns should be unloaded and out of reach of children.

Poisonings from 1 year through 4 years of age are common. Insecticides, detergents, and cleaning agents do not belong under the sink in the kitchen within the child's reach but rather on a high shelf. The tops of bottles or jars containing these materials should be well fastened so that, even if the toddler climbs up and reaches his hand to the shelf, he cannot open them. Medicines should be out of reach, but the 3- or 4-year-old child can also be taught that medicines are swallowed when a person is sick. The preschool child wanting to play "hospital" with her doll should be given some pink and white peppermint candies to use as pills. Since baby aspirin comes in pretty colors and tastes good, the child might use that if no substitute were given.

Medical supervision

Physical examination. The child needs a physical examination by a physician at least yearly during this period to see if he is growing and developing in the expected routine pattern of development. Any defects not picked up previously could be identified and treated. He can be given immunization as necessary (Tables 9-3 and 9-4). The mother can be given guidance with any problems in the routine of eating, sleeping, elimination, play, and prevention of accidents as necessary.

As previously stated, prompt medical attention is necessary when the child is ill. The mortality rate from influenza and pneumonia is high in this period of life.

Testing of vision. Since poor vision influences the child's behavior, development, and adjustment to others, it should be tested at least prior to entering school. If the nurse sees the young child at home and there is a question of whether he can see well, she should urge that he be taken for a physical examination by a physician. The child may have congenital cataract or other abnormal condition. The nurse should particularly look at the eyes of a child who has other congenital deformities.

A Snellen chart with the letter E or with pictures is used for screening purposes in some child health conferences or at the physician's office.

If he cannot focus both eyes on an object at one time, but one eye seems to wander either in or out, the child needs to have medical help. If the condition is not corrected until later in school age, he may lose part of the vision in the affected eye since he only uses the good eye to see.

Dental supervision and care. Since the child's teeth have erupted by 2½ years, he should visit the dentist by 3 years of age.

The purpose of the first trip to the dentist is primarily to become acquainted with the dentist and familiar with the appearance of the office and to get used to sitting in the chair there. Since the child should be seen by the dentist every 6 months of his life, it is extremely important that his first trip to the dentist be pleasant. Possibly, besides looking at them, the doctor may clean the teeth. If there are cavities, another appointment should be made. Thus the cavities are not filled on this first dental visit.

Cavities of deciduous teeth need attention since, if the tooth becomes so decayed that it has to be removed, the other baby teeth can drift and cause malocclusion. Eating, speech, and facial expression would then be affected. Early and constant dental care avoids serious problems. If a tooth is lost, a space maintainer has to be placed in the child's mouth to keep a space for the permanent tooth to erupt.

Aids to dental health other than periodical visits to the dentist include fluoridation of the water, topical applications of fluoride to the teeth by the dentist, brushing the teeth for 2 minutes after eating, and a well-balanced diet. Restricting sugar in the diet—such as candy, sweetened beverages, jams, and jellies—helps to prevent decay.

The child can be taught to use a small soft toothbrush if he has a small mirror hung low enough for him to see what he is doing. The teeth should be brushed away from the gums.

Summary

Assessment of the child's health gives the nurse a clue to whether medical help is needed and/or what further education the parents may need in helping the child toward optimum health. The factors of particular importance that promote health are those of general hygiene— eating, sleeping, bathing, and toileting. Routines are also important to the young child. Play in this period is the child's work. It is essential for him. This implies the need of a safe place to play (especially for the toddler), play materials, and companionship. The beginnings of sharing, taking turns, and participating are part of guided social behavior during his play.

Discipline is perceived as teaching the child acceptable ways of behavior.

Periodic visits, at least yearly, to the physician to see if the child is growing and developing as he should or if there are any defects to be remedied are just as important as seeing that the child receive necessary immunization to prevent certain diseases. Also, periodic visits to the dentist are essential.

As accidents rank first as a cause of death in this age period, the need of anticipatory guidance of parents can be seen. Poisonings are frequent in this age group. Accidents from fire and drowning are preventable.

Other factors in the mental and emotional health of the child include the knowledge that he is loved. A chance for both achievement and independence and providing ways for self-expression are important. Attitudes toward sex, although begun in infancy, are further formed during these years.

PROMOTION OF HEALTH IN MIDDLE CHILDHOOD
Health problems

Death from accidents still ranks as the first health problem in this age group and continues to do so through the entire adolescent period. Influenza and pneumonia, which ranked third as a cause of death in the preschool period, drop to fourth place in children 5 to 14 years of age. Malignant neoplasms rank second; the majority of deaths from this cause are due to leukemia. Congenital malformations remain a problem, ranking in third place. (In the preschool period they ranked second.) It is impossible to tell from this table whether most of the deaths due to suicides were in the teenage group (13- and 14-year-olds) or whether they occurred at an earlier school age.

Possibly these mortality figures point up the need of a careful assessment of health when periodic examinations are done; also they point to the need of an awareness of the child as a person by everyone coming in contact with him.

Accidents are preventable. At this age it is the child who can be taught safety, whereas in the earlier years the parents or caretakers were primarily responsible for the safety of the child.

Table 9-6. Deaths and death rates for children 5 to 14 years, both sexes*

Rank	Cause of death†	Number	Rate‡
	All causes	16,847	41.3
1	Accidents (E800-E949)	8,203	20.1
2	Malignant neoplasms, including neoplasms of lymphatic and hematopoietic tissues (140-209)	2,429	6.0
3	Congenital anomalies (740-759)	901	2.2
4	Influenza and pneumonia (470-474, 480-486)	651	1.6
5	Homicide (E960-E978)	360	0.9
6	Diseases of heart (390-398, 402, 404, 410-429)	344	0.8
7	Cerebrovascular diseases (430-438)	272	0.7
8	Benign neoplasms and neoplasms of unspecified nature (210-239)	165	0.4
9	Suicide (E950-E959)	132	0.3
10	Bronchitis, emphysema, and asthma (490-493)	129	0.3

*Modified from Facts of life and death, Public Health Service, Rockville, Md., 1974, U.S. Department of Health, Education, and Welfare (Table 28).
†According to International classification of diseases, eighth revision, 1965.
‡Per 100,000 population in age group.

Identification of any malformation should be done early and help obtained. Children who have leukemia or a malignant disease need supportive care since they have remissions.

Role of the nurse

Although the office nurse and hospital nurse also see the child at this age, it is the school health nurse who is in the best position to contact frequently both the child and those who guide him—school personnel as well as parents. Except in large cities, the public health nurse usually has the responsibility for the schools in the particular district in which she works. It is possible that through her home contacts she knows the child in school. Sometimes she acts as a go-between for the home and the school. The nurse can actively participate in the school health program of each school she visits. She should be able to assess the child's health and give appropriate health guidance. Factors

Text continued on p. 221.

SECTION 1: PHYSICAL EXAMINATION

Directions: Fill in blanks with appropriate information.

MEASUREMENTS

Height _____ Weight _____ Respirations _____ Blood pressure _____

Circumference: Head _____ Chest _____

SKIN

Color _____ Tissue turgor _____ Bruises _____ A_____ _____

Dryness _____ Other _____

SENSORY DEVELOPMENT

Eyes

General observations: Color _____ Expression: Dull _____

Inflammation: Eyes _____ Eyelids _____

Discharge: Right _____ Left _____

Dried secretions on eyelids: Right _____ Left _____

Pupils react equally to light: Right _____ Left _____

Strabismus (Observe position of light reflected in cornea; should be in center of each pupil.):

Right _____ Left _____ (Cover one eye at a time and have child fixate on distant object

straight ahead. Note if uncovered eye moves in either direction.): Right _____ Left _____

Visual acuity: Test with Snellen chart.

Ears

(Use otoscope as necessary.)

Normal configuration and position _____ Other _____

External ear normal _____ Cysts, malformations _____

Pain: Right _____ Left _____

Canal: Clean _____ Wax _____ Discharge _____ Lesions _____ Foreign

body _____ Other _____

Tympanic membrane color (normally gray) _____ Handle of malleus visualized _____

Concave eardrum _____ Cone of light reflex (from otoscope) fans out externally _____

Hearing (Audiometer may be used.): Right _____ Left _____

NOSE

Nostrils patent (Close one nostril with finger and observe breathing through other.): Right _____

Left _____

Dried secretions _____ Discharge (describe): Right _____ Left _____

Fig. 9-19. Guide for health assessment of school-age child.

Continued.

SECTION 1: PHYSICAL EXAMINATION—cont'd

Mouth and throat

(Use tongue depressor and flashlight as necessary.)

Lips: Moist _____ Dry _____ Cracked _____

Mouth breathing _____ History of snoring when asleep _____

Condition of gums _____ Buccal membrane _____

Teeth: Number _____ Condition _____ Date of last dental visit _____

Pharynx clearly visible _____ Exudate on tonsils _____

Tonsils: Inflamed _____ Obstructing view of pharynx _____

Soft and hard palate intact _____

HEAD

Shape: Symmetrical _____ Unusual (describe) _____

Scalp: Smooth _____ Dry _____ Scaly _____ Sores _____

Hair: Texture (fine, coarse) _____ Dandruff _____ Nits _____ Pediculosis _____

Face: Symmetrical _____ Other _____

    Expression: Dull _____ Alert _____ Rash _____ Anything unusual _____

NECK

Supple (full range of motion) _____ Symmetrical _____

Cervical lymph nodes (palpable, tender) _____ Occipital _____

CHEST

Lungs (Use stethoscope as necessary.): Expand symmetrically _____

Quality of respirations: Breathing quiet _____ Grunting _____ Wheezing _____

    Other _____

Bruises _____ Scars _____ Rash (describe) _____

Protrusions _____ Hair on chest _____ Breast development _____

HEART

(Use stethoscope.)

Quality of heart sounds _____ Rate _____ Itensity _____ Rhythm_____

    Murmur _____ Unusual sounds _____

ABDOMEN

(Palpate gently.)

Contour: Symmetrical _____ Protuberant _____ Flat _____ Distended _____

    Hard _____ Tender _____ Masses _____ Scars _____ Protrusions _____

Bowel sounds _____

Umbilicus: Clean _____ Protruding _____ Discharge _____ Other _____

Fig. 9-19, cont'd. Guide for health assessment of school-age child.

SECTION 1: PHYSICAL EXAMINATION—cont'd

EXTREMITIES

All joints

Full range of motion _____ If not, explain _____

Arms and hands

Edema _____ Color _____ Unusual warmth or coolness __ _____

Nodules _____ Rash _____ Other _____

Nail beds. Color _____ Circulation (Apply pressure and see if color returns quickly.) _____

Clubbing of fingers _____

Presence of axillary hair _____

Legs

Edema _____ Color _____ Unusual warmth or coolness _____

Nodules _____ Rash _____ Equal in length _____ Straight _____

Other _____

Hips

Test for dislocated hip (see p. 342).

BACK

Scapulae equal _____ Vertebrae straight _____ Scoliosis _____ Lordosis _____

Kyphosis _____ Other _____

Moles _____ Protrusions _____ Swelling _____ Other _____

Iliac crests even _____

GENITALIA

Female

Presence of pubic hair _____

Labia symmetrical _____ Clean _____ Inflammation _____

Discharge (describe) _____

Presence of clitoris _____ Vaginal orifice _____ Urinary meatus _____

Onset of menarche (date) _____ If present, duration of menstruation _____ Dysmenorrhea _____

Male

Penis with urethral opening at end _____ If not, describe _____

_____

Testes in scrotum: Right _____ Left _____

Circumcised _____ If not, foreskin easily retracted _____ Clean _____

Discharge (describe) _____ Pubic hair _____

ANUS

Patent _____ Fissures _____ Hemorrhoids _____ Other (describe) _____

Continued.

Fig. 9-19, cont'd. Guide for health assessment of school-age child.

SECTION 1: PHYSICAL EXAMINATION—cont'd

NEUROMUSCULAR DEVELOPMENT

First (olfactory) cranial nerve

Identification of familiar odors (oranges, peanut butter, etc.) _____

Second (optic) cranial nerve

Visual acuity: Snellen test _____

Peripheral vision (Have child focus on object such as examiner's nose; move finger through all hemispheres; ask child when he can first see the finger.): Nasal side (should be 100 degrees) _____

Vertical (should be 130 degrees) _____

Third (oculomotor), fourth (trochlear), and fifth (abducent) cranial nerves

Unequal movement of pupils (Have child follow examiner's finger moving through all quadrants.):

Right _____ Left _____

Pupillary light reflex in corresponding spots on pupils: Yes _____ No _____

Nystagmus _____

Sixth (trigeminal) cranial nerve

Motor division: Symmetry of strength of muscles of jaw (Try to pull tongue blade away as child bites

hard on it.) _____

Sensory division (Touch forehead, cheeks, and jaw with point of pin.): Sensation present _____

Sensation absent _____ Symmetry of response: Right _____ Left _____ Corneal

reflex (Touch cornea with wisp of cotton.) _____

Seventh (facial) cranial nerve

Motor division: Symmetry _____ (Have child wrinkle forehead, smile, and raise eyebrow; have

child close eyes while examiner tries to open them by pushing upward on eyebrows.) Equality of

strength: Right _____ Left _____

Eighth (acoustic) cranial nerve

Test hearing with audiometer.

Ninth (glossopharyngeal) and tenth (vagus) cranial nerves

Hoarseness of voice _____ Ability to swallow _____ Gag reflex _____

Eleventh (accessory) cranial nerve

Strength and symmetry of sternocleidomastoid muscle (Turn child's head against opposing pressure

on one side, then the other): Right _____ Left _____

Strength and symmetry of trapezius muscle (ability to lift shoulders simultaneously against opposing

pressure): Right _____ Left _____

Twelfth (hypoglossal) cranial nerve

Have child press tongue against each cheek: Right _____ Left _____ Symmetry _____

Fig. 9-19, cont'd. Guide for health assessment of school-age child.

SECTION 1: PHYSICAL EXAMINATION—cont'd

Cerebral function

Use psychometric examinations; note general behavior and levels of consciousness.

Cerebellar function

Touches nose with index finger with eyes closed (Repeat once or twice, note consistent past pointing.) _____

Pats knee with palm of hand, then with back of hand (Repeat several times.) _____

Twists both hands as if screwing a light bulb (Child should copy twisting motion demonstrated by examiner.) _____

Stands straight with feet together and eyes open _____ With eyes closed _____

Walks heel to toe several steps _____

Stands on one foot _____

Runs in place _____

Motor system

Muscle size: Normal _____ Hypertrophy _____ Atrophy _____

Tone: Good _____ Flaccid _____ Hypotonic _____ Spastic _____

Symmetry (Measure muscles in calf of leg and compare with similar muscles of other leg.) _____

Muscle strength (Have child push against resistance from the examiner.) _____

Symmetry of resistance in arms (Have child extend arms out straight; try to push them apart.) _____

(Try to push them together.) _____

Other groups of muscles tested same way _____

Abdominal muscles (ability to do several sit-ups) _____

Abnormal muscle movements: Twitching _____ Tics _____ Tremors _____ Choreiform movements _____ Jerking involuntary movements _____

Sensory system: primary sensation

Superficial tactile sensation (Test symmetrical areas of body with wisp of cotton. Have child close his eyes and point to the spot he felt sensation.) _____

Superficial pain (Test symmetrical parts of body with sharp and blunt ends of pin. Have child close his eyes and tell whether pin is sharp or blunt.) _____

Temperature (Fill one test tube with hot water and one with cold. Have child close eyes and touch him with alternate tubes.) _____

Vibration (Use large tuning fork. Ask child to tell when vibration stops. Places tested for vibration include sternum, elbows, knees, toes, iliac crests.) _____

Continued.

Fig. 9-19, cont'd. Guide for health assessment of school-age child.

SECTION 1: PHYSICAL EXAMINATION—cont'd

Cortical and discriminatory sensation

Two-point discrimination (Ask child to close eyes and tell if one or two points are pressing on skin.

Test several areas.) _____

Point localization (Have child close his eyes and ask him to point to spot where object touched him.

Use wisp of cotton, test tube, or pin.) _____

Extinction phenomena (Test of parietal lobe in child older than 6 years. Touch child simultaneously

in two homologous parts; ask child where he was touched; he should feel two places.) _____

_____

Reflexes*

Plantar grasp reflex _____ Biceps reflex _____ Triceps reflex _____

Brachioradialis reflex _____ Achilles tendon reflex _____ Patellar reflex _____

Globular reflex (Tap bridge of nose and eyes will close; check for symmetry.) _____

Blink reflex (Shine light suddenly in eyes.) _____

Babinski reflex† _____

SECTION 2: GENERAL CARE

GENERAL HYGIENE
Bathing

Daily _____ Other _____

Sleep

Usual bedtime _____

Elimination

Stool daily _____ Other _____ Characteristics (amount, color, consistency) _____

_____

Voiding (number of times): Daytime _____ Nighttime _____

NUTRITION

Describe food eaten in last 24 hours: Breakfast _____

Snacks _____

Lunch _____

Dinner _____

*The following infant reflexes should have disappeared: Moro reflex, tonic neck reflex, rooting reflex, and stepping reflex. Their continued presence is abnormal.
†Should be negative after 18 months.

Fig. 9-19, cont'd. Guide for health assessment of school-age child.

SECTION 2: GENERAL CARE—cont'd

DENTAL CARE

Brushes teeth _____ When? _____

INTERESTS AND DISCIPLINE

Education

Grade placement _____ Likes school _____ Passing all subjects _____ Uses public

or school library for personal nonrequired reading _____

Recreation

Activity most enjoyed _____

Membership in special group: Y.M.C.A. _____ Scouts _____ Sunday school _____

Other _____

Plays after school with one friend _____ Several _____ Other _____

Skills: Jumping rope _____ Musical instrument _____ Bicycle riding _____ Skating _____

Ballet dancing _____ Swimming _____ Horseback riding _____ Other _____

Recreation with mother _____

With father _____

With whole family _____

Discipline: Are there definite rules? Explain _____

Is child ever punished? _____ How? _____

Home responsibilities _____

TOPICS FOR HEALTH GUIDANCE

Recreation, need of group play

Prevention of accidents: bicycling, swimming, crossing street

Sex education: preparation for menstruation and adolescent changes

Drugs

Smoking

Sleep

Nutrition

Dental care

Fig. 9-19, cont'd. Guide for health assessment of school-age child.

pertinent to children's health of this age are discussed in detail in the pages following a description of the physical examination.

Assessment of health

Signs of good health include an animated expression, good posture, clear skin of good color, and bright eyes. The well child increases steadily in weight and height. He has a good disposition. A child who is constantly irritable or who does not enjoy activities with other children needs help.

See Fig. 9-19 for a general assessment guide for physical health, hygiene, interests, and possible topics for health guidance. Physical examination and assessment of a toddler and preschool child are described on p. 192. The chief differences in the physical assessment of the school-age child and the toddler and preschool child are increased motor coordination as shown in the neurological examination, the development of sinuses, and the beginning of eruption of permanent teeth. In some females signs of puberty may be present before 12 years. Menarche could have begun. It is a period of less rapid growth than the preceding one.

If the school child has pain or discomfort anywhere in the body, he is fully able to communicate this. In general it is a period of good health. Children have few physical complaints during this time, although some girls of 11 and 12 years of age suffer from dysmenorrhea. If a school child has an overbite or underbite or gives any signs of permanent teeth deviating from the normal, a referral to an orthodontist should be made.

In general in the health promotion of the child who starts school it is important to see that he is adequately immunized to tetanus, diphtheria, pertussis, poliomyelitis, rubeola, and rubella. Health instructions should include knowledge concerning nutritionally balanced meals and the physiological value of good food. Oral hygiene becomes increasingly important because of the eruption of permanent teeth. Teaching school-age children swimming and water safety will help avoid water accidents. Preparatory information about physiological changes in adolescence should be given by 10 or 11 years of age before adolescent changes begin.

From the mother the nurse can learn the child's grade placement and whether he is having any difficulty in schoolwork. The nurse should be cognizant of available community resources for children with learning disabilities. Also the mentally retarded child has difficulties in school achievement. Again, the nurse needs to have knowledge of where and how the child can be evaluated and helpful guidance can be given to the parents. The emotionally disturbed child may have difficulty with schoolwork because he cannot give it his attention. He is concerned and worried over other matters. The nurse's interest in the child can be of help to both the school personnel and to the parent.

Behavior characteristics

For the convenience of the reader, a brief discussion of some of the characteristics of children in middle childhood is given. Usually the well 6-year-old child is aggressive. His emotions tend to fluctuate. He has difficulty in accepting criticism or blame. The 7-year-old child is more withdrawn. Often he complains that he is "picked on." He wants to play and be with other children rather than adults. At 8 years children are cheerful and active—in fact rather exuberant. School is a novelty no longer. Learning to read and write gives the child a sense of power and prestige. He seems more able to relax. He may join scouts or a similar organization. At 9 years the child is more independent of his parents. He worries about school if he is not doing well and may complain of physical illness in order to stay at home. The 10-year-old child is fairly stable. His peers become increasingly important to him. The 11-year-old child is critical of his parents and rebels against them. He is restless. He wants to be involved in activities of his own age group. The 12-year-old child is more stable than in the previous years. His interests are broader. He desires adventure and excitement in company, of course, with his peer group of the same sex.

Health factors in the home
Emotional needs

When a child enters school his world enlarges. There are more adults, more children, new activities, and big buildings. The more secure the child feels at home (because of affection, achievement, recognition, and a feeling of belongingness), the freer he is to give his attention to school. If the child has accepted authority at home, he will accept the authority of the teacher at school. Also, if he has learned to play with others, manage clothing with little help, and be happy with adults other than his parents for short periods of time, his adjustment in school is much smoother than that of the child who still has these things to learn.

The 6-year-old child who has started school needs opportunity to talk about his new experiences in school and to role-play authority figures. Because of the emotional strain of going to school, an hour's rest on his bed when he comes home may help him to relax. Even if he does not sleep, his metabolism will slow down if he actually lies down on his bed.

The 7-year-old child needs to feel the warmth of adult approval and acceptance. Although he wants to play with other children, he wants approval from both his parents and his teacher.

If a child complains of physical illness as an excuse to stay home from school, the parents need to talk with the teacher and see if there is a learning problem or if there is a problem in relationship with other children or possibly with the teacher; on the other hand, perhaps the parents have too high expectations for their child and the child cannot meet them. The school nurse might be of assistance to the teacher, the parents, and the child. Whatever the problem is, it should be cited and available community resources used to their advantage.

From 9 or 10 to 15 years of age being part of a certain play group or club can give the child a further feeling of confidence. This is the "gang" age, when children enjoy most of all being with children of their own age and sex. The opinion of the group means more to them than the opinions of adults. Belonging to various groups such as a Sunday school class, a scout troop, or a swimming class contributes to the security of the child. He identifies with these groups and receives a feeling of belongingness. Also, learning skills like bicycle riding or doing stunts on a jungle gym gives the child a sense of self-confidence.

The child who is not well accepted by others is a child who especially needs a chance to succeed at school. He needs recognition from the teacher, the nurse, and other adults with whom he comes in contact. Not every child receives affection at home; for one who does not, the school personnel and the parents of his friends often provide an affection that he lacks but craves. A child has to experience friendliness before he is friendly to others. The child who misbehaves may be a child who feels that he is not loved or accepted; he is misbehaving to get attention. Recognition should be provided so that misbehaving to get attention is unnecessary.

Physical needs

Eating. The eating habits learned in early childhood will continue to be a major factor influencing the foods selected by the school-age child; however, new influences from outside the home will become increasingly more significant as the child goes to school, establishes relationships with other children from different backgrounds, and learns to accept the authority of adults other than his parents.

Nutritional needs. The food needs of the school-age child differ from those of the preschooler only in quantity. The same variety of foods from the Basic Four food groups needs to be provided to supply adequate calories, protein, vitamins, and minerals to allow for slow but steady increases in height and weight. Children from 7 to 10 years of age need 2,400 calories and 36 gm. of protein a day.

In the years immediately preceding puberty the child begins to store protein, calcium, and iron. These reserves will be drawn upon to meet increased requirements for these nutrients during the adolescent growth spurt. The body's ability to efficiently use nutrients during adolescence is therefore partly conditioned by the child's diet during the elementary school years.

Since girls ordinarily reach puberty before boys, their nutrient needs begin to differ from those of boys in the preadolescent years. It is especially important that a girl enter adolescence with good body stores of iron; otherwise the onset of menstruation with resultant blood losses can lead to anemia. The 11- to 12-year-old girl needs 18 mg. of dietary iron a day compared to 10 mg. for boys of the same age. Since the calorie requirement for the 11- to 12-year-old is lower for girls than boys (2,400 and 2,800 calories, respectively) the preadolescent girl needs counseling in food selection to help her meet her special dietary needs.

Although growth rates of school-age children are quite variable, each child can best meet his individual potential when the diet includes 3 to 4 cups of milk, at least two servings of meat or other good-quality protein food, one egg, four servings of fruits and vegetables, and three to four servings of enriched breads and cereals each day.

Food habits. As the child begins to spend more time away from home, it becomes more difficult for the mother to control his diet. After-school activities, parties, "lunch swapping," etc., make it very hard for the mother to always know exactly what her child is eating; however, there are some things a mother can do to help ensure proper nutrition.

First, of course, she should make sure that the meals the child receives at home are well balanced. The morning routine for getting ready for school must include time for eating a good breakfast. Children who do not eat breakfast are certain to be hungry at midmorning recess. If they have nothing to fill up on then but candy, potato chips, soda pop, and other "empty-calorie" snacks, they will not be hungry at lunchtime. When they come home from school, they will be hungry again and will want to snack before dinner. Such irregular eating habits shortchange the child on nutrients. The poorly nourished child is more susceptible to minor infections that keep him home from school; he lacks energy and the ability to concentrate on his studies. Excessive consumption of sticky sweets also contributes to dental caries and childhood obesity. If such patterns persist, normal growth and development are ultimately affected.

This does not mean that snacks cannot be a part of the child's diet. If they are planned to provide nutritious foods at reasonable intervals, small snacks can significantly contribute to the quality of the diet. For example, the child sent to school with a piece of fruit or cookies made of peanut butter, oatmeal, raisins, or nuts to be eaten at recess has an excellent supplement for energy, protein, vitamins, and minerals.

Too many extracurricular activities and lack of sleep might also interfere with good eating habits and nutritional status. Whereas sports, scouting, music lessons, and other after-school events are all desirable activities for the school-age child, parents should be warned not to overemphasize them to the point that the child is constantly on the go with little time for proper meals and relaxation.

Social needs

As the child becomes older, he is no longer satisfied to play with an adult as he was during the preschool period but wishes the companionship of another child. Parents have the responsibility of seeing that other children are invited to play with him. The beginning concepts of social behavior were learned in preschool years. These concepts are modified and further developed in the elementary school years by the child's being with children in school, playing with them after school, and belonging to groups such as the scouts.

For the child between 6 and 9 years of age, games of chase that include a great deal of running are popular. Examples of these are tag, hide-and-seek, and blindman's bluff. These games have few rules, and any number can play. A game having many rules requires a degree of social maturity that is not expected until teenage.

A jungle gym, swings, and slide all provide wholesome recreation, as do a bicycle, sandbox, and tree house.

Checkers and games like Sorry and Candy Lane hold his attention, as do simple puzzles, toy animals, Tinker Toys, blocks that are of different sizes and shapes, clay, cars, and trucks. Dolls and doll equipment usually appeal to girls, but the dolls must be more lifelike than in the preschool period. They should have eyes that open and shut, hair that can be combed, and several changes of dresses. Coloring books are popular. The child of this age can stay within the lines in the picture. He has better control of his finer muscles than the preschool child. Cutting out paper dolls and their clothes is of interest.

The child from 9 or 10 to 12 years of age is in a stage of rivalry. He wishes to do better than anyone else a particular skill he enjoys. For this reason he may spend considerable time practicing bicycling, swimming, skating, throwing, stunts, and the like. As with children who are 6 to 9 years old, parents should encourage participation in physical activities so that the children will not be left out. Also, development of a particular skill leads to feelings of self-confidence. These feelings may well carry over into nonphysical activities.

Children in the last part of elementary school (those in the fourth, fifth, or sixth grade) increasingly enjoy adventure. Camping, hiking, fishing, and trips to the country supply fun and excitement.

Boys do enjoy woodwork and various mechanical devices. Helping to build a tree house that can be headquarters for a club or gang finds favor. Boys like to play war. In contrast, girls like domestic activities such as playing house, sewing, and cooking. Reading is enjoyed by both sexes, as is watching television programs. As children grow older, between 6 and 12 or 13 years of age the interests of boys and girls become increasingly divergent. Girls play more with other girls, and the boys play with boys. This is particularly true of children from 10 to 15 years of age, at which time girls and boys are attracted to one another.

Pets are popular with both sexes. Boys and girls can show affection and love to animals at times when displaying affection in such ways as sitting on parents' laps or kissing them in public is simply not done.

Provision for and supervision of activity. It is a parent's responsibility to see that children in the primary grades (one, two, and three) have a space in which to play, companions with whom to play, and materials with which to play. If there is no back yard, taking children to a park where there is recreational equipment can meet the child's needs. As children grow older in the fourth, fifth, and sixth grades, they begin to take more responsibility for inviting other children to their homes. Children continue to come to visit, depending on how they are greeted by adults, the manner in which they are supervised, and whether there is anything interesting for them to do.

The children in primary grades need more supervision in their play than the older ones because of their lack of social development and understanding of acceptable social techniques. Hitting each other, slapping, hair pulling, and failing to take turns are not acceptable behaviors. The right supervision helps children to grow socially. If a parent has difficulty with a child guest who does not accept explanation or guidance, the wise action of the parent is to send the child home. Children still need protec-

tion from one another when they are 6, 7, and 8 years old. Parents should let children themselves settle their differences as much as possible. If children's parents interfere and fuss, their own quarrel may continue long after the children have forgotten the episode. If two sets of parents are cool in their relationship, the relationship of the children is affected.

It is usually easier for one child to maintain a smooth relationship with *one* other child than with two others at the same time. Either two or four children can play together more easily than three.

Clubs and camps

The height of interest in gangs is usually from about 10 to 15 years of age. Of course, there are individual variations. Since children wish to be with others at this stage, provision should be made for group activities like those in organized camps, scouts, and recreational groups such as the Y.W.C.A. In cities, settlement houses may have planned programs for children. The ability of children to get along with each other is furthered in supervised groups. Energy, imagination, initiative, and independence are well utilized under supervision.

If children attend overnight camps, their parents should be sure the camp meets at least the minimum requirements specified by the American Camping Association. These include safe water supply and sewage disposal, and adequate diet, medical attention, provision for water safety, acceptable sleeping arrangements, and adequate supervision of the children. At all times the camp personnel should know how and where to reach parents or those responsible for the child.

Providing group experiences for children, especially those in fourth, fifth, sixth, and seventh grades, is a neighborhood and community responsibility. If suitable recreation is not supplied for children in the gang period, children may seek adventure in ways that may be harmful to them and to others.

Discipline

Discipline has been discussed in relation to the health of the preschool child. It is necessary in the elementary school years to continue teaching the child acceptable ways of behaving. To the previous discussion can be added the general concept that as children grow older they tend to discipline each other. The child increasingly wishes to gain the respect of his peer group (especially in the gang age between 10 and 15 years); therefore he conforms to what he believes is considered right by his peers. If a parent wishes to change the behavior of her growing young girl or boy, she will have to influence the child's friends also in order to be successful. Adequate supervision of recreation and activities of the children after school and on weekends helps in teaching right ways of behavior. The standards of the child are influenced by the school he attends as well as the ethical and religious beliefs of his family.

As the child becomes older, he can begin to participate more in family conferences about general rules for happy family living. He learns democracy this way. He can better appreciate the reason for having mealtime set at certain hours, the need for housekeeping chores, and the like. Knowing exactly what is expected of him gives him added security and helps to lessen friction between parents and child. After conferences are held and decisions made, parents need to be consistent in holding the child to those decisions.

Medical supervision

The child of school age should continue to have physical examinations yearly, visual and hearing examinations every 2 to 3 years, and dental supervision every 6 months.

School health program

Whether the school has a sound health program depends upon the interests of those connected with the school. Someone has to take the initiative to start a school health council or committee that can make general policies for the program. This person may be the school principal, a teacher, a nurse, a parent, a doctor, or anyone who wants to promote the health of the children.

In order to direct and implement the school health program there should be a school health council or committee made up of a member of the school board, the school principal, a representative from the county medical society, a local dentist, a county health nurse or a school nurse, a nutritionist, a health officer, a physical education teacher, a classroom teacher, a representative from the parent-teacher association, and representatives from local health organizations.

The school health council or committee should make policies about the health program. Depending upon the size and locality of the school, a steering committee also may be necessary. This is more likely to be true in a large city. The school administrator should be the head of a steering committee. A large metropolitan area might well have a central health council with representatives from individual schools.

There are three phases of a school health program: healthful school living, health services, and health and safety instruction.

Healthful school living

Conditions of the school should be conducive to healthful living. This includes the school lunch, the provisions for sanitation and safety, the health of school personnel, and the mental and emotional health of pupils.

Minimum standards for sanitary facilities are listed in the building codes of state departments of health and education. To see that these are maintained is the responsibility of the sanitarian from a local health department. He makes periodical visits to look into the safety of the building and the playground and to inspect the ventilation, lighting, rest rooms, sewerage, water supply, and methods of storing and handling food. Stairways should be "fireproof," and there should be adequate exits for use in case of fire. Doors should open outward. Lavatories, handwashing facilities, and drinking fountains should be adequate in number and of approved design. Good housekeeping standards should be maintained.

An important factor in the health (physical and emotional) of the students is the physical, mental, and emotional health of their teachers. If teachers are coughing and sneezing, a respiratory infection can easily be transmitted to the children. The mental health of the children is affected by the personality of the teacher. A friendly but firm teacher who truly enjoys children as well as teaching a particular subject is a big factor in the children's school adjustment and their further social and emotional growth.

To maintain standards after they have been instituted is important. In a sense this is everyone's responsibility. Since the nurse, however, belongs to a health profession, she has certain special responsibilities for this.

When the nurse visits the school, she should be aware of safety factors such as school zone and speed limit signs. She should notice what provision there is for safety of children crossing the streets near the school. She should be aware of the safety of the playground and the physical plan of the school. She should note the ventilation, lighting, and general housekeeping, particularly in the bathrooms. If no soap or towels are available in the bathrooms, desirable health habits are obstructed.

Doors that open inward are a hazard.

The nurse should inquire about fire drills and the result of them. How quickly do the children leave the building? Have any accidents or unforeseen problems occurred? The nurse should inquire also at the beginning of the year about safety rules and regulations concerning school bus transportation. She should scan the school records of accidents to see if ways of prevention might be better taught and maintained. (A safety program does not imply that all hazards can be eliminated, but rather it teaches how to live safely with unavoidable hazards.)

The nurse is in a position to recommend equipment for the first-aid room and also to help in establishing school health policies for emergency situations or accidents.

The nurse should try to be present at a teachers' meeting and to know the teachers. Her presence at a parent-teacher meeting is also desirable. The nurse should make a special effort to establish and maintain a good relationship with all school personnel in order to best contribute and participate in the school health program.

School lunch. The National School Lunch Act, approved in 1946, has made it possible for thousands of school children to receive nutritious meals at minimal cost throughout the school year. The program is administered by the United States Department of Agriculture, which provides surplus food commodities and grants-in-aid to state and local school authorities. In return for this assistance the schools must meet certain standards outlined by the Secretary of Agriculture.

1. No child can be denied a lunch because he cannot afford to pay—upon approval of local authorities the child is served meals without cost or at a reduced cost.

2. There must be no discrimination against the child who cannot afford to pay.

3. The meals served must meet nutritional standards. The Type A pattern has been devised as a guide for menu planning. It includes meat or an alternate, fluid whole milk, two sources of fruits or vegetables, enriched or whole grain bread or cereal, and margarine or butter. Meals planned around the Type A pattern provide one third of the total daily nutrient allowances for the school-age child set by the National Research Council.

4. The meals must be attractive, and they must be prepared in accord with state health department regulations.

5. The school must provide suitable dining facilities.

6. The program must be run on a nonprofit basis.

If properly supervised, the school lunch can aid in the development of good eating habits. In some situations the school lunch may be the only opportunity the child has for receiving a nutritious meal throughout the entire day.

Health services

Physical examination. Some school systems employ a school health physician who gives periodical examinations to children, but the trend is to have each child go to his own private physician. If a child is taken to a private physician, the family is more likely to follow his recommendations.

Examination by a physician is usually required at the beginning of school (the first grade). Any recommendations that he makes should be known to the school. In most states a successful vaccination also is required before entrance to school. The public health nurse must be familiar with the requirements of the state and county in which she is working. Ideally the child should have a physical examination every year.

Testing vision and hearing. The frequency of eye examinations may be somewhat different in various counties and states. It is preferable that an eye examination be made before a child first goes to school. After school entrance an examination may be done yearly or every 3 years. The Snellen chart is used in school for eye tests. This chart picks up defects of near-sightedness but not farsightedness or astigmatism. Mothers frequently assist with this eye examination. In such cases the nurse has the responsibility of teaching the parent how to give the test, which is really a screening test. The nurse also explains to the teacher that the children should be told in advance about the test and why it is given. If the child fails to have 20/20 vision, he is referred to an ophthalmologist, but a child before 8 years of age (a third grade child) may normally have vision of 20/30.

Hearing tests are done with an audiometer. In some cities personnel from a speech and hearing center may take the responsibility for giving the tests. The frequency with which these tests are given varies in different school systems.

Speech correction. Speech is the chief means of communication. The speech of a child influences his adjustment in school, at home, and on the playground. Later in life it could affect his vocational adjustment.

Difficulties in articulation constitute the most common type of speech defect. The teacher and the nurse should be alert to them and refer a child with these difficulties to the proper resource in the community for correction. Nasality and poor speech patterns due to organic defects such as cleft palate also need correction.

Daily observation. The nurse can be helpful to the teachers in explaining what daily observations should be made relative to the health of children. A child who is inattentive and a troublemaker in class may be bored because he is superior in intelligence and the lesson is not challenging to him, or he may not be able to hear. Another possibility is that he is unable to see well and therefore is limited in his ability to read books or words on the blackboard. Normally children in the first and second grades are farsighted. The teacher who sees a child either leaning close to his paper and book or squinting should realize that he may have a visual problem. Also, eyes can become irritated if the child is straining them.

Constant pallor and listlessness could denote anemia or even the beginning of rheumatic fever. In addition, the anemic child in certain regions of this country may be one who has hookworm or some other intestinal parasite.

A child with intestinal parasites frequently has nervous mannerisms. Peculiar posture may mean something is wrong, and the child should be referred to the nurse.

The child who constantly stays by himself or one who is overly aggressive needs thoughtful consideration. A child with constant clumsiness or twitching should be watched because that child may be developing chorea. A child with nervous habits may need more sleep. Cruelty to other children or pets, constant irritability, attention-getting behavior, or clinging to an adult is not a sign of good health.

The child who has a nasal discharge or cough should be sent home promptly so other children will not be infected. By resting at home for 1 or 2 days he will probably get over his illness more promptly than if he tries to remain in school.

The nurse should have ready access to the health records of the children. There should be a cumulative health record on every school child, beginning with his preschool examination and continuing through the twelfth grade. The nurse should follow through any recommendations that a doctor has made for an individual child. Many times the county nurse already knows the family of the child who has a health problem.

Referral to community resources. The nurse must know community resources and agencies so that she can best help children. Communities may vary, but the nurse can find a directory of official and voluntary agencies in the local health department. The nurse should also be cognizant of local and state resources for special education for the slow child, the hard-of-hearing child, the visually defective child, and other handicapped children. If a nurse is in a city, it is important for her to know the available recreation centers. Sometimes these are located in settlement houses. Also, there are community organizations such as the Y.W.C.A. and Y.M.C.A. Both the county public health nurse and the school health nurse in the city need knowledge of the nearest camps for handicapped children as well as the availability of summer camps for well children.

Health and safety instruction

Many state departments of education have a recommended health instruction curriculum for different grades. The school nurse or the county health nurse should be familiar with what is recommended by the state in which she is practicing as well as know what health textbooks her schools use. The nurse does not do the teaching herself, but she has the opportunity of acting as a consultant to teachers. How much the nurse can accomplish depends on her relationships with the teachers and her own interests.

Much of the health teaching in the elementary grades should be related to daily activities such as eating, hand washing, and play. For example, Why should hands be washed before eating? Why is rest important? Play? The nurse should know what movies and slides relative to health and safety instruction can be obtained from the state health department, university, or other source.

Nutrition. The emphasis of nutrition teaching in infancy was on learning to enjoy food; for the preschool child it was on increasing his ability to feed himself and to accept a variety of foods. In the school years, as the child assumes more responsibility for selecting his own diet, he needs to know which foods are important and why. Nutrition education can be integrated throughout all the elementary school years. The nurse and the nutrition consultant from the state or local health department can be helpful to teachers as they plan units of instruction.

Children in the primary grades learn about activities of daily living at home, at school, and in the community. Their interest in food centers around knowing how it tastes and where it comes from and helping mother to shop and cook. Suitable activities for nutrition education include visits to markets, dairies or farms, tasting parties, playing store, etc. Children in rural areas may like to grow a new vegetable at home, bring it to class, and tell the others what it is and how it grows. The class can learn to cook the vegetables and taste them. A project for the year might be learning to classify foods according to the Basic Four food plan and keeping a scrapbook of cut-out or colored pictures of foods the class has studied and learned to like.

In the intermediate grades children can learn that the kind of food they eat makes a difference. Animal experiments are popular learning activities in the fifth or sixth grade. In these experiments two white rats are generally used; one is fed a good diet and the other a poor one. During the year the children see that rats need certain foods to maintain proper growth, appearance, and activity. At the same time they also learn that boys and girls need certain foods to grow and stay healthy. The children keep track of their own height and weight and record their daily food intakes. The teacher can use these records to determine where further nutrition education is needed, and the nurse can use them in evaluating the health status of the elementary school child.

The school lunch should be used as an example of what a nutritious meal should be. Children in the later elementary grades may even be able to plan menus for the school lunch.

Sex education. As previously stated, children's interest in sex varies at different ages. During the school years children should be prepared for the physiological changes that take place prior to their occurrence. They then have a more objective attitude. Girls should know about physiological changes that are normal in boys during adolescence and vice versa. Children mature at different age levels. Not later than the sixth grade—and preferably in the fifth—they should be given explanations relative to secondary sex characteristics and other bodily changes that will take place.

The term *sex* is not very acceptable to school authorities, but the term *family living* may be. There are some excellent films available at state health departments, which can be used to supplement teaching in schools. Many pamphlets also are available from the same service.

Before showing films it might be well for the nurse to suggest to the teacher that parents be invited to view the film at the same time that the children do.

Accident prevention. In the elementary school years, just as in the toddler and preschool period, accidents reign as the first cause of death. Being run over by an automobile, drowning, and fire also remain the three chief offenders; however, between 5 and 9 years of age drowning is more common than death by fire. For children in the age group of 10 to 14 years, accidents that result from being a passenger in a car rather than a pedestrian are the first cause of death, drowning remains second, and death by firearms is third.

Relative to automobile accidents, parents' attention should be called to the importance of their adhering to rules of safe driving. Possibly in a parent-teacher meeting a film on safe driving could be shown, followed by a discussion on safety measures that prevent automobile accidents. Children, especially those in the primary grades, are safer riding in the back seat than in the front seat. Also, children can be taught to fasten their seat belts in a car.

Parents should be urged to have children learn to swim and to teach them not to go swimming alone. The presence of a lifeguard at a pool or lake is helpful.

Prevention of fire should be taught both to parents and to children. In school this could be in connection with fire drills. A parent-teacher meeting is the easiest way to reach parents with regard to fire prevention at home. If firearms are kept at home, bullets should be removed. Firearms should not be handled by children except under supervision. Explicit direction in use of firearms may eliminate some accidents.

Since sports and recreational activities may contribute to the number of fractures, sprains, and strains found in the 10- to 14-year-old group, specific direction as to the use of equipment and knowledge of a particular sport may lessen accidents. This includes instruction in bicycle safety.

Safety education might well be correlated with the time of year. For example, water safety could be emphasized in May and safe conduct in the gymnasium, corridors, stairs, and the school bus in September. In October or November fire prevention could be stressed. In January or February prevention of accidents in crossing an icy street or in coasting or prevention and treatment of frostbite could be stressed. What safety education needs to be emphasized must be considered also in reference to the location of the school in its community and the geographical setting.

Summary

The 6-year-old child enters a new world as he starts school. He sees new people, has new experiences, and as time goes on in the elementary school years he should be encouraged to belong to special interest groups, such as scouts, arts and crafts groups, and the like. He needs reasonable explanations, requests, room for rough-and-tumble play at home, play experience with other children of the same sex after school, and a minimum of nagging. Learning skills such as swimming, roller skating, and bicycle riding help develop self-confidence. Sympathetic interest in his school problems is important since going to school is a new achievement. The ability to read and write gives him a sense of added power.

During the preschool period the child needed protection from accidents such as ingestion of poisons, fire, and drowning, while in the school-age period the child needs further education about the prevention of accidents, especially from water, fire, and automobiles. The family and the community have a responsibility to see that there are safe places in which the child can play after school and on weekends. Periodical health assessments and dental visits remain important—both to see that he is developing and to detect any deviations from good health. Booster shots for various immunizations are vital. If the child's vision and hearing have been tested before entering school, testing again by the third grade and at periodical intervals thereafter is advisable unless there is a problem that needs more frequent supervision. The degree to which the school health program and all its aspects (healthful environment, health instruction, health services) influences a particular child depends upon the interest of the school personnel, the parents, and the school nurse.

PROMOTION OF HEALTH
IN ADOLESCENCE
Health problems

The health problems of the young adolescent (12 to 14 years of age) are included in Table 9-6. Interestingly enough, accidents rank highest as a cause of death in both elementary and junior and senior high school students. In the school-aged child deaths from congenital malformations and from influenza rank third and fourth, respectively, while in later adolescence homicide and suicide rank second and third (Table 9-7). In both groups, diseases of the heart rank fifth. Prevention of accidents through safety education relative to motor accidents, drowning, and firearms is important in these years plus continuing periodical medical supervision. The incidence of both homicide and suicide points to the fact that preparation for adolescence begins in the cradle and continues through the formative and school years. Attitudes toward authority and values including the

Table 9-7. Deaths and death rates for children 15 to 24 years, both sexes

Rank	Cause of death†	Number	Rate‡
	All causes	45,261	127.7
1	Accidents (E800-E949)	24,336	68.7
2	Homicide (E960-E978)	4,157	11.7
3	Suicide (E950-E959)	3,128	8.8
4	Malignant neoplasms, including neoplasms of lymphatic and hematopoietic tissues (140-209)	2,931	8.3
5	Diseases of heart (390-398, 402, 404, 410-486)	1,054	3.0
6	Influenza and pneumonia (407-474, 480-486)	866	2.4
7	Congenital anomalies (740-759)	739	2.1
8	Cerebrovascular diseases (430-438)	553	1.6
9	Complications of pregnancy, childbirth, and the puerperium (630-678)	303	0.9
10	Nephritis and nephrosis (580-584)	286	0.8

*Modified from Facts of life and death, Rockville, Md., 1974, Public Health Service, U.S. Department of Health, Education, and Welfare (Table 28).
†According to International classification of diseases, eighth revision, 1965.
‡Per 100,000 population in age group.

meaning of life and finding a vocation all become increasingly important. The use of alcohol, drugs, and tobacco may be crucial health problems in the life of the adolescent. They tell something of his adjustment.

Role of the nurse

The role of the office nurse becomes increasingly important when the adolescent girl or boy comes to a doctor's office for an examination. Some pediatricians have a special time for seeing adolescents. In some areas there may be clinics just for the adolescent. If the nurse treats a person of this age with the respect accorded an adult, it makes the adolescent feel important. Also, if the nurse can tactfully suggest that the adolescent boy see the doctor alone without his mother, the adolescent will be appreciative. The same is true of the adolescent girl; the nurse, of course, will be with her when she is examined by the doctor. The adolescent boy or girl is sensitive to his or her bodily changes. The examining physician has a better chance to talk with the adolescent and establish favorable communication if the mother or parents remain in the waiting room. The adolescent then feels more free in talking with the doctor. Sometimes it is the office nurse, in taking a history, who establishes such a good rapport that a girl speaks freely to her.

The school health program gives the public health nurse or the school health nurse an opportunity to have contacts with the preadolescent and adolescent boy and girl. Each should understand his role in maintaining good health. (Refer to pp. 226 and 238 for an explanation of the school health program.)

The hospital nurse begins to direct her teaching to the adolescent girl or boy. With the younger children she has directed her teaching more to the parents. Junior and senior high school students should be given increasing responsibility for their own behavior and health. The nurse should help them to understand the "why" of certain health recommendations.

The camp nurse also has a unique opportunity to guide the health of children.

In some child health conferences, the nurse may be the one who examines the child and does a health assessment.

SECTION 1: PHYSICAL EXAMINATION (See Fig. 9-19.)

SECTION 2: GENERAL CARE

Directions: Fill in blanks with appropriate information.

BATHING
Daily _____ Other _____

SLEEP
Usual bedtime _____

ELIMINATION
Daily stool _____ Other _____ Characteristics (color and consistency) _____

Voiding (number of times): Daytime _____ Nighttime _____

NUTRITION
Describe food eaten in last 24 hours: Breakfast _____

Snacks _____

Lunch _____

Dinner _____

DENTAL CARE
Brushes teeth _____ When? _____ Date of last dental visit _____

INTERESTS AND DISCIPLINE
Education
Grade placement _____ Plans to complete high school _____

Special interest clubs in school _____

Special academic clubs _____

Interests in college _____

Vocation
Part-time jobs _____

Desired vocation as adult _____

Church
Attends church _____ Sunday school _____ Church clubs _____

Recreation
Activity most enjoyed _____

Membership in teams (explain) _____

Skills: Swimming _____ Tennis _____ Singing _____ Clubs _____ Musical in-

struments _____

Fig. 9-20. Guide for health assessment of adolescent.

SECTION 2: GENERAL CARE—cont'd

Recreation—cont'd

Recreational interests with companions _____

Special friend: Same sex _____ Opposite sex _____

Dating: Double date _____ Alone _____

Recreation with father _____   _____

   With mother _____

   With whole family _____

Discipline: Are there definite rules? _____ Explain _____

Home responsibilities _____

TOPICS FOR HEALTH GUIDANCE

Recreation	Nutrition
Alcohol	Dental hygiene
Vocational interests	Bathing
Smoking	Sleep
Drugs	Relationship with parents
Sexual behavior	Driving education

Fig. 9-20, cont'd. Guide for health assessment of adolescent.

Assessment of health

See Fig. 9-19 for suggested guide to physical assessment (Section 1) and Fig. 9-20 for general care of adolescents.

The chief differences in physical assessment of the school-aged child and the adolescent are in their growth and development, which include signs of puberty—some earlier than others. There is usually a preadolescent spurt of growth in height followed by a gain in weight in adolescent years. (Because of rapid growth, teenagers' appetites should be very good.) In general the young teenager is tall and slender, while the older one has a more mature figure. The physical appearance of the face, nails, and hair tells something of teenagers' feelings about themselves since teenagers are interested in their personal appearance. Some teenagers (both boys and girls) have trouble with acne or skin eruptions on their face. The sebaceous glands are more active in this period and help to account for this condition. Body contour is changed. There is further growth of the lower jaw that changes the shape of face. The circumference of the legs and arms increases in both sexes. Physiological changes of puberty in girls include breast development, growth of axillary and pubic hair, onset of menarche, and broadening of hips due to subcutaneous fat deposition and growth of pelvic girdle. In general menarche begins about 13 years of age. In boys physiological changes include voice changes, seminal emissions, and growth of facial, axillary, and pubic hair. Girls mature physiologically sooner than boys. Permanent teeth have errupted by 14 years of age except for third molars. Special attention should be given to the ausculation of the heart since the incidence of heart disease increases during this period. Careful examination of breasts of girls as well as a Pap smear after 15 years of age is worthwhile.

The trend is for the pediatrician to assist the adolescent through the critical stages of growth and development when emotional impacts exert a profound influence. The older adolescent girl should be encouraged to make regular visits to the pediatrician or gynecologist. Since this is a rapid period of growth a hemoglobin count is one indication of whether the nutrition of the adolescent is adequate. Poor posture may indicate undue fatigue. There should be careful scrutiny of the spine for scoliosis, kyphosis, or lordosis.

Because of the increased incidence of gonorrhea, any discharge from the vagina should be especially noted as well as any signs of abdominal pain.

In general health guidance attention should be given to adjustment problems of adolescence. Attention to adjustment problems could prevent the occurrence of alcoholism and drug abuse. Again, it is essential for the nurse to be aware of community resources, including counseling, that are available to the adolescent.

Teenagers in senior high school evidence their maturity by taking an interest in making plans for the future concerning college and a vocation and by indicating interest in community affairs through volunteering their services in hospitals, settlement houses, or special interest groups.

Behavior characteristics

Before thinking about the needs of teenagers, it might be well to review some of their characteristic behavior. The 13-year-old tends to be very self-absorbed. He often worries and cannot immediately go to sleep at night because of this. He is critical of himself and of others. He wants more independence and freedom and goes into his own room for privacy.

In contrast to this behavior the 14-year-old has more self-assurance and is exuberant and more congenial with everyone although still rather hypercritical of his parents. He likes team games and sports. Both boys and girls are beginning to take an interest in the opposite sex, and both are concerned about their body image.

The 15-year-old adolescent is a more complex person than he was in the previous year.

He has increasing self-awareness. He feels he is growing up and wishes increasing independence. At times he is quiet and thoughtful, usually mulling over his own feelings about everything. He may acknowledge that at times he feels "mixed up." At other times he is restless and rebellious against authority. He enjoys peer age gatherings and can be quite gregarious with his peers.

At 16 years the teen-ager has more self-assurance and a sense of independence. There is less friction with parents and siblings. The 16-year-old young person is more stable than previously. He exhibits more friendliness and more of an outgoing behavior. He is particularly interested in people and enjoys informal parties. Both boys and girls think about marriage and college and a vocation. They begin to plan for the future.

Guidance toward health
General hygiene

Eating. The healthy adolescent is characterized by a healthy appetite. The foods selected will still reflect patterns learned early in life, but even to a greater extent than the elementary school child, the adolescent will be swayed by influences outside the home. Social activities, concern about appearance, and food habits of friends will all play a role in determining teenage eating behavior.

Nutritional needs. The adolescent growth spurt serves as the physiological basis for nutritional requirements. Rapid gains in height and weight in early adolescence suggest an increased need for calories and protein to maintain tissue synthesis. The National Research Council recommends an intake of 2,100 calories and 48 gm. of protein for girls and 3,000 calories and 54 gm. of protein for boys between the ages of 15 and 18 years. In addition to these recommendations the allowances for all the major vitamins and minerals are substantially increased during adolescence. For boys there is no other time during the life cycle when nutrient needs are so high. For girls only pregnancy and lactation equal or surpass the adolescent requirements. When the accelerated phase of growth begins to taper off in late adolescence, rapid muscle development and bone mineralization continue the body's demand for nutrients so that requirements for good-quality protein, vitamins, and minerals remain high throughout all the teen years. A quart of milk, a serving of meat or other protein food at each meal, four or more servings of fruits and vegetables, and four or more servings of breads and cereals are to be encouraged daily.

The increase in skeletal size makes the intake of calcium especially significant. The recommended dietary allowance for calcium is 1,200 mg. for girls and boys. After 18 years of age the calcium allowance for both girls and boys drops to the adult level of 800 mg.

A number of investigators have studied the ability of adolescents to utilize dietary calcium. A study of particular interest by Stearns examined calcium absorption in two groups of teenage girls. The girls in one group were considered to have consumed adequate diets over a period of several years. They were immediately able to absorb the recommended amounts of calcium when given a little less than a quart of milk a day. The second group had previously been malnourished; their diets had been inadequate in all nutrients except total calories. It took 6 months of a step-by-step increase in milk to more than 2 quarts a day before these girls were able to absorb the recommended amounts of calcium. The study indicates that inadequate nutrition during any considerable part of childhood can clearly affect nutritional status during adolescence.

Likewise, poor nutrition during adolescence will be reflected in later life. In evaluating the obstetrical performance of women in Aberdeen, Scotland, Thomson and Billewicz concluded that insufficient calcium intake during adolescence was probably one of the most significant factors in the incidence of cesarean section. It is conceivable that lack of calcium at the critical time in a girl's life when her pelvic bones enlarge in preparation for reproduction can result in an inadequate structure, which precludes normal delivery. Poor calcium intake during adolescence and the reproductive years is also considered to be a possible cause of osteoporosis in elderly women.

Thus the nutritional status of adolescents must be viewed as the crux of a continuum that encompasses the entire life-span, conditioned by the nutritional experience of childhood and determining the nutritional potential of the adult. The relationship between nutrition and health becomes even more apparent when some common nutrition problems of adolescence are considered.

Nutritional problems. The incidence of overt nutritional deficiency diseases among teenagers in the United States is low. With the exception of iron deficiency anemia the easily identifiable consequences of poor nutrition are seldom seen. However, statistical indices of common disorders mong adolescents suggest underlying dietary factors.

Poor eyesight, poor dentition, and a high incidence of tuberculosis are generally recognized health problems that are associated with improper nutrition. Dietary surveys show vitamin A, vitamin C, calcium, and iron to be the nutrients most frequently deficient in the diets of adolescents. The roles of vitamins A and C in maintaining the body's resistance to infection have been established. Calcium and vitamin C are necessary for tooth formation and resistance to decay. Vitamin A is instrumental in the maintenance of proper vision.

Examination of adolescent food habits provides an answer as to why these particular nutrients are often deficient. It is a foregone conclusion that snacking is the teenager's way of life. Frequent visits to the hamburger stand and pizza parlor may allow him to consume adequate amounts of protein and calories, but they offer little opportunity to maintain the recommended intake of fruits and vegetables— especially the dark green and yellow vegetables, which are major sources of the aforementioned four nutrients. Skipping breakfast in favor of a doughnut and coffee and missing dinner because of social events and after-school activities make it extremely unlikely that the teenager is able to supplement these nutrients from meals at home.

The high calorie content of typical snack foods is also a factor in the incidence of adolescent obesity. An individual is classified as obese when his weight is 20% above that which is considered desirable for his age, sex, height, and body build. By this criterion it is estimated that nearly 3 million adolescents in the United States are sufficiently overweight to be considered obese. The incidence is slightly higher for girls than for boys. Obesity adds to the social and emotional problems of adolescence; it also is generally true that the fat teenager becomes the fat adult, with all of the inherent complications of overweight—increased risk of diabetes, heart disease, gastrointestinal disorders, problems of pregnancy, etc. It is for these reasons that obesity among adolescents is a growing health concern.

Underactivity rather than overeating is sometimes the cause of obesity. In fact, some obese teens actually consume less food than their nonobese peers. Ill-advised efforts to reduce often cause these teenagers to place themselves on unduly restrictive diets that strain nutrient requirements. An understanding of the mechanisms of weight gain and loss coupled with a sensible diet and exercise program can be expected to result in greater long-range health benefits than any crash regimen.

Another significant nutritional problem is encountered in the teenage girl who becomes pregnant. The pregnant adolescent, already an obstetrical risk, is in even a more precarious situation if her nutrition is poor. The fact that pregnancy imposes additional nutrient demands on a body still requiring a large supply for its own growth and development makes diet consultation extremely important. Although specific food needs for pregnancy have been discussed in Chapter 3, here it is important to remember that the teenage girl, who normally requires from 100 to 400 calories more than the mature woman, will need yet another 300 calories if she is pregnant. Vitamin and mineral requirements that are generally higher than those of an adult also are increased in pregnancy. Meeting the needs of both pregnancy and adolescence without incurring obesity requires careful food selection. Pregnant teenagers should be encouraged to choose foods according to the basic four recommendations for pregnancy and supplement extra calories from the milk and meat groups.

Rest and sleep. At the very time recreational interests and social life increase, a young teenager needs more rest and sleep. The incidence of tuberculosis increases in this age period. Rest and sleep also influence the mental state, and, as has been mentioned, the rate of suicide increases in adolescence. Rest helps emotional stability.

If the adolescent seems tired, does not wish to get up in the morning, and is irritable, he may not be getting enough sleep or rest. Sometimes there are so many extracurricular activities that there is not time for relaxation. The adolescent is on the go every minute of his waking hours. This is wrong. Every afternoon should not be taken. In the evening, except when there is no school the following day, the teenager should be in bed at a reasonable hour.

Calling attention to the health rules of a varsity football team or a basketball team helps to show that sleep is important. Summer months spent as a junior counselor in camp are beneficial because of regular hours of sleep and activities plus exercise in the open air.

Rest must not be interpreted to mean sleep necessarily. A quiet activity, as opposed to a strenuous tennis game, or lounging in a chair watching television is resting. The adolescent is often accused of being lazy. This is unjust since many times he is tired.

Emotional, social, and intellectual needs

The word *adolescence* is used to denote that period of time between puberty and adulthood.

During these years, the family remains important but in a different way. As the elementary child goes into the junior or senior high school, he needs to be given increasing responsibility and helped toward social and intellectual independence. He should take part in family conferences and decisions such as when and how to spend a vacation, which evening he can stay out late, and at what hour he must be home. Setting reasonable limits to a teenager's activities and privileges gives him a sense of security. Asking the adolescent boy or girl to telephone when he or she cannot be home at the designated time relieves parental anxiety and lets the teenager know his parents have confidence in him. It also helps him to develop a sense of responsibility. Participation in family conferences gives the adolescent a feeling of belonging and recognition.

During adolescence there is a rapid spurt of growth, and the high school boy or girl may be as tall as or taller than his (or her) parents. He wishes to be treated with the respect and courtesy due an adult (even though he does not have the judgment of an adult). What the adolescent says should be taken seriously. He needs to voice his opinions and ideas. At the legal age, allowing the adolescent to have a driving permit and drive the car gives his self-image a boost.

The parents may believe the teenager is unduly critical of them as he gets older, but this is part of a process whereby he is separating himself from his parents in order to feel emotionally independent rather than stay a dependent child. He has to sell himself as a person in his own right. He goes through this stage to one of later identification of himself as a man like his father or a woman like her mother.

In spite of this critical attitude, the adolescent needs to be aware that he is accepted and loved at home. If he rebels at limitations and at questions about where he is going, the parents can point out that it is because they love him that they are concerned about him. Sometimes the adolescent feels lonely, different from others, perhaps even adopted. The world of the adolescent becomes increasingly larger and sometimes it is bewildering. He needs to feel not only that he is accepted and loved at home but also that he has certain possessions and friends. Parents should respect his privacy. His particular possessions should not be touched by others. If possible, he should have a room to himself. Friends should be welcomed by his parents, and they should be able to enjoy and use the home. The home belongs to him as well as the parents. If parents do welcome these friends of their adolescent boy or girl and provide them with suitable recreational diversion, the teenager will often remain in the home rather than seek adventure, excitement, and understanding away from home. Card games, Scrabble, Monopoly, and Ping-Pong are popular. Listening to records and dancing are enjoyed especially by the older teenager.

In the junior and senior high school, young people show an interest in the opposite sex. The gang age (9 or 10 years to 15) gives way to dating or double dating by senior high school. Often there are informal social gatherings. If a group of teenagers feel welcome in a home and diversion has been provided, they will probably return. Social interaction with the opposite sex is necessary since the world is not composed of all men or all women. On the other hand, "going steady" has a disadvantage since it limits the social contacts of a boy or girl.

Conferences and discussions between parents and teenagers concerning their friends and social activities are profitable and possible if each is able to listen as well as talk. In view of the increasing incidence of venereal disease and the use of drugs and alcohol, the teenager needs help in forming values.

Hunting, fishing, golfing, or camping overnight with his father gives a boy a certain feeling of identity with his own sex. Some project on which father and son could work together does the same thing, if within the child's ability, as does playing competitive games such as chess or pool.

The courtesy and protectiveness shown by the father to the mother is equally important. Companionship of a mother and daughter has significance for the daughter's development.

The adolescent needs and wants increasing responsibilities. He does not wish to be treated as a child. Arranging his room the way he wishes, having responsibility for its appearance, spending his allowance as he wishes, and working in summer vacations are methods of giving desired independence. All of this aids the teenager toward self-reliance.

In senior high school the adolescent wishes to choose his life work. Parents can help by finding out educational requirements needed for various types of work. It may be wise for parents to visit colleges in which their son or daughter may wish to enroll to get the necessary preparation for their life work.

Physical education teachers, ministers, counselors, community organization leaders, and teachers play important roles in character building and in the formation of ideals and philosophies of young people. Many times young people enjoy counseling and guidance from adults outside the family group. A 15-

year-old adolescent may even seek out a counselor to whom he can express himself.

Up to adolescence, religious beliefs of the family are usually accepted, but in the period of adolescence these may be questioned. Young people want a better understanding of religion and world religions. Membership in young people's organizations in churches does much to help the adolescent in this area.

The older adolescent is in quest of intellectual knowledge. This should be handled constructively. It is an excellent time to interest him in plays, travel, books pertinent to his interests, visits to industries, discussions of politics, and visits to historical points of interest. Explanations and visits to the office or work of the teenager's father or parents also open new vistas to the growing young person.

Social activities at school, at church, and in the neighborhood increase in junior and senior high school, but there is a real need for the adolescent to utilize some of his energy in wholesome outdoor exercise and in team games. Sports also act as an outlet for feelings of aggression. The girl who has not learned skills such as skating or tennis and the boy who cannot swim or show skill in any form of athletics will begin to be onlookers. They are handicapped socially and physically.

By high school the teenager should be ready to relinquish individual supremacy for the good of the group. Team games furnish increasing fun. Participation in sports helps to increase learning to share, to play fairly, to be loyal, and in general to live and work with others. Recreation provided by a community center or "teen town" helps fulfill the recreational needs of the teenager.

The interest that girls have in their body image suggests why specialized classes in the use of cosmetics, in care of the hair and hairdos, and in modeling are popular. These are sometimes sponsored by an organization such as Y.W.C.A. or by a large department store. Some girls enjoy special gym classes in physical fitness.

School health program
Healthful living

For discussion of the school health program, refer to p. 226. In addition to the discussion of safety and healthful living as part of the school health program, mention should be made of student organizations for safety at the high school level. Students could assist faculty in developing suitable policies regarding safety in play areas, gymnasiums, hallways, and stairs. A student organization or committee could urge students to practice self-discipline in observing safety rules. Any accidents in school or on school grounds could be reviewed by the group, and better preventive measures might be instigated.

Health services

As stated previously, the number of physical examinations and the examinations done vary in each county and state. Ideally the growing child should continue to have a semiannual dental checkup and an annual physical examination. Because the majority of children do not have physical examinations annually, the teacher's observations of untoward symptoms and her referral of children to the nurse are still of utmost importance. (See Table 9-3 for the recommended immunizations and vaccinations.) Booster injections for tetanus must not be neglected in view of the frequency of cuts and injuries. If the child is going camping or vacationing where there is any question about contaminated water, a typhoid booster injection is advisable, even though there is a specific drug for typhoid fever.

Sometimes the school health nurse is a confidante of the junior and senior girls, and they may wish to discuss menstrual hygiene, boy-girl relationships, and dating with her. The nurse must be careful to be a good listener and to judge when information will be accepted. If she is too eager to talk, she may lose the interest of the girl.

Sometimes, if a girl becomes pregnant, the nurse may be the first consulted by the school authorities. To see that the pregnant girl receives medical supervision is the nurse's responsibility and to work cooperatively with the hospital or private doctor in plans for her care. The nurse must make every effort to let the teenager know that she accepts and likes her as a person. To be judgmental of the illegitimate pregnancy is not the function of the nurse; nor is it her function to urge that the unborn child be adopted or kept. This is a decision of the family. A social worker at the hospital will help to make plans for the unborn child. If the family is known to the department of public welfare, they too will participate in plans. If the teenager keeps the infant, the county health nurse may in turn have the infant on her case load.

Health instruction

Four areas of health instruction need particular emphasis in the adolescent period: nutrition, safety education, personal hygiene, and education for family living. Whether education relative to smoking, drinking, and the use of drugs should be part of school health instruction and/or the family's responsibility is a moot question.

Nutrition instruction. Teenagers frequently complain that nutrition is a boring subject. They say they have heard it all before. To many of them nutrition means eating what you dislike and giving up everything you do like. In some cases their complaints are justified. If nutrition at the junior and senior high school level is merely repetition of material learned in the elementary grades and is unimaginatively presented as a list of do's and dont's, the teenager has every right to be rebellious and bored. By the time a child leaves grade school, he should know the names of the nutrients, in which foods they can be found, and why he needs to eat them each day. In high school he is ready for a more sophisticated approach to the qualitative and quantitative aspects of diet.

Traditionally nutrition content has been relegated to specific courses in health, home economics, or family living; but nutrition concepts can be easily integrated into nearly every course in the curriculum. For example, biology can be used to demonstrate the physiological dependence of all living organisms on an adequate diet and to introduce basic principles of food sanitation by studying food- and water-borne agents of disease. In chemistry students can learn to identify basic elements contained in food and simple reactions that occur when the body uses food. Physics offers the opportunity of demonstrating the manner in which the body converts the potential energy of food to energy for performing physical work. Here students can learn to calculate their own energy requirements and compare them to the caloric value of the foods they eat. Economics can be employed to study factors influencing the cost of living and the price of food. A project might be meal planning on an economy budget. History and social science can illustrate the meaning of food for man and his society, cultural food patterns, the force of food in shaping the history of the world, and future expectations in regard to population and the food supply.

Such an innovative approach to the teaching of nutrition first requires education of the educators. The school or community health nurse who takes part in the planning of the health curriculum can see to it that teachers are made aware of the need for including nutrition content in a wide range of courses so that more students can be reached. She can serve as a resource for teachers who need their own background in nutrition strengthened by direct counseling or by actually taking part in classroom teaching.

Meanwhile the nurse must make her influence felt among the students themselves. She can provide reliable answers to questions about diet, weight reduction, and food fads. In some schools nurses organize diet and exercise programs for obese teenagers under medical supervision and counsel individual students with special nutrition problems. As in elementary school, the school lunch should be used to advantage in nutrition education.

Safety education. Specific safety education, exclusive of participation in a school committee for safety, includes driver education and knowledge of safety programs in the community or nearby city.

Prevention of automobile accidents through knowledge of traffic laws, avoidance of mechanical car difficulties, handling a car in bad weather, backing a car, and knowledge of how to drive a car are all part of driver education. Motor vehicles are the chief cause of death from age 15 to 24 years.

Excursions to an industry to see a safety program or to a farm to study principles of accident prevention give a realistic appreciation of safety. Also, attendance at 1-day institutes on safety stimulates interest.

Instruction in water safety is still important in this age period. The number of deaths from drowning increases as children get older. Death rate for boys is higher than for girls. Older children participate in swimming, boating, and other water sports more frequently than younger children.

It is an unusual school that has a swimming pool, but the school could seek cooperation with a community organization such as the Y.W.C.A. and Red Cross to have junior and senior high school students participate in swimming instruction and could ask members of such community organizations to be guest speakers to a safety class.

Personal hygiene. As children go from junior high school to senior high, they are increasingly interested in personal appearance. They are aware of their bodily changes, and how they look is important to them. Also, they wish to look attractive to the opposite sex. A class in personal hygiene is useful to them; such a class should include instructions in care of the hair and nails, proper use of cosmetics, and appropriate clothing. This might be one unit in a course that also includes ways to keep healthy: medical examinations, nutrition, cleanliness, rest, and recreation.

Education for family living. Another area of instruction needing attention is education for family living. A topic such as "choosing a mate" should include a discussion of factors that make for a successful marriage such as similar religion of both parties, similar educational level, common interests and goals, etc. The reason health of each partner is important needs discussion; how much it costs for two people to live together and keep house (rent, utilities, groceries, clothes, transportation, medical care, etc.) are an essential part of knowledge for family living. How much money does it take for a man to support a wife? The cost of having a baby could be investigated by a class. It should be pointed out that medical supervision throughout pregnancy is necessary for the sake of both the mother and the unborn baby. The availability of such resources as family planning clinics needs mentioning. A representative from a family planning clinic might be asked to speak to a class. Knowledge of the care of infants and children is essential not only for future parenthood but for teenagers who baby-sit.

Of course, knowledge of one's own body as well as that of opposite sex is essential as well as an understanding of human reproduction. Ways of giving each partner in marriage happiness and pleasure from coitus is all part of education for successful marriage (Masters and Johnson).

Since both venereal disease and illegitimacy increase in the adolescent period, the adolescent needs a better understanding of these conditions. The price of illegitimacy to the individual (the unborn child and members of the family), to the community, and to the taxpayer should be thoroughly discussed.

An interested county health nurse or school nurse could contribute as a consultant in planning classes in health education. She might be instrumental in seeing that such classes are given if she is on the school health committee. How much the nurse does will depend on her insight into the young people's needs, the philosophy of the school health committee, and her relations with the teachers.

Availability of community resources

Each community differs, and the nurse needs to know the location of near family planning clinics, prenatal clinics, child health conferences, child abuse centers, drug abuse centers, mental hygiene clinics, community facilities for recreation, etc. This knowledge is essential for her to have as she helps to guide the adolescent with whom she comes in contact.

Summary

In guiding the health of the adolescent, it is essential to be aware of him as a person. He needs to feel he is a worthy person. Many times he needs someone to listen to his views and someone to whom he can express himself. Knowing resources to which he may be referred for educational, physical, or mental health is important for the nurse to know. Health problems that have increased during the adolescent period are the use of drugs and alcohol and venereal disease.

The adolescent needs more than periodic physical examination. He needs a complete health assessment; then problems can be cited early and help given. The adolescent has to be taught to gradually take the responsibility for his own health.

• • •

An infant is entirely dependent on adults for his care and survival. After progress through infancy, through the toddler and preschool period, through middle childhood, and finally through adolescence, the child has grown into a young man or woman who should be able to care for himself. The question that every nurse has to ask herself is whether she contributed to his development the very best she could when she saw him or his parents—whether that was in the newborn nursery, the child health conference clinic, the home, the school, the camp, or a hospital.

REFERENCES

Alexander, M., and Brown, P.: Pediatric physical diagnosis for nurses, New York, 1974, McGraw-Hill Book Co.

Aliss, A. S.: Bridging the concept gap in work with youth, Children **18:**13, January-February, 1971.

Ames, L., and Chase, J.: Don't push your preschooler, New York, 1974, Harper & Row, Publishers.

Anderson, L., and Creswell, W. H., Jr.: School health practice, ed. 6, St. Louis, 1976, The C. V. Mosby Co.

Barnes, L. A.: Manual of pediatric physical diagnosis, ed. 3, Chicago, 1966, Year Book Medical Publishers.

Barnett, E. M.: Pediatric occlusal therapy, St. Louis, 1974, The C. V. Mosby Co.

Barnett, H., et al.: Pediatrics, ed. 15, New York, 1972, Appleton-Century Crofts.

Caghan, S.: The adolescent and nutrition, Am. J. Nurs. **75:**1728, October, 1975.

Chinn, P. L.: A relationship between health and school problems; a nursing assessment, J. School Health, **43:** 85, 1973.

Chinn, P. L., and Leitch, C. J.: Child health maintenance: A guide to clinical assessment, St. Louis, 1974, The C. V. Mosby Co.

Coakley, J. M., and Parker, J.: Education for school nursing, Am. J. Nurs. **65:**84, November, 1965.

deCastro, F. J., Rolfe, U. T., and Drew, J. K.: The pediatric nurse practitioner: Guidelines for practice, ed. 2, St. Louis, 1976, The C. V. Mosby Co.

Eisenson, J., and Ogilvie, M.: Speech correction in schools, ed. 2, New York, 1963, Macmillan, Inc.

Effects of a balanced school lunch program on growth and nutritive status of school children, Nutr. Rev. **23:**35, 1965.

Fox, V.: Alcoholism in adolescence, J. School Health **13:**32, January, 1973.

Fredlund, D.: Juvenile delinquency and school nursing, Nurs. Outlook **18:**57, May, 1970.

Gimbel, H.: Group work with adolescent girls, Nurs. Outlook **16:**47, April, 1968.

Giuffra, M.: Demystifying adolescent behavior, Am. J. Nurs. **75:**1724, October, 1975.

Goda, S.: Speech development in children, Am. J. Nurs. **70:**276, 1970.

Haggerty, R.: Preventive pediatrics. In Vaughan, V. C.,

III, and McKay, R. J., editors: Nelson's textbook of pediatrics, ed. 10, Philadelphia, 1975, W. B. Saunders Co.

Harmer, S. L.: The role of the nutritionist in the adolescent clinic, Children **13:**217, 1966.

Heald, F., editor: Adolescent nutrition and growth, New York, 1968, Meredith Corp.

Hubbard, C. W.: Family planning education: Parenthood and social discase control, St. Louis, 1973, The C. V. Mosby Co.

Jackson, C.: The eye in general practice, ed. 5, London, 1969, E. & S. Livingstone.

Jenne, F. H., and Greene, W. H.: Turner's school health and health education, ed. 7, St. Louis, 1976, The C. V. Mosby Co.

Kitzman, H.: The nature of well child care, Am. J. Nurs. **75:**1705, October, 1975.

Knaff, L.: A community gets a health center, Am. J. Nurs. **70:**1498, July, 1970.

Kosidlak, J.: Improving health care for troubled youths, Am. J. Nurs. **76:**95, January, 1976.

Leverne, M.: The pursuit of wholeness, Am. J. Nurs. **69:**93, January, 1969.

Masters, W. H., and Johnson, V. E.: Human sexual response, Boston, 1966, Little, Brown & Co.

Miller, B., editor: The modern encyclopedia of baby and child care, New York, 1966, Golden Press.

Miller, M.: Sunday's child, New York, 1968, Holt, Rinehart & Winston, Inc.

Miner, J.: Wyoming school nurse, Am. J. Nurs. **65:**954, September, 1965.

Moore, M. V.: Diagnosis: Deafness, Am. J. Nurs. **69:**297, February, 1969.

Oberst, B.: Practical guidance for office pediatric and adolescent practice, Springfield, Ill., 1973, Charles C Thomas, Publisher.

O'Brien, M.: A nurse in school—why? Nurs. Clin. North Am., June, 1969.

Patton, R. G., and Gardner, L. I.: Influence of family environment on growth: The syndrome of "maternal deprivation," Pediatrics **30:**957, 1962.

Payne, P., and Payne, R.: Behavior manifestations of children with a hearing loss, Am. J. Nurs. **70:**1718, August, 1970.

Prior, J. A., and Siberstein, J. S.: Physical diagnosis: The history and examination of the patient, ed. 4, St. Louis, 1973, The C. V. Mosby Co.

Redl, F.: Pre-adolescent—what makes them tick? New York, 1969, The Child Study Association of America.

Salk, L.: Preparing for parenthood, New York, 1974, David McKay Co., Inc.

United States Department of Agriculture: National School Lunch Program, Washington, D.C., 1968, U.S. Government Printing Office.

Watson, L.: Child behavior modification: A manual for teachers, nurses, and parents, New York, 1973, Pergamon Press.

Wayne, D.: The lonely school child, Am. J. Nurs. **68:**774, April, 1968.

Williams, S. R.: Nutrition and diet therapy, ed. 2, St. Louis, 1973, The C. V. Mosby Co.

10

PSYCHOLOGICAL ASSESSMENT OF CHILDREN

Physical health is greatly influenced by mental health; therefore it is essential for the nurse to understand the interaction between these two systems to deal effectively with the whole child. Understanding the whole child involves knowledge not only of his developmental and medical history but also of his cultural, cognitive, and socioemotional adjustment. Much information on each area is gained through observational techniques, interviews with the child and with his parents, teachers' comments, and records of the family physician. These are all excellent sources of information. Sometimes this information is not enough, or data from some sources may be missing. Additional information can be supplied through psychological assessment, which typically involves interviews and psychological testing. Psychological assessment is so widely utilized with young persons that it is essential for professionals in the nursing field to have some understanding of this procedure, the rationale behind its use, and the bases on which referrals for assessment are made, especially since nurses are typically primary referral sources for psychological evaluations. In some settings nurses may be part of the decision-making team. Therefore it is necessary that they be familiar with the kinds of information available through assessment and how such information can be utilized in their child care planning.

Until recently there were only two main contributors to the attempt to divide the measurement of behavior into logical units: Bloom (Bloom, 1956; Bloom, Hastings, and Madaus, 1971; Krathwohl, Bloom and Masia, 1964) and Buros (1959, 1965, 1972). Buros' measurement yearbooks are the best known and most comprehensive references on tests and measurements.

In the past few years two newly published guides to tests and measures have appeared. Johnson and Bommarito (1971) have divided unpublished child development measures for ages through 12 years into 10 categories, many of which are overlapping. Hoepfner, Stern, and Nummedal (1971) have provided a reference containing published tests for preschool and kindergarten-age schoolchildren. A brief survey of the existing classification schemas reveals a major difficulty for the person who does not have intensive training in assessment. All of the existing schemas or outlines vary according to the authors' purposes and interpretations of the uses of a measure. There is a great deal of overlap in each schema because a child's development cannot be divided accurately into discrete parts. On the contrary, a child's development should be seen as one dynamic process that matures through the interaction of his biological makeup with his environment. Therefore it should be kept in mind that the classification of measures into the following schema, a modification of Walker's (1973), is simply a convenience in discussing assessment and should not be interpreted as a natural division of a child's behaviors. No such division exists.

INDIVIDUAL AND GROUP TESTS

In the measurement of behavior, tests may be divided into two broad categories on the basis of the nature of the test administration. First, tests may be administered on an individual basis, as is most often done in the clinical evaluation of children. Individual tests permit careful observations of reactions and require verbal responses from the child being tested. This procedure involves the investment of a substantial amount of time on the part of the child and the psychologist and consequently an increase in the cost of testing. Some examples of individual tests are the Wechsler Intelligence Scale for Children–Revised (W.I.S.C.-R.), the Stanford-Binet Intelligence Scale (Revised Form L-M), and the McCarthy Scales of Children's Abilities (M.S.C.A.). The examiner records correct and incorrect responses and the method the child uses to solve various problems. Thus on the block design subtest of the W.I.S.C.-R. the examiner notes whether the child constructs the design from the model by means of a trial-and-error method, a part-whole method, or some idiosyncratic method. *How* the child solves the problem may be more important than whether or not he does solve it.

Because of the necessity of making careful observations in individual tests, it is important that the psychologist be well trained and experienced both in the test and in the knowledge and observation of human behavior. It is also necessary for him or her to have specific knowledge of the age group with which he or she works because the typical behaviors of children and of adults may be, and often are, two very different things. The information gained from the test depends on the knowledge, skill, and integrity of the user. Therefore one limitation of individual tests as compared to group tests is the reduced objectivity of scoring and interpretation. However, this limitation is more than offset by the greater depth and accuracy of the information provided. Only a psychologist or other professional intensively trained in the use of individual tests for children should be permitted to interpret them.

The second type of test administration is on a group basis. Group tests are designed primarily for mass testing and are widely used in the educational assessment of children. Since many children can be tested by a single examiner in a single testing session, the amount of time and the cost involved are less than for individual tests, but the amount and quality of the information obtained from group tests are reduced. Some examples of group tests often used with children are the California Test of Mental Maturity, the Otis Quick Scoring Mental Ability Test, the Iowa Test of Basic Skills, the Lorge-Thorndike Intelligence Test, and the S.R.A. Primary Mental Abilities Test. All of these tests are used for school screening and assessment; they are primarily objective tests and usually consist of multiple-choice items.

Besides efficiency of time and cost, another way in which group tests facilitate mass testing is in the simplification of the examiner's role. Most group tests require only that the examiner read simple instructions and keep accurate time. Thus less detailed training and experience are required of the examiner administering group tests, although it is required that he follow a standardized procedure.

Because of their ease of administration, of scoring, and of use with groups of any size, group tests tend to be highly popular. However, these tests have several limitations. One of these is the restricted opportunity for the examiner to establish rapport with and obtain cooperation from the child. Also temporary conditions such as fatigue and special problems of the child such as reading inability are less readily detected. Finally, group tests provide little opportunity for careful observation of the children's behavior and thus reduce the opportunities to identify the causes of poor performance. Within these limitations group tests can serve a very useful function in situations requiring screening of large numbers of children for an *estimate* of their performance. However, when important decisions are to be made about individuals or when there is any doubt about the validity of the results, these group measures should be supplemented either with individual examinations or additional information from other sources or both.

MULTIPLE TESTS, TEST BATTERIES, AND PROFILES

Because tests are not perfect instruments of prediction and assessment, it is best to administer multiple tests to increase reliability among the findings rather than to rely on the results of only one test. These should be viewed as giving *specific* information, not unique information. That is, tests should be used to obtain concrete information about a child's strengths and weaknesses, and the greater the agreement of such findings across several tests, the greater the confidence in the validity of such findings. Results that are idiosyncratic or unique to a particular test should be questioned.

Persons with the same general competency usually have different patterns of abilities. It is sometimes difficult to assess these patterns adequately from a single test because of the problems in obtaining a test that is high both in internal reliability (the consistency with which it measures the abilities it sets out to test) and in construct validity (the degree to which the test as a whole measures the abilities or traits that it purports to measure). The ideal solution to this problem is to administer a test battery composed of several tests, each of which measures a different component of the total competence to be assessed. Each of the individual tests should be reliable, and the battery as a whole should be valid in assessing competency in some area.

Since batteries consist of several tests, the amount of time required for their administration is considerable, and consequently their use with young children is limited. However, a type of battery that is often used with children, especially in the schools, is the multilevel battery. This is a series of overlapping tests, each covering a restricted range of difficulty suitable for the particular age, grade, or ability level for which it is designed. A child is tested only with the level appropriate for him, but other levels can be used for retesting him in subsequent years or for comparative judgments of various age groups. Multilevel batteries provide a reasonable degree of continuity with regard to content or intellectual functions covered. Some representative multilevel batteries are the California Test of Mental Maturity (C.T.M.M.), which covers grade 4 through adulthood, the Cooperative School and College Ability Tests (S.C.A.T.), which cover grade 4 through college, the S.R.A. Short Test of Educational Ability (S.T.E.A.), which covers kindergarten through grade 12, and the Analysis of Learning Potential (A.L.P.), which is among the most recently developed, is directed explicitly toward the prediction of academic performance and reflects a growing emphasis on the measurement of prerequisite intellectual skills for schoolwork and other daily activities.

Test batteries yield information expressed as multiple scores that can be plotted on a profile. A profile is a chart that depicts the child's pattern of performance on the test battery in the various areas (verbal, motor, numerical reasoning, etc.) that are thought to be components of some larger concept (such as intelligence). A profile of a child's performance has far more practical value than a single score such as an I.Q. score. By observing a child's profile, one can immediately determine in which areas a child is strong or weak. This kind of information allows the nurse or anyone else involved in child care planning to come to grips with the needs of the individual child in all his unique socioemotional complexity. A single score completely obscures a child's individuality. Although such individual tests as the Wechsler tests and the McCarthy Scales of Children's Abilities (M.S.C.A.) are not batteries (because the component subtests do not measure relatively independent abilities), the subtest scores may be plotted on a profile or otherwise expertly analyzed to obtain a more meaningful and detailed picture of a child's performance than the I.Q. score alone would yield.

MEASUREMENT

In measuring a child's behavior different kinds of information are obtained, depending on the type of measurement techniques employed. For the nurse making referrals some knowledge of these techniques and their limitations can facilitate her role both in providing and in requesting the type of information that would be most useful in developing a health care program for a child. This knowledge can provide a basic framework for selection of the appropriate techniques for the goals the nurse has in mind.

Measurement techniques vary mainly in terms of the objectivity and structure involved. Objectivity refers to a uniform method of administration and scoring, whereas structure refers to the power of items to call forth a specified response. In practice these two characteristics often overlap considerably, although they need not do so. Highly objective, well-structured tests are powerful in that variations in children's responses must be due largely to characteristics of the children and not to differences in the way the tests are administered. However, such tests may have serious drawbacks when one considers the wide range of motivation and prior test experience that a population of children has. This is especially true of children of preschool age, of different socioeconomic levels, and of different cultures—a topic that will be considered later in this chapter. In many cases more subjective and unstructured tests yield more accurate information when administered by experts. The following is a brief summary of some of the more common measurement techniques employed. A more extensive survey is given by Walker (1973).

Standardized testing

A test may be standardized in two ways. First, a test may be standardized in that the procedures, apparatus, and scoring have been fixed so that the same testing procedures can be followed by different examiners at different times and places. Second, a test may be standardized in the sense that it is provided with a table of norms specifying the range of scores earned by representative groups of subjects. The process of gathering normative data is called standardization. Reliability and validity data are provided in an accompanying manual.

Most standardized tests tend to be psychometric in nature; that is, they provide a numerical evaluation of performance by emphasizing the measurement of individual traits or abilities rather than emphasizing a global assessment of the child. Included in the category of standardized tests are the major intelligence and educational achievement tests.

Projective methods

Projective tests require that the individual being tested respond to the test stimulus in his own idiosyncratic way, which reflects his personality and individuality—his socioemotional adjustment. Thus the name, *projective:* the subject *projects* upon the relatively unstructured material his own unique perceptions, interpretations, and way or organizing his world. There are no right and wrong answers as on an intelligence test or other psychometric instruments.

As was stated at the beginning of this chapter, it is essential for adequate care of the child or of any individual that the nurse understand as much as possible about the patient as a whole person in his unique difference from all other persons. Group tests give us averages or means and the range of variation among groups. Through statistical manipulation they point out how closely the individual under consideration conforms to the norm or how widely he differs from it. The profile of test results shows in which areas tested the individual excels, conforms, or is weak in relation to the average. Individual tests such as the Stanford-Binet Intelligence Scale or Weschler Intelligence Scale for Children–Revised (W.I.S.C.-R.) give a better picture of the child if specific responses are analyzed.

However, if one wishes to understand the individual personality of the child, more is required. Personality may be considered "as a dynamic process, the continual activity of the individual who is engaged in creating, maintaining, and defending that 'private world' wherein he lives" (Frank, 1948, p. 8). Projective testing provides one of the best methods available "from which a useful description of the uniqueness of the person can be gleaned" (Exner, 1974, p. xi).

Although the expert clinician finds the projective test a valuable aid in understanding the individual, there has been and still is a great deal of criticism of projective tests by psychologists and others. They do not lend themselves easily to statistical analysis or to routine studies of reliability and validity. It can be readily understood that group norms are difficult to apply to a descriptive account of the individual as he is now, and many research studies have been equivocal or negative. Also many results have been positive when the investigator was an expert in the use of the instrument in addition to having a knowledge of research design and statistics.

It should be remembered that projective tests should be used only for the purposes for which they are intended, not routinely, and only by professional persons, usually psychologists, who have had extensive training in their use. When properly used they can provide valuable information not otherwise readily obtainable. They can give the nurse an understanding of the individual child patient that can significantly increase her efficiency in working with him.

One more point must be borne in mind. The psychologist who deals with children should have had special training in child psychology. Knowledge of adults is not enough. Dr. Louise Bates Ames, Co-Director of the Gesell Institute in New Haven, Connecticut, is an outstanding expert in the use of projective tests (especially the Rorschach) with children and has written extensively on the subject (Ames et al., 1952).

There are many projective tests. Some of the more widely used will be briefly described later in the chapter. They are used primarily in personality assessment along with other diagnostic tools. Projective tests are impractical in the average classroom situation because of their cost, time to administer, and need for specialized personnel to administer and interpret them.

Unobtrusive measures

Unobtrusive measures include the use of physical traces (such as replacement and repair rates of toys and supplies and areas of the room most used) as well as archive records (such as school records of the number of days absent from school). The advantage of these measures is that they are usually generated without the knowledge that anyone will use them as a measurement index and therefore avoid such problems as awareness of measurement, interviewer effects, and the bias that comes from the measurement itself. There are relatively few unobtrusive measures at present because they have not been used consciously or systematically in the past to assess development of young children. However, one such measure is the Nursery School Adjustment Scale.

Observational procedures

Observational measures range from intensive coverage of long-term sequences such as a diary report or description to more narrowly circumscribed, shorter, and more highly controlled observations such as time sampling (a record of behaviors during several short observational periods). Observational techniques are widely used, especially with preschool chil-

dren. At present they are the best measures of socioemotional growth in young children because they minimize incorrect assumptions by allowing one to observe spontaneous behavior as it occurs in a natural setting. Some behavioral observations include those on play interactions, peer interactions, social participation, leadership, nurturance, dependency, aggression, and affection.

Frequently mentioned but not insurmountable problems with observational procedures are observer influence, reliability between raters, instrumental aids, definition of categories, cost, and time. Some examples of observational methods can be found in the Stevenson Behavioral Unit Observational Procedure and the Affectional and Aggressive Observation Checklist.

Situational measures

Situational measures cover a wide range of situations from highly structured to almost totally unstructured. These techniques place the child in a situation closely resembling or simulating a real-life situation and are designed to reveal to the observer something about the child's socioemotional adjustment. Some examples are the Character Education Inquiry (C.E.I.), designed to measure such behaviors as honesty, self-control, and altruism in a realistic but disguised situation, and the McCandless-Marshall, Minnesota, and Dunnington sociometric status tests, which enable the tester to locate isolates, cliques, and other aspects of group interrelationships by asking the child to select from a large board of pictures those peers he would most like to be with for a particular task.

Despite past extensive use of sociometric techniques as a research tool in analyzing group structure and social behavior, they are still in the process of development.

Rating scales

Broadly speaking, rating scales are a type of observational measure and are used to measure the impression a child makes on a particular judge, usually a parent or teacher. Rating scales focus on describing a child's behavior in terms of personality traits such as study habits, punctuality, task orientation, obedience, friendliness, conformity, hyperactivity, and with-drawal. Some examples are the Behavioral Classification Project—Children's Form, the Behavior Rating Scale, the Classroom Behavior Inventory, and the Emmerich Classroom Observation Rating Scale. More generally rating scales include ranking lists, checklists, descriptive rating scales, and numerical rating scales. Although rating scales are a quick and inexpensive way of evaluating behavior, especially socioemotional behavior, they involve subjective judgment, the categories are often ambiguous and biased, and the evaluations they provide are not as broadly based as those provided by other methods already described. Nevertheless, they are helpful when properly interpreted.

Self-report measures

Self-report measures are self-rating questionnaires that focus on an individual's personal feelings. Most of the self-report measures used with children are semi-projective in that the child is asked to respond to pictures or drawings. Self-report measures assess characteristics ranging from achievement motivation and self-concept to racial attitudes. Included among these techniques are the Color-Meaning Picture Series, the California Test of Personality, the Preschool Academic Sentiments Scale, and the Self-Concept and Motivation Inventory.

There are many problems in use of self-report techniques, especially with young children. The reliance of these measures on verbal and reading skills makes them particularly difficult to use with most young children.

Interviews

Interviews, both structured and unstructured, concentrate on data gathering from the child's history. The interview also provides the opportunity for the examiner to make behavioral observations of the child. The ultimate value of the interview procedure rests on the interviewer's knowledge of child development and ability to relate to children.

CHOICE OF TEST

The various techniques of measurement are simply tools used in assessing a child and describing his behavior in several domains. The kind of test used depends upon which domain one wishes to investigate. As mentioned earlier, one scheme of conceptualizing a child's behavior is in terms of four major categories: cognitive, socioemotional, psychomotor, and developmental.

Cognitive domain

By far the major emphasis of assessment in the cognitive domain has centered around two types of tests: achievement tests and intelligence tests. Achievement tests surpass all other types of standardized tests in sheer number. These tests are designed to measure a relatively standardized set of antecedent experiences such as a specific program of instruction or training. Achievement tests are used primarily in educational settings because of their heavy dependence on fairly specific and uniform prior learning; they represent a terminal evaluation of the child's status on the completion of such learning. Although administration and scoring of standardized achievement tests usually require only that the examiner be able to read, explain, and understand instructions and keep accurate time, the interpretation of such tests depends on knowledge of the training program and its goals as well as some understanding of the child's motivation and emotional readiness. Included among the commonly used achievement tests and batteries are the California Achievement Tests, the Iowa Tests of Basic Skills, the Fundamental Achievement Series, the S.R.A. Achievement Series, the Sequential Tests of Educational Progress (S.T.E.P.), and the Stanford Achievement Test, which includes a pre-primary level.

Although the pediatric nurse will not often be in need of the kind of information made available through educational achievement tests, it is important that she understand the nature of the achievement test because it is often contrasted with the aptitude test. This distinction is often a hazy one, and persons obtaining information through psychological tests should be cautious of applying this distinction too rigidly.

The term *aptitude test* is a misnomer; aptitude tests do not measure "innate capacity." Rather aptitude tests are intended to reflect the cumulative influence of a multitude of experiences in daily living and can give the expert valuable indications of capacity. Thus, whereas achievement tests measure the effects of learning under partially known and controlled conditions, aptitude tests measure the effects of learning under relatively unknown and uncontrolled conditions. Aptitude tests also differ from achievement tests in their general purpose. Achievement tests are used as a terminal evaluation of performance; aptitude tests are used to predict future performance in some area. This distinction is also vague since achievement tests are sometimes used as predictors of future learning. Probably one of the most useful concepts that can be employed is that of developed abilities. This concept describes all ability tests in terms of the level of development attained by the individual in a particular ability and avoids the achievement-aptitude problem.

Intelligence tests are in reality a form of aptitude test. They range from group paper-and-pencil tests of intelligence, which provide a quick estimate in as short a time as 5 minutes, to the highly complex and individually administered tests that last for 1 to 2 hours and require a skilled psychologist to give the test and interpret the results. Between these extremes there are many group and individual tests that measure intelligence, both verbal and nonverbal. Each of the tests is built on the concept that people are different and that these differences can be measured.

Intelligence tests for infants and preschool and early school–age children

Intelligence testing of very young children is not always carried out on a one-to-one basis. Persons who assess the intellectual abilities of young children in hospitals or day care centers can get important clues from the nurse in attendance. The nurse may report a series of highly pertinent and important observations about a child's activities that help the psychologist in assessing the intellectual behavior of that child. In making a referral the nurse should include such observations as sensory and motor behaviors, responsiveness and interactions with peers and with adults, language behavior, and comprehension of instructions as well as any special problems that the child may have.

The Bayley Infant Scale of Mental Develop-

ment and the Cattell Infant Intelligence Scale are individual tests often used with infants to appraise such abilities as exploratory alertness, goal-directed attention, sensory and motor responses, and social responses. Items demand deliberate and complex behavior so that for a child of 1 year these tests are truly mental tests. With a child younger than 1 year they reflect primarily attentiveness and responsiveness of the infant. Unfortunately scales for use with infants and young children tend to have a low level of reliability. That is, measurements made at very early ages do not predict with any great degree of success the intelligence scores that will be attained at later periods of time. In most instances they are able to screen out those children who are severely retarded as compared with others. They are much less successful in differentiating between the normal and the very bright. An important factor about these scales that limits their accuracy of prediction is that infant tests are made up of sensory-motor tasks. Also premature infants or those who have lacked normal stimulation from the environment are likely to test too low when chronological age since birth is the criterion.

At the preschool level the Stanford-Binet form L-M, the Wechsler Preschool and Primary Scale of Intelligence (W.P.P.S.I.), and the McCarthy Scales of Children's Abilities (M.S.C.A.) are among the most popular intelligence tests. These tests may also be used with early school–age children. (More details will be given about the Stanford-Binet test in the next section.)

The W.P.P.S.I. is a new scale for the preschool child of 4 years to the beginning school 6½-year level. Like the other Wechsler scales, it provides both verbal and performance intelligence scores (IQ's) based on a series of subtest scores. Both size and composition of the normative sample represent a considerable advance over earlier preschool tests. The M.S.C.A. is the most recent addition to this group of tests and is appropriate for children from the 2½- to 8½-year level. The M.S.C.A. provides a general cognitive index score based on verbal, perceptual-performance, and quantitative subtest scores. Subtest scores on memory and motor functions are also provided along with information on eye and hand dominance. Like many intelligence tests, these tests are heavily weighted with verbal items and are validated against measures of academic achievement; thus, while obscuring or minimizing other aspects of intellectual development, they are good predictors of school success.

Other scales used for testing the mental development of the very young are the Griffiths Mental Development Scale for Testing Babies from Birth to Two Years, the Merrill-Palmer Scale of Mental Tests, the Minnesota Preschool Tests, the Northwestern Intelligence Test, the Kuhlmann-Binet Scale for Infants, the Slosson Intelligence Test, and the Quick Test.

Intelligence tests for children and adolescents

For many years the two most popular individually administered tests for measuring intelligence in children and adolescents have been the Wechsler Intelligence Scale for Children (W.I.S.C.) and the Stanford-Binet Intelligence Scale. Both have undergone revisions in recent years to reflect more effectively regional and minority populations and to eliminate biases that were a part of early standardizations. The W.I.S.C.-R. and the Stanford-Binet form L-M represent the most recently revised forms of both scales.

The W.I.S.C., unlike the Stanford-Binet, consists of both verbal and performance scales that provide a series of subscores of different aspects of intelligence. I.Q.'s are derived from subscores for verbal and performance levels, and these are combined to obtain a total, or full-scale, score. The Stanford-Binet provides only a single I.Q. score, although the subtests include both verbal and performance items, and responses should be analyzed individually and by topic. These tests measure in varying degrees such abilities as verbal ability, memory, conceptual thinking, reasoning and comprehension, numerical reasoning, visual-motor coordination, and social intelligence.

Tests used in assessing other cognitive functions

Other individual tests are available that were developed for specific problems in intellectual assessment and for assessment of other cognitive functions. Several tests have been developed to assess intellectual competency in children whose special problems make the use of most standardized intelligence tests infeasible. The Hayes variation of the Binet is used for testing children with visual problems. The Arthur Point Scale of Performance Tests, Revised Form II, has been used extensively with children with hearing losses, those with reading disabilities, those with delayed or deviant speech, and non-English-speaking children. It is used with children and adolescents between 5 and 15 years of age. Tests such as the Hiskey-Nebraska Test of Learning Aptitude, the Porteus Mazes, and the Leiter International Performance Scale have had extensive use with children who have physical or motor problems.

The Peabody Picture Vocabulary Test (P.P.V.T.), the Illinois Test of Psycholinguistic Abilities (I.T.P.A.), Developmental Sentence Scoring (D.S.S.), and the Environmental Language Inventory (E.L.I.) are used to assess language development. The E.L.I. is the most recent and most promising addition to this group.

Piagetian tasks of conservation and imagery are used to determine more fundamental cognitive abilities than are tapped by the typical intelligence tests. Conservation is the concept that relevant dimensions of amount or quantity remain the same, or are "conserved," despite changes in the size or shape of an object; imagery refers to such tasks as visualizing through imagination the changes in shape of a liquid that are caused by, for example, tilting its container. These tasks were developed by the outstanding Swiss cognitive and developmental psychologist Jean Piaget. Piagetian tasks represent *cognitive universals* to a large extent. Cognitive universals are basic cognitive processes found in all children everywhere. Cross-cultural studies support the idea that the basics of cognitive functioning as described by Piaget are similar in a variety of cultures throughout the world (Ginsburg, 1972). Piaget's work deals with the basic categories of mind: concepts of space, time, and causality. Because these tasks do not emphasize verbal skills and academic achievement, they are not as useful as predictors of school success as are the typical intelligence tests but may have more to do with basic capacities.

Socioemotional domain

The term *socioemotional* is a newly coined comprehensive term including all areas from subjective states of feeling (emotional) to behaviors that are evoked and modified by the presence of another person (social). Encompassed by this category are tests of general personality and emotional adjustment, self-concept, behavioral traits, social skills, attitudes, interests, and preferences.

A socioemotional test may lead to insights into what types of reward a young person responds to, what forms of control work most effectively for him, and what his major sources of fear are. These little bits of information can be carefully assembled and make for much more successful ward management and a much happier hospital stay for even the very young child. It is true that quite often this information is gained through a trial-and-error method. Consider, however, the advantages gained and the time saved when this information can be systematically provided and not patiently "dug out" by the busy pediatric nurse.

Socioemotional adjustment is the result of interaction between the inherent characteristics of the individual and the influences of the environment and has traditionally been referred to as personality. Its characteristics are not static. They undergo constant change throughout an individual's life. They are developed and elaborated upon by maturation, learning, limitations inherent in the organism, and experiences that may act to limit or change earlier behavior. Not only does the equipment that an individual has at his disposal differ from age to age but the responses required of him are very different at each stage of development. The school age child is required to make a wide variety of responses and to behave in highly specialized ways in a series of specific situations: in school, in church, in the presence of adults, with other children, and with regard to parents. By the time adolescence or early adulthood is reached, many additional and often contradictory de-

mands have been placed on a person. He is expected to have reached a balance between dependence and independence, conformity and individuality, aggressiveness and reserve. There is a normal range of behaviors expected of each person at each given stage.

The expected behavior has physiological, developmental, and socioemotional origins and forms the basis for much of the measurement of what we call personality. Personality tests are probably the most popular type of socioemotional test, and the number of available personality tests run into several hundred. Most of these are of the paper-and-pencil questionnaire variety, but there are also projective tests, the most widely used of which will be briefly discussed here.

The Bender-Gestalt test is a visual-motor test in which a child or adolescent is asked to copy several geometrical designs. By examining such things as distortions of shape, rotations and integrations of figures, and perserverations (compulsion to perform a motor act repeatedly and mechanically), the expert can obtain an indication of a child's emotional adjustment and disturbances, his developmental level, and the possibility of brain damage or retardation. The Goodenough Draw-A-Person Test (D.A.P.) is another projective test often used with children and adolescents. The child or adolescent is asked to draw a picture of a person, then draw a person of the opposite sex, and then to construct a story about the figures. The figures are rated by clinical psychologists on such factors as realism, detail, fluency, flexibility, and composition and can reveal a great deal about the child's self-concept.

Three other popular projective tests used with children and adolescents are the Thematic Apperception Test (T.A.T.), the Children's Apperception Test (C.A.T.), and the Rorschach Inkblot Test. The T.A.T. consists of a series of pictures about which the child is asked to invent a story, telling what is happening, what led up to the scene, and what the outcome will be. An experienced psychologist assesses the stories according to various categories, which include the main theme, main hero, needs of the hero, conception of the environment, significant conflicts, and anxieties. The C.A.T., devised by Leopold Bellak, is similar but consists of pictures considered more suitable for children. It can be obtained in two forms; in one form the characters are portrayed as animals. This appeals to younger children, but for older ones human characters bring forth more revealing stories.

The Rorschach test consists of a series of 10 cards with bilaterally symmetrical inkblots; some are black and white only, some have touches of bright red, and some have pastel shades. It is the most widely known and most frequently used of the projective tests, not only in the United States but throughout the world. Inkblots are ambiguous stimuli and can pick up differences among cultures as well as among individuals. The subject is asked to report what the figure represents to him or what he sees in it. No two protocols are alike. Responses are scored and analyzed according to approach to the task, location on the blot, determinants of the response, content, and originality. The data reflect "a complex specimen of behavior" (Exner, 1974, p. 20) that, when related to other data, "can be translated into a series of statements which describe the subject."

Again it must be stressed that projective tests are difficult to interpret and require not only intensive study of the particular instrument but a sound knowledge and understanding of personality development and of psychopathology. Otherwise faulty interpretation may do more harm than good. Nevertheless, when there is a serious personality problem, projective tests properly given and interpreted can enable the nurse or other professional therapist or counselor to gain an understanding of the patient or client that might otherwise take months to uncover. Proper writing of reports is all important; they should be in standard English and written in a style readily understandable by an intelligent reader.

Play techniques are often useful with very young children. Some of these are the Driscot Play Kit, the Free-Play Method, the Structured Doll-Play Test, and the Toy World Test.

Self-report techniques, rating scales, and observational techniques are common in socioemotional assessment. Among these are the California Personality Inventory (C.P.I.), the California Personality Questionnaire (C.P.Q.), the Behavioral Classification Project—Children's Form (B.C.P.), the Hyperactivity and Withdrawal Rating Scales, Heather's Emotional Dependence-Independence Measure, the Hartup-Keller Nurturance and Dependency Measures, the Anxiety Scale, and the Affectional and Aggressive Observation Checklist.

Psychomotor domain

Psychomotor is a term referring to the motor aspects of the psychological development and growth of a child whose coordination and fine muscular skills increase in complexity as he grows. Many tests have been devised to measure psychomotor functions, ranging from purely observational and descriptive assessments of motor sequence development in infancy to actual performance tests of speed, coordination, and dexterity. Most infant tests rely almost exclusively on the description of sensory and psychomotor behavior. This is true of infant tests whether they are labeled intelligence test, personality test, or developmental test. Consequently there is considerable overlap among these categories in discussions of infant tests.

As predictors of later intellectual competency infant tests of psychomotor ability are poor instruments because of their low reliability, as mentioned earlier. However, as tests of strictly psychomotor coordination and ability they are much more accurate, as is true of the rotary pursuit task and the two-hand coordination task. In most cases we are not interested in a child's motor coordination for its own sake. We attempt to use this function as an index of more complex mental processes. Accordingly, psychomotor tests will be discussed under categories for which their predictive value is intended.

Developmental domain

The term *developmental* implies the use of normative data. That is, we compare a particular child's development to the norms, or average development for his age. Therefore virtually all tests to assess cognitive, socioemotional, or psychomotor development are developmental tests in a very real sense. It is not known to what extent developmental signs are related to cognition, but it is well established that children who are delayed physiologically and neurologically in their development are typically delayed cognitively, socioemotionally, and motorically.

Most of the scales labeled developmental are concerned with assessing gross motor development, fine motor coordination, adaptive behaviors, cognitive and language development, development of personal and social skills, and emergence of individual developmental skills. As mentioned earlier, there is a heavy reliance on sensory and psychomotor items to assess these behaviors, resulting in a great deal of overlap among the test of various functions of infant development. Included among the developmental scales are the Gesell Developmental Schedule (recently revised), the Cattell Infant Intelligence Scale, the Bayley Infant Scales of Development, the Lincoln-Oseretsky Motor Development Scale, the Griffiths Mental Development Scale, the Vineland Social Maturity Scale, and the Pediatric Neuropsychological Battery used to detect and assess developmental dyslexia (Flick, 1972).

Up to the present time developmental research has produced relatively gross measures in prediction of cognitive functioning and neurological development. Nonetheless, research is constantly being done in this area. Some of the more recent developmental screening tools show great promise and are especially valuable to nurses and others in the health care fields since they are often the ones called upon to make such assessment. Among these are Brazelton's Neonatal Behavioral Assessment Scale, the Carey Tool Assessment of Infant Temperament, the Denver Developmental Screening Test, the Developmental Profile, and the Graham/Rosenblith Neonatal Test.

The Neonatal Behavioral Assessment Scale is an observational technique designed to assess early signs of maturation, integration, and organization of the central nervous system in the newborn. The specific behaviors that are rated include visual tracking, sensory adaptation, attention span, auditory and visual discrimination and habituation, muscle and motor development, visual-motor coordination, social respon-

siveness including affectional responsivity, and individual temperamental characteristics such as activity level. The Neonatal Behavioral Assessment Scale is not used for predictive purposes but rather for current assessment of a child's developmental status. The nurse or other health care person should get training and experience before administering and interpreting this scale.

The Carey Tool Assessment of Infant Temperament, used to assess development between the ages of 4 and 8 months, is a questionnaire designed to obtain information about a mother's perceptions of her infant. The mother rates her infant according to several categories including activity, rhythmicity, adaptability, approach, sensory threshold, intensity, mood, distractibility, and persistence.

The Denver Developmental Screening Test, based on the work of Gesell, is a standardized test with which a child's performance is assessed in terms of four categories: gross motor performance, fine motor performance, personal-social skills, and receptive and expressive language abilities. The test covers the age range of 2 weeks to 6 years with a preponderance of motor items at the early age levels. Optimal ages for its use have been suggested (Werner, 1972). Because of the standardized procedure involved, training and experience are needed by the examiner. In many cases the nurse may be called upon to fill this role.

The Developmental Profile is used to assess the following categories of abilities: physical abilities, self-help skills, social behaviors, academic skills, and receptive and expressive communication skills. The ratings may be obtained from anyone who is knowledgeable about the child, such as a parent, teacher, or sibling.

The Graham/Rosenblith Neonatal Test measures maturation, irritability, muscle tone, and vision to help identify high-risk newborns.

Rather than being used only for predictive purposes, the information obtained from all of these instruments has implications and usefulness for counseling and training of those persons who interact with the child. The examiner can use the information to develop concrete programs of health care, environmental stimulation, and behavioral management. Once the nurse has obtained information about the developmental status of the child, she may wish to consult a psychologist, speech therapist, or teacher about the kinds of techniques or activities that could facilitate carrying out such programs in the hospital or that could be recommended to the parents for use in the home.

INTERPRETATION OF TESTS

Most of the improvement needed in psychological assessment is not so much in the construction of new and better tests as in the interpretation of test scores and the orientation of test users. As mentioned earlier, a test is only as effective as its user. For this reason emphasis is placed on the proper training and experience with a particular assessment tool and with the population one is going to be assessing. This is true whether the examiner be a clinical, educational, or developmental psychologist or registered pediatric nurse. The extent of training and experience differs among individuals doing psychological assessment. The examiner should seek guidance and information from authorities before attempting to use any assessment tool with which he is not thoroughly familiar.

A second problem of test interpretation is the testing situation. The question always arises as to whether or not the behavior observed in the testing situations is representative of behavior observed outside the testing situation. In many ways the testing situation is an artificial setting for the child. This presents problems of test anxiety and test-taking motivation. These problems may be a characteristic of the child and will be discussed as such later, but there are also problems built into the test itself.

The third problem of interpretation of tests is the appropriateness of the test for a particular population. Very few instruments have adequate standardization norms that are representative for a wide range of children of varying ethnic groups, competency levels, and socioeconomic backgrounds. The problem of testing minority children with tests standardized for white, middle class, Anglo-Saxon children has gained recognition in recent years. However, the problem of testing across cultures has been recognized since the beginning of the twentieth century, when attempts were made to develop "culture-free" and "culture-fair" tests. These tests are designed to rule out one or more parameters along which cultures vary. One such parameter is language. This alone has caused major problems with the testing of black, Indian, and Spanish-speaking children in American culture. It is only recently that acknowledgment has been given to the fact that many black Americans and white Americans have different dialects. Many blacks speak black nonstandard English, whereas many whites speak standard English (Dale, 1972). Each of these dialects is grammatically and culturally rich and complete in expressing the ideas of the culture it represents. The problem is that they are different and that most tests are standardized on the basis of speakers of standard English. It is easy to see how misunderstandings and lack of communication and comprehension can occur on the part of both the examiner and the child being tested.

This provides a built-in mechanism for children from minority groups to score low on most tests, and indeed they do. Although they have I.Q.'s essentially equal to those of white children in infancy, black children and other minorities do increasingly poorly on intelligence tests as they grow older. That is, their average I.Q. scores decrease as they mature. The attempts to develop culture-free and culture-fair tests have not been successful because of the failure to recognize that performance on an intelligence test is in part the summation of the learning experiences of an individual within a particular culture and in part the result of motivation to excel in those tasks that are viewed as valuable to a particular culture. The learning experiences and the cultural or social class values of white, black, Spanish-speaking, and Indian children differ; it is only reasonable to expect these differences to appear on tests that are designed to reflect these differences. The fallacy exists in interpreting these performance differences on intelligence tests as indicators of differences in intellectual competency and adequacy. If one recognizes the problem, however, valuable information about the child's adjustment can be gained from his responses and general behavior.

Nonverbal tests are also not culture free. Actually nonverbal tests appear to be more culturally "loaded" than verbal tests. In addition there remains the questionable assumption, on which culture-free and culture-fair tests are based, that verbal and nonverbal tests are measuring the same functions. For these and other reasons culture-free and culture-fair tests have not been very successful assessment tools (Anastasi, 1972; Sattler, 1974). One solution to this problem is the establishment of separate norms for various sociocultural groups. Until such norms are gathered the examiner should be cautious in the interpretation of test results and select assessment instruments that will give the most accurate information about the individual child being assessed. This may sometimes mean the substitution for or addition to standardized tests more open-ended observational techniques such as observing a child's play or interaction with others on the ward or in the school.

Early researchers hoped to find physiological factors that were related to high or low intelligence. They studied such characteristics as strength, reaction time, sensory discrimination, head size, cranial capacity, and other physical characteristics of individuals—factors that may have a slight relationship to intelligence but do not allow for test items of any appreciable validity in the measurement of intelligence. Whereas we are able to say that most bright children are healthier, better looking, and larger than children who have low intellectual competency, we cannot say simply because a particular child is larger than others of his age that he definitely will be brighter.

The disappointing results of using physiological factors led to work with memory, problem solving, and judgment. These elements were found to be much more closely related to what we have defined as intelligence by using school success as the measuring stick. Therefore among the many definitions of intelligence that have been proposed the most commonly recurring are those that characterize intelligence as the ability to deal with abstract symbols and relationships and the capacity to adapt to new situations or profit by experience. Nevertheless, difficulty persists in defining intelligence precisely.

Many of the same problems in attempting to define intelligence exist in trying to define socioemotional adjustment or personality. It is a nebulous quality that on the one hand is of an enduring and persistent nature—coloring every aspect of a person's behavior—and on the other hand is of a dynamic and changing nature—developing through interactions of a person's biological makeup and his environment.

THE WELL CHILD

The most important goal of assessment in all its aspects is to provide a description of the individual child as he is at the time of testing with his assets and liabilities and his unique personality makeup. Most of the children seen for psychological assessment are ones who would be termed well or normal. Psychologists are interested in how the normal mind works and in why children and adolescents behave, think, and function as they do. It is only through a comprehensive knowledge of how the normal child functions that one can deal effectively with problems and limitations. Assessment of the well child extends far beyond personality evaluation and intellectual assessment. Of concern also are the child's social values and his aptitudes, perceptions, achievements, and interests. Instruments have been devised to assess individual characteristics in each of these areas. Measurement itself is not the end product of the psychological evaluation of the well child. When the instruments used to assess personality, interests, aptitudes, and intelligence are then used to predict future behavior, they become of vital importance in the total developmental process. They permit families, schools, and others to engage in long-range planning for the child.

Consider the case of the child of interested parents who hope that he can go on to college but are concerned because his marks in grade school are just average. Through a series of tests it is possible to determine whether the child is slightly underachieving, is working up to capacity, or is more interested in subject matter not included in his current curriculum. Should the parents learn that their child is working up to capacity and is of just average abilities, their planning may expand to include some alternatives to a 4-year college program, such as a 2-year technical program in a junior college or some form of apprenticeship training after completion of high school. These worthwhile and meaningful activities may provide a positive outlook toward education for the child rather than force him into a straight academic college program where his modest abilities may cause him to fail. Thus better planning becomes one of the major assets gained in evaluating the well child.

Prediction is one major goal of assessment and helps in preventing long-term difficulties of adjustment. Through intellectual and socioemotional assessment, relevant variables affecting a child's development can be discovered. Factors that impede a child's progress can be minimized and those that facilitate his progress can be cultivated to aid in developing a mature individual. Society will ultimately reap the benefits of assessment since it aids in producing individuals who are developing their capacities as fully as possible.

In our discussion we should not neglect the "supernormal" child. A fortuitous set of circumstances provides such a child with an intellectual endowment that is far above that of the average child. In nearly every instance the gifted child's talents extend far beyond one single, narrow area. These children tend to show above-average abilities across a wide range of subjects and interests. Quite frequently they will do well in such widely separated fields as mathematics, art, music, social leadership, sports, science, and literature. Often it is possible for a gifted child to choose any one of many areas and be successful in it.

Gifted behavior is not limited to the highly intelligent person. It is possible for a normal child whose intellectual abilities are average or just a little better to be gifted in a special area. Frequently children and adolescents whose abilities in a wide variety of subjects are within the average range may possess unusual musical ability, artistic talent, or skill in one of the crafts. The development of gifted behavior or talent is a combination of motivation, training, and some predisposing ability such as excellent motor coordination, high intelligence, or sensitivity to tones, colors, etc.

Identifying the normal child

Normality includes a wide range of behaviors, both desirable and undesirable. However, the undesirable behaviors are not so marked that they interfere with a child's adequate daily functioning. Most often the well or normal child is assessed informally and without the use of special testing instruments, at least during his formative years. In some school systems his "normality" is determined by readiness tests or preschool evaluations that indicate to educators that he indeed is ready for the school experience on both an emotional and an intellectual basis. In many instances it is his normal performance in the classroom, his bringing home acceptable grades each term, and his regular progression through school that indicate to parents and educators that the child is functioning in a normal manner. Through her constant contact with him, the teacher is able to note areas of proficiency and areas of deficit and report these to the parents or attempt to deal with them directly through the educational process. That this pattern of evaluation and training has been successful is demonstrated by the fact that each year increasing numbers of persons are graduated from high schools and that these persons go on to achieve adequate records in colleges and universities throughout the country.

This may lead to the conclusion that tests for the well or normal child are not really necessary. Tests are of great value in uncovering exceptional talents or discovering "hidden" weaknesses of very bright and capable children who perform on just an average level. After learning the range of their ability the psychologist can often determine through extensive evaluation why they are underachieving and take proper steps to bring them up to a more acceptable level. There are many factors that can cause a child to perform less well than might be desirable. Cultural backgrounds, emotional problems within the family, and slight physiological handicaps may lessen effective performance. In the next section we will look more closely at some of the special problems of evaluation that psychologists face. Most often the subjects are quickly and easily identified because the handicap is severe. In only a few instances are these cases hidden from view by the child's use of compensating behaviors to hide his defect and thus appear normal.

More than 50% of the children the nurse will encounter in schools, in hospitals, or simply walking on the street fall into the category we have just described. Although test scores differ according to the instrument used, normal intelligence generally ranges upward from an I.Q. of 90 to 119. Those whose I.Q.'s are above 120 are considered of superior abilities; those whose scores range in the 130's and above may be classified as exceptional or gifted. In spite of high intellectual ability, in their social behavior they may bear a strong resemblance to other "normal" individuals. By their very normality such children pose no special problems for the psychologist who would evaluate them. To be sure, many children and adolescents in this normal group will have anxiety about being evaluated. They may be concerned about the outcomes, they may be eager to please parents, or they may be slightly less mature under stress than others within the group. However, none of their behaviors is so deviant as to pose special testing problems.

Since the normal group forms the baseline for understanding any group at any age, its members have been studied intensively from earliest infancy until later life. There are, of course, special evaluation problems for this group that are peculiar to evaluating persons at given stages of development. We know, for example, that it is quite difficult to assess intellect and personality to infancy. As a result infants who by definition are normal are difficult to test and evaluate because of distractibility and a lack of verbal communication. This situation is expected, and psychologists make a wide range of allowances for the normal problems encountered and the difficulties of evaluation of the very young. Similarly at other stages of development they anticipate other types of problems. In evaluating the normal 3- or 4-year-old the psychologist can expect a great deal of motor activity and a short attention span on many of the tasks he or she would attempt to have the normal child perform. As a result, tests are organized for a short testing period, with tasks requiring no more than a few moments' atten-

tion to complete. In this way the examiner overcomes many of the potential hazards and handicaps in evaluating children in this group. As the child grows older and becomes more verbal in his behavior, tests take on increasing complexity and are specifically concerned with tasks of a verbal nature.

It is the normal child's way of approaching tests, both of intelligence and of personality, that sets the pace or provides a baseline of knowledge for evaluation of the child with special problems.

Problems in assessing the well child

One of the greatest problems encountered by psychologists in evaluating children, whether they do this in the hospital, in the school, or in their office, is the lack of structure or the type of structure that parents give the children prior to testing. In some cases seeing the psychologist is simply identified as "a trip to the doctor." This frequently sets up in the mind of the child, even the most normal and healthy child, the image of someone who will give him a shot or perform some unpleasant medical procedure. The fact that the parents say that the psychologist will see him merely to do some tests is little appeasement for the child. This term frequently makes a child think of blood tests or other medical tests increasingly used today.

In other instances the parents will explain that "you will play games," or "it is something like going to school." The instructions provided by most parents are not adequate to describe the situation to the child.

The biggest limitation is that the child is not informed as to exactly where he is going and for what reason. This tends to place the psychologist doing the assessment at a distinct disadvantage. Fortunately psychological evaluations are sufficiently interesting and nonproductive of anxiety for most children that subsequent visits may be handled quite readily and easily. First visits, however, require a great deal of time for acquainting the child with the why of the evaluation and how it will be accomplished. This is less true for the child who operates on a preverbal level. Most tests used with him are of a motor type and take the form of observing developmental characteristics and social behaviors. When children are functioning on a verbal level, there will be much curiosity and interaction regarding the nature of the evaluation itself.

A great deal of the anxiety seen in normal children who are being evaluated is a direct result of their recognition of parental concern and anxiety. One sure way to produce resistance, concern, uncooperativeness, and anxiety in the child is for the parent to show apprehension and concern about the situation. Parents frequently will place fear and concern about a situation in the mind of the child simply by statements like "This is not going to hurt you at all," or "Don't be worried that we'll go away and leave you; we'll be in the next room." In both examples parental concern and anxiety about the experience and about separation may make testing nearly impossible even in the healthy, well-adjusted child. The normal child who hears the expression that something is not going to hurt him has through past experience learned to expect something disagreeable and unpleasant although not basically harmful to his existence. With his guard up the child evaluated under these circumstances may perform at less than an optimum level.

There is no simple way to overcome this. It is not possible to provide a complete system of parental education before the child is brought in for a psychological evaluation. It is possible when setting up appointments to structure circumstances sufficiently that overconcern should not be present. A simple structuring of the amount of time involved, the persons who will be seen, and the physical setting may relieve much parental apprehension. Quite frequently parents are brought into contact with the psychologist in a session before the child is seen. In this way the parents can size up the situation, look over the persons involved, and develop some personal reassurance about the total process. They can thus create less anxiety for the child in his subsequent visit.

As we have indicated, these are normal problems in dealing with normal children. When evaluation procedures are complicated by additional stress and strain or handicaps in either parent or child, the situation becomes even more complex and delicate. We will look at the child with special problems in the remainder of this chapter.

THE CHILD WITH SPECIAL PROBLEMS

We have discussed some of the problems that face the psychologist attempting to assess the well child in a well child conference, in the office, in the school, or even in the home. It is vitally important for the examiner to know how the normal child functions so that he can then look at the child with problems in a clear and realistic manner. Judgments of a child's behavior are formed against a baseline of normality as determined by the behavior and actions of normal children. Actually the behavior of the normal falls along a continuum that, as noted earlier, includes a wide range. Realistic appraisals can be made by determining where a particular child falls on this continuum of competency and socioemotional adjustment in relation to his peers. A child with special problems is distinguished from the normal child only by the degree to which the problems interfere with normal daily functioning. Even though the child with special problems may fall below the normal child in current levels of functioning, this does not mean that he cannot receive training and education that will allow him to compete effectively with normal children. The efforts of many professionals in child care and health today, particularly in research, are directed toward seeking ways to increase efficiency in learning and training for both normal children and children with special problems. This, of course, represents a second stage beyond the assessment of behavior, intellectual competency, and socioemotional adjustment. Children with problems in one or more of the sensory modalities may be trained to develop effectively their particular skills and talents. The discovery of new training techniques has done much to reduce differences between the normal child and the child with special problems. So revolutionary have been some of these approaches that they have even modified the training and teaching of normal children as well.

Since we have already detailed many problems of assessment under varying conditions, we will not repeat these in the following section except where they are applicable to special problems. In turning our attention to the assessment of the child with special problems, we will consider the following major types of problems: (1) behavioral problems, (2) learning problems, (3) sensory problems (auditory and visual), (4) motor problems, (5) chronic medical problems, and (6) emotional problems. Such problems increase the difficulty of assessing a child satisfactorily and increase the importance of providing experts to do the examination. There is a general tendency among the public to emphasize the limitations of children with special problems; conversely parents of these children may overestimate their hard-won gains and accomplishments.

Reality lies somewhere between in most instances. The evaluation team must sort out reality from wishful thinking and behavioral stereotypes. This team must somehow sift through both public opinion and parental exaggeration and define and describe the true potential of the child. They must do this in terms of widespread knowledge about the meaning of their instruments as applied to these children. The usual measures such as educational achievement, I.Q., and motor dexterity must be considered in terms of whether they represent maximal levels of attainment or whether the very nature of the instruments used in assessment may work against reaching an accurate measure of functioning or potential. Many of the tests, as we have already learned, are heavily weighted in cultural factors. Frequently the child with special problems, even though he has good potential, may suffer on such tests because he lacks the meaningful interaction with his environment that is available to the well or normal child. Whereas the limitations for each type of problem may be different, they all operate to decrease social interaction. Let us now consider the special problems of these children.

The child with behavioral problems

Behavior problems are characterized as behavior that, although it has no obvious organic, sensory, or emotional basis, serves to interfere with the child's daily performance. By and large this behavior is learned. Although on a superficial level such behavior may appear maladaptive, on further investigation it is usually found to be based on an adaptive attempt by the child to cope with a difficulty in the environment. This can be found in children labeled hyperactive, aggressive, or acting-out in the classroom. Many of these children come from minority cultures in which higher activity levels and more aggressive behaviors are cultural norms and quite adaptive to survival in such settings. In addition, many children with behavior problems may come from abnormal home environments in which one or both parents are missing, mentally ill, or suffering from a personality disorder. The child is faced with chronic abnormal conditions, and his "problem" behavior may be useful in helping him cope with such conditions. This behavior becomes a problem only when it is carried over into other settings in which the behavior is no longer functional. What such children need is not to relinquish such behavior but rather to learn to discriminate environments to employ the appropriate behavior for a particular setting. This may be done through behavior modification techniques that involve providing clear and discrete guidelines for the child and rewarding (with rewards that are particularly meaningful to him) conformity with such guidelines. Some alterations in the environment may also be called for and should be made wherever possible.

Of a less chronic nature may be the behavior of a child who develops problems in response to an acute crisis such as the birth of a sibling, the loss of a loved one, or a change in schools and peers. In such cases attempts should be made to help the child adjust to his new circumstances. Often this can be done by giving him special responsibilities on the ward or in the classroom, such as cleaning the blackboard or running an errand. These activities, while serving to distract him, also give him a place of prestige in his new situation. What is needed is an assessment of environments to help children with behavior problems develop more appropriate methods of interacting with their environments.

Assessment of the environment applies also to the testing situation. The examiner has a responsibility to determine what aspects of the environment motivate a particular child and should use this information in making the necessary modifications to assess the child accurately. This examiner accountability both to normal children and children with special problems has been lacking in many cases.

The child with learning problems

The term *learning problems* encompasses a vast range of problems from mental retardation to learning disabilities. The American Association on Mental Deficiency offers a fourfold classification system of mental retardation. Children with the first three types of retardation are most often found in institutional settings; the classes are moderate retardation, severe retardation, and profound retardation. Mild retardation, the fourth category, is most often satisfactorily dealt with in the community and through the use of special education classes. Children in this group have I.Q.'s generally from the low 50's to approximately 70. These four groups comprise roughly 2% of the population. For purposes of adequate understanding we must also include an additional category, which has been called borderline retardation and which extends roughly to an I.Q. level of 85. This brings in a considerably larger number of persons, somewhere between 14% and 16% of the population depending upon which assessment scale is used. Some educators have believed that cutting off at this point fails to describe adequately the child in this group. It is their opinion that many children whose I.Q.'s are below 90, again adding another part of our population (about another 10%), suffer in all activities requiring intellectual skills. Rarely do these children finish high school or develop the economic security and stability available to brighter persons in the population.

In viewing the characteristics of retardation, we are impressed with two factors. One is the number of medical characteristics—genetic syndromes and physical abnormalities or changes—that produce mental retardation. There are also behavior patterns that separate one form of retardation from another. These categories are not mutually exclusive, and combinations may exist in many children. It is not possible to provide an adequate diagnosis of mental retardation without a thorough knowledge of both aspects, medical and behavioral.

Assessment and diagnosis are especially important if we view mental retardation as symptomatic behavior rather than a final statement about an individual. It is quite conceivable that in certain types of retardation (as measured by psychological tests), enriching the environment, altering the care, or applying certain medical techniques may result in changes in the measured I.Q. of the individual. Such changes are not uncommon. The result is not that the severely retarded individual becomes normal but that such changes may allow for programs through which retarded individuals can develop compensatory areas of skill and reduce the differences between their behavior and that of others in the world around them.

Other children may have learning problems of a more specific neurological nature. The term *dyslexia* is used loosely to account for many problems of this nature. Two types of dyslexia may be distinguished. The first is acquired dyslexia and is usually found in older children and adults. Acquired dyslexia is caused by a lesion of the left side of the brain, an area that is important in verbal comprehension and functioning. A fairly well–delineated category of similar symptoms is included in what is known as Gerstmann's syndrome. This syndrome includes left-right confusion or disorientation, finger agnosia (inability to visually differentiate one's fingers in space), agraphia (inability to write, spell, or express thoughts in writing), acalculia (inability to do simple arithmetical calculations), and other visual perception problems. This is not to be confused with aphasia, which is a much broader term for a disturbance in symbolic formulation and comprehension of language. Dyslexic symptoms may also be present in the individual having this broader language disorder.

A second type of dyslexia is specific developmental dyslexia, defined by the World Federation of Neurology as a condition found in children who fail to develop normal reading ability despite normal educational instruction, normal socioeconomic opportunities, average or above average intellectual competency, and freedom from gross sensory, emotional, or neurological handicaps. This definition does not exclude the possibility of neurological causes but merely states that no specific evidence of such a cause has been demonstrated.

Early identification of children with dyslexia is essential in adapting the education process to their needs, thus facilitating prevention. Unfortunately children with this disability have often been labeled as retarded because of poor academic performance, or they have developed "behavior problems" or "short attention spans" caused by the frustrations they encounter in trying to make sense of a distorted page of print or a "simple" arithmetic problem.

The group most likely to benefit from good assessment and diagnosis includes culturally deprived individuals who, because of lack of experience and contact with the world around them, fall short of other persons in measured ability. (This definition excludes the child from a different culture or from a minority culture since there is no substantial evidence to support the idea that these cultures are deprived simply because they are different. However, when a child attends school in a culture different from that of his home, he may appear deprived to his teachers.) A deprived child's scores may indicate that he is functioning in the retarded range of abilities. Yet more complete knowledge—that he has lacked so many of the enriching experiences of life—may suggest that his abilities might be improved by programs of training and enrichment. Had the evaluators simply looked at scores without looking into causal factors, this type of child might have been written off as hopeless. These problems emphasize how important it is to have an examiner who is expert in interpreting test results, who can differentiate between obtained scores and probable potential, who does not overemphasize the I.Q., and who can estimate what might be expected of a particular child if he is given proper guidance, encouragement, and instruction. Significant changes in I.Q. scores are not uncommon under these circumstances.

Environmental factors

It is not always possible in the hospital situation to fully recognize the impact of the child's home environment on his behavior and ability. In the case of a deprived child this information may frequently be obtained through the referral source, who quite often is the public health nurse. She can provide the evaluation team with many important insights into the background of a child with learning problems. As the child matures, other sources of information become available: the schools, social agencies, community organizations, etc. These influences will not only affect how a child learns but will also have a major part in the shaping of his personality. Anyone growing up in a neighborhood that provided no higher level role models than delinquency, crime, and prostitution might have goals in life that would fall far short of those expected of "normal" persons within our society. Handicaps are placed upon the child both intellectually and in the personality realm when he has exposure to little else than this type of environment during his formative years. In evaluating all children it is necessary to go beyond the reported test scores.

This stresses the vital importance of having a thorough history of all persons to be evaluated. You have already been drilled in the importance of the history in arriving at a proper medical diagnosis and case appraisal. The history is no less vital in looking at the intellectual and personality development of each person. Without that information we can talk only about the person as he is now. We have no idea as to causal factors or the modifiability of these factors unless we have a complete picture. Rarely is it possible for a single individual to obtain all of this information. Understanding of all cases, particularly of a child with learning problems, requires coordinated efforts of the whole team.

Motor abilities

The evaluation of motor ability in a child with learning problems is important. We have many sayings in our culture that suggest that the individual who does not do well in academic subjects works well with his hands. How true is this? Is it possible for a child to show normal motor abilities yet be retarded in his verbal abilities? There certainly is evidence to support the fact that, barring physical abnormalities or genetic disorders, many children with learning problems develop physically at the same rate as normal persons. However, physical growth is not an assurance that motor abilities will be adequate. Most investigators have found that, whereas differences are not grossly obvious, some children of lesser intellectual abilities tend to be smaller and shorter, weigh less, and do less well on tests of manual and motor dexterity than do children considered to be of above-average intelligence. This is not a striking difference, but it is a low, consistent variation that coincides with the concept that very bright children tend to be healthier, better looking, stronger, and taller than individuals of lesser intellectual abilities. These distinctions become quite sharp when we consider children in the lower ranges of mental retardation. Quite frequently their lack of growth and development is genetically determined or limited by malfunction of glandular systems.

One reason for the belief that children who do not score well on tests of language skills may do well on nonlanguage tests is that children with learning difficulties may come from homes in which English is not the basic language or in which standard English is not spoken. Such children are not retarded and can do as well on nonverbal tasks as other children, but the lack of skills in standard English hinders them in school and often leads to faulty evaluation and diagnosis or even to delinquency. Bilingual instruction in the primary grades, now being widely advocated, should help to minimize this misinterpretation.

Socioemotional assessment

We have already indicated many of the handicaps in assessing socioemotional adjustment in the very young. Socioemotional adjustment is an emerging characteristic. Instruments designed to tap this in normal chidlren are only moderately successful. When we add the problems of dealing with an individual who has learning problems, difficulties in socioemotional assessment increase even further. In the case of the most severely retarded individuals much of the behavior is nonverbal, and only the most primitive form of behavior patterns will appear. Frequently they are unable to engage in even the basic components of self-care; they may not be able to feed themselves, dress themselves, etc.

With mildly retarded and borderline individuals measurement of personality becomes less a problem than with other groups. Early measurement is difficult because they are frequently much slower in reaching a verbal level of interaction than normal children. However, when they do reach a verbal level, they generally can be assessed by use of the same instruments that are applied to normal children. The stereotype that these individuals are insensitive and unaware is frequently in gross error. Many children on the borderline and mildly retarded levels are quite aware of their differences from brighter children and those who are more able to compete physically, and they may be quite sensitive about it. Socioemotional assessment of children in this group has been revealing and informative.

It has been generally found that, if it is possible to keep the child in the home and to supply proper training there, the results tend to be more satisfactory. The effects of long-term hospitalization or institutionalization can exact a high price from the child in terms of his social adjustment, self-concept, and ability to make his way in the world independently of others.

A lack of sensitivity does exist in some children, but this seems to operate on a level of abstract thinking. Many of our higher and more sophisticated social interactions are of an abstract nature, and the retarded child may be insensitive to them. However, in most social interactions that are quite concrete he possesses full awareness and understanding. Thus socioemotional assessment, even for the retarded child, can shed important light on his potential and be significant for his program planning, both in the hospital and in his home environment.

The child with less severe forms of learning problems than retardation, such as learning disabilities or dyslexia, may be detected and assessed with tests designed for such a purpose. Some of these instruments have been discussed.

The child with sensory problems
The child with auditory problems

Impaired hearing is a highly complex problem. It is not simply a case of a person's being able or unable to hear. Only a small percentage of persons with hearing losses are totally deaf. Many others have some degree of residual hearing. These are individuals who have a congenital absence of structures or surgical or traumatic destruction. In most instances of impairment, there is residual hearing ability although, for purposes of everyday communication by verbal means, the individual may be described as functionally deaf. Some persons have impairments in certain frequency ranges, whereas others may have a general loss over a wide range. The involvement may be bilateral or present in only one ear. Hearing impairments may be conductive, sensorineural, or mixed in nature, depending upon the site of lesion in the auditory system. However, all persons with impaired hearing share a common problem: a reduced ability to respond to verbal communications and to benefit from auditory information in the environment. If the hearing impairment is adventitious, occurring later in life after critical language learning has taken place, a groundwork has been laid for verbal communication. But in the child with a congenital hearing impairment the ability to learn language by normal auditory means is obviously limited, depending on the child's remaining hearing capabilities.

Early detection of hearing impairment is critical. Fortunately, advances in clinical audiology permit accurate assessment of very young children. Subsequent early treatment, either by surgical or prosthetic means, and special educational programs may greatly enhance the opportunities for language learning in the hearing-impaired child. Because of the increased availability of speech pathology and audiology centers, it is now much less likely that a child would grow to school age and beyond with an undetected hearing problem.

Like any other problem, impaired hearing involves the operation of many social and cultural factors. These consist of family attitudes toward deafness, the individual's desire to overcome or deal effectively with this problem, and the presence of other limiting factors accompanying the hearing loss (brain damage, emotional disorders, etc.). In many instances highly motivated and bright children learn to rely on secondary cues in compensating for their loss. In

many instances formal training is provided by school systems or in residential centers for those with severely impaired hearing.

Let us now turn our attention to some of the techniques that have been used in assessing the ability or intellectual potential of the child with hearing problems.

Intellectual assessment. Evaluation of the child with a hearing loss presents many problems since only limited verbal communication may be available. However, in the presence of reasonably normal vision the problems are much less complicated. Most of the tests relied on are of the nonverbal or performance type and can be explained to the child through the use of pantomime or demonstration. For some tests this works quite well. However, it is difficult to convey effectively the concept that the subject should work as fast as he can. Where possible in testing deaf children power tests (tests without fixed time limits) are most desirable. Each of the major tests of intelligence has a series of items that can be used with the child who has a hearing loss. Adaptations have been made of the Stanford-Binet, Wechsler, Peabody Picture Vocabulary, and other tests to conform to the accessible areas of measurable ability in the child with a hearing loss. Total I.Q.'s derived on all subtests in this manner are virtually meaningless, of course, and should usually not be used. Examiners tend to rely most strongly on those scales that are of a nonverbal type and that can be pantomimed or given to the subject without verbal instructions. In this way they are able to form some concept about the potential level of functioning of a child and make recommendations for appropriate training.

The problems of testing the very young child with hearing problems are probably less complicated than those of evaluation at later stages. As you recall, testing the very young involves the use of developmental scales and tests of motor coordination. Since this area is less likely to be affected by deafness during early development and since the child is usually preverbal and would not understand verbal commands at this stage, there has been some success in early evaluation.

There is no question that a severe loss of function in this one vital sensory modality results in a lowered ability to cope with the environment. Children with a hearing loss learn less efficiently and less rapidly than those with normal hearing. This deterence could pose potential socioemotional problems if not detected early and prevented by adjustments in the child's environment.

Much of what we must rely on for judging adjustment in the young child is the observation of his behavior. When he is older, it will be possible to use some of the standardized paper-and-pencil tests to seek out his feelings, attitudes, and opinions.

The use of projective tests of personality is somewhat limited in that it is difficult to convey instructions to the child with severe hearing problems and difficult for him to convey his answers to the examiner. Again, as with the paper-and-pencil tests, the problem is lessened when the child is able to read or communicate through a nonvocal medium. Unfortunately by the time he reaches this stage diagnosis may well be of only minor importance. Early detection and diagnosis are as important in working with deaf children as for any other group.

Lacking successful communication with the child, professionals interested in the emotional interplay within the child may resort to observing him in a play situation or in his daily routine. Valuable information and impressions can also be gained through conferences with the parents, although this source of information must be carefully evaluated since parents can rarely be totally objective. It is probably better that they should not. The detached attitude of an objective observer rarely permits the imparting of the warmth and love so necessary in dealing with any child.

Personality evaluations made by using the methods available to the psychologist often produce an evaluative report suggesting poor adjustment. This is partly because adjustment is often rated in terms of the ability to engage in a wide range of activities and in a variety of situations and circumstances. By the very nature of his problem the child with hearing losses is unable to engage in many of these activities. Play activities are limited because of the importance of verbal commands and directions. Roaming freely about the community is limited because of the necessity to detect warning sounds: automobile horns, ringing bells, etc. The child with hearing problems can look forward to a life in which he may not be able to obtain a driver's license and cannot utilize self-propelled objects except in very limited circumstances—a life in which he will be dependent upon others for many of the important verbal cues necessary to adjust in a world of sound.

There are several patterns of development that may occur among children with severely impaired hearing. One such pattern is a way of life that is entirely outside the world of the hearing. A child may spend his early years in an institutional setting and his later years in a small colony centered around a sheltered workshop. In this way there would be a nearly complete break with the world of the hearing. Another pattern is denial of the hearing loss completely in a series of compensatory behaviors and acts in an attempt to convey the impression that his hearing is normal. Perhaps most satisfactory is the life of the individual who as a child is permitted to remain in the home and develop to his full capacity activities and interests that are a part of the larger community. Although he may be forced to avoid certain areas and types of activities, he can be educated, play, and finally work with others in situations in which effects of his hearing loss are minimized.

Assessment of the child with a hearing loss plays a vital role in determining what course of action may be taken for his education and for his future. Early detection and planning can help to shape realistic parental attitudes and guide parents through the difficult adjustment to having a child who is different from the others around him. Too often children have been subjected to an environment in which parents have attempted to deny or to hide their problem and thus have created even greater difficulties for the child. The nurse with a growing awareness of the many facilities available to help children with special problems can be a successful guide in helping parents seek out educational and training facilities. Hearing loss, although a serious medical problem, need not be a serious socioemotional problem. Both medical advances and new concepts in education and training have acted to decrease the differences between the normal child and the one with a hearing loss.

The child with severe visual problems

No single problem so much sets a child apart from others as does severely impaired vision. His problems may be classed under several major headings: the problems of physical mobility, the problems of learning and communication, and personal-social problems. In each of these categories there are features unique to the child with visual problems. Each of these features also produces problems for the individual who would evaluate the intelligence and personality of a child with severely impaired vision. Before investigating each of these aspects and their generalized effects, let us discuss the characteristics of the child with visual impairment.

Psychologists and educators usually classify as visually impaired a child whose visual fields are defective, color vision is impaired, or visual acuity is significantly decreased. Traditionally individuals with visual acuity of less than 20/200 are considered blind. Distortions or losses of function in parts of the visual field may also result in a severe handicap and an inability to function successfully in a sighted world. Color blindness, although not as restrictive as some forms of visual impairment, can result in a limiting of mobility and a failure to detect vital color signs in a variety of situations.

These visual impairments may come from a variety of sources. Chiefly they appear to be caused by some form of known prenatal influence. This accounts for more than half of the cases of visual impairment. Some other causes are quite well known, however. Infectious diseases, injuries, and poisoning such as use of excessive oxygen in care of premature infants account for roughly 30% to 35% of cases. Other sources such as tumors and residuals of other diseases account for much of the remaining percentage. Of course, there will be a big shift in accounting for future cases of blindness since the discovery in 1954 that retrolental fibroplasia has been caused by high oxygen concentrations. Since 1954 the incidence of this condition has been considerably decreased.

As with any form of loss, the range in impairment of vision is quite large. The handicap may range from total blindness from time of birth in extreme cases to varying degrees of partial sight. There are even some reported examples of children who were born with cataracts and in adolescence gained sight. These individuals, too, have partially impaired vision, not because the vision was restored partially but because of a lack of early learning experience, which seems to produce a profound effect on the ability to learn or to perform some visual activities.

We are fortunate as compared with some cultures: the incidence of blindness in the United States, Canada, and nothern Europe is less than 1 in 2,000. With recent advances in medical technology and greater understanding of the action of certain toxic substances on prenatal development, we can anticipate a further decrease in this number.

Intellectual assessment. One of the most difficult problems in evaluating the visually impaired child is that fact that his learning experiences are drastically different from those of most normal individuals. His only contact with the world around him is through other sensory modalities. Thus any talk about color, motion, shape, and other form qualities of objects or situations is usually vague or distorted for the person with severely impaired vision. Although he may hear motion and experience tactile sensations associated with things that have a particular color (such as fire), his ability to form a meaningful concept about any of these objects is greatly decreased. Such common visual experiences as implied in the term *high* have very little meaning for the individual who can form the limited concept that high is something out of his reach but cannot think of high in the sense of a tall building or "reaching to the sky." The sun, the stars, the moon, or an airplane flying overhead may register with him in terms of warmth or sound, but it is nearly impossible for him to comprehend their vastness. Thus such words, which take on common meanings in our everyday language, can mean little or nothing to the person with severely impaired vision. This is especially important to the examiner who would use verbal tests of ability with this person. Vocabulary, considered one of the most important tests in intellectual measurement, can be considerably depressed in total score by the fact that the individual has not had the necessary visual experiences to support his definition. Imagine the difficulties in trying to define some of the following words without having had a visual experience upon which to base a definition: umbrella, horse, microscope, or even icicle. We should not be misled, then, by thinking of the child with severely impaired vision as one who has access to the same verbal experiences that a sighted person does. Even those who are trained to overcome some of their visual loss by means of braille or other training devices still are unable to conceptualize the world around them as others do. To be sure, other sensory modalities tend to be relied on to a greater degree, but they cannot supply the form and structure or the color of objects effectively.

This all results in the lowering of measured intelligence in a child with severe visual problems. Whereas the distinction on the verbal level is not as obvious as it is on the performance level, the lack of certain verbal information that can be understood fully only through vision does act as a depressor of measured intelligence. Even on tests especially designed for blind children (the Hayes-Binet test), although there is a lessening of difference, the differences do still exist.

Similarly achievement rests reflect lower levels for a severely visually impaired child. Many of these factors are due to the less economical methods for communicating available to such a child. For example, reading in braille takes much longer and requires much larger and more difficult-to-handle books than reading for sighted persons. Time factors work against the visually impaired individual in many other situations. Similarly his lack of freedom in moving about in his environment can affect both his intellect as measured by available tests and his achievement, just as it operates to cause a profound effect on his personality. Many blind persons develop some facility in moving about their environment, but it is an infinitesimal movement when compared with that available to any sighted person. The severely visually

impaired infant can learn much of his own small home environment, but, unlike other children, he will never fully experience the greater stimuli of the world around him. Because of his severe visual problem he will not be exposed to interactions with other children frequently, and his decreased mobility will exact a further toll on his development.

Socioemotional assessment. We have already detailed many of the potential problems facing the blind individual in his social and personal life. Each of the factors mentioned in relation to his acquisition of learned materials will operate against him. The result may be that the child has emotions and experiences almost totally unlike those of sighted persons. We should not overlook certain other aspects of developmental problems for the child with severe visual problems—the attitudes of other persons toward him because of his handicap. His experience with other people who may show only pity, sympathy, or concern might well add further adjustment problems.

In gathering information about the socioemotional development of the child with visual problems, parental attitudes become especially important. In studying the very young child it has been found that parents react in a variety of ways to a visually impaired child; each has importance for the evaluation of his personality. In some cases parents are accepting. In many other cases there is a great tendency to overprotect the child or a subtle rejection or denial reaction in which parents seek a magic cure from medical sources; in nearly every instance the search is a complete failure. Most difficult to cope with in assessing potential for the child has been the parental attitude as to causal factors. Many parents feel extreme guilt or shame about their child, thinking that somehow their behavior may have accounted for his difficulty. Some of these parental attitudes can produce serious adjustment difficulties for the child. Socioemotional evaluation becomes a problem of evaluating more than the child; it becomes one of evaluating also the parents' adjustment to the disorder.

As a child matures, it is more and more possible to work directly with him and with his attitudes. Most of the tests involving visual stimuli cannot be used with him; however, verbal communication and sometimes the administration of paper-and-pencil tests by reading the questions to the child can provide the examiner with needed information. In exploring any adjustment difficulties of the blind or severely visually impaired child it becomes apparent that in many ways his life is immeasurably different from that of individuals with better vision. His concepts of sexual attractiveness, love, and meaningful interaction with others as well as his fantasies may be formed in a way quite different from that in normal children. One special problem for the evaluator is to determine the normality of certain behaviors within the visually impaired population. What is normal sexual development for such a child? What stages of emotional development will he go through? Will he ever be able to develop and maintain an adequate relationship with a member of the opposite sex? To these and many other questions the answers are only poorly formed. With partially sighted individuals the chances of normality are greatly increased. With the totally blind, however, especially those who have never been sighted, these questions take on added significance.

Assessment of each child thus is completely unique. Not only may the instruments necessary for evaluation be quite different but the goals, the hope of the future, and even the training of the child will be dependent upon the complex interaction of his measured abilities, parental attitudes, the attitude of the environment in which he must live, and the resources within him, which may seek to grow and develop to their full potential or may perhaps prefer retreat to a sheltered environment where he will be completely dependent upon the care of others.

The child with motor problems

The discussion of children with motor problems includes children who have problems in motor development caused by neurological and orthopedic handicaps. As a group they have much in common with children with chronic medical disorders. However, for the purposes of psychological evaluation they have many different characteristics; therefore they will be discussed separately. Our discussion thus will cover children with disorders ranging from cerebral palsy to congenital deformities and to diseases such as poliomyelitis or osteomyelitis and their residual effects.

Many of the factors that affect children with other special problems are also important to the child with motor problems. Not only must he face and deal with the normal difficulties at each stage of development but he must likewise cope with his special physical problem. A motor disorder may limit drastically a child's ability to attain the rewards of this culture, set him apart from others, prevent him from attending regular classrooms, or in less severe instances curtail his activities so that he cannot take part in many of the sports and social activities that are part of the usual life of infants, children, and adolescents. These blocks or barriers to social interaction can and do mold an individual's personality as well as limit his functional intelligence. Here, too, other persons' perceptions of his disability change and shape his self-concept and self-esteem. Most persons in our culture grow up with some feelings of inferiority or unworthiness. Consider the implications of a severe physical handicap that makes an individual not only feel different but also appear greatly different from his peers. The feelings of inferiority and lack of personal worth generated by these problems can be tremendous.

It is possible for an individual to develop normal patterns of interaction by adopting realistic personal goals and by developing meaningful social relationships. However, the family's perception of his handicap and what they feel they should do for him may block any attempts he may make toward stable, meaningful interaction with others.

In evaluating both the intelligence and the socioemotional adjustment of the child with motor problems the psychologist must be able to assess a number of important factors. He or she must be able to determine, either independently or in consultation with medical experts, whether the individual is making maximal use of his unimpaired motor abilities or is responding to treatment and training for impaired areas that may be developed for partial usage. These factors must then be weighed against his intellectual potential, the environmental potentials, and his own insights and motivation.

Few persons are able to have such ideal consultation and guidance. As a result most of the available information about children with motor problems shows that their adjustment is far below that of normal children. Before considering some of the methods used in assessing this level of adjustment we will turn our attention to the intellectual assessment of the child with motor problems.

Intellectual assessment

The nature of a crippling disorder may well result in lowered intellectual abilities. Brain damage that produces cerebral palsy may be so extensive as to destroy some of the higher brain centers and thus drastically limit the intellectual potential of the individual. As a result many children with cerebral palsy are also intellectually retarded. Most studies suggest that about 40% of cerebral palsied children are intellectually impaired, whereas only 26% are average or above in intelligence. This appears to be a result of tissue damage.

Testing of such persons is not a simple matter. In many instances they have impaired speech so that verbal communication is limited. In other instances the speech problems are linked with a lack of motor control, preventing the use of nonverbal tests of intelligence to assess ability adequately. In still other cases a child with brain damage may be so hyperactive that he is unable to focus his attention for sufficiently long periods of time to be satisfactorily evaluated. This is true regardless of the test utilized. None of the individually administered tests is sufficiently free of verbal or motor aspects to provide a real measure of intellectual potential. They are valuable in assessing what the child can do at the moment, but they may fail to indicate what the proper training and education would permit him to attain. All of the tests utilized reflect about the same results. The child with motor problems does less well than the normal child on all forms of testing.

Often the conditions under which testing is done will greatly modify the ability to obtain a "good" test result. This is why it is so important to have the child examined by an expert.

Properly trained psychologists often undertake examination of a child with brain damage with or without motor disorders in a room where there are minimal distractions. All objects, toys, pictures, and other stimuli that might draw the brain-damaged child's attention away from the task at hand are eliminated. With the sensory input thus restricted the child is often able to demonstrate scores much higher than would be possible if he were tested in a typical setting with many distracting stimuli acting upon him.

Power tests (untimed tests) take on special meaning for children who have severe motor impairment. The timed test is often handicapping in that the concentration necessary for some children to overcome their physical handicap and gain sufficient motor control to perform some of the tasks is not taken into consideration. The standardizing of timed tests is invalid for this group.

Children whose physical condition has affected only the extremities are, of course, accessible to evaluation by means of verbal tests. Although such a child has quite likely had only limited experiences as compared with other children, today's modern teaching techniques and the availability of television, radio, and other sources of sensory input can make possible for this child a high degree of awareness of what goes on in the world around him. Whereas this may not be an ideal situation for personality development, it does decrease the formerly great differences between normal children and children who are quite limited in their mobility.

Socioemotional assessment

We have seen that a child with motor problems often has other problems as well. He may have difficulties in both verbal and nonverbal communication. If he has cerebral palsy, he may be unable to write or speak in an intelligible manner. This is a great detriment to any verbal form of communication with him. For such children socioemotional assessment, like intelligence testing, may rely on objects of exaggerated size and shape so that the effects of motor impairment may be minimized. For example, a child may be required to make an X in a block to respond to a personality questionnaire. If the blocks are of the usual size for children his age, he may not be able to place a proper sign in it. However, if the size of the square is increased to four or five times its former dimensions, even a child with severe motor handicaps may be able to respond properly. In many cases this is, of course, not possible. Suitable responses can be gained through verbal interaction with children who are able to speak effectively. Standardized personality tests may be read to the child and his responses gained, or he may be tested by using projective techniques that also provide for a verbal response. Many psychologists go to great lengths to obtain personality data from such children. A child's self-concepts, his attitudes toward others, and his aspirations, hopes, and dreams are all especially important to the psychologist who may use knowledge about these characteristics as stepping-stones to build and plan for the child's future. Without this information effective plans cannot be developed. A child who might have an elaborate program developed for him may fail to achieve in it because of socioemotional factors working against him or because of limitations in intelligence. Similarly many parents have been discouraged in working out plans for children with motor problems whom they thought to be intellectually limited or dull. Subsequent evaluation has sometimes revealed that these children, far from being dull, had above-average intellectual potential. We recall quite vividly the case of a boy whose speech was almost unintelligible and who had virtually no motor control but who possessed above-average intelligence. Carefully tutored by his family, he had gained the equivalent of several years of college education and was highly informed on a wide variety of subjects.

Adequate evaluation of children with motor problems can often be achieved only with long periods of assessment. These children may appear to have extremely limited abilities intellectually and socioemotionally. It is only after they have remained in an enriched training program that adequate understanding of their intellectual potential is attained. Nevertheless, a psychologist who has worked extensively with organically impaired children often is able to make a remarkably accurate prognosis of a child's good potentials when superficially he appears to be badly handicapped.

The child with chronic medical disorders

The psychological evaluation of the child with chronic medical disorders also poses special problems. In many cases the very nature of his disease requires extended periods of hospitalization. In some instances this hospitalization may terminate in the death of the child. Conditions such as tuberculosis, heart disease, diabetes, epilepsy, asthma, and cancer may all require extended hospitalization. In some instances this requires a complete disruption of the family situation with only limited contact permitted. In other instances hospitalization may be for shorter periods of time with home care being the most desirable situation.

Assessment of the newborn or very young with a grave illness may be quite difficult and provide very limited information. In cases of a chronic medical disorder in a child and or adolescent, evaluation is of prime importance. Intellectual evaluation in this group is usually much more successful than for the groups we have discussed previously. In most instances there are no blocks to verbal or motor tasks. The subject generally has a more limited range of experiences, and this must be taken into account in prediction, but the need for special tests is considerably less. In almost no instance are the tests so strenuous that they would overtax any individual with a chronic disorder. Thus at any given age tests appropriate for normal children can be used.

Similarly, when evaluating the personality structure of the child with a chronic disorder, the testing problems are essentially those found in normal children. However, evaluation of test results takes on a special character and deserves additional mention.

Psychological factors in chronic illness

A matter of prime importance in the psychological evaluation of the child with a chronic illness concerns the meaning that the illness may have to the child and to his parents. When illness affects a child who has previously had normal development, it acts as an overlay or an additional factor in the ever present problems of the developing child and adolescent.

It is possible through extended interviews and testing of these children to learn many of the attitudes that they have regarding their illness. In many instances they feel that they are sick because they have not followed parental directions, they were bad, or they have done something wrong. It is much like the small behavioral incident in which a child does something outside the guidelines of the parents, receives some minor hurt, and is told by the parent, "You got what you deserve," or "I told you that would happen." It is a human characteristic to seek explanations for the occurrence of events, particularly those that will affect our lives significantly such as a chronic medical disorder. In seeking these explanations both parents and child may attempt to provide a rational explanation for the circumstances in which they find themselves. Their explanations may have nothing to do with the reality of the situation and yet may serve them as explanatory concepts.

Among the commonly observed reactions in parents and children with chronic medical disorders are symptoms such as regression, extreme dependency, denial, and rebelliousness. Of course, there are more positive reactions to the illness in which the child and parents work together to provide the most active and meaningful environment possible under the circumstances. It must be stressed that these are symptoms that are expected to show up in personality testing and should not be considered atypical for persons with chronic medical disorders. Although many of these reactions are not particularly desirable, they do occur commonly and will be seen by the nurse in the home, in the hospital, and in the office. When such children attempt to carry on relatively normal school activities in spite of their disorders, the problems will also confront the school nurse.

Although exceptions do exist, it is the rule to find adjustment problems in persons with chronic medical disorders. It is virtually impossible to escape this. Denial simply does not work and may even be fatal. Hospital records are full of cases in which persons denied the presence of diabetes or heart conditions, for example, and continued to attempt to function as normal. Not infrequently this has resulted in further impairment or even death. The purpose of psychological evaluation in many instances is to learn of the dynamics and motives of the child with a chronic disorder so that some way may be discovered to reach this child and help him to develop more constructive future planning and activities.

The realistic evaluation of hospitalized children is always complicated by the very real presence of pain, discomfort, and fear. Counseling, psychotherapy, and other remedial efforts work particularly well when the fears are psychologically induced and concerns can be lessened by slight changes in the environment. These techniques are much less effective in dealing with pain, discomfort, and fear of separation or death. There is some evidence to suggest that children as young as 5 years have some understanding and anxiety about death (Melear, 1973). The painful task of comforting the dying child in his last hours frequently falls into the hands of the nurse.

Often educative procedures and counseling can communicate to the child that present discomforts may lessen as times goes on, and this may even work to help the child accept things that cannot be changed. These approaches, however, are frequently only partially successful. It is dependent on the personality makeup of the child, but quite often in conditions with a grave prognosis a return to his home may be the only "medicine" that the child can successfully respond to. Young children particularly, who draw most of their emotional support from members of the family, may make their greatest progress when they are able to function as day patients in the hospital or when some "live-in" arrangement can be made for one or both of the parents during the hospital stay. These variations are being provided more and more by modern hospitals. However, for most situations the present autocratic conditions, limited staff, and lack of awareness of such problems make this approach difficult if not impossible.

Psychological tests can provide valuable information, frequently indicating when and how children can rejoin the normal community to some degree. In some instances this will be in the form of attending regular schools but in a special class setting where their particular disorders may receive special attention.

Each chronic medical disorder has its organic component but also possesses a strong psychological overlay. The mere fact of the presence of the disease, the reaction of other persons to the condition, and the child's feeling about himself, knowing that he has a particular illness, interact to produce adjustment difficulties. Careful planning requires a balancing of all factors involved. Career planning, educational procedures, and family conditions must take cognizance of the disease itself and of the limitations that it places on the individual when suitable educational and occupational roles are being considered. When these various physical, psychological, and socioemotional conditions are assessed and controlled, adjustment can be positive and successful. Guidelines can be laid down only when a thorough knowledge of the personality dynamics is obtained and the ability level of the child is understood.

The child with emotional problems

Understanding the behavior of the child with emotional problems is intimately linked with understanding the normal child. It is through study of the differences that occur in the intellect and socioemotional adjustment of a child with emotional problems as compared with the normal child that the dimension and form of problem areas can be seen. Evaluation of the child with emotional problems is principally concerned with intelligence and socioemotional adjustment but is by no means restricted to these areas alone. It is quite possible that interest patterns, aptitudes, and achievement all suffer or are distorted as a result of problems in socioemotional adjustment. Results obtained with testing instruments that point up problems in social adjustment, social awareness, and interactions with others are almost always at variance with patterns found in normal children. Attitudes about self, about others, and about the world in general take on many different dimensions in a child or adolescent with emotional problems. There may be a pattern of

great deviancy indicated by inconsistency, unconventionality, insensitivity, rigidity, or disregard for the rights and feelings of others. This is true of the child with autistic-like behaviors. In other cases it may take the form of setting personal requirements and standards for self and for others at so unrealistically high a level that no person could possibly live up to them. These represent only a few of the many areas that are assessed.

Evaluation of the very young

The assessment of very young children is quite difficult. A major problem at this age, particularly in the preschool group, is one in which verbal communication is at best limited. Thus assessment of this age group most often relies on observations of behavior such as bed-wetting, aggression, hyperactivity, head banging, rocking, inattention, withdrawal, and disobedience, to mention a few. Since each of these behaviors may also be caused by an organic condition, diagnosis becomes a matter of diagnosis by exclusion. That is, once physical causal relationships for the problem behavior have not been found, children are frequently referred by prediatricians for evaluation of a possible psychological basis. It thus becomes a problem of "since it does not appear organic, it must be functional or psychological." Although this undoubtedly is a logical course of action, there is always the nagging point that merely the fact that no organic relationship was established does not completely eliminate the possibility that one exists.

Further complications are added to the already muddy issue by the fact that for young children wide ranges of behaviors are permitted that would not be tolerated at later stages of development. Imaginary playmates, extremes of fantasy, and whopping lies are part of the normal repertoire of behavior. It is only when these take on extreme forms and interfere with reality contact that they are cause for concern. However, should they persist beyond this preliminary period of development, they are considered quite deviant.

Some of these characteristics may seriously impede the adequate assessment of intellectual functioning and adjustment in young children.

Quite frequently, hyperactivity is so great that children cannot focus even on the short-term, quickly performed tests used with individuals of this age. This does not completely defeat the psychologist. As has already been indicated, many of the scales for the very young child are developmental in nature and can be obtained through observation. To be sure, this method is crude and only a rough indicator of ability, yet the appearance of certain coordinated and skilled behavior in a child who is otherwise inaccessible to testing will provide the information that he is at least as able as others who function on the observed behavioral level. Should this seem difficult to understand, consider the small child who refuses to cooperate with the examiner in performing coordinated activities with blocks. Perhaps he prefers instead to play with them completely on his own and ignore the instructions provided. If the psychologist notes that this child in his play is able to stack blocks to a certain height, build toy bridges, or in other ways demonstrate coordination and organizing activity, he may also take note that these activities appear only in children who are at least 2 years of age. He can thus learn that this child is able to do some things as well as normal 2-year-old children, even though he has been unable to directly test the child's ability. If a child has severe emotional problems and is suspected of being intellectually deficient, having such information might be vital to arriving at a more positive diagnosis. Perhaps this child is only 2 years old at the time of testing. Finding that he is able to do some things on a level normal for his age is highly indicative of the fact that the child is in all probability not retarded but suffering from some disturbance that interferes with his testing.

Evaluation of older children and adolescents

Only in children with the most extreme emotional problems are serious difficulties encountered in assessment during the preadolescent or adolescent period. Although hostility, aggression, and uncooperativeness are frequently encountered, they only rarely are sufficiently intense to prevent any sort of personality or intellectual evaluation in this older group. Even the varied forms of resistance and the refusals encountered often provide important diagnostic clues about the type of disturbance present, its intensity, and its modifiability. Since psychologists are not bound to arrive at their conclusions during one single interview, it is frequently the practice to have repeated visits with persons who are extremely disturbed and presently uncooperative. Some evaluations have been known to require a period of many weeks or months. In such cases a child so severely disturbed that he is almost completely inaccessible may be gradually won over to evaluation by the development of a positive relationship with the child and then a gradual introduction of testing or evaluation material at later stages of the relationship. In the extreme cases evaluation is somewhat less important because the very gravity of the emotional problem almost diagnoses itself. It is the borderline case of the child who may be disturbed or may be suffering from some other form of handicap that requires special diagnostic skills and investigation. Examples of this are the child who hides guilt, concern, anxiety, and feelings of unworthiness under a superficial veil of indifference and unconcern. Were the evaluator to simply accept the child's overt behavior, he might conclude that the child was poorly motivated, socially unconcerned, and perhaps even developing initial signs of sociopathic behavior. However, through his use of subtle testing instruments that are aimed at reaching deeper levels of personality less easily covered by superficial attitudes and manners, he may learn of the true feelings of the child being evaluated. In these and many other cases the child may then be led to a more open recognition and expression of his feelings and ultimately away from the area of severe disturbance.

REFERENCES

Allison, J., Blatt, S. J., and Zimet, C. N.: The interpretation of psychological tests, New York, 1968, Harper & Row, Publishers.

Alpern, G. D., and Boll, T. J.: Developmental profile manual, Indianapolis, Psychological Development Publications.

Ames, L. B., Learned, J., Metraux, R., and Walker, R.: Child Rorschach responses, New York, 1952, Paul B. Hoeber, Inc.

Anastasi, A.: Differential psychology, ed. 3, New York, 1958, Macmillan, Inc.

Anastasi, A.: Psychological testing, ed. 3, New York, 1972, Macmillan, Inc.

Baley, N.: Development of mental abilities. In Mussen, P. H., editor: Carmichael's manual of child psychology (Vol. 1), ed. 3, New York, 1970, John Wiley & Sons, Inc.

Bloom, B. S., editor: Taxonomy of educational objectives: Handbook 1, cognitive domain, New York, 1956, Longmans, Green & Co., Inc.

Bloom, B. S., Hastings, J. T., and Madaus, G. F., editors: Handbook on formative and summative education of student learning, New York, 1971, McGraw-Hill Book Co.

Brazelton, T. B.: Neonatal behavioral assessment scale, London, 1973, William Heinemann Medical Books, Ltd.

Buros, O. K., editor: The fifth mental measurements yearbook, Highland Park, N.J., 1959, Gryphon Press.

Buros, O. K., editor: The sixth mental measurements yearbook, Highland Park, N.J., 1965, Gryphon Press.

Buros, O. K., editor: The seventh mental measurements yearbook, Highland Park, N.J., 1972, Gryphon Press.

Carey, W. B.: Clinical applications of infant temperament measurements, Behav. Pediatr. **81:**823, 1972.

Cronbach, L. J.: Essentials of psychological testing, ed. 3, New York, 1970, Harper & Row, Publishers.

Cruickshank, W. M., editors: Psychology of exceptional children and youth, ed. 3, Englewood Cliffs, N.J., 1971, Prentice-Hall, Inc.

Dale, P. S.: Language development: Structure and function. Hinsdale, Ill., 1972, Dryden Press.

Exner, J. E., Jr.: The Rorschach: A comprehensive system, New York, 1974, John Wiley & Sons, Inc.

Flick, G.: Dyslexia, New Orleans, 1972, Lecture presented at University of New Orleans.

Frank, L. K.: Projective methods, Springfield, Ill., 1948, Charles C Thomas, Publisher.

Frankenberg, W. K., Dodds, J. B., and Fandal, A. W.: Denver Developmental screening manual, Denver, 1970, University of Colorado Medical Center.

Ginsburg, H.: The myth of the deprived child: Poor children's intellect and education, Englewood Cliffs, N.J., 1972, Prentice-Hall, Inc.

Guilford, J. P., and Fruchter, B.: Fundamental statistics in psychology and education, ed. 5, New York, 1973, McGraw-Hill Book Co.

Hoepfner, R., Stern, C., and Nummedal, S. G., editors: CSE-ECRC preschool/kindergarten test evaluations, Los Angeles, 1971, Center for the Study of Evaluation and Early Childhood Research Center, Graduate School of Education, University of California, Los Angeles.

Johnson, O. G., and Bommarito, J. W.: Tests and measurements in child development: A handbook, San Francisco, 1971, Jossey-Bass, Inc., Publishers.

Krathwohl, D. R., Bloom, B. S., and Masia, B. B.: Taxonomy of educational objectives: Handbook 2, affective domain, New York, 1964, David Mckay Co., Inc.

Melear, J D.: Children's conceptions of death, J. Genet. Psychol. **123:**359, 1973.

Rosenblith, J. F.: Prognostic value of neonatal behavioral tests, Early Child Dev. Care **3:**31, 1973.

Sattler, J. M.: Assessment of children's intelligence, Philadelphia, 1974, W. B. Saunders Co.

Senna, C.: The fallacy of the I.Q., New York, 1973, Joseph Okpaku Publishing Co., Inc.

Walker, D. K.: Socioemotional measures for preschool and kindergarten children, San Francisco, 1973, Jossey-Bass, Inc., Publishers.

Werner, E. E.: Review of the Denver Developmental Screening test. In Buros, O. K., editor: The seventh mental measurements yearbook, Highland Park, N.J., 1972, Gryphon Press.

Williams, G. J., and Gordon, S.: Clinical child psychology; Current practices and future perspectives, New York, 1974, Behavioral Publications, Inc.

PART II

Nursing care of the handicapped and ill child

11

General nursing care of
THE HOSPITALIZED CHILD

IMPACT OF THE HOSPITAL
ON THE CHILD

Whether the effect of hospitalization will be a negative or a positive one, a socializing or a traumatizing one, depends on many factors, including the personality of the child himself. Research studies regarding effects of hospitalization are not conclusive (Yarrow). On the other hand, it is certain that the child will, at the end of his hospitalization, have some attitude toward medical and nursing personnel, the hospital, and his stay there. Nursing personnel can help to make the attitude a positive one. True, physical illness itself is unpleasant and treatments for it may be painful, but what can be done to offset physical discomfort with its accompanying emotional distress and possible bewilderment at strange sights and sounds?

Physical setup

As the child is admitted to the pediatric unit, the general appearance of the unit may frighten him if it resembles the usual adult unit. Pastel-colored walls, pictures, a goldfish bowl, or plants help to make the child feel less apprehensive. Some pictures painted on the wall at the eye level of a preschool child may arouse his interest and curiosity, especially pictures of things that he knows such as kittens, ducks, or cartoon characters. Pretty curtains and bedspreads can brighten a room. Provision of a junior bed rather than a crib for a child over 4 years of age may give him a feeling of reassurance.

The sight of play materials on open shelves in the recreation room or the presence of a rocking horse may reassure the young child. Doll equipment (doll, doll bed, doll carriage) is familiar to most preschool children. A card table with a game such as Sorry, Monopoly, or checkers may help to make the hospital less awesome for the elementary school child. A record player has an appeal for children of various ages. A few easy chairs for adults may look inviting to the mothers. A bookcase with low shelves that the young children can reach and higher shelves for the older ones has a place in meeting the diversional needs of a child whose physical activity is limited. A toilet located near the recreation room is convenient.

If rooms for the children have two beds rather than four or eight, the child has fewer people with whom to adjust. Having a bathroom between every two rooms is helpful. For the 3- or 4-year-old child there should be an adjustable seat for the toilet plus a footstool on which he can stand to reach the toilet seat. Some pediatric units have a small toilet chair. Each child's bedside stand should be provided with individual equipment for him: his towel, washcloth, bath basin, bedpan, and emesis basin. There should be a special place provided for the bath blanket and for the rest hour blanket that can serve also as a night blanket in cold weather. Each toddler and infant should have a bib at the bedside as part of his equipment. (Preschool and older children like to act grown-up and use napkins.)

Suitable clothing should be available: colored pajamas for bed patients and play clothes for ambulatory children. The use of hospital gowns should be reserved for the very sick child who needs to wear something that can easily be slipped on and off with little disturbance to him.

Preparation for hospitalization

When possible, it is helpful for the child at home to have an explanation of his forthcom-

275

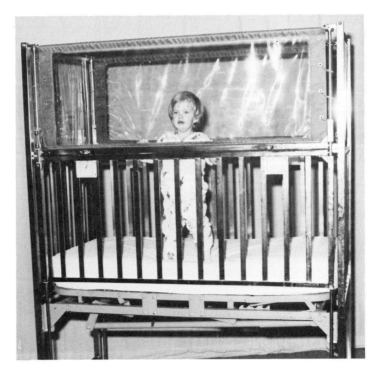

Fig. 11-1. Pediatric hospital bed. Note plastic siding that prevents child from climbing over bedside but permits him to see his surroundings.

ing hospitalization, why he is going to the hospital, and something about a hospital. For a child who is going to have elective surgery performed such books as *Linda Goes to the Hospital* or *Johnny Goes to the Hospital* are informative and interesting at both preschool and elementary school levels.

The office nurse, the nurse in a crippled children's clinic, or the nurse in an outpatient department who knows the date of the child's hospitalization has a chance to say something to the child and to his parents. Pertinent literature might be made available in a waiting room. The nurse may have the opportunity to suggest to the mother that the child be allowed to take to the hospital some favorite toy or doll. The presence of something familiar is always helpful in new surroundings. The child may enjoy helping to pack a suitcase to go to the hospital. Details of an operation are neither necessary nor desirable; however, the child should know he will be sleeping when the doctor "fixes his foot" or "takes out his tonsils." He should

know that he is going to stay in the hospital several days, that other children are there too, and when he will see his parents, if they do not remain with him during the whole hospitalization. There may be, as Abbott et al. (1970) write, a "dress rehearsal" for the hospital. The child and his parents and siblings can all enter a play about the child going to the hospital and returning home again. In addition, it may be possible for the child and his parents to visit the hospital and pediatric unit before he is admitted.

Younger children sometimes enjoy playing "hospital" with dolls and toy doctor and nurse equipment. It is wise to suggest to the mother that, in preparing an older infant or toddler for hospitalization, she let a babysitter or someone outside the immediate family care for the child for short intervals (2 or 3 hours) to permit the child to get accustomed to people other than just his mother caring for him.

Unfortunately, many children are admitted when acutely ill and there is no time for anything but the briefest of explanations, so the child has both physical discomfort and new surroundings to which to adjust.

Orientation to the hospital unit

When a new child is admitted to the pediatric unit, the nurse should introduce herself, other children, and/or adults who happen to be in the room. Since the younger child especially is influenced by his mother's (or parents') behavior, the nurse should make every effort to put the mother at ease. She should avoid making the mother feel that she (the nurse) is taking the child from her. The mother can assist in undressing a child and putting him in bed (that is, if the child is not allowed to ambulate). For a young child who is wearing a brace on one leg it may be very distressing to have this removed immediately, especially if he cannot walk at all without it. His brace is, in a sense, part of him; without it he cannot assert himself and be independent. Judgment is needed as to whether the child has to be completely undressed and placed in bed right away or whether he can remain out of bed.

The nurse should inquire what name the child wishes to be called. He may want to be addressed by his given name or he may prefer a nickname. The name or nickname he likes should be indicated both on the identification band on his wrist and on the name card on his crib or bed so that this information will be readily available.

The nurse can inquire from the mother if there is anything special she would like to tell about his care: whether the child is toilet trained or is not, what words he uses to communicate his toilet needs, what fluids he particularly likes, what particular toys he likes to play with, whether or not he feeds himself, whether he uses cup or bottle, and what he understands about the reason for his admission to the hospital. Anything that seems pertinent to the mother is important for the nurse to know. Asking the mother of a young child to supply information about him serves to let her know both the nurse's desire to take good care of the child and the nurse's respect for the mother's care at home. This may help the mother to be less tense. A good relationship with the mother aids the nurse in having a good relationship with the child.

If the child is not acutely ill, he should be given some diversional activity. The nurse can suggest to the child's mother that he may like to have his favorite toy brought from home to be with him if the child now has none of his own play materials. The presence of something familiar in a stressful environment helps lessen fear.

An explanation of a routine day in the hospital should be given to the child. This routine may vary in different hospitals, but the young patient should know the general sequence of events in a day: that there will be breakfast, dinner, and supper; that rest hour follows dinner; that doctors usually see children both morning and afternoon; that at night when children sleep a nurse is there to watch over them as well as during the day. That there are three shifts of nurses is of interest to the child: Some work in the day, some work in the evening, and some work all night.

The nurse should also reassure the parents that she will be back from time to time to see the child.

Although many mothers remain with young children, this is less true with older children. The latter should know when to expect a visit from mother or parents.

Kind of care

The child's adjustment to the hospital and his new surroundings is influenced by the kind of care he receives: the skill with which intramuscular injections or a bath is given, the mechanical ability the nurse shows in regulating a Croupette* or oxygen tent, the manner in which he is physically handled, the kind and preparation of food he is offered, and the adeptness with which he is made comfortable. Physical care when the child is in discomfort or acutely ill contributes to his emotional support. The nurse may be a gentle and kind person, but unless she has both an understanding and knowledge of the child's needs and the technical skill involved in meeting those needs, the comfort and care she can offer the child are limited.

---

*Air Shields Co., Hatboro, Pa.

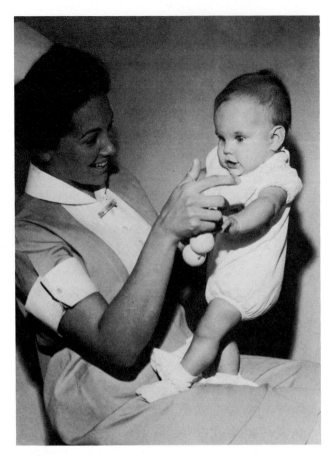

Fig. 11-2. Infants need sensory stimulation as well as mothering.

New nurses assigned to the pediatric unit need an orientation not only to the general policies and physical setup of the unit but also to the nursing procedures and measures used on that unit. This is true of nursing aides and assistants also if they are to function in an optimal way. Nursing procedures and routines should be written, kept up-to-date, and made available to everyone on the unit.

Since babies cannot talk and young children are limited in verbal communication and since older children seldom complain as adults do, the nurse needs to make rounds frequently to see the children assigned to her, being observant at the same time of their nonverbal communication. The posture of a child and his behavior, facial expression, and activity all have meaning just as do the quality of the pulse, the color of the child, and/or the presence of dyspnea.

The importance of the manner of the nurse toward the mother when the child is admitted has been discussed. The way the nurse behaves toward the child in the days after he is admitted is equally important. What should be her approach to him?

Need for attention and affection

Even though the nurse is busy, she should make the most of every contact with the child to show him she likes him. The infant can be cuddled when he is fed. The nurse can talk with children as she cares for them. One child confided to an instructor, "My new nurse doesn't like me." The instructor inquired why the child believed this. The child's reply was, "She gave me a bath. She made my bed, but she didn't say nothin'."

In addition to words a smile says a great deal. Answering a child's needs quickly, giving a child something with which to play before she leaves him, or even putting her head in the door of the child's room just to call, "Hello, Johnny!" indicates recognition of the child.

The child who is pretty and appealing often receives the most attention, but it is the less attractive infant or child, the child with eczema, or the malnourished infant with diarrhea, who really needs the additional attention. Also the child who is quiet and good needs watching, since he may be more frightened of his new environment than the one who cries and misbehaves.

The child who has a physical disorder such as hydrocephalus or a mental disorder such as Down's syndrome may be hard for some nurses to accept, but these children need special loving care also.

Belonging

The possession of his own individual bedside equipment and crib or bed helps the child to develop a feeling of belonging, especially if he is left in the same room and not transferred to another. Having the same nurse on each shift for a period of time and having a particular doctor also contribute to the sense of belongingness.

Achievement and recognition

Attention, a sense of belonging, achievement, and recognition are all important psychological needs of children. Achievement means different things at different ages. For a toddler to help wash his hands or pull on his sock is an accomplishment. Putting a jigsaw puzzle together or constructing something with Tinker Toys is an achievement for an older child. Ambulating or taking a few steps alone in a new brace or on crutches needs to be rewarded by praise and recognition for a child of any age.

Child's routine

Programs during the child's stay in the hospital should be planned to coincide as much as possible with his routine at home. The routine day of the child should be posted in the nurses' station so that all personnel can easily refer to it. Everyone should know what is done when

the child first awakens, at what hours his meals are served, the time and length of his rest hour, the time for recreational or diversional therapy, visiting hours, and bedtime. Older children who are in the hospital for a long period may go to school in the hospital or have the schoolteacher come to their bedside. The nearer the routine can be kept to what the child does at home, the less the child has to adapt to a new situation. The kind of clothes worn in the hospital, the physical appearance of the pediatric unit, and the recreational activity offered either hinder or help the child's adjustment in accordance with what they are. This has been discussed under physical setup.

Administration of the pediatric unit

The relationship of personnel to one another creates a certain atmosphere that makes itself known to the child and to his parents. This does not mean that there should be a "country club" type of relaxed atmosphere. Rather it should be one that is professional, is friendly, and shows the goodwill of the staff—toward each other, toward the patients, and toward the visitors. There are sure to be problems from time to time between nursing service and medical or housekeeping or dietary personnel, but there should be a planned means of communication at stated intervals to discuss problems involved. This need may be met in different ways at different hospitals. In one situation there may be a committee for the improvement of nursing care of pediatric patients, in which there are representatives from other departments. Another hospital may have regular weekly meetings between the resident and the head nurse. Problems with other departments may be solved as they arise through conference with the head of the department concerned. In another hospital there may be nursing meetings scheduled with representatives of both aides and staff nurses from each tour of duty to discuss possible ways to improve nursing care.

In order that all can work together for the best care of the patient, there has to be not only a definite philosophy but also ways to constantly keep alive that philosophy.

Leadership is expected of the head nurse. Tangible evidence of her interest in maintaining high standards is needed daily. The duties of the professional nurse, the practical nurse, and the aide should be clearly understood by all, as well as the difference between the duties of the head nurse and those of the team leader. The staff nurse must not forget, no matter how many aides are helping her or are on her team, that it is she who is expected to have the know-how in observing and judging the condition of the patients assigned to her.

With a smooth organization and functioning of personnel the child may feel less confused and more secure because the personnel are more self-confident when they know exactly what should be done and how to do it.

Nursing care plan

To make an effective care plan the nurse needs first to assess the child, then to make a plan, to implement the plan, to evaluate it after trial, and then to modify the plan in accordance with the patient's treatment, adjustment to the hospital, and general progress. Daily evaluation of the care plan and its effectiveness is necessary. Methods of planned communication between each shift of nurses is essential for continuous implementation of the care plan.

The nurse needs to *know the child,* his problems, and possible *measures of nursing intervention* that would be of assistance in bringing a given child back to a more optimum state of health. Suggested physical assessment forms for various age levels are shown in Chapter 9, Promotion of Health. The nursing care of common medical problems is discussed in the following chapters.

Medical records

As to the child as a person, there is much the nurse can learn from the child's medical record. Knowing his race and religion helps to establish his cultural and ethnic background. If the address of the child's home is familiar to the nurse, this may give her clues to his socioeconomic status or whether he comes from a rural or an urban community.

If the child is functioning in a milieu different from the one to which he is accustomed, the nurse who understands his background may be able to anticipate some of the difficulties the child is likely to encounter and thus be better equipped to guide his adjustment. For example, the child may reject unfamiliar hospital foods. If the nurse is aware of the child's cultural food patterns, she may be able to make arrangements with the dietary department to serve the child foods he is more likely to accept. If the nurse knows that the child comes from a family where there are strong religious ties, the child may feel more comfortable if the nurse arranges for a member of the clergy to visit him. When the nurse realizes that the child will be hospitalized at the time his family celebrates an important traditional holiday or feast, feelings of loneliness and ''missing out on the fun'' can be allayed if the nurse is able to duplicate some form of the festivities for the child on the ward. All these efforts on the part of the nurse will reduce the child's anxiety and tension in adjusting to the new and unfamiliar hospital setting. They will produce a more stable emotional outlook, which will contribute to the speed of the child's physical recovery.

It is worthwhile for the nurse to note the age and marital status of the parents, their occupations, and their health. Certain occupations such as physician, lawyer, police officer, or army officer may carry special prestige values for the child and give him a sense of security. On the other hand, if one or both of the parents is disabled or unemployed, the child may be aware that his hospitalization causes the family considerable financial strain. He may be concerned about his being a burden on the family for fear they may cease to love him. In a single-parent family the nurse should know who is responsible for the child when the parent goes out to work or whether they live on funds from welfare. This will establish what sort of practical arrangements can be made for the child if he should require extended health care after discharge from the hospital.

The child's position in the family in relation to siblings might also affect his hospital stay. If there are other children in the family, the child may adjust more readily to other children in the hospital than if he is an only child. Isolation from other children would only intensify his feelings of loneliness.

From the child's record the nurse can usually

ascertain the child's grade placement in school. Is this grade appropriate for his age? Perhaps he is an exceptionally bright child who has skipped a grade. Possibly he is a slow learner or in a special education class for the mentally retarded. Intellectual ability will influence the way the nurse communicates with the child and how well he understands her teaching.

After having studied the child's medical record for significant data, the nurse can turn to the child's day sheet (nurse's notes) to read the record of his admission history. The nurse who admitted the child should have made some pertinent comments about the appearance and behavior of the parents (or other persons) who brought him to the hospital as well as about the parent-child relationship at that time. True, the hospital admission of the child may be stressful for both parents and child, but even so, some valuable clues can be discovered: Did the child cling to his parents, ignore them, converse with them? Did the parents seem unduly solicitous or domineering? Did they threaten to punish the child if he "didn't mind the nurse"? Did they give the child assurances that they would be back to visit him soon?

Observation

When the nurse cares for the child during the days after his hospital admission, evidence of the socioeconomic, cultural, and family home environment may still be observed. As the nurse cares for the child, it is important that she note his interaction with her, with other hospital personnel, and with other children. The child who feels secure at home makes a better hospital adjustment. He relates and communicates better than others. It is normal for the youngster to show signs of separation anxiety, but, if he is used to people coming and going in his home and has experienced stable relationships with his parents, brothers, and sisters, the strangeness of the hospital may wear off soon. The "good" child who is very quiet and cooperative may well need as much reassurance and affection as the obviously unhappy child who cries and rebels at everything.

It is significant to note whether the child talks about his home and family or whether he never mentions them at all. If the parents do not come to visit the child, the nurse should not necessarily conclude that they are indifferent. They may be unable to arrange transportation to the hospital or baby-sitters to care for the other children in the family. When the family does visit the child, the nurse can talk to them about the child's responsiblities and interests at home.

When the parent visits the child, the nurse can observe the consistency, frequency, and sensitivity of the parent's response to the child. This is important in evaluating the parent-child relationship. Further insights about the parent's attitude toward the child can be gained from noting the parent's behavior toward the nurse: Does the parent want to talk to the nurse about the child's care? Is he or she cooperative in giving accurate information, or does the nurse sense that the parent is trying to cover up facts that would create an unfavorable impression regarding his ability to raise the child? Is the parent possessive of the child and hostile toward the nurse when she attempts to touch the child or do anything for him? The nurse's estimate of the parent's attitude toward her in relation to the child will determine the degree of rapport that she is able to establish. This in turn will influence how well her health teaching is accepted and carried out by the parents.

Meeting the child's needs

Again, to make a nursing care plan it is necessary to make an assessment of the child, make a plan for care, implement this plan, evaluate it, modify it in accordance with its effectiveness, and reevaluate it constantly. The nursing intervention measures taken into consideration are the child as a person, his parents, his home environment, and his medical problems. The plan includes care of the child's present problems, health teaching for the child and parents in the present situation, and teaching for the promotion of health in the future.

Summary

The child's adjustment is dependent not only on his preparation for hospitalization and the adjustment of his parents to his hospitalization but also on many factors and events that happen daily while he is in the hospital. Whether the impact of the hospital can be used constructively depends a great deal on the kind of care he receives. This complex subject includes not only the general administration of the unit but also the nursing care plan for him. This plan, of necessity, might undergo several modifications in accord with the child's total condition and progress.

SKILLS IN THE NURSING CARE OF CHILDREN
Techniques in approaching children

In her contacts with children there are certain general principles that are helpful for the nurse to know.

1. Remember the child's age and interests in talking with him.
2. Treat the child with respect and courtesy.
3. Explain treatments before doing them. (Puppets can be utilized effectively in explaining treatments, operations, cardiac catheterizations, etc. What will be done to the child is done by one puppet to another puppet, with a real person supplying the dialogue.)
4. Use every contact with the child to show him your interest and affection.
5. Provide suitable recreation and diversion in accord with his age, physical activity, and interests.
6. Have a sense of humor, but laugh with him and not at him.
7. Avoid commands. Give positive statements: "It's time to put away toys" instead of "Put your toys away."
8. Expect obedience. People tend to live up to what is expected of them. The nurse *expects* the child, for example, to take the oral medication.
9. Give choices when possible; for example, a child likes to choose what he wants for morning nourishment.
10. Realize that wholesome companionship with children of the same age can be pleasant.
11. Do not expect as high a standard of behavior in the evening as during the morning.
12. Give approval for anything done well. Do not make an issue of failures.
13. Avoid talking about the child's condition in his presence. It is confusing and upsetting to the child.
14. Try to arrange for each child to have adequate attention. The presence of his parents, help from a recreational therapist, celebration of his birthday by means of parties, and individual recognition by a charge nurse on each tour of duty all contribute toward this goal.
15. When behavior problems do occur, try to analyze the cause and prevent it from occurring again.

In addition to these general principles some special attention needs to be directed toward the toddler and the infant. Much of the communication with these children is on a nonverbal level. An infant reacts to facial expressions, tones of voice, and the way he is handled. Abrupt and sudden movements frighten him. A more deliberate approach is necessary with infants. The infant over 6 months of age (and sometimes younger) distinguishes between strange and familiar people. On admission to the hospital it is well to let the mother undress the infant and the toddler while the nurse stands near the mother. The nurse should not make the mistake of taking the infant quickly from the mother's arms. She should let the infant or toddler get used to her before she tries to hold him and cuddle him. On the other hand, an infant who goes easily to other people must have had very pleasant contacts with people other than his parents.

The presence of a favorite toy such as a doll or teddy bear is often very helpful to the child. If the nurse is caring for a toddler and wishes, for example, to change a colostomy dressing on the toddler, she might put a dressing on the teddy bear, show it to the child, then gently remove the teddy bear's dressing and place a fresh dressing on the teddy bear prior to changing the child's dressing. The teddy bear is a live animate person as far as the toddler and preschooler are concerned. If the nurse abuses the teddy bear, it is like abusing him (the child).

The young child is often accused of negativism. A withdrawal or refusal to do something may indicate fear. Other times it may indicate his desire for independence. To walk around (rather than being carried) is still a novelty to a toddler. He feels himself a person separate from his mother or father. Let the toddler do as much for himself as possible. Often he will eat more if allowed to feed himself, even though he spills a lot. Avoid issues and conflicts with the toddler by making his necessary routines such as preparing for nap time and bathing pleasant and fun to do.

The child who is hospitalized for a period of time with rheumatic fever may be depressed in the early morning when he awakens. This is a difficult time of day. The nurse should not expect him to be responsive to her friendly overtures when she enters the room in the morning. Such attentions as washing the child's hands and face, lifting him up in bed, and making him physically comfortable let the child know the nurse's concern and affection for him. By the time the child has had his breakfast and then his bath he may be able to respond to another child if one is brought into his room to play cards or some game. The child who feels thoroughly secure with the nurse may even show hostility toward her by the middle of the morning.

During visiting hours or when the child's parents are present, the child enjoys having ''his'' nurse come to see his parents and speak with them. He also likes to show his parents his nurse.

The nurse at all times must remember that talking is part of social behavior, and during the time the child is ill he does not feel particularly sociable. For this reason a good deal of the communication between the nurse and the child, no matter what the child's age, is on a nonverbal level. At the time the child is talkative it is time for him to be discharged because he is well.

Because it is difficult for a preschool child to express his feelings about treatments or operations that he has had, it is necessary that the nurse provide him with some means of nonverbal communication so that he can express his feelings—perhaps through the use of clay, crayon and pencil, doctor's and nurse's kits, or other types of play material. The older child can verbalize his feelings sometimes, and then again sometimes it is rather hard for him to express his feelings verbally. Two children of a

similar age in a hospital will often talk to each other about their experiences when they do not feel like talking about them to an adult.

In understanding a child's feelings as well as his physical condition, it is essential for the nurse to be observant of the child's facial expression, his eyes, his posture, what he does with play materials, and all his activity. The child who begins to eat better and is more active is a child who is feeling better physically. The majority of children act the way they feel, and a notation should always be made on every shift as to the general behavior of the child since it is one indication of his physical condition.

The exception, of course, is the good little child, whom everyone believes is no trouble. Actually such quietness should be a cause for greater concern than the aggressiveness and misbehavior of another child. We do not know what the child is thinking when he is so quiet. In her encounters the nurse should take considerable pains to try to learn more about the quiet child's adjustment.

General hygiene
Mealtime

Children. The sick child does not have as good an appetite as the well child; therefore psychological aspects of eating (p. 204) are of particular importance. During illness and fever there is an increased need for calories and protein due to the increased metabolism and tissue destruction.

On the pediatric unit the ''Routine Day of the Child'' should be posted so that hospital personnel may see it and know the times the child's meals are served. This helps nursing personnel to prepare him for meals. At noon and in the evening, personnel should go to lunch and dinner prior to the patients' mealtime so there will be enough personnel on hand to help and supervise all the children. The medical staff should be aware of the child's schedule so that medical procedures and venipunctures can be done at another time. Pain and discomfort are not conducive to enjoyment of mealtime; in fact, they may not only take away the appetite of the child who is in pain but also affect the appetite of other children who hear him cry.

Preparation for mealtime helps children to be

in a state of readiness to eat. In the morning the child should be offered the urinal or bedpan and then have his face and hands washed. Combing and brushing hair before breakfast is more consistent with the pattern of living at home. In addition, some children may like to brush their teeth prior to breakfast. The lower bedclothes should be dry and comfortable, and the upper ones sometimes need a little straightening. The head of the bed should be rolled up. If the child is in a crib, a small sturdy tray can be put in position for him.

At noon and at night when meals are served, again the child should be made ready first. Toys should be put away, toilet needs should receive attention, and children should be made physically comfortable.

Every effort should be made to have mealtime pleasant. Children should be taken into the playroom for mealtime when possible. Company with meals is enjoyable; also, being in an attractive room, with table and chairs of the right size, adds to the comfort of the child.

If a nurse sits at the table and eats with children, she can supervise them at the same time. She can also help to make the mealtime sociable. She can see that small servings are given and that the needed seconds of some foods receive prompt attention. If a child dislikes one food such as his cereal, perhaps another cereal can be substituted. She should avoid nagging the children but should let them see that she expects them to eat. Sometimes, foods children can pick up with their fingers—like oranges cut in fourths, whole apples, or bananas—can be eaten more readily by toddlers than a food for which they have to use a spoon. The emphasis is not neatness but enjoyment of food.

Sweetened fruit juices and simple cookies might be offered the children in the middle of the morning and afternoon. Sometimes chocolate milk or warm cocoa at night before bedtime is a diversion as well as a method of getting children to take more fluids.

Infants. (For the technique of bottle-feeding see p. 68.) If for any reason the infant cannot be held in the nurse's lap for feeding, then the head of his bed should be elevated to lessen the danger of aspiration. Feeding bottles should never be propped, nor should an older infant be handed his bottle to hold while the nurse leaves the room. If the infant is interested in holding his bottle completely, then it is time to get him interested in holding a cup instead. In no case should the nurse leave the infant alone with his bottle.

When the infant has solid foods as well as his bottle, he should be offered the solid foods first, then his bottle. As the infant grows, he needs solid food more than milk. At 1 year of age, if he is taking adequate amounts of solid food, he cannot possibly consume a whole quart of milk a day.

When the nurse is uncertain how well the infant takes cereal, she should make the cereal very thin with milk. The small infant tends to suck the cereal off the end of the spoon. He cannot handle a very thick cereal. Solid foods such as cereal, fruit, and vegetables should be offered prior to the formula. He may accept them better when he is hungry.

Some children are still on the bottle even when they are 2 or 3 years of age. When the infant is acutely ill, no effort is made to change his method of taking fluids. That can be done when he is well again. On the other hand, a toddler is sometimes admitted with severe anemia because the mother gave him mostly milk in a bottle and insufficient solid food. It is necessary to encourage these toddlers to eat solid foods. If the toddler awakens at nighttime, water or fruit juice should be given instead of milk to make sure the child will be hungry enough to accept his breakfast.

Bathing

Purposes. Bathing has several purposes, whether it is for an infant or a child. It is a time when the nurse and child can get better acquainted. Also, the bath furnishes the nurse a splendid time to observe the child. The bath stimulates circulation and certainly provides an excellent opportunity for the infant to get exercise. The child has the entire attention of the nurse during the procedure. She can easily let the child see her interest in him. The relationship of the child and the nurse should be strengthened during this time together. The nurse wishes the child to be clean, but that is not the child's desire; his interest is in the en-

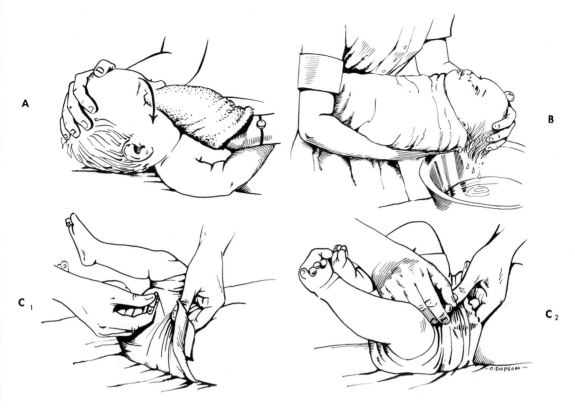

Fig. 11-3. A, Bathing the infant. Note that the nurse is wiping from the inner canthus outward. Infant is not undressed until the face and hair have been washed. **B,** Nurse uses the palm of her hand rather than her fingertips in shampooing the infant's head. This is more soothing. **C,** Diapering the infant with a contour or square diaper. Diaper should fit snugly around the waist of the infant. Nurse holds her hand between the infant's skin and the diaper to prevent sticking the infant with the pin.

joyment of the water and the procedure. That he does enjoy bath time is important in the formation of his attitude toward cleanliness and bathing.

Special points. The hospital tradition is to give baths in the morning, but ambulatory children and selected other children may be more benefited by a bath in the evening. The older child can be bathed in the same manner as the adult. The nurse needs to ensure the privacy of the patient, especially the adolescent, during bath time. Many children, even in the preschool age, are sensitive to exposure of that part of the body that is usually covered by clothing. The child should be well covered by a bath blanket during the procedure so that he does not feel unduly exposed. If the room is cool, he may need two bath blankets over him or the bath

blanket plus his bed blanket. The younger children enjoy putting their feet and hands into the basin of water, and almost all children enjoy a good back rub after the bath.

Children who are old enough and well enough like to help bathe themselves. In that case the nurse can arrange the bath equipment and then return to the bedside to bathe the child's back and buttocks and give him a back rub, the same as for the other children.

In bathing infants the exact procedure followed varies with the child and with his condition. A soft washcloth should be used. In general the face, ears, and hair should be washed before the infant is undressed to avoid the possibility of chilling him. In undressing the infant the diaper can be unpinned but left in place until the genitals are to be bathed. The upper part of the body (both anterior and posterior surfaces) can be bathed and the baby's undershirt replaced; then the legs are washed and finally the diaper area. If the infant is small, the nurse may find it easier to soap him with her hands instead of using a washcloth. First she soaps the neck and then, with long movements, each arm. She can then rinse these areas with a washcloth and wipe. The chest and other parts of the body can be done likewise. The infant responds better to long stroking motions than he does to short quick ones. If the infant is large, his body can be bathed in the same way as that of an older child, but the shirt should be put on after the upper part of the body has been bathed to avoid letting the child become cold.

Some small infants may enjoy being soaped all over and then placed in a bath basin to have the soap rinsed off. This can only be done, of course, if the room is warm and the infant's physical condition permits.

Clothing

Infants and children who are acutely ill need clothing that can be easily slipped on and off with a minimum of motion and irritation to them. Although by tradition hospital gowns are white, might not a soft pastel color be more relaxing and soothing to a child?

For children who are not in acute physical distress, pretty pajamas should be supplied. It is necessary that the cloth be durable so that the pajamas can stand the wear and tear of frequent washing and ironing. In summer, short pajamas are more comfortable than long ones. The ambulatory child should have play clothes or other suitable clothing.

Clothing for the preschool child should be made in such a way that the child can easily put it on and take it off by himself. Openings in the front or side rather than in the back are conducive to self-help and may add to the child's sense of achievement.

Different-sized undershirts should be available for the infant. In place of a nightgown, a flannellike bed jacket, which ties in the back and thus keeps his chest covered, is suitable for infants. A bed jacket does not need changing each time the infant's diaper is wet, since the bed jacket reaches only to the waist.

If hospital funds are not available for suitable clothing for children, sometimes women's clubs or other organizations will help. Clothing for hospital children may be regarded as a special project.

Sleep and rest

Rest and sleep slow metabolism, relax muscles, and promote emotional stability.

Rest hour. Rest hour is an important treatment in helping toward recovery. Toys and play materials should have been put away prior to nap time. The doll or teddy bear that the child holds can be patted by the nurse and put down comfortably so the child can see that it, too, is resting. Bedpans and urinals need to be offered. Sticky hands need washing or wiping off with a wet washcloth. Drawsheets should be tightened and crumbs should be brushed out. A light blanket can be placed over the toddler and upper bedclothing adjusted on the older children. A back rub and skin care to bed patients aid relaxation. The room should be darkened but well ventilated.

In order to see that rest hour is maintained a nurse needs to supervise the children in the pediatric unit. After 1 or 2 days of being quiet in rest hour, children often fall asleep at that time.

The infant under 1 year of age usually has a morning and an afternoon nap. Information given by the child's parents when he is admitted will let the nurse know his particular habits.

Night sleep. At night the routine of getting the children ready for sleep is the same as that used for rest hour, except that sometimes quiet music is helpful and suggestive of rest. In addition, teeth should be brushed and hands and face should at least be wiped with a warm washcloth. Some children like to say a prayer as they do at home.

There should be a definite time established for lights to be turned off in the rooms, and a dim light should be used in the hall. Noise should be kept at a minimum. After getting the children ready for the night a nurse needs to make rounds frequently to make sure the children are comfortable and to meet any special needs they may have.

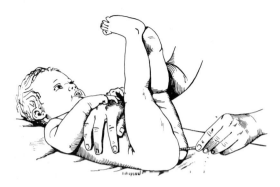

Fig. 11-4. Taking rectal temperature. For safety one hand of the nurse is holding the thermometer while the other is on the infant so he will not turn over suddenly.

Nursing procedures
Taking vital signs

Temperature. Rectal temperature is usually measured for infants and children up to 6 years of age, at which age an oral temperature is taken. As children object to intrusive procedures, some thought might be given as to the feasibility of taking axillary temperatures of children who are over 2 years of age until they can hold an oral thermometer in the mouth and under the tongue.

In taking the rectal temperature of an infant, the thermometer should be well lubricated. The infant may be on his side or back. The nurse separates the buttocks, sees the anus clearly, and then gently inserts the thermometer. One hand should be kept on the thermometer while the other hand is placed over the hips of the infant so that he will not turn suddenly and possibly break the thermometer. As long as the nurse has a firm hold on the thermometer, it does not matter if the infant waves and kicks his legs.

In taking an axillary temperature, the bulb of the thermometer should be placed in the axilla of the child, anterior to the arm. There seem to be varied opinions concerning the accuracy of axillary temperatures, as well as the length of time required for its measurement. Nursing research appears to be needed. The American Academy of Pediatrics recommends that the thermometer be left in place for 1½ minutes (Committee on Fetus and Newborn).

An axillary temperature reading is commonly used in caring for premature infants, for infants and children who are dyspneic, and for those with diarrhea or abnormal pathology of the rectum. Hospitals vary in their routine in the nursery for newborn infants as to whether an axillary or a rectal temperature is taken.

Pulse and respirations. In infants and toddlers under 2 years of age both the pulse and respirations vary in accordance with whether the child is sleeping, crying or awake. Sometimes the hospital routine is not to take the pulse and respirations of infants unless they are specifically ordered, as they would be, for example, if the patient was an infant who had an abnormal condition of the heart. If the infant's pulse and respirations are to be taken, it is best for the nurse to take them prior to taking the temperature since that procedure, if the infant is sleeping, may awaken him and then it will be more difficult to take his pulse and respirations.

In certain conditions it is important for the nurse to describe the quality of the pulse: in severe illness, in the immediate postoperative period, and in any case in which the child has an abnormal heart condition. At any time when the nurse taking a child's pulse finds that it is irregular or weak, this fact should be reported. If irregular, the pulse should be counted for a full minute. Any great change in either the pulse or respirations of a child should be recorded in the bedside notes and reported to the physician.

Blood pressure. For taking the blood pressure of a child the nurse should first be sure to get a cuff of the right size. Too wide a cuff may give a low reading and too narrow a cuff would give a high reading. In general the width of the cuff should be two thirds of the length of the upper arm. There should be cuffs of several sizes on every pediatric unit.

Before his blood pressure is taken the child should see and handle the equipment. The nurse can explain in simple terms what she is going to do.

In taking the blood pressure the nurse should remember several significant points. The child should be in a comfortable, relaxed position. The blood pressure is higher if the child is sitting rather than lying down. The correct-sized

Table 11-1. Average pulse rates at different ages*

Age	Lower limits of normal		Average		Upper limits of normal	
Newborn	70		120		170	
1-11 months	80		120		160	
2 years	80		110		130	
4 years	80		100		120	
6 years	75		100		115	
8 years	70		90		110	
10 years	70		90		110	
	Girls	**Boys**	**Girls**	**Boys**	**Girls**	**Boys**
12 years	70	65	90	85	110	105
14 years	65	60	85	80	105	100
16 years	60	55	80	75	100	95
18 years	55	50	75	70	95	90

*From Kaplan, S.: The cardiovascular system. In Nelson, W. E., editor: Textbook of pediatrics, ed. 9, Philadelphia, 1969, W. B. Saunders Co.

Table 11-2. Average blood pressures of children*

Age	Systolic	Diastolic
4	85	60
5	87	60
6	90	60
7	92	62
8	95	62
9	98	64
10	100	65
11	105	65
12	108	67
13	110	67
14	112	80
15	115	72
16	118	75

*From Kaplan, S.: The cardiovascular system. In Nelson, W. E., editor: Textbook of pediatrics, ed. 9, Philadelphia, 1969, W. B. Saunders Co.

cuff should be placed snugly around the child's arm, about 2.5 cm. above the antecubital crease.

The manometer should be on a level surface so that the observer's eye can be on the level of the meniscus of the mercury column.

The lower arm should not be hyperextended but slightly bent, or the diastolic reading may be falsely low. The nurse should locate the artery by palpation, then close the air valve and inflate the cuff. The air valve should then be released gradually so the mercury column will descend slowly. The systolic pressure is judged by the first sound heard and the diastolic pressure by the last sound heard. The air valve should be opened, the cuff deflated, and the blood pressure taken a second time to assure an accurate reading. After the blood pressure has been measured and the cuff removed, gentle massage will add to the child's comfort.

Crib making

For infants. The mattress should be protected with a rubber or plastic covering. The bottom sheet should be sufficiently long so that it can be tucked under the head and foot of the mattress. Sometimes fitted sheets are available. For practical purposes it is wise to have a rubber and cotton drawsheet at the head of the bed, over the bottom sheet, so the latter need not be changed if the infant drools or vomits. The rubber with the cotton drawsheet over it should be tucked under the mattress at the head of the bed. It should cover approximately one third of the head of the bed. If the infant is not yet in the crawling stage, a pad can be placed in the center of the bed under the infant's buttocks. If the infant is crawling, it is a waste of linen to put a pad in the bed.

Each infant should have his own top bed blanket or quilt. This is placed over him when he is sleeping and resting. The blanket should be comfortably tucked around the infant rather than tucked under the mattress. Top sheets and spreads can be omitted unless a pretty spread is used to cover an empty crib.

When the nurse makes the crib with the infant in it, she may move the infant to the farther side of the crib, make up the side of the crib nearest her, raise the side rail (testing to make sure it is secure), and cross to the other side of the bed. She can then lift the infant onto the clean side and complete the bed.

For children. The entire mattress for the child needs to be protected with a covering used in the same way as in the infant crib. Whether a drawsheet or rubber is used over the center of the bed (the same as in an adult's bed) depends on the child. If the bed is likely to become soiled in the center, whether from dressings or from other sources, the bed should have a drawsheet and rubber. Many times a crawling infant or toddler in a crib moves around and, if he soils the sheet, it may not be at the center. For this reason a drawsheet placed routinely on a crib is a waste of linen. The bottom sheet has to be changed anyway.

In general top bed clothing (sheet, blanket, and spread) is used for children 3 years of age or older. The toddler has a blanket placed over him when he is resting, just as the infant does.

Administration of medications

Drug dosage. There are several formulas to estimate the dose for a child, such as Clark's rule,* but Shirkey believes that if the surface area is used, there is greater accuracy.† He gives two suggested formulas. The first assumes that the adult dose is known and that the average surface area of the adult is 1.7 square meters:

$$\frac{\text{Surface area of patient (in m.}^2) \times \text{Adult dose}}{1.7} =$$

Approximate dose for patient

The second formula assumes that the dose of a given drug per square meter is known:

Surface area of patient (in m.^{2}) $\times$ Dose per m.^{2} =

Approximate dose for patient

---

*Clark's rule: Patient's weight in pounds $\times$ Adult dose $\div$ 150 = Approximate dose for patient.

†Shirkey, H.: The dose of drugs. In Vaughn, V. C., III, and McKay, R. J., editors: Nelson's textbook of pediatrics, ed. 10, Philadelphia, 1975, W. B. Saunders Co. (Chapter 5).

Nelson's Textbook of Pediatrics (Vaughn and McKay, 1975, p. 1713) lists the commonly used drugs for children together with the dosages per square meter and per kilogram of body weight. This can be used as a reference, as can *Pediatric Therapy* (Shirkey, 1975, p. 1187).

Before administering a medication the nurse should know the desired action and possible side effects. Medicine cards should be checked against the doctor's original order to make sure the dose was copied correctly and also to ascertain whether the order for the medicine was changed. If the medication order is not fully understood by the nurse, she should ask the physician about it. Except in an emergency situation, all orders for medications should be written. This avoids the possibility of any misunderstanding.

Oral administration. In pouring medications the nurse should read the label of the medicine before she takes it from the shelf, reread the label before she pours it, and then read it again as she is replacing the medicine on the shelf. If there are special notations on the bottle, such as "Shake well" or the expiration date, these should be noted and followed. Certain drugs have directions for refrigeration.

If the medication is a liquid, the medicine should be poured from the side opposite the label. The bottle should be wiped off with a paper towel before it is replaced. Liquid vitamins should be measured by the dropper in the bottle and then placed in a medicine cup, the same as other medications.

Medications should be given with accuracy. For an oral medication of less than 5 ml., a minim measuring glass should be used. Scored pills can be cut but not unscored ones such as aspirin.

Medicines should not be mixed with food or placed in an infant's formula. The infant or child may not finish the food, in which case all the medicine will not be taken; also, the medicine may change the flavor of the food and cause the child to dislike the food.

When the nurse administers medications, she should take with her two different kinds of fruit juice, straws, and drinking cups (possibly paper ones). After the child takes his medicine he can have a choice as to which juice he wishes and

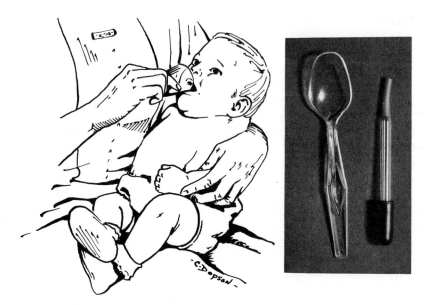

Fig. 11-5. Oral medications (including vitamin preparations) can be given to the infant in a medicine cup, a small spoon, or by a medicine dropper that has a rubber tip extending ½ inch beyond the glass dropper. (Courtesy Medical College of Georgia, Augusta, Ga.)

whether he wishes to drink from a straw or cup.

If the nurse does not know the child, she should check his identification band before giving him his medicine. Her approach in presenting the medicine to the child should be a positive one. She should let him believe that she expects him to take it. The infant (and sometimes the toddler) should be held in the nurse's lap. In holding him, the nurse should place one of the infant's arms behind her and hold his other hand with her left hand. She holds the medicine cup with her right hand. Vitamins and liquids the infant can drink out of the cup. He often shows less resistance to this than to medicine that is put on a spoon. Most of the medicines (especially the antibiotics) are rather bland in flavor or are sweet tasting. They are not objectionable in odor and taste. An exception to this is phenobarbital, which is bitter.

Before administering any sulfa drug, it is wise for the nurse to see if the child has voided since the last time it was given.

Good hydration with adequate renal function is important in a child taking a sulfa drug; therefore fluids should be offered frequently to help prevent the complications of crystalluria, hematuria, and renal shutdown.

Intramuscular injections. Intramuscular injections are common procedures given by nurses. In infants and young children the sites of preference are the vastus lateralis muscle (the midlateral muscle of the thigh) and the rectus femoris muscle (the midanterior muscle of the thigh). The gluteal muscles are not well developed in infants, and an injection given in the buttocks could inadvertently be injected in a layer of subcutaneous fat; moreover there is danger of injuring a nerve, especially the sciatic nerve. Permanent disabilities such as paralysis of the leg can occur from injury to the sciatic nerve. In older children the upper outer quadrant of the gluteal muscle can be used.

In administering an intramuscular injection, a 2 cc. syringe with a No. 22-gauge needle is used. For an infant or a thin child a 1-inch needle is long enough. No more than 2 cc. should ever be injected in one site. If a dose of less than 5 minims is going to be injected, for accuracy, a tuberculin syringe should be used rather than a 2 cc. syringe.

There are several methods to lessen discomfort in injecting the medication. The nurse should use a sharp needle (without a burr), allow the antiseptic that was used to cleanse the site of the injection to dry, make counterpressure with the thumb and finger on each side of the injection site, allow the solution to go into the muscle slowly, rapidly withdraw the needle after the injection is given, and rub the area with a dry cotton ball afterward.

The nurse should explain to the child what she is going to do and that it will hurt for a minute but that is all. A second nurse may be needed to hold the toddler or younger child for safety's sake.

To avoid having the child thereafter associate the discomfort of injections with a particular nurse, the latter should speak pleasantly to the child, give him play materials, or do something that is cheerful before leaving him. The more skillful the nurse is in giving the injection, the less discomfort the child will have.

Eye instillations. The nurse should draw up into the eyedropper only the amount of solution she needs, since excess solution has to be discarded. The eye should be gently wiped from the inner canthus to the outer canthus by means of a cotton ball moistened with saline solution before drops are instilled. With one finger of her left hand the nurse pulls down the lower lid. Pressure should not be put on soft tissue in pulling down the lid but rather on bony structure. With her right hand she holds the eyedropper in a horizontal position over the bridge of the nose and allows a drop of solution to fall on the center of the everted lower lid. She can then repeat the procedure for the other eye, using opposite hands. If the patient is an older child, the nurse can ask him to look up while she instills the drops.

It may be necessary in instilling drops in the eye of the newborn to use a piece of gauze to help hold the lower lid down because the vernix is so slippery. The nurse should avoid letting the solution drop directly on the cornea.

Nose instillations. For an infant or young child who has a thick nasal discharge, often the physician prescribes use of nose drops prior to the child's feeding. The older infant may need to be restrained for this. If gentleness is used and if the toddler is allowed to hold a cotton ball or a cotton applicator and/or help with the procedure, he is usually cooperative.

Each nostril should first be cleansed gently

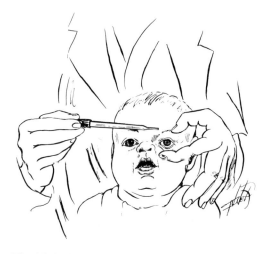

Fig. 11-6. Nurse putting eyedrops in child's eye. The drop should fall on the everted lower lid. Nurse's thumb and finger rest on the bony orifice around the eye.

with a cotton applicator to remove crusts and dried secretions; then a pillow or folded blanket should be placed under the child's shoulders so his head is tilted back. As the nurse instills the drops of the solution in the right nostril, she should hold the child's head to the right side for a few minutes; then she does likewise for the left nostril. If the nurse does not turn the child's head to the side on which the drops are instilled, the solution may slide directly through the nose and into the back of the throat.

After instilling the drops the nurse should wait a few minutes, then use a rubber bulb ear syringe to see if she can suction any secretions and thus relieve the child's breathing during feeding time. It is difficult for the child to eat if he cannot breathe through his nose.

Suctioning with a rubber bulb ear syringe. In using a rubber bulb ear syringe to suction it is important for the nurse to first deflate the syringe, then introduce the tip of the syringe into the nostril or cavity to be irrigated. The syringe quickly becomes inflated again by itself, sucking secretions in as it inflates. It should be withdrawn from the cavity, emptied of secretions, wiped on waste tissues, and reintroduced. This procedure should be repeated as often as necessary. It is less traumatic to tissues than use of a rubber catheter attached to a suction machine (Fig. 11-7).

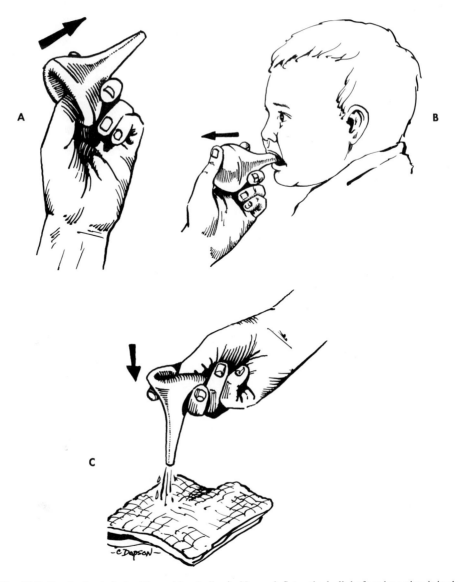

Fig. 11-7. Suctioning infant with a rubber bulb. **A,** Nurse deflates the bulb before inserting it in the infant's nose or mouth. **B,** With tip of the bulb in the infant's mouth the nurse is releasing her thumb to aspirate mucus. **C,** Nurse deflates the bulb to expel the mucus.

Temperature-reducing measures. When a nurse discovers that the child to whom she is assigned has a temperature of 100° F., she should retake the temperature in an hour to see if it has risen higher. Often children's temperatures rise quickly. A physician should be notified if the temperature continues to rise because there is a possibility that the infant or child may have febrile convulsions.

There are several nursing measures that

sometimes aid in reducing fever. If an infant or child has an elevated temperature, some of his bedclothing might be removed. Clothing such as the infant's undershirt can also be taken off; however, in removal of clothing and bedclothing the warmth of the child's feet needs to be felt. If they are cold (and often they are), a small blanket might be put around them. The child's room should be cool, and fluids should be offered frequently. Since the child feels hot from his elevated temperature, usually these are accepted readily. If he does not care for one fluid, another should be tried.

An icecap might be placed on an older child's head, and a diaper or towel wrung out of cold water could be folded and placed around the younger child's head like a turban. The head of an infant is the first part of his body to get warm and the last to cool.

A tepid sponge bath (temperature about 100° F.) may be effective in reducing an elevated temperature. Gentle friction to the part sponged helps to bring the heat to the surface where it can be evaporated. A cotton bath blanket can be placed over the child during the bath. The child's temperature should be taken a half hour after the sponge bath to see if the temperature has fallen. Cold sponges are avoided since they may cause vasocontriction, cyanosis, and then an elevation of temperature.

Wrapping the child in a cool wet sheet, in such a manner that no two body surfaces are touching, is another manner of reducing elevated temperatures. The sheet should be removed in 20 minutes and gentle friction applied.

Aspirin or acetaminophen (Tempra) drops may be ordered. When oral aspirin is given to an infant, the tablet should be placed in one spoon and crushed and then a little water added to the spoon with the aspirin. This should be stirred with a second spoon and given to the infant.

After the medication has been given, the infant should be offered sterile water from a bottle.

NURSING CARE IN SPECIAL SITUATIONS
Child in an oxygen tent and/or with high humidity

Young children may receive oxygen if they have respiratory infections, congestive heart failure, or postoperative respiratory difficulties. After a bronchoscopy or a tracheotomy a child may be in oxygen with high humidity. Oxygen supersaturated with water helps to loosen tenacious secretions. It helps to relieve inflammation and edema of respiratory passages and can be used for relieving anoxia.

In the crib of the child who will receive oxygen a rubber or plastic covering should be used over the mattress. Next to the bottom sheet should be a cotton blanket. Also, a cotton blanket should be substituted for the top sheet. Bedding becomes moist from the humidity, so a cotton blanket is more comfortable for the child.

The infant and child would be comfortably warm if the sewing room of a hospital could make flannelette pajamas with feet in them and with the end of the sleeves sewed together. Extremities of little children get cold early, and it is a problem to keep them covered.

Before the child is placed in the tent, the tent should be flushed with oxygen; 10 to 20 liters per minute for 5 minutes or possibly less should be adequate. The oxygen content of the tent should be analyzed. The physician should always specify the concentration he wishes. Usually the concentration desired is not over 40%.

In order to maintain the desired concentration the oxygen content of the tent should be tested at 4-hour intervals. To get a 40% concentration in a Croupette the oxygen flow should be 5 to 8 liters per minute; in a tent for larger children it should be 10 to 12 liters per minute (Smith).

If the toddler or older infant has a particular pet toy, this should go into the oxygen tent with the child. It is frightening not to be able to breathe well, and the tent itself may alarm the small child. It is new and unfamiliar to him. Once the child in respiratory distress has been in the tent for a while, he often falls asleep. Respirations should become slower. The nurse should return frequently to see how he is and note his color and rate of respiration. Also it may be reassuring to the toddler to see a familiar person when he is in this new environment.

In caring for the child the nurse should offer him fluids, change his position, and change wet clothing or bedding about every 2 hours. At the same time she can see if both the flow of oxygen and the humidity are regulated correctly. Distilled water is added to the water jar of the Croupette, and ice is added to the container if necessary. The types of oxygen tent used may vary somewhat. The nurse should make sure

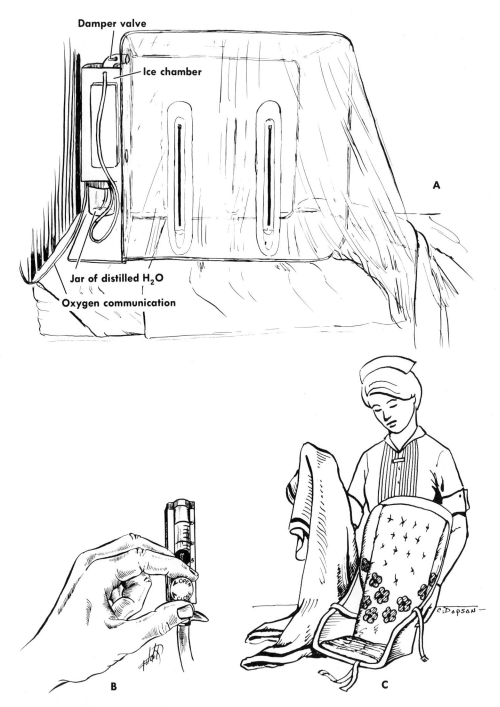

Fig. 11-8. Croupette. **A,** Nurse fills the ice chamber, puts distilled water in the special jar for it, opens the damper valve, and connects the tent to the oxygen outlet. **B,** Next, before the infant is placed in the tent, the nurse turns on the oxygen and makes sure that all openings in the tent are closed. **C,** Nurse adjusts the blanket on the infant carrier. (Infant carrier is used for dyspneic infants. Carrier is placed in Croupette; then infant is placed in carrier in tent.)

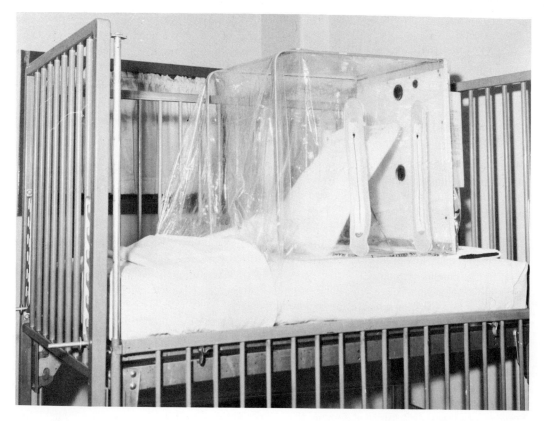

Fig. 11-9. Croupette with infant seat. (Courtesy Medical College of Georgia, Augusta, Ga.)

she understands the regulation of the tent being used for a particular child before she assumes responsibility for his care.

If the infant is having dyspnea, it is better to feed him while he is in the tent. When the bed is made, it is best to get a second person to assist. This is easier for both the infant and his nurse.

As the child's nurse visits him at the beginning of each shift, she should note both his color and the quality and rate of respiration first of all; then she should look at the rate of oxygen flow and actually place her hand at the inlet opening for oxygen in the tent to see that it is coming through all right. The temperature of the tent needs investigation. If it has become warm, the child's respirations will have increased and the tent will be lacking in effectiveness as a treatment. Regulation of the temperature may need immediate attention before the nurse fusses with changing the child's linen and

bathing him. That the child's position be conducive to his comfort and breathing is essential. An infant is often placed in an infant carrier since an upright position makes breathing easier. An older child may rest well with a pillow. In that case the pillow should be kept away from both the inlet and the outlet opening of the tent.

When the physician enters the child's room to examine the child, the nurse, wishing to please the physician, may turn back the entire front of the tent canopy. This is a sad mistake. If the physician cannot examine the child through the opening provided in the tent, it is better to remove the child from the tent and quickly put the tent canopy down so the oxygen concentration will not be lost. Even so, every time the tent is opened the oxygen flow should be increased for a few minutes afterward in order to maintain the desired oxygen concentration. Oxygen therapy is just as important as a medication to the child given orally or intramuscularly.

When oxygen therapy is discontinued, the tent should be thoroughly washed and cleansed; otherwise it could act as a reservoir of infection.

Preoperative nursing care
General care

The psychological aspects of preoperative nursing care are discussed on p. 415. This section will be devoted to physical aspects of the child's care.

Prior to operation the nurse should see that a specimen of urine is sent to the laboratory for routine analysis and that an operative permit is signed by the parents or guardian of the child. Depending on the child's age, the nurse may need to assist the physician when he takes blood for blood chemistries on the child. Also, the nurse should be present when the physician examines girls of school age. The top bedclothes should be turned back and a cotton blanket or sheet placed over the child. The nurse should place a towel over the child's chest when the physician examines the child's abdomen. If a schoolage child is having elective surgery, the nurse has time to teach him how to cough and deep-breathe so he will know what to do postoperatively. The child should practice this several times. If he is going to have chest surgery, the nurse can show him how she will support the operative area with her hands when he coughs.

The patient's nutritional status and general condition are checked carefully by the physician. Every effort is made to see that an infant is in electrolyte balance prior to surgery. Frequently a cutdown intravenous infusion is begun in an infant just prior to any major surgery. A vein is kept open in case the infant needs parenteral fluids (as he usually does) during an operation. It is this attention to fluid balance that aids in the prevention of shock.

If gastric suction is going to be used, a nasogastric tube may be passed through the child's nose and into his stomach before he leaves the unit for surgery. Gastric suction during the operation lessens the possibility of aspiration and of vomiting and also lessens distention.

The nurse must be sure to report any sign of respiratory infection in the child, such as a nasal discharge, a cough, or either one combined with an elevated temperature. If the surgery is elective, the surgeon will postpone the operation. If a child develops a rash of any nature, this too should be reported. The child may have a communicable disease.

In some hospitals the anesthetist checks the child's mouth to see if there are any loose teeth—a condition that should be known prior to the operation.

Immediate preoperative care

In the immediate preoperative care on the day of surgery, the nurse makes sure the child is clean (including the umbilicus) and that toenails and fingernails have received any necessary attention, that the child has some form of identification on his arm or leg, that he voids prior to surgery, and that he receives his preoperative medication on time. If the child is wearing fingernail polish, it should be removed from the index finger so that the anesthetist can note the color there if he wishes.

Fluids and food are usually withheld from children for about 6 hours prior to surgery. The infant may be allowed to have a 2 A.M. feeding on the day of the operation. Then fluids should be omitted if he is going to have an early-morning operation. Nurses are so accustomed to adult patients having nothing by mouth after midnight that they often forget to ask if the early-morning feeding of the infant may be given. The infant cannot tolerate long periods without fluids.

If the operation is scheduled early in the morning, the child's bath may be given the previous evening. When the preoperative medication is given at 6 or 7 A.M., the child should be asked to void and then be allowed to go back to sleep. Awakening a child at 5 or 6 A.M. to be bathed before his operation at 8 A.M. does not seem particularly kind. If the operation is not until late in the morning, the child's bath might be given while the other children are having breakfast. This helps to distract his attention from mealtime.

When the preoperative medication is given, the nurse should try to have the child's room quiet and reduce stimuli in general. Venetian blinds might be closed to darken the room. Conditions should be conducive to the child's going to sleep. The child can be asked to void after the medication is given so that he will not be disturbed again.

Postoperative nursing care
Immediate postoperative care

Immediate postoperative care by the nurse includes attentions to the patient himself, any special equipment involved, and medications that may be ordered.

Position. Whether the child returns to the recovery room or to the unit following his operation, the nurse should turn him on his side to minimize the possibility of aspiration of vomitus. There are certain common exceptions to this rule: For example, the child with generalized peritonitis is usually ordered to be in semi-Fowler's or Fowler's position. Also, if a child has had cardiac surgery, the surgeon may specify a particular position in which he wishes the child to be placed. If a patient with chest surgery has any difficulty breathing, he should not be on the untreated side. He should either be on his back or be turned toward the operative side so that the good side of his chest has a chance to expand. A child who has had a brain tumor removed should lie on the unaffected side; pressure on the operative site should be avoided. After a tonsillectomy the child should be placed in a prone position with a pillow under his chest and upper abdomen to prevent possible aspiration of vomitus. The infant has a weak cough reflex; aspiration of vomitus could very easily occur if the infant is on his back.

Care of special equipment. If the child needs any special equipment such as Foley catheter or gastric or chest suction, it should be connected at once with the aid of the physician. Drainage tubes should be well secured, especially with toddlers. Any drainage bottles should be placed in a special holder or fastened to the bed in a holder where there is no danger of its being kicked over on the floor.

Infants and toddlers who have had endotracheal anesthesia are often placed in a Croupette for 24 hours so that they can have cool, moist air. Some edema of the trachea may result from use of the endotracheal tube, and breathing in an atmosphere of cool air is helpful.

The infant or child might have an intravenous infusion as he goes to the recovery room or returns to his unit. (Refer to p. 301 for a description of the responsibilities of the nurse in caring for a child with an intravenous infusion.) After operation on the chest the total amount of fluids prescribed for an 8-hour or 24-hour period is usually less than it might be for the same child if he had another type of operation. The physician wishes to prevent the possibility of pulmonary overload and congestive heart failure.

Observations. Vital signs are taken every 15 minutes until they are stable. (See Tables 11-1 and 11-2 for average values of blood pressure, pulse, and respiration of children at different ages.) In addition, the nurse should note the child's color and the character of the pulse and respiration.

In an infant the rate of the pulse, the character of the respirations, and the color should be particularly watched, as they are excellent indications of his condition. The nervous system is immature in an infant, so the vital centers controlling respiration and temperature are not well developed; hence there is irregularity in breathing and in body temperature. Also, since his metabolism is more rapid than an older child's, the infant is more susceptible to hypoxia. He uses more oxygen than the older child. An unobstructed airway is essential to the infant.

Shock results when there is insufficiency of circulating blood volume. Pallor, coldness, a rapid pulse, and irregular respirations are signs of shock in children of all ages; in an older child, however, in addition to the foregoing, a lowered blood pressure and sweating are seen. Delayed shock can be caused by hemorrhage.

Increased understanding of fluid and electrolyte balance and greater recognition of the special problems of pediatric surgery are factors that help to account for the lower incidence of shock in patients postoperatively; however, an infant or small child's condition can change rapidly, so that frequent observations are essential.

Postoperative medications. When a child recovers from the effects of his anesthetic, he may profit from medication not only for physical reasons for discomfort but for emotional reasons also. Rest and sleep may help him to feel better. Restlessness may be a sign of pain or may be a sign of hypoxia, so the child's condition needs evaluation before a medication is given. The presence of a familiar person (such as the mother) or a certain favorite toy may help toward relaxation.

General postoperative care

When the child has recovered from the anesthesia, important factors in his general care include continual watchful observation, attention to diet and fluids, recording of intake and output, prevention of infection, and promotion of good hygiene, comfort measures, and exercise.

Observations. On every tour of duty the nurse should observe and record the child's behavior, color, quality of pulse and respiration, condition of the dressing (if there is one), and whether any special apparatus being used for the child is in good working order (drainage tubes, oxygen tent, intravenous infusion, etc.). Signs of dehydration should be noted if present, such as dryness of the skin and mucous membranes, sunken eyes, poor tissue turgor, and sunken fontanel (if the latter is still open).

The behavior of a child is very significant. If he is cheerful and responsive, he is progressing well toward recovery. If he is quiet and listless, he feels, and is, sick. A restless and whining child may be one who is in pain.

Recording intake and output. Oral intake, urinary output, and gastric and chest drainage all need to be measured and recorded. The need for parenteral fluid therapy in the postoperative period is largely gauged by a record of these factors plus the general appearance of the child. If a child is dehydrated, the urinary output is decreased. The nurse should be careful to record the amount of urine the child voids. The preschool child should be placed on a bedpan or given the urinal about every 2 hours when he is awake. Each time the nurse changes the infant's diaper she should chart that the diaper is wet. A check (✔) in the urine column of the nurse's bedside notes is adequate; however, the nurse must be conscientious in doing this.

Diet and fluids. After an operation on the child the nurse should be sure there are specific orders given by the physician in regard to diet. There appears to be a growing trend toward the physician's writing "Diet as tolerated." This gives the nurse leeway to offer small amounts of clear fluids frequently and then fluids with milk and a soft diet. The infant can be given glucose water, then half-strength formula, and then his usual diet. Some pediatric units have a special postoperative regimen for infants. Instead of half-strength formula, a formula low in fat may be prescribed prior to returning them to their full diet. The sooner the child is taking and retaining liquids, the sooner the intravenous can be discontinued.

Prevention of infection. There seems to be a growing trend to place small infants who have had surgery in an intensive care unit along with premature infants. This practice, besides affording them a better opportunity to be closely observed, protects the infants from infections, since rigid techniques are carried out in these nurseries.

After surgery children should be kept away from children with any respiratory infection. Also, personnel with colds or any sign of respiratory infection should not participate in their care.

The position of children should be changed frequently: every 2 hours when awake and every 3 hours during the night. Older children can be taught to cough and deep-breathe several times daily. Infants should be well propped on one side and then the other in such a manner that they will not roll and lie flat on their backs.

General hygiene. The nurse should handle the infant or child with surgery gently. He does not express himself verbally like the adult. The tenseness of the child's body as the nurse touches him tells her something about how the child is feeling.

As he feels better, he will participate more in his own care. A daily bath, plus special care to back and bony prominences several times a day helps to keep the skin in good condition as well as stimulate the general circulation.

Proper nutrition, sleep and rest, and suitable diversion are all factors that promote healing and recovery. If a child is physically comfortable and happy, he eats well, so it is difficult to make a clear dividing line between psychological and physical factors in the child's care; they are interrelated.

Exercise. As the child feels like it, he will move around in his bed. Usually children become more active sooner than adults in the postoperative period. When confined to bed, it is possible the child may like his bed taken to the playroom; other children may prefer to be in their own room with some suitable type of recreation.

When the physician specifies that the child may ambulate, the nurse should let the child dangle his legs first as he sits on the side of his bed. His pulse should be taken. The first time he is up it should be for a brief period of only 10 or 15 minutes. The child's pulse should be taken again as he is put back to bed to see if it has increased greatly. If so, this should be reported. The time out of bed should be increased gradually and in accord with the physician's plan of care for the child. Also, the child is allowed up in order to ambulate, not to sit down.

Before the child is discharged the nurse should be sure that his parents understand if there are limitations to the child's activities.

Child with a Foley catheter

Sometimes a child comes back from the operating room with an indwelling Foley catheter. This can be attached to a drainage bottle by means of a glass connecting tube and rubber tubing (Fig. 11-10).

The Foley catheter is held in place in the bladder by a small balloon, which has inflated after the catheter has been inserted. To make sure the tube will not slip out the nurse should fasten the tube securely to the child's thigh and also to the bed.

Urinary output should be measured at specified intervals; every 8 hours is usually more practical than every 12 hours. From this the 24-hour amount of urine output can be totaled.

In irrigating the catheter tube, the nurse

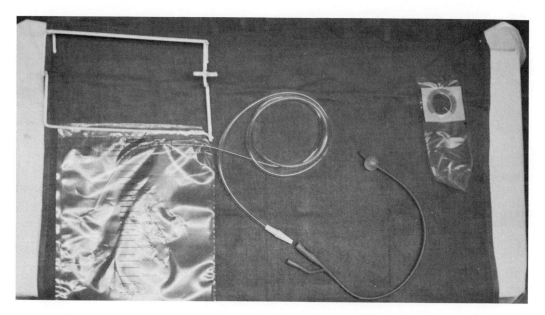

Fig. 11-10. Foley catheter with one end in the plastic urine bag, which can be fastened to the side of a bed. The tiny balloon at the other end of the catheter is inflated after the catheter has reached the bladder. The inflated balloon helps to keep the catheter from slipping out. To the right of the Foley catheter is infant urine specimen collection bag for a single specimen. (Courtesy Medical College of Georgia, Augusta, Ga.)

should allow the fluid (saline or other solution) that is used to flow by gravity rather than force. She should pour the prescribed amount of solution into the sterile container, disconnect the Foley catheter from the glass connecting tube, and insert the end of an aseptic syringe into the tube. The irrigating solution can then be placed in the aseptic syringe and, as just advised, allowed to flow by gravity. The amount of solution used by the nurse should be charted so that it can be subtracted from the total output at the end of 24 hours.

The nurse should be aware that some physicians do not wish a Foley catheter to be irrigated. They believe that such irrigation is a possible means of infecting the bladder.

Child with a tracheotomy

Some of the same general principles in the care of an adult with a tracheotomy are true of a child. A tracheotomy is associated with a patient who has an obstruction of the airway, such as a child with acute epiglottitis or diphtheria. The object of the operation is to get air into the lungs. After an opening is made in the trachea a tracheotomy tube is inserted. The tube should be held firmly in place by tape fastened to each side of the tube and tied together on the side or back of the neck of the child. The child who has had a tracheotomy should have special nurses so that he will not be alone at any time.

Equipment. At the bedside there should be a tray with a complete tracheotomy set as well as a duplicate tracheotomy tube. In addition, there should be a suction apparatus with a rubber catheter that has a Y attachment, a container of sterile physiologic saline solution in which the suction catheter can be rinsed, and equipment for cleansing. (Fig. 11-11 illustrates a tracheotomy tube. Note that it has two parts: the outer part, which is fastened to the neck of the child, and the inner one.) The solution used to cleanse the inner cannula may be saline solution or a 3% solution of hydrogen peroxide. The catheter used for suctioning should have an open end.

Suctioning. Suctioning should be done frequently, especially when the child coughs, is very dyspneic, or is very cyanotic. Before suctioning, the nurse should remove the inner

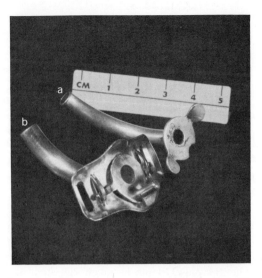

Fig. 11-11. Tracheotomy tube for a young child. The inner cannula, *a*, is removed at intervals to be cleansed while the outer one, *b*, remains in the trachea. (Courtesy Medical College of Georgia, Augusta, Ga.)

cannula and drop it into the solution of either physiologic saline solution or hydrogen peroxide. The rubber catheter should be open at the end and have a Y tube attachment. The suction should be turned on. The rubber catheter should be gently passed as far as it will go; then, while the open part of the Y tube is covered with a finger, the tube should be pulled back slowly and steadily. This should be repeated until the child is breathing more comfortably. If the secretions are very tenacious, the physician may suggest that a few drops of saline solution be put into the tracheotomy tube prior to suctioning. This helps to loosen secretions. The inner cannula should be cleansed with a pipe cleaner. Crust and secretions on the outside of it should be wiped off before the tube is replaced in the outer cannula and fastened.

Observations. The nurse should note the child's color and the quality of the pulse and respiration frequently as well as record the rate of the pulse and respiration.

Humidity. The child who has a tracheotomy is usually placed in oxygen with high humidity. Cool moist air is needed. (Refer to p. 293 for a description of the nurse's responsibilities in the care of a child in an oxygen tent.)

Child's reaction. The older child should be

reassured that he will be able to talk again. He should have an explanation of his treatment. A calm, deliberate approach is helpful with the toddler and young child. The experience of dyspnea and the tracheotomy is anxiety provoking. The child needs reassurance and emotional support.

Child with an intravenous infusion

Oral fluids. Some children have an intravenous infusion begun or continued because their oral intake is poor. A sick child seldom takes much fluid at one time, so the nurse needs to be persistent in her efforts to increase his intake of fluids. She must offer fluids frequently. She needs to use ingenuity to make it fun for the child to take another swallow. Although a large cup or glass might be brought into his room, a small glass of the fluid should be offered. It can be refilled from the larger glass. Other times, the child can have nothing by mouth, so he is unable to take oral fluids.

Composition of body fluids. Water makes up about 80% of the body weight in infants as compared to 60% in adults. The proportion of extracellular to intracellular water is greater in infancy than in later childhood and adulthood.

The extracellular fluid is composed of (1) blood plasma, which contains a fair amount of protein but is proportionately higher in sodium and chloride, and (2) interstitial fluid, which also has large amounts of sodium and chloride and small amounts of protein, potassium, calcium, and magnesium.

Intracellular fluid contains a large amount of protein and potassium.

The infant has a large surface area in proportion to his weight. The smaller the body the greater is the proportion of water in the body and the sooner the baby suffers from dehydration in certain situations. In addition, his kidneys are immature in infancy so there is less ability to concentrate and conserve fluid.

Dehydration. How is dehydration judged? Sunken eyes, depressed fontanel, dry skin and mucous membranes, and a loss of skin elasticity all aid in communicating the fact that the infant needs more fluids. In addition, the dehydrated infant voids less often. If he is severely dehy-drated, the circulation is affected and the child may have cold extremities, pallor or ashen gray color, collapsed peripheral veins, low blood pressure, and increased pulse.

The report of blood chemistries reveals whether the child is in electrolyte balance. (See Appendix B.) The nursing supervisor of the pediatric unit of a hospital should secure a copy of normal blood values from the chemistry laboratory in that hospital and post it on the bulletin board on the unit.

Infants become dehydrated faster than adults. Normally there is loss of fluid content from the body via the skin, respiratory system, urine, and stools. When an infant has diarrhea, the amount of fluid he loses increases, and if he is vomiting, still more is lost. At the same time often the intake is decreased. If an infant or child has an elevated temperature, the dehydration is further increased. In conditions such as burns there is increased loss of fluid from the skin.

Parenteral therapy. If an insufficient amount of fluid or no fluid can be given orally, the fluid is administered parenterally to improve the circulation and renal function. The physician has the responsibility of calculating and deciding the plan of parenteral therapy. He takes into account clinical signs of dehydration of the child, reports of blood chemistries and gases (Appendix B), and the maintenance needs of the child plus any replacement needed for both past deficits and concomitant losses. The amount of urine voided or the number of times the infant has voided is also considered. The physician should write the rate of flow desired for the intravenous infusion; he usually will require it over a period of 24 hours or even several days.

Site of injection. Frequent sites of injection are the ankle and the scalp vein; sometimes the arm is used. The sites of injection should be rotated to prevent phlebitis of the vein used.

Role of the nurse. The nurse's role is to assist the physician in starting the intravenous infusion, to monitor the rate of flow, to see that the child is comfortable, to look for any untoward symptoms, and to make sure the fluids are going into the vein rather than the tissues.

If the physician uses an ankle vein or an arm

Text continued on p. 306.

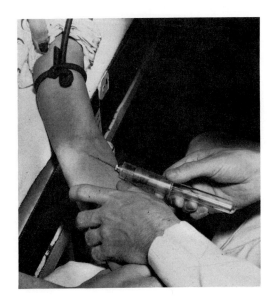

Fig. 11-12. Antecubital vein puncture using Vacu-tainer syringe. (From Varga, C.: Handbook of pediatric medical emergencies, ed. 4, St. Louis, 1968, The C. V. Mosby Co.)

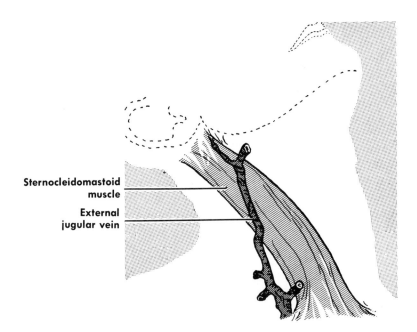

Sternocleidomastoid muscle

External jugular vein

Fig. 11-13. Superficial anatomy and course of the external jugular vein. (From Varga, C.: Handbook of pediatric medical emergencies, ed. 4, St. Louis, 1968, The C. V. Mosby Co.)

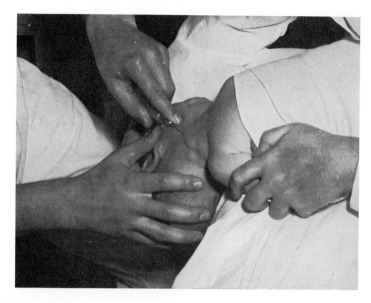

Fig. 11-14. External jugular vein puncture (using finger as guide to palpate landmarks). (From DeSanctis, A. G., and Varga, C.: Handbook of pediatric medical emergencies, ed. 3, St. Louis, 1963, The C. V. Mosby Co.)

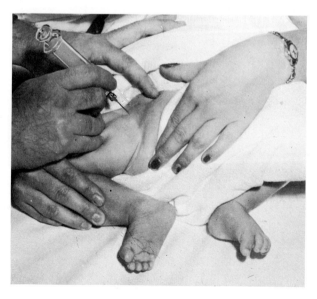

Fig. 11-15. Femoral vein puncture. (From DeSanctis, A. G., and Varga, C.: Handbook of pediatric medical emergencies, ed. 3, St. Louis, 1963, The C. V. Mosby Co.)

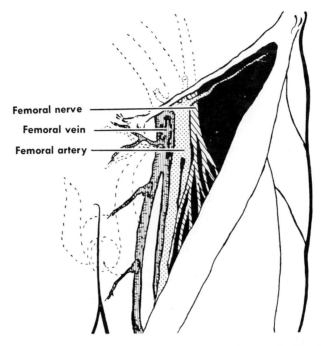

Fig. 11-16. Anatomical relationships of femoral vein. (From Varga, C.: Handbook of pediatric medical emergencies, ed. 4, St. Louis, 1968, The C. V. Mosby Co.)

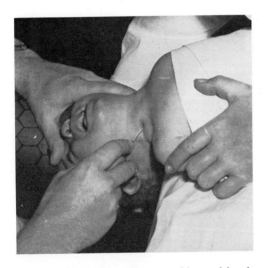

Fig. 11-17. Position for puncture of internal jugular vein. (From DeSanctis, A. G., and Varga, C.: Handbook of pediatric medical emergencies, ed. 3, St. Louis, 1963, The C. V. Mosby Co.)

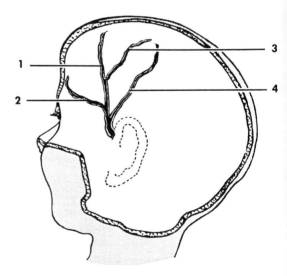

Fig. 11-18. Anatomy of superficial temporal veins: *1, 2, 3,* and *4* are common tributaries of the superficial temporal vein. (From Varga, C.: Handbook of pediatric medical emergencies, ed. 4, St. Louis, 1968, The C. V. Mosby Co.)

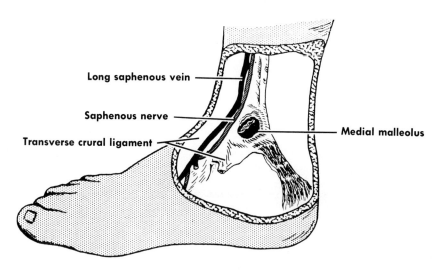

Fig. 11-19. Anatomical relationships of the grcat (long) saphenous vein at the ankle. (From DeSanctis, A. G., and Varga, C.: Handbook of pediatric medical emergencies, ed. 3, St. Louis, 1963, The C. V. Mosby Co.)

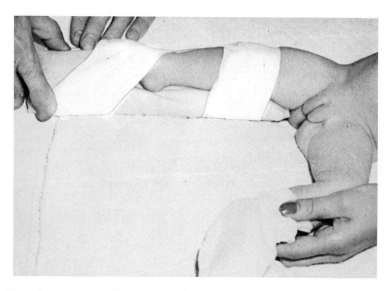

Fig. 11-20. Proper restraint of leg for cannulization of the long saphenous vein—step 1. (From DeSanctis, A. G., and Varga, C.: Handbook of pediatric medical emergencies, ed. 3, St. Louis, 1963, The C. V. Mosby Co.)

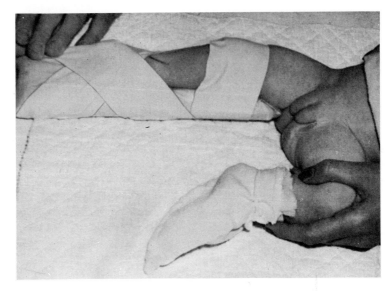

Fig. 11-21. Proper restraint of leg for cannulization of the long saphenous vein—step 2. (From DeSanctis, A. G., and Varga, C.: Handbook of pediatric medical emergencies, ed. 3, St. Louis, 1963, The C. V. Mosby Co.)

as the site of the intravenous injection, the arm or foot should be restrained against an armboard or sandbag for safety's sake. Thus anchored, there is less danger of the needle's coming out of the vein.

The infant or young child should be placed in a comfortable position in bed. If not too sick, he may like to hold a cuddly teddy bear or doll. If the infant is on nothing by mouth, a pacifier might be offered him. Also, his lips should be moistened with water.

The number of drops per minute of the intravenous infusion should be counted and regulated according to the specific order by the physician. The intravenous infusion is as important as any medication. If there is any question as to the rate of flow desired, the physician should be called.

Children's hospitals and many pediatric units in general hospitals have a special chart on which to record pertinent data about the intravenous infusion. This record is usually the result of the combined thoughts of pediatric medical and nursing personnel. It is important that at any given time the amount of fluids absorbed should be known. Flasks may be added or changed, and unless there is a special record, it is difficult to know exactly how much fluid the

child has had. Too much fluid could result in congestive heart failure.

The rate of the flow should be counted at least hourly and recorded because intravenous infusions often, of their own accord, speed up or slow down. There are various types of intravenous infusions. The nurse should be aware of the number of drops per cubic centimeter (cc.) and be able to estimate the rate of fluid flow per minute. The pediatric micro-drip is calibrated so that there are 60 drops per cubic centimeter. The nurse should record the rate at which she finds an intravenous flowing and the rate to which she adjusts it. Also, she should record each hour the amount absorbed within the past 60 minutes and, in another column on the chart, add that amount to what has already been given to the patient so that the physician will see the total amount absorbed at any one specific time. A new fluid chart should be begun on each 8-hour tour of duty of the nurse.

When there are many infants and young children with intravenous infusions, it takes one person's attention to monitor them adequately. Sometimes the treatment room nurse does this; sometimes the nurse who is assigned a particular patient takes care of her own.

If the intravenous infusion is running too

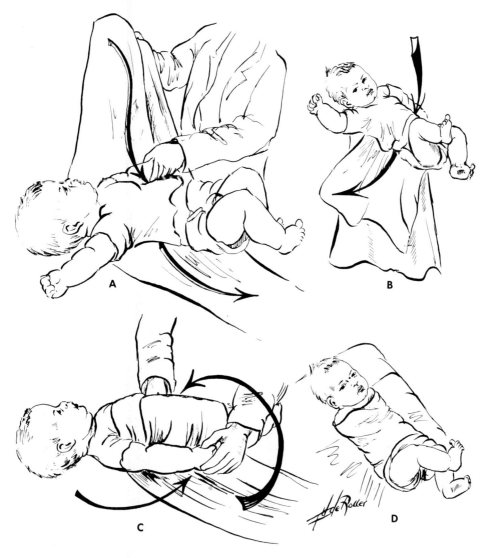

Fig. 11-22. Nurse restraining an infant who is going to have an intravenous infusion started in the ankle. Sheet is removed after intravenous infusion has been started.

slowly, even though it is not clamped, the pole on which the flask is hanging might be raised. The leg of the infant or young child can be elevated on a folded blanket if the site of the injection is the ankle. Changing the position of the child so that the area of the site of the intravenous infusion is uppermost may help. The nurse should be sure that nothing is pressing on the intravenous tubing. The vein of the infant is small and the needle may be against the wall of the vein. This would result in poor fluid flow.

When the rate of flow has been adjusted, the nurse needs to make sure the intravenous infusion is not entering the tissues. Any edema around the site of the injection should be noted. If there is a *little* edema, it might be caused by the adhesive used to anchor the intravenous tubing. The physician should be called if there is any doubt, and the intravenous infusion slowed but not turned off. If the tubing were clamped completely, the blood would coagulate and occlude the needle. If the needle were in the vein, it would then have to be taken out and restarted in another vein.

Beside checking the rate and whether the intravenous infusion is infiltrating the tissues, the nurse should see if there are any untoward signs such as dyspnea, cyanosis, hyperirritability, lethargy, twitching, or restlessness. She looks to see if there has been any significant change in the patient's condition. If a change is negative, the nurse's observation should be reported promptly to the physician.

Before leaving the patient she should make sure he is comfortable. The position of the child should be changed frequently. If the patient is an infant, he might be gently and carefully held in the nurse's arms when he is fed. Younger children often like to be held while their beds are being made.

When changing the flasks, the nurse must be careful not to let air inside the tube. As a first precaution, she must not wait until all the solution has run out before changing flasks but make the change while the tubing is still filled with solution; otherwise there is danger of an air embolism.

If the infant is going to the operating room, a cutdown intravenous infusion often is started before he leaves the unit. The cannula is held in place with a suture. A cutdown intravenous set should be changed after 3 to 4 days to avoid the possibility of infection. The responsibility of the nurse is the same as for any intravenous infusion.

Blood transfusion. The responsibility of the nurse for a blood transfusion that is given intravenously is the same as for any intravenous infusion, except that a rectal temperature is taken every half hour while the blood is being infused.

The different types of reactions to a blood transfusion are as follows:

1. *Allergic reactions:* Allergic reactions are most commonly manifested by urticaria, wheezing, or arthralgia. The mechanism of these reactions is not certain, but they may be due to allergenic substances in the donor plasma. Therapy with antihistamines and corticosteroids is effective in treating this type of reaction.

2. *Febrile reactions:* The use of disposable plastic equipment has eliminated most external pyrogenic substances. Use of antipyretics may modify this reaction.

3. *Hemolytic transfusion reactions:* These reactions result in massive intravascular destruction of red blood cells, which is manifested clinically by fever, chills, headache, and back pain. Hemoglobinemia and hemoglobinuria are usually observed. Whenever any of the symptoms of a reaction are suspected, the flow should be stopped and the physician notified. The nurse should realize that the young child who cannot verbalize his discomfort will manifest the symptoms of a reaction by changes in his behavior. He may grow restless and cry. Close observation probably will show changes in color, temperature, respiration, and heart rate.

Assisting with treatments
Lumbar puncture

The physician does a lumbar puncture, or spinal tap, to get a sample of spinal fluid for diagnostic study. The responsibility of the nurse is to first explain to the child in simple terms (if the child is conscious and able to understand) what is going to be done: He has to lie on his side with his knees flexed and his head down. An older child may be told to grasp his hands together under his knees. He must stay very quiet. The nurse will have to hold him in this position. He will feel the one spot on his back being bathed to make it clean, then the needle prick when the doctor puts the medicine into his skin. After the one prick he will not feel any more pain, but he does need to be very quiet. The doctor gets a specimen of spinal fluid, and then the child can straighten out his legs again and be put back in his own bed.

A pediatric lumbar puncture tray should be set up, holding whatever size of needle or special equipment the medical staff desire. A spinal needle for infants is considerably shorter than that for adults. A special sterile drape for an infant may have to be made for the pediatric unit. A large towel that has a hole in the center of it might serve much better for a drape than would a combination of two or three sterilized towels, which tend to fall off. Usually three sterile test tubes, spinal needles, sponges, and a manometer for measuring spinal pressure together with a three-way stopcock should be on the tray. A 2 ml. syringe with the solution used for local anesthetic is not usually in the tray.

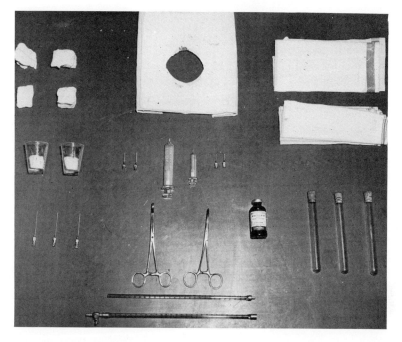

Fig. 11-23. Equipment for lumbar or subdural puncture. (From DeSanctis, A. G., and Varga, C.: Handbook of pediatric medical emergencies, ed. 3, St. Louis, 1963, The C. V. Mosby Co.)

The nurse should position the child before the physician begins. She must be sure not to bend the hips of the child either toward her or toward the physician. They should be vertical to the table, and the spinal column should be horizontal. Since crying increases the spinal pressure, a small infant may be given a pacifier to suck to keep him happy.

The physician often draws an imaginary line between the two iliac crests and introduces the needle between the third and fourth lumbar spinous processes.

If there is increased pressure, the fluid comes out more rapidly. The fluid usually is measured, but not always in infants. Sometimes the nurse is asked to compress the veins in the neck together, first on one side, then the other. This compression normally raises the spinal pressure. After a lumbar puncture the child remains recumbent for several hours, although some children do not need this. The child should be watched for any untoward reaction.

Diagnostic measures of the digestive tract

General comments. A simple explanation of any x-ray diagnostic measures should be given to a child so he will know what to expect. If possible, the nurse should remain with the child, especially a preschool child, during the test since strange-looking equipment might frighten him.

While waiting to get an x-ray film made the child might be given diversional play materials. While other children have breakfast, he might have his bath. The infant might be given a pacifier to suck when his feeding is delayed until after the test is done.

The infant should be taken to the x-ray department in a crib rather than in the nurse's arms. The latter method is a potential hazard since, if the nurse fell, the infant would be injured. The older child can be taken by stretcher, but the preschool child will probably be more comfortable if he goes in his crib or in a wheelchair to the x-ray unit. A stretcher is unfamiliar to him.

Barium swallow. The barium swallow procedure is done when there is a question of abnormalities of the upper gastrointestinal tract such as pyloric stenosis. It has to be scheduled in advance with the x-ray department. The physician leaves special orders for the preparation of the child. Usually nothing is allowed by

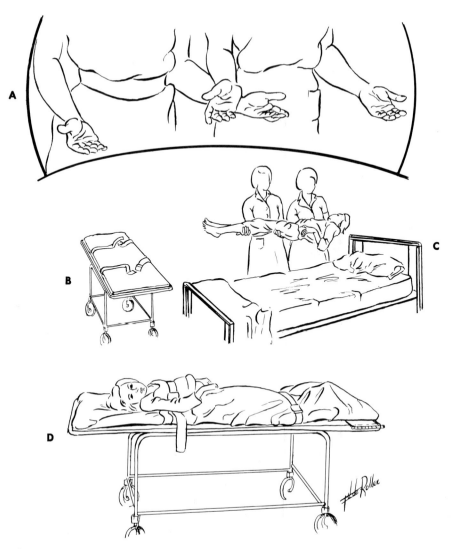

Fig. 11-24. Lifting child onto stretcher for x-ray film. **A,** Nurse crossing hands with second nurse before picking up child. **B,** Stretcher is at right angles to the bed for convenience. **C,** Child is lifted to the stretcher. **D,** Child is covered with sheet; for safety, two straps are placed around the child to prevent his falling off the stretcher.

mouth for several hours prior to the barium swallow.

Just prior to taking of the film the infant is given the barium by bottle; the child is given it by a glass or cup, as an adult is.

When the patient returns to the unit, no food should be given until the radiology department indicates it is all right to do so. If films are unsatisfactory, more may need to be taken.

Barium enema. The barium enema proce-

dure is used when there is a question of abnormalities in the large colon. The physician will write any special orders relative to the preparation of the patient for the test. When the child is taken to the x-ray department, barium is introduced into the colon via a small rectal tube. Several films are taken with the child lying first on one side, then flat on his back, and finally on the other side. The barium outlines the colon and helps to indicate abnormalities.

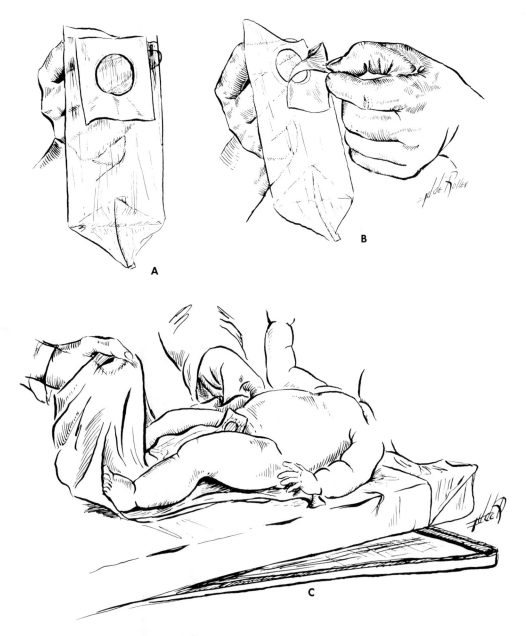

Fig. 11-25. Nurse putting urine collector on infant. **A,** Urine collector. **B,** Nurse removing protective paper before applying it to the infant. **C,** Urine collector in place. Note that the head of the bed is raised. (Courtesy Medical College of Georgia, Augusta, Ga.)

Diagnostic measures of the genitourinary tract

Renal function studies

Collection of urine specimens. Every child who is admitted to the hospital has a routine urinalysis. It is done to detect the presence of disease in the kidney. The specific gravity and the pH are especially important. Specific gravity is a measure of the solids in the urine; it is a measure of the kidney's ability to concentrate fluids. A child who is ill and who has taken little fluid has concentrated urine if his kidney is functioning normally.

Obtaining specimens of urine for admission routine urinalysis presents no particular problem in the older child, but sometimes the preschool child does not wish to sit on a bedpan or care to cooperate with a stranger immediately on admission. If at all possible, the help of the child's parents might be sought at the time of admission for these procedures. The nurse can explain to the parents (or parent) what is wished and then perhaps leave the room for a few minutes. The mother is often successful in having the child void.

Sometimes small toilet chairs are more readily acceptable to young children than a bedpan. A special receptacle to catch urine might be placed in the vault in the bathroom and the child carried into the bathroom to sit on the toilet there. (The latter method of collecting urine is often used in a private pediatrician's office.)

In collecting urine specimens from infants, a special urine collector is utilized (Fig. 11-25). As infants usually void during a feeding, the urine collector should be placed on the infant just before the nurse gives him a bottle. By the time the infant has finished his feeding the urine is in the collector and it can be removed.

If the nurse is unsuccessful in obtaining the urine specimen during the feeding, she can leave the special collector on the infant, elevating the head of the infant's crib or bassinet so the urine will go into the bag by gravity. Giving the infant plenty of fluids will, of course, aid him in voiding.

Laboratory data. Besides urinalysis, laboratory tests that are done on children with renal diseases or malfunction include blood urea nitrogen test, Addis count, phenolsulfonphthalein test, urea clearance test, bacteriologic culture, renal scan, and renal biopsy. Information about the procedure for doing each one can be obtained from the laboratory in the hospital. There should be a file on each hospital pediatric unit that contains specific information as to the details of each procedure.

1. A blood urea nitrogen test is a blood test. It measures the level of the blood urea nitrogen. When kidneys are unable to excrete the end products of protein metabolism, the blood urea nitrogen level is increased. In general, the normal values are 8 to 16 mg. per 100 ml. of urine.

2. The Addis count tests for the presence of active renal disease. It tells the number of cells and casts excreted in the urine over a given period of time (usually 12 hours). A timed urine specimen is collected. The child is asked to void. This specimen of urine is discarded; then the timed collection is started. Just before the end of the collection period the child is also asked to void. This voiding is added to the timed specimen in order that all the urine during the period of collection is obtained.

3. The phenolsulfonphthalein test measures tubular excretion function. Again, a timed urine specimen is necessary. Results are usually reported in terms of the percentage of dye (phenolsulfonphthalein) that is excreted. Within a 2-hour period of time 85% to 100% of dye is recovered.

4. The urea clearance test tells the rate at which kidneys clear urea from the blood. A blood sample is taken at the midway point in the timed urine collection. It is a measure of both the glomerular and tubular function. The range of normal is 60 to 90 ml. per minute.

5. Bacteriological culture of urine requires careful preparative cleansing of the genital area and collection in a sterile container. A midstream collection is most reliable but frequently impossible to obtain in young children. Suprapubic puncture of the bladder may be performed to obtain urine for culture. Catheterization for culture should be resorted to only after equivocal results have been obtained on two or more "clean catch" specimens and should be done by the physician.

6. Renal scans can be used to demonstrate renal tubular function by injecting radioactively tagged mercury or technitium.

7. Percutaneous renal biopsy is a valuable tool in the evaluation and management of selected renal patients. It is usually performed in children whose renal disease is atypical or chronic. The information obtained may help to indicate future course of the disease and influence decisions regarding drug therapy.

Intravenous pyelogram. For the child with urinary tract infections, an intravenous pyelogram may be done to see if there is any anatomical abnormality in the kidney and ureters. This test has to be scheduled in advance. The physician writes orders for the preparation of the child. Usually nothing by mouth is given for a number of hours prior to this procedure. The nurse taking the infant to the x-ray department may be asked to bring with her a bottle of carbonated beverage. The carbon dioxide released on ingestion of the beverage results in a large air space in the stomach. The beverage is given to the infant or young child so that projection on the intravenous pyelogram will permit better visualization of the renal pattern.

A radiopaque dye is injected intravenously. Since the patient may be sensitive to the dye, the physician often waits several minutes after a little has been injected, to see if there is any reaction such as urticaria before injecting the remainder of it. A film is then taken at 3-, 5-, and 10-minute intervals. After the child voids, another film is taken to see if all the dye has been excreted.

Cystoscopy. Cystoscopy is a procedure in which the physician visualizes the bladder by means of a cystoscope. The nurse in the operating room assists the urologist. In addition to visualization of the bladder, cystoscopy makes it possible to see uretral openings. A cystoscopy is helpful in diagnosing bladder neck obstructions.

Retrograde pyelogram. At the time the cystoscopy is done, a retrograde pyelogram may follow it. Specimens of urine from each ureter are usually collected by means of threading a catheter through the cystoscope. Then a radiopaque dye is usually instilled into both ureters. By this means abnormalities in the kidney or ureters can be visualized.

REFERENCES

Abbott, N. C., Hansen, P., and Lewis, K.: Dress rehearsal for the hospital, Am. J. Nurs. **70**:2360, 1970.

Azarnoff, P. Mediating the trauma of serious illness and hospitalization in childhood, Children Today **3**:12, July-August, 1974.

Barnett, C. R., et al.: Neonatal separation: the maternal side of interactional deprivation, Pediatrics **45**:197, 1970.

Beardslee, C.: The interaction between a failure to thrive infant and his mother, Maternal-Child Nurs. J. **1**:129, Summer, 1972.

Begue, M. T. A.: Play: The hospitalized child's best friend, Hosp. Topics **51**:45, April, 1973.

Blake, F. G.: Immobilized youth, Am. J. Nurs. **69**:2364, 1969.

Blom, G.: The reactions of hospitalized children to illness, Pediatrics **22**:596, 1968.

Brittingham, T. E., and Chaplin, H., Jr.: Febrile transfusion reaction caused by sensitivity to donor leukocytes and platelets, J.A.M.A. **165**:819, 1957.

Brown, M. J.: Pre-admission orientation for children and parents, Canad. Nurse **67**:29, February, 1971.

Condon, M. R., and Peters, C.: Family participation unit, Am. J. Nurs. **68**:504, March, 1968.

Cooke, R.: Disturbances of fluid and electrolyte equilibrium. In Vaughn, V., III, and McKay, R. J., editors: Nelson's textbook of pediatrics, ed. 10, Philadelphia, 1975, W. B. Saunders, Co.

David, N.: Play: A nursing diagnostic tool, Maternal-Child Nurs. J. **2**:49, Spring, 1973.

Davidsohn, I., and Stern, K.: Diagnosis of hemolytic transfusion reactions, Am. J. Clinc. Pathol. **25**:381, 1955.

Davis, V.: Through the bars of a crib, Am. J. Nurs. **71**:1752, September, 1971.

Dolan, M. B.: Shelly was angry, so was the staff, Nursing '74 **4**:86, June, 1974.

Erickson, F.: Reactions of children to hospital experience, Nurs. Outlook **6**:501, September, 1958.

Erickson, F.: When 6 to 12 year olds are ill, Nurs. Outlook **13**:48, July, 1965.

French, R.: Nurses' guide to diagnostic procedures, New York, 1975, McGraw-Hill Book Co.

Glenn, E. K.: Erick's hospital story, Am. J. Nurs. **75**:838, May, 1975.

Grant, M., and Kibo, W.: Assessing a patient's hydration status, Am. J. Nurs. **75**:1306, August, 1975.

Geolat, D., and McKenney, N.: Administering parenteral drugs, Am. J. Nurs. **75**:788, May, 1975.

Gurevich, I.: Some new concepts in tracheostomy suctioning, R.N. **35**:52, September, 1972.

Hardgrove, C., and Rutledge, A.: Parenting during hospitalization, Am. J. Nurs. **75**:836, May, 1975.

Holt, J.: RX: Play PRN in pediatric nursing, Nurs. Forum, **9**:288, 1970.

Issner, N.: The family of the hospitalized child, Nurs. Clin. North Am. **7**:5, March, 1972.

Jackson, C. W., et al. Sensory deprivation as a field of study, Nurs. Res. **20**:46, January-February, 1971.

Johnson, B.: Before hospitalization: A preparation program, Children Today November-December, 1974.

Kreiger, D.: Therapeutic touch: The imprimator of nursing, Am. J. Nurs. **75**:784, May, 1975.

Laire, C. A.: Meeting parents' concerns, Children Today **2**:2, May-June, 1973.

Mahaffy, P. R.: Admission interviews with parents, Am. J. Nurs. **66**:506, March, 1966.

Millar, T. P.: The hospital and the preschool child, Children **17**:171, September-October, 1970.

Mitchell, G.: A child's response to consistent care, Canad. Nurse **66**:47, March, 1968.

Mollison, P. L.: Blood transfusions in clinical medicine, ed. 4, Philadelphia, 1967, F. A. Davis Co.

Oakes, A., and Morrow, H.: Understanding blood gases, Nursing '73 **3**:14, September, 1973.

Oliver, P., et al.: Tracheotomy in children, N. Engl. J. Med. **267:**631, 1962.

Petrillo, M., and Sanger, G.: Emotional care of hospitalized children, Philadelphia, 1972, J. B. Lippincott Co.

Pinney, M. S.: Postural drainage in infants, Nursing '72, **2:**45, October, 1972.

Plank, E.: Working with children in hospitals: a guide for the professional team, Cleveland, 1962, The Press of Case Western Reserve University.

Robson, A.: Parenteral fluid therapy. In Vaughn, V., III, and McKay, R. J., editors: Nelson's textbook of pediatrics, ed. 10, Philadelphia, 1975, W. B. Saunders Co.

Rubin, R.: Body image and self-esteem, Nurs. Outlook **16:**20, June, 1968.

Rundels, J. C.: Iron deficiency in children, Nurs. Care **6:**16, September, 1973.

Schneider, G. M.: Oliver in the pediatric ward, Am. J. Nurs. **68:**2598, December, 1968.

Shirkey, H. C.: Table of drugs. In Shirkey, H. C., editor: Pediatric therapy, ed. 5, St. Louis, 1975, The C. V. Mosby Co.

Smith, R. M.: Anesthesia. In Shirkey, H. C., editor: Pediatric therapy, ed. 5, St. Louis, 1975, The C. V. Mosby Co.

Vaughn, V., III, and McKay, R. J., editors: Nelson's textbook of pediatrics, ed. 10, Philadelphia, 1975, W. B. Saunders Co.

Vernon, D., Foley, J., Sipowicz, R., and Schuliman, J.: The psychological responses of children to hospitalization and illness, Springfield, Ill., 1965, Charles C Thomas, Publisher.

Yarrow, L.: Separation from parents during early childhood. In Hoffman, M. L., and Hoffman, L. W., editors: Review of child development research (Vol. 1), New York, 1964, Russell Sage Foundation.

Young children in the hospital Nurs. Times p. 92, January, 1971.

West, C. D.: Parenteral fluid therapy. In Shirkey, H. C., editor: Pediatric therapy, ed. 5, St. Louis, 1975, The C. V. Mosby Co.

12

Nursing care of
THE INFANT WITH CONDITIONS PECULIAR TO THE NEWBORN

PREMATURITY AND LOW BIRTH WEIGHT
Definition

The words *premature infant* designate an infant born less than 37 weeks after the beginning of the mother's last menstrual period. *Low birth weight* infants weigh 2,500 gm. or less at birth. These infants have generally been called premature. The low birth weight is caused by either a shortened gestational period or a retarded rate of intrauterine growth or both. Prematurity and low birth weight usually occur at the same time, particularly among infants weighing 1,500 gm. or less at birth. These definitions are in line with the recommendations of the World Health Organization and American Academy of Pediatrics.

The problem

In the United States 6% to 15% of live-born infants weigh 2,500 gm. or less; the incidence varies in different areas and populations. Approximately half of the low birth weight infants have a gestational age of 37 weeks or more. About 4% of the infants who weigh more than 2,500 gm. have gestational ages less than 37 weeks. Premature and low birth weight infants account for the second largest percentage of infant deaths in the neonatal period.

Many factors, both fetal and maternal, are associated with variations in birth size. In general *premature birth* is associated with conditions in which there is inability of the uterus to retain the fetus, premature separation of the placenta, interference with the course of pregnancy, or a stimulus to effective uterine contractions prior to term. *Low birth weight for gestational age* is associated with conditions that interfere with the circulation and efficiency of the placenta, with the development of the fetus, or with the general health and nutrition of mother. Low birth weight is more common in black than white infants, in female than male infants and in infants of young primiparas. Other maternal factors include low socioeconomic status, residence at high altitude, illegitimacy, cigarette smoking, and poor nutrition. Long-range research studies to determine other causes of prematurity and low birth weight are essential because the majority of these infants are born to women who show no symptoms of physical disease.

Prevention

The prevention of prematurity should begin in the junior or senior high school with health teaching that points out (1) the importance of parents' being in good health prior to marriage and (2) the necessity of continuous medical supervision for the mother throughout her pregnancy and the postnatal period (Chapter 2). The school health nurse should use her position as health consultant to the best of her advantage (pp. 16, 226, and 238).

The public health nurse should utilize every opportunity she has in her home visits to notice whether women she sees may be pregnant and, if so, to urge that they attend prenatal clinics or see a private physician if they are not doing so already.

The cause of premature birth is not known in many instances, but since it is often associated

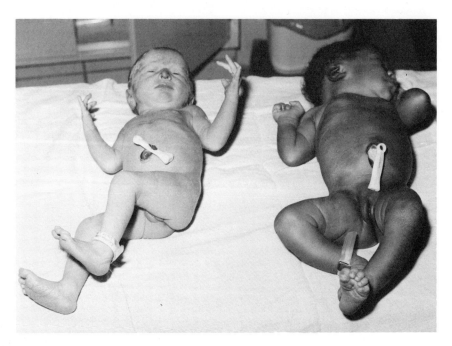

Fig. 12-1. Gestational age of these two neonates is 38 weeks. The infant on the left weighed 5 pounds and is a low birth weight infant; the infant on the right weighed 7 pounds 11 ounces, normal for this age.

with mothers who have diabetes, multiple births, complications of pregnancy such as toxemia and bleeding, infections, chronic malnutrition, and chronic conditions such as kidney or heart disease, the nurse in the prenatal clinic needs to focus her attention particularly on the expectant mother with any of these conditions. Besides getting instruction in general hygiene, including nutrition, these mothers should be taught to return to clinics or seek medical help if they have any bleeding, visual disturbance, severe headache, or swelling of feet, hands, or face. Possibly mothers with any complications of pregnancy or those who have chronic conditions should be referred to the public health nurse for further home visiting.

Syphilis of the mother was formerly an outstanding cause of death of infants, but a blood test of the mother and treatment if that test is positive lessen the likelihood of syphilis as a cause of premature birth. If expectant mothers go into premature labor, every effort should be made to get them to the hospital while the infant is still in utero.

Care in mother's labor

When the mother of an expected premature infant is in labor, the physician usually avoids the use of any drugs that are likely to depress the infant's respirations. He is trying to avoid possible anoxia and asphyxia of the premature infant, who, even if no depressant drugs are given to the mother, still has a harder time breathing than does the full-term infant. Sufficient anoxia can cause brain damage.

A pudendal block may be done so the muscles of the vulva and perineum will relax. The premature infant has more fragile blood vessels and may easily hemorrhage. For this reason, also, the smaller the infant, the wider is the episiotomy done. The infant's head is usually lifted out with forceps.

The mother in premature labor is in special need of someone to stay with her throughout her labor, especially if it is her first infant. She is usually anxious about the birth and whether the infant will be all right and anxious, too, about herself. The nurse is in a position to be very supportive to the mother. For general nursing

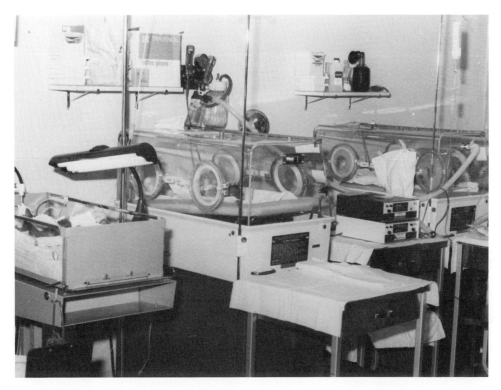

Fig. 12-2. Newborn in a modern neonatal intensive care unit. Note assisted ventilation and continuous monitoring of vital information on the infant's condition.

care of a patient during labor and delivery consult any standard textbook in obstetric nursing.

When the physician delivers the infant, the nurse will note that he suctions the infant as soon as the head is born; if the infant were to aspirate mucus in taking his first breath, it could be fatal. There is some controversy about when the umbilical cord should be clamped—whether at once, or later, after it stops pulsating. Some physicians believe that a delay in clamping the cord is detrimental to the infant since he already has an overloaded pulmonary circulation. Other physicians may delay cutting the cord while they give the mother 100% oxygen.

A warmed bed or incubator, oxygen, and resuscitation equipment should be readily available. (Refer to Chapter 4 regarding essential equipment and also regarding the prophylactic care of the eyes of the infant.) An intramuscular injection of 1.0 mg. of water-soluble vitamin K_1 is given after birth to correct any coagulation defect related to vitamin K deficiency and to prevent the usual neonatal decrease in plasma prothrombin level.

Intensive care unit

Since 1960 there has been development of intensive care units in which nurses, physicians, and paramedical personnel with special skills and training can care for the newborn infant who is having difficulty in his adaptation to extrauterine life or to some untoward circumstance. Methods for the evaluation of numerous crucial parameters of fetal and neonatal illness are readily available.

Electronic equipment to continuously monitor cardiorespiratory function is obtainable as well as mechanical respirators to assist ventilation. Laboratory microtechniques are frequently utilized for multiple biochemical tests of minute quantities of blood. Radiant heaters and servocontrolled incubators are used to help conserve body heat of the neonate. These intensive care units have succeeded in reducing the mortality as well as improving the quality of the survivors.

Handicaps of the premature infant

To understand the reason the premature infant needs special care, the nurse needs to know the physiological handicaps of the infant. The more immature the infant, the greater will be the handicaps; conversely, the nearer the infant is to term, the fewer will be the handicaps.

The infant is susceptible to respiratory difficulties such as primary atelectasis (lack of complete expansion of the lung) because of weak respiratory muscles, poor development of lung tissue, flexibility of the thoracic cage, and poorly developed respiratory center. The infant's breathing may be dyspneic and irregular, and he may have periods of apnea and cyanosis.

The nervous system is more immature than that of the full-term infant. The premature infant is slow to respond to stimulation. Centers that control vital functions are poorly developed. The temperature of the infant may be very unstable. He gets chilled and overheated easily. It may be hard to stabilize his temperature. The swallowing and sucking reflex may be weak or absent, so that the small premature infant may need to be fed by means other than a bottle. The cough reflex may be weak or absent. This predisposes the infant to aspiration of mucus or fluids.

The retina of the eye is immature so that the eyes have to be protected from overexposure and high concentrations of oxygen to prevent the infant from developing retrolental fibroplasia.

As indicated earlier, the premature infant has a tendency toward hemorrhage. The prothrombin in the blood is lower than that of the term infant, and there is increased fragility of the capillary walls of blood vessels. The premature infant is particularly susceptible to intracranial hemorrhage.

The fact that the blood sugar level is lower than that of a full-term infant helps to account for the sluggishness and listlessness of the small premature infant. Also, it implies there is a greater need for more calories per pound or per kilogram (kg.) of body weight than in the full-term infant. The infant has a tendency toward hypoglycemia.

The premature infant has a lower gamma globulin level than the full-term infant, and therefore he has even less resistance to disease. Also, because the hemoglobin level decreases steadily after birth and rises slowly, the premature infant is likely to be anemic after a few weeks of life. He needs additional iron.

The premature infant's digestive system is immature. His stomach is smaller than that of the full-term infant, and there may be impaired ability to absorb fat. This is the reason for many physicians' belief that the formula for the premature infant should be low in fat. His need for additional calories has already been mentioned.

Although the kidneys are large in proportion to the body of the term infant, they are still immature in the premature infant. There may be a retention of water caused by difficulty of the kidneys in excreting sodium and chloride. This together with anemia and hypoproteinemia helps to account for the edema often seen in the premature infant after birth. If the edematous tissue becomes hard, the condition is called scleredema. In addition, dehydration can occur easily if there is vomiting or diarrhea because of the kidneys' inability to concentrate urine.

The premature infant's temperature is subnormal for several possible reasons. The infant is less active, he has little subcutaneous tissue, and he has a relatively greater body surface than the full-term infant.

There are other differences between the full-term newborn and the premature infant, but they are not particularly significant in the nursing care of the infant except in interpreting the appearance of the infant to the parents. The testicles of male infants may still be in the abdomen, whereas in female infants the labia majora are undeveloped, and the labia minora are temporarily the larger. The premature infant has more lanugo hair than the full-term infant, his fingernails are softer, and his skin is more red and wrinkled. The circumference of his head and that of his chest are both smaller than in the full-term infant.

Role of the nurse

The aims of nursing care of the premature infant are to maintain respirations, conserve energy, provide and maintain nutrition, maintain a stable environmental temperature, prevent infection, and meet the infant's psychological needs. Methods of achieving these aims vary in different hospital situations. The nurse needs to work closely with both the obstetrician and the pediatrician.

Admission to the nursery

The infant should be transported in a heated bed or incubator to the nursery as soon as possible from the delivery room. He should have some identification on him, prophylactic measures against ophthalmia neonatorum should be started, and 1 mg. of water-soluble vitamin K_1 (AquaMephyton) should be administered.

The responsibility of the nurse in admitting the premature infant to the nursery is the same as outlined for a newborn infant in Chapter 4, except that the nurse should be particularly aware of the activity, muscle tone, respirations, and heart rate of this infant. The limp and listless infant needs even more careful watching than another of the same weight and size who moves his body and extremities. Respirations consistently over 40 per minute may indicate respiratory distress, and a persistently high heart rate may indicate circulatory difficulties.

After weighing the infant and taking his rectal temperature, the nurse should place him in an incubator or heated bed and leave him there until his temperature is stable. No attempts should be made to bathe or cleanse him until temperature stability has been achieved, the infant has recovered from the birth process, and the nurse has had an opportunity to further observe his condition.

There are various types of incubators. The nurse should be very familiar with the management of incubators before she cares for the infant who is in one. Information about the incubator should be part of the nurse's orientation to the premature and/or intensive care unit.

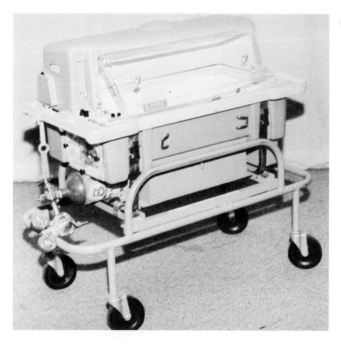

Fig. 12-3. Transport incubator. The infant can be moved from one location to another with assurance of a controlled protective environment. (Courtesy Earl K. Long Hospital, Baton Rouge, La.)

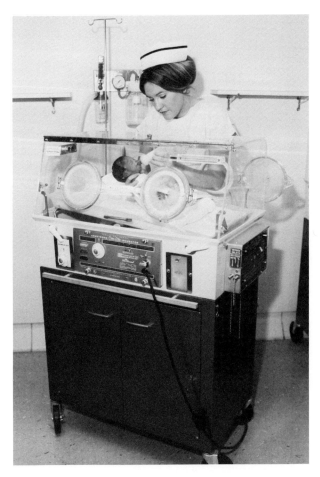

Fig. 12-4. Incubator provides a protective environment for the infant. This premature infant is being bottle-fed.

Since new models are constantly being put on the market, only a few general principles about them will be discussed here. For the smallest infant a temperature of 90° F. is suggested, whereas the larger premature infant may do well with a temperature of 85° F. Heat should not be used without regulation of humidity. A 55% to 65% humidity is usually acceptable unless the physician specifies differently. In general, the smaller the infant, the higher should be the prescribed amount of humidity. A large premature infant is better with less humidity.

One type of incubator is now equipped with a device known as a Servo-Probe thermometer, which can be fastened to the groin or abdomen of the infant. This records the infant's temperature. When the temperature falls below or rises above the temperature that is set, the heating mechanism of the incubator automatically adjusts itself to the desired temperature.

Daily care

Each infant should be considered as an individual and a separate plan of care made for him. Because two infants are of the same weight does not mean that the plans for them are the same.

Techniques for bathing, feeding, handwashing, and the like should be decided upon by the nursery of each hospital. There is sure to be some variation since different approaches can be used to achieve the same goals. General guidelines for many of these procedures in nursing care are briefly given here.

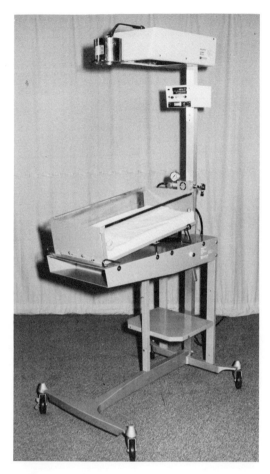

Fig. 12-5. Type of overhead radiant heater that provides a safe, controlled heat source for the exposed infant. It provides immediate access for efficient infant care.

Careful observation of the infant on each tour of duty together with knowledge of his medical care plan is basic to the nursing plan of each infant. Observations that the nurse needs to make frequently on each tour of duty include quality and rate of respirations, color of skin, activity and behavior, quality of cry, bleeding, vomiting, edema, distention, character of stools, voiding, signs of dehydration, tense or bulging fontanel, twitching or seizures, and anything unusual. The nurse should bear in mind that congenital defects often occur in a premature infant; some growth defects can be seen and others can be internal. The sucking movements of his lips and how the infant takes his feeding, as well as his behavior both before and after the feeding, are all important to know.

Maintaining respirations

For emergency use oxygen, suction, and a resuscitation tray should be readily available. A rubber ear bulb syringe for suction purposes should be at each infant's bedside. During the first hours of his life the infant should be placed on his abdomen so that mucous secretions can drain freely from his mouth. In this position there is no chance of aspiration. Some physicians prefer that the infant's head not be lowered during his first hours of life. This position might increase intracranial pressure and cause more respiratory embarrassment since the liver pushes against the diaphragm, which in turn may crowd the lungs. After the first few hours of life the infant's position should be changed every 2 or 3 hours to prevent hypostatic pneumonia. In an emergency situation the nurse should remain with the infant and signal for help.

If oxygen is given to the infant for a continuous period of time, the oxygen content should be analyzed at least every 4 hours. Unless specified differently, the oxygen content should not be over 40%. If cyanosis of an infant is not relieved by oxygen concentration at this level, the oxygen content may be increased.

Conserving energy

The nurse should assemble materials she needs for the infant, do what she needs to do, and then let him rest. Often the infant takes his feeding better if he has a rest between his bath and his feeding. If the infant is in poor condition, possibly only the face and the diaper area should be cleansed daily. On the other hand, if he is in fairly good condition, placing the infant in a basin of water after soaping him may tire him less than a sponge bath. The bath, of course, should be given inside the incubator. (The infant whose cord has not yet come off should have a sponge bath.) After the bath the infant can be placed on a soft blanket or towel and be patted dry. To conserve his energy feedings are small and given frequently. If sucking tires the infant, he can be fed with a cup or medicine dropper. The infant under 1,000 gm.

is too immature to having a sucking reflex and often needs to be gavaged. If the infant is in severe respiratory distress, the energy he has may be conserved, relative to eating, by a gastrostomy.

Nutrition

As indicated in the discussion of handicaps of premature infants, the infant's digestive system is immature; his stomach is small. He needs a formula high in calories and low in fat. Breast milk or a commercially prepared formula with 24 calories per ounce instead of the usual 20 calories per ounce is often ordered.

Method. The method of feeding depends on the infant, his maturity, and his condition. Some infants, although premature by definition, are able to breast-feed or take the bottle. If bottle-feeding is too fatiguing or if the infant is too immature to have developed a sucking reflex, he may be fed by cup, medicine dropper, or most frequently by gavage. (Of course, if the infant has respiratory distress or is seriously ill, no *oral* feedings are given.)

Each time the infant needs a feeding, a gavage tube can be passed through one nostril or through the mouth down to the stomach (intermittent gavage). The tube can be left in place and taped to the infant's face (an indwelling catheter). If this is done the catheter should be changed every 48 to 72 hours. Sometimes an indwelling catheter is connected to a flask and drip chamber. An indwelling catheter has one particular advantage. The small infant is disturbed very little for frequent feedings. The disadvantages are (1) obstruction of one nostril and thus the infant's airway, (2) possible rhinitis, (3) collection of mucus in the nostril, and (4) possible irritation of the mucous membrane lining of the nose and the upper gastrointestinal tract.

As soon as it is possible infants are fed by bottle or cup since even intermittent feeding by gavage carries with it the disadvantage of irritation to mucous membranes as well as the danger of aspiration of milk if there is incorrect placement of the gavage tube.

Whatever method is used for feeding, the infant should have his head and shoulders *elevated* during the feeding. In cup feeding he sits almost upright (Fig. 12-6). After the gavage the infant can be gently sat up and burped in his

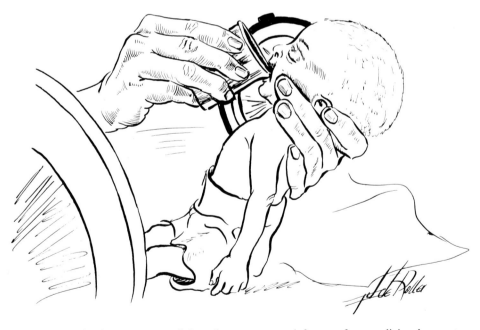

Fig. 12-6. Cup feeding a premature infant. Some premature infants prefer a medicine dropper to a cup.

incubator. The infant's back should *not* be patted but should be rubbed gently from the lower part upward toward his neck. After feeding the infant is placed flat in bed on his right side and propped that way. Some nurses prefer to place the infant on his abdomen after feeding to prevent the possibility of aspiration from regurgitation of the feeding. Whether the infant was hungry before his feeding and whether he was satisfied after his feeding should be noted on the chart. If he made sucking movements of his lips or resisted the gavage procedure, this should be charted, too. The latter helps to denote his readiness to progress from gavage feedings to feedings with a medicine dropper or bottle. The amount of feeding given and the type and size of catheter should be charted.

Gavage technique. The nurse needs a size 5 or 8 French catheter with a rounded tip, a syringe with an adapter, the feeding, a small basin or medicine glass, a stethoscope, and a small piece of tape.

The infant is placed on his back or side. The distance the tube is to be passed for the gavage is measured from the bridge of the nose to the lobe of the ear, then down to the xiphoid process at the end of the sternum. The distance on the tube is marked with tape. This measurement will take the tube past the lower end of the esophagus, past the cardiac sphincter, and into the stomach. The tube may be lubricated with sterile water. The tube is inserted into either one nostril or the mouth and passed gently but continuously until the tape mark is reached.

There are several ways of testing to see if the gavabe tube is in the stomach. The free end of the tube can be submerged in a basin or cup of water to see if bubbles rise. If there is bubbling, then the tube is in the respiratory tract and should be removed at once.

Another method is to place a stethoscope over the infant's stomach and listen while introducing a small amount (0.25 ml.) of air by means of a syringe (Behramen, 1975). There should be a sound of rushing air if the tube has been placed correctly. This air should then be aspirated; if no sound is heard, then the tube, of course, should be removed.

Another method is to pull back gently on the syringe to see if any stomach contents appear.

After ascertaining that the tube is in the right position, the nurse should wait a minute to let the infant get used to the feel of the tube. If the infant is fussy, the feeding will not digest as well. The nurse can speak soothingly to the infant and stoke him with one hand. The other hand holds the tube in place. The feeding should be allowed to run in slowly by gravity. Chinn (1971) suggests it takes 5 to 10 minutes for 5 ml of fluid to flow into the stomach.

The nurse should not remove the tube until the last drop of the feeding has disappeared; then she should pinch the tube and withdraw it quickly and smoothly. If all of the formula has not left the tube, there is danger that might drop into the respiratory tract as the gavage tube is pulled out.

If an indwelling catheter is used, then 1 or 2 ml. of sterile water should be injected to clear the tube.

The burping, positioning, and charting have been already discussed.

Maintaining stable temperature environment

If the temperature of the nursery can be kept stable by air conditioning in the summer, it is helpful to the infants in the incubators to graduate to a bassinet before they are discharged. It has been suggested that 75° F. is a good room temperature (Gluck, 1975). Comfort of the personnel of the nursery also needs consideration.

The temperature of the incubator should be kept stable. The nurse should set the dial for the desired temperature and then leave it; she should not keep swinging the dial back and forth. As stated on p. 320, the smaller infant's incubator might be regulated at 90° F. and the larger infant's at 85° F. As the infant grows and develops, the temperature of the infant will increase and the temperature of the incubator can be lowered accordingly. The temperature of the incubator needs to be checked and recorded at frequent intervals (every 2 to 3 hours).

To maintain an even temperature the porthole of the incubator *must* be kept closed. The plastic arm cuffs on the incubator *must* fit the nurse's arm snugly as she handles the infant. In caring for the infant the nurse needs to get her equipment together and place what needs to be kept inside the incubator in it, thus minimizing the number of times she will have to open and close the portholes. Opening the portholes frequently will keep the temperature of the incubator unstable.

Prevention of infection

The nurse needs to be cognizant of the recommendations of the American Academy of Pediatrics. Particular attention is drawn to the need of handwashing before touching the infant. Also, no personnel should be in the nursery who have an infection of any kind.

Careful cleansing of each incubator and bassinet and the small parts that go with the incubator should be done when the infant is discharged. The incubator is cleaned with a damp cloth daily to catch any dust particles.

Meeting psychological needs

The premature infant is a human being just as any other infant is. Because he is so small and special equipment is used for him, some nurses are afraid of the infant. Although minimal handling of the infant is encouraged to conserve his energy, this does not mean that while the nurse is caring for him she should not talk to and caress the infant. Stroking and gentle handling provide essential sensory stimulation. The nurse needs to remember that for many weeks the infant has been confined to a small area where, if he reached out a hand or foot, he touched something. The amniotic fluid can be likened to a blanket around him; then suddenly the infant is evicted from his snug home. He can stretch and move in any direction yet feel nothing except the mattress under him. It is interesting to see how the premature infant manipulates his body until he is next to the side of the incubator. Sometimes a diaper or light blanket tucked around the infant or even placed over him will eliminate a certain amount of restlessness.

Possibly the infant suffers from loneliness in the incubator. The nurse should utilize every contact she has with the infant to show him affection, such as at bath and feeding times and when giving him medications.

When the premature infant is no longer in the incubator but has been moved to a bassinet, he should be held for his feedings, the same as any other infant. Suitable music may be utilized to good advantage in a nursery and provide further sensory stimulation, as may a toy tied to the crib.

Parent teaching

Parent education is part of meeting the infant's psychological and physical needs for good care.

The various attitudes of the parents should be considered. There is possible disappointment of both parents that the excepted infant is different from most infants, is smaller and weighs less than the average, and needs special care. There may also be resentment. There may be anxiety about his health. In addition, the longer the infant remains in the hospital, the greater is the expense to the parents. When parents see the infant and see also the special equipment used in his care, they may be afraid of him. Perhaps they fear they may hurt him when he finally gets home. Because the infant must be in the hospital for so long, parents may lose interest in him. While the mother is still in the hospital she should be encouraged to come to the premature unit to see her infant. An explanation of the incubator and other equipment for her infant should be given her. The father also should be made welcome. Both should be encouraged to telephone the hospital to see how the infant is if they cannot come to see him. The nurse should use every means to help them continue their interest in the infant.

Before the infant goes home the mother should be given the infant to hold and cuddle so she can become better acquainted with her son or her daughter. Facilities such as a special room should be provided for parent teaching. The mother can be shown how to feed her infant. By the time he is ready to be discharged he may be eating fruit, cereal, and formula. The mother can feed the infant under the nurse's supervision. The emotional needs of the infant should be interpreted to the mother and/or father just as is done for the normal newborn (p. 73). At first the most important teaching the nurse can do is to have the mother and infant get to know one another. Formula making and other topics can be done in relation to the mother's knowledge and previous experience with infants.

Planning for home care

Before the infant is discharged a referral should be made to the public health nurse so she can visit the home and see that all is in readiness for the infant. If any members of the household are ill, the discharge of the premature infant may be delayed.

When the infant is finally discharged, the public health nurse again calls on the mother and supplements the teaching done in the hospital. It is important that the nurse help the mother feel adequate concerning the responsibility of caring for the premature infant. Other siblings may wish to hold the infant, the same as they might if he were full term and just coming home. The nurse can explain that, as long as the children are free of infections, they may participate in the infant's care.

The public health nurse may visit the infant over a period of months to interpret the needs and care of the infant to the family. To treat this infant differently from other siblings might lead to behavior problems later in his life. He should receive the same kind of care at home that any normal newborn infant receives.

Prognosis

It is not possible to state the prognosis of a small neonate except to note that it is not as good as that of large newborn infants. Only a small number of those who weigh less than 1,000 gm. survive, and of those who survive 80% have permanent central nervous system damage. Infants whose birth weights are over 1,500 gm. have a good outlook for the future, and those weighing 2,000 gm. or more have nearly as good a prognosis as full-size neonates. The most common handicaps in premature infants are mental retardation, spastic diplegia, growth retardation, emotional problems, hearing losses, and school failures.

POSTMATURITY

The term *postmaturity* is used for infants whose gestation exceeds the normal by 7 days or more (Fig. 12-7). About 5% of newborn in-

fants are postmature. The cause will remain unknown until the mechanism of onset of labor is fully understood.

The postmature infant has the appearance and behavior of an infant 1 to 3 weeks of age. He is prone to have long nails and hair, have no lanugo, and be more mentally alert than the normal neonate. The skin may be parchment-like with desquamation because of diminution of vernix caseosa beyond term. When postmaturity exceeds 3 weeks, there is a significant increase in mortality. The induction of labor or a cesarean section may be done in certain selected cases, but such treatment may be riskier than postmaturity itself.

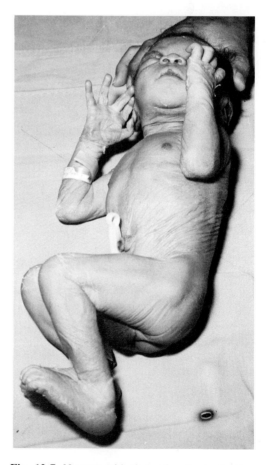

Fig. 12-7. Neonate with signs of postmaturity (dysmaturity). Note presence of desquamation of skin, especially of hands, feet, and face.

PLACENTAL DYSFUNCTION SYNDROME

Placental dysfunction syndrome has been postulated to be the result of degenerative changes in the placenta that result in progressive reduction of oxygen and nourishment for the fetus. As a result the fetus does not grow properly. About 80% of these infants are premature or born to elderly primigravida or toxemic mothers. The other 20% of infants having this syndrome are *postmature*.

The vernix, umbilical cord, skin, and nails are bile stained by the amniotic fluid containing meconium. In mild cases the staining is green; in more severe forms it is bright yellow. The presence of meconium-stained amniotic fluid suggests a lack of oxygen in utero.

When the complications of cerebral anoxia and meconium aspiration pneumonia occur, they are treated symptomatically. Many of these neonates have severe respiratory symptoms, apparently from aspiration of amniotic fluid containing meconium. The morbidity and mortality vary according to the severity of the placental dysfunction; nevertheless, they are significantly higher than in normal newborns.

PHYSIOLOGIC JAUNDICE OF THE NEWBORN

The terms *physiologic jaundice* and *hyperbilirubinemia of the newborn* usually refer to the slight degree of jaundice that is clinically visible 48 to 72 hours after birth. The bilirubin that is formed in the fetus in utero can cross the placenta and be excreted through the liver of the mother. However, immediately after birth the only means for ridding the infant of bilirubin is through the infant's own liver, which for the first week or so of life still functions poorly and is incapable of conjugating significant quantities of bilirubin for excretion into the bile. Consequently the plasma bilirubin level rises from a normal of less than 1 mg. per 100 ml. to an average of 5 mg. per 100 ml. during the first 3 days of life and then gradually falls back to normal as the liver becomes more mature in function.

Clinically the neonate develops yellow coloration (jaundice) of the skin and bulbar conjunctiva.

No special treatment is required for physiologic jaundice except to make certain that none of the other serious causes of neonatal jaundice is present. The nursing care should center around determining the age of onset of jaundice because erythroblastosis fetalis must be suspected when jaundice is observed within the first 36 hours of life. The nurse should notify the physician whenever jaundice is suspected in a newborn, especially when the infant also shows signs of an illness or infection.

HEMOLYTIC DISEASE OF THE NEWBORN (ERYTHROBLASTOSIS FETALIS)

Erythroblastosis fetalis is a disease characterized by progressive destruction of erythrocytes (hemolysis) and increased efforts to form new ones (erythroblastosis). This condition may occur when an Rh-negative woman (with no antibodies against Rh antigen) is pregnant with a fetus whose blood contains the Rh-positive antigens inherited from the father. Minute amounts of fetal blood enter the maternal circulation through breaks in the placental villi that usually occur when the placenta separates from the uterine wall. The immunological response is initiated by the foreign antigen, which stimulates the production of anti-Rho antibodies. Sensitization of Rh-negative women can be effectively prevented by the intramuscular administration of Rho immune globulin (RhoGAM) within 72 hours of delivery of an Rh-positive infant. As an added measure of prevention, Rho immune globulin should be administered to nonsensitized Rh-negative women following abortion and amniocentesis; it is not effective in women who are already sensitized.

During pregnancy in women who have been sensitized and whose fetuses are Rh positive, there is increased production of anti-Rho antibodies, which cross the placental barrier into the fetal bloodstream. These antibodies react with the Rh antigen on the fetal erythrocyte causing hemolysis and severe anemia. For the first few weeks of life many of these immune antibodies from the mother remain in the infant's body, destroying the red blood cells as quickly as they are formed. The rapid destruction of the red cells releases extremely large quantities of bilirubin into the plasma, causing severe hyperbilirubinemia. This condition occurs either mildly or seriously in 1 of every 200 to 250 newborn infants.

The clinical manifestations of this disease vary greatly. The newborn is usually jaundiced and anemic at birth, and the anti-Rh agglutinins from the mother usually circulate in the infant's blood for 1 to 2 months after birth, destroying more and more red blood cells. Therefore the hemoglobin level of the erythroblastotic infant often falls below 8 gm. per 100 ml. The liver and spleen enlarge greatly because they are attempting to replace the red blood cells that are being hemolyzed. In the affected infant jaundice is usually evident within the first 24 hours of life. The plasma bilirubin concentration may reach extremely high levels (20 to 50 mg. per 100 ml.). At these high levels precipitation of bilirubin crystals in the basal ganglia and other nuclei of the brain may occur. The destruction

of the neuronal cells by the precipitation of bilirubin is called *kernicterus.* This damage is clinically manifested by lethargy, poor feeding, a high-pitched cry, and loss of the Moro reflex. Children who survive kernicterus exhibit permanent mental impairment or damage. In the severely affected infant cardiac decompensation may result in massive anasarca and the clinical picture of *hydrops fetalis.* Hydrops fetalis almost invariably results in death in utero or shortly after birth.

When hemolytic disease of the newborn is suspected, blood grouping and Rh typing of the mother should be done early in pregnancy. If the mother is Rh negative, the maternal anti-Rh antibody titer should be tested frequently during the latter part of the pregnancy. If the physician considers the antibody levels to be sufficiently high to do possible injury to the fetus, the progress of the disease in utero may be followed by amniocentesis. Measurement of the bilirubin

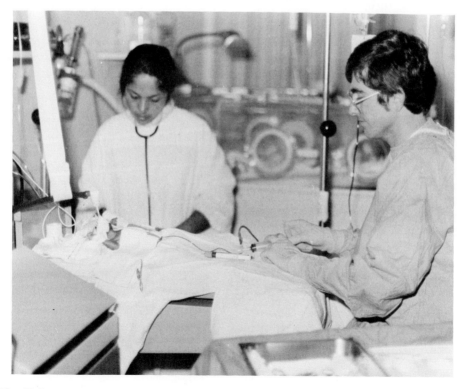

Fig. 12-8. Exchange transfusion being performed on a neonate who had hyperbilirubinemia secondary to Rh erythroblastosis. A plastic catheter is inserted into the umbilical vein of the cord, where blood is withdrawn and replaced in 10 to 20 ml. increments until approximately 500 ml. of blood has been exchanged.

pigment levels in the amniotic fluid is accomplished by special laboratory tests. Intrauterine blood transfusions have been successfully administered to severely affected fetuses in an attempt to improve the hemoglobin level. Induction of premature labor of the mother is delayed as long as possible because of the many handicaps that accompany prematurity.

Immediately after birth blood should be drawn from the infant for Rh and ABO typing, determination of hemoglobin level, and a reticulocyte count to evaluate the severity of the hemolytic process. Total and indirect bilirubin determinations to establish the serum level and a direct Coombs test to check for the presence of anti-Rh antibodies are also ordered. After the diagnosis is confirmed, the child is followed by careful clinical observation and repeated determinations of hemoglobin and indirect bilirubin levels in the blood.

The treatment of the mildly affected neonate can be accomplished by the use of phototherapy (bilirubin-reduction light). An exchange transfusion should be carried out as soon as severe anemia is diagnosed or the indirect serum bilirubin is rising rapidly or at any time the indirect bilirubin level is 20 mg. per 100 ml. or above (Fig. 12-8). About 100 ml. of Rh-negative blood per pound of body weight is infused over a period of 1 to 2 hours while the infant's own Rh-positive blood is being removed. Once the Rh-negative blood is in the infant, red blood cell destruction decreases, and second transfusions are usually unnecessary.

During the exchange transfusion the nurse may be asked to monitor the child's temperature, pulse, heart rate, respiration, and color. A record of the venous pressure readings as well as the amount of blood withdrawn and injected should be kept. After the procedure the infant should be observed by the nurse for hemorrhage from the transfusion site as well as his overall general activity and condition. Any changes in the infant's condition should be immediately reported to the physician.

HEMOLYTIC DISEASE CAUSED BY ABO INCOMPATIBILITY

Hemolytic disease caused by ABO incompatibility is a mild form of hemolytic disease in the newborn. Usually the mother's blood is type O and the infant's is type A or B. The anti-A and anti-B isoagglutinins are not as severe as the Rh isoagglutinins; therefore erythroblastosis secondary to ABO incompatibility is milder than Rh erythroblastosis.

Clinically the infant becomes jaundiced 24 to 36 hours after birth. The jaundice may reach high levels, but usually the bilirubin level crests under 20 mg. per 100 ml. The occurrence of kernicterus, hydrops fetalis, or severe anemia is extremely rare. The most important laboratory findings are (1) ABO incompatibility between mother and infant, (2) usually a normal hemoglobin level, (3) elevation of the bilirubin level (in 15% of cases it may increase to 20 mg. per 100 ml. or more), and (4) a positive direct Coombs test.

Therapy is directed at preventing the indirect bilirubin level from rising about 20 mg. per 100 ml., thereby preventing kernicterus. Phototherapy (bilirubin-reduction light) is used to prevent the slow rise of the bilirubin level. If the indirect bilirubin level reaches 20 mg. per 100 ml. in a term infant or 18 mg. per 100 ml. in a premature infant, an exchange transfusion is performed using group O blood of the appropriate Rh type.

Care of a newborn with hemolytic disease requires skillful nursing. The usual supportive measures for a newborn should be maintained with special attention paid to the respirations, pulse, temperature, color, and activity. If an exchange transfusion is performed, any untoward reaction or change should be reported to the physician. Neonates who develop kernicterus may be weak and have a poor sucking reflex and therefore should be fed with a soft nipple with a large hole or by a medicine dropper or gavage.

INFANTS OF DIABETIC MOTHERS

Infants born to diabetic mothers tend to have more difficulties than the normal neonate. Infants of diabetic mothers have a high incidence of associated hydramnios and a high neonatal mortality rate.

The infants tend to be large and plump with edematous and plethoric facies. They also have excessive secretions of mucus from the pharynx

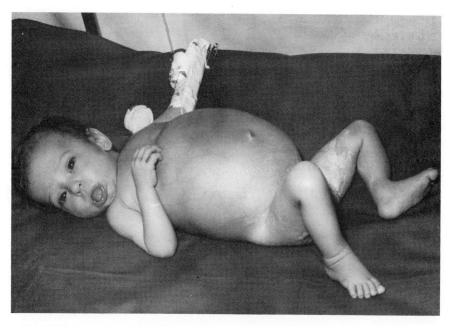

Fig. 12-9. Biliary cirrhosis with ascites in a 1½-year-old girl. At 6 weeks of age the child was diagnosed as having hyperbilirubinemia secondary to biliary atresia.

and stomach. Idiopathic respiratory distress syndrome and unexplained cyanotic attacks are common. Convulsions associated with hypoglycemia are occasionally observed, or the infant may become *trembly* after the first 18 hours of life.

Treatment

The blood sugar levels of these infants should be monitored every 2 hours after birth until stable. Blood glucose levels of 20 mg. per 100 ml. with or without symptoms of hypoglycemia should be treated with 50% glucose or glucagon infusion.

Oral formula feedings are recommended 3 to 4 hours after birth to help decrease the hypoglycemic state.

IDIOPATHIC RESPIRATORY DISTRESS SYNDROME (HYALINE MEMBRANE DISEASE)
Definition and problem

Idiopathic respiratory distress syndrome is a syndrome of neonatal respiratory distress in which pulmonary hyaline membranes with atelectasis are the main findings at autopsy. It accounts for 25,000 to 40,000 deaths in the United States per year, making it the commonest cause of death among premature infants. It is observed in 10% of all premature infants. Approximately 50% of all infants of diabetic mothers develop the disease.

The etiology of respiratory distress syndrome is still not known after years of research. The hypoperfusion theory is frequently used to attempt to explain the pathogenesis of the disease. This theory proposes that the pulmonary blood flow is decreased because of increased pulmonary vascular resistance, atelectasis, and acidosis. Another factor that may contribute to the pathogenesis of this disorder is deficiency of a surface tension–reducing film of lipoprotein (surfactant) that is normally present in the alveolar wall. In the absence of surfactant, lung expansion is almost impossible.

Nature of condition

Clinically the symptoms of respiratory difficulty develop at birth; many infants need resuscitation at time of delivery. It begins with rapid, shallow respirations that usually increase to 60 or more per minute within 2 hours of birth. Expiratory grunting, flaring nostrils, and retraction of the suprasternal and intercostal

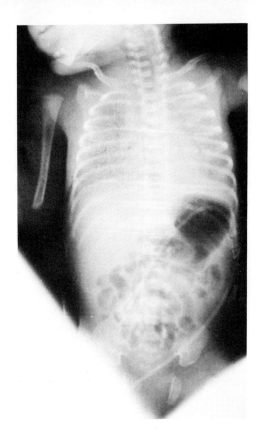

Fig. 12-10. X-ray film of infant with respiratory distress syndrome. Note the reticulogranular (ground-glass) pattern and decreased aeration of the lungs.

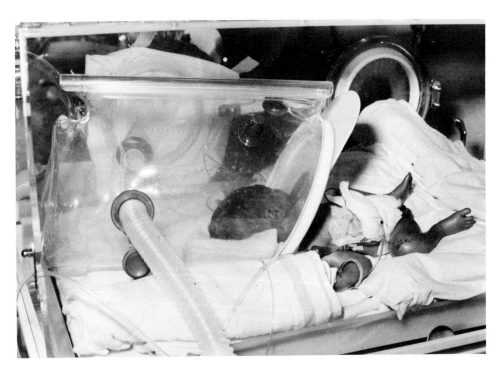

Fig. 12-11. Continuous positive airway pressure (C.P.A.P.) being administered to a newborn infant with respiratory distress syndrome. Note the use of the umbilical vein catheter for administration of intravenous fluid and drugs.

spaces with mild cyanosis are characteristic of the early stages of the disease. As the disease progresses, there is increasing hunger for air, cyanosis, and exhaustion from excessive respiratory effort.

Spontaneous recovery often occurs beginning at 36 to 48 hours of age, whereas most deaths occur before 72 hours of age. Chest roentgenograms reveal a reticulogranular (ground-glass) appearance and decreased aeration (Fig. 12-10).

Treatment

Treatment is somewhat unsatisfactory. The infant is usually placed in a humidified incubator with sufficient oxygen to overcome or prevent cyanosis and adequate heat to maintain normal body temperature. Appropriate intravenous fluids and drugs are given to prevent or control dehydration, hypoglycemia, acidosis, and hyperkalemia. Antibiotics are administered if any evidence of infection is found in the mother or infant or if many procedures are performed on the infant. Assisted ventilation with a mask and bag resuscitator or patient-cycled positive pressure respirator with a nasotracheal tube has been widely used. Also, continuous positive airway pressure (C.P.A.P.) may be administered by the use of a ventilatory apparatus that maintains pressures above zero at the end of expiration, thus preventing alveolar collapse by forcing retention of alveolar air (Fig. 12-11). By providing this continuous positive airway pressure much of the atelectasis that is characteristic of respiratory distress syndrome is overcome. The oxygen and carbon dioxide tension and the pH of arterial blood must be monitored periodically to determine the effectiveness of the therapy. The blood may be obtained from an indwelling catheter in an umbilical artery or blood drawn from the temporal artery.

A record of the amount of blood withdrawn should be kept to prevent anemia. If anemia does develop, a blood transfusion is recommended. Care should be taken to prevent contamination of the indwelling umbilical vessel catheter.

Prevention

Since the respiratory distress syndrome often accompanies prematurity, every effort should be made to prevent prematurity. The nurse should be diligent not only in case finding of pregnant mothers to see that they do receive medical supervision early and throughout pregnancy but also in using all available opportunities to teach the importance of medical supervision in pregnancy. Such teaching should also be part of the health education in school health programs in both junior and senior high schools.

Nursing care

In caring for newborn infants the nurse needs to be particularly observant of the premature infant, the infant born by cesarean section, and the infant born of the diabetic mother. Difficulty in respiration is shown by retractions, poor color, and rapid respirations. The infant generally appears normal at birth but within a few hours (and rarely as long as 24 hours) begins to show signs of respiratory distress.

The nurse should be sure there is an open

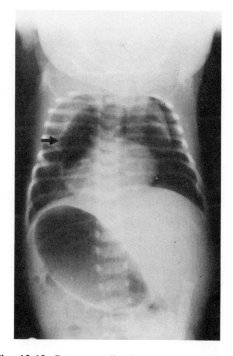

Fig. 12-12. Pneumomediastinum in a newborn infant. Note accumulation of air trapped in mediastinum (end of arrow) probably secondary to too vigorous resuscitation at birth.

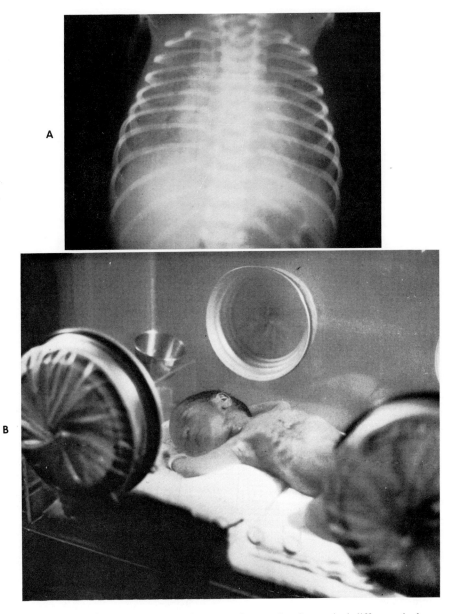

Fig. 12-13. A, Infant with hyaline membrane syndrome, showing typical diffuse reticulogranular pattern. **B,** Infant with respiratory distress syndrome, showing marked sternal and intercostal retractions. (**A** from Cook, C. D.: N.Y. J. Med. **58:**372, 1958. **B** from "Resuscitation of the Newborn," motion picture by Smith, Kline & French Laboratories, Philadelphia, Pa.)

airway. The infant born by cesarean section often has more mucus than other infants and needs frequent suctioning. He should be propped on alternate sides. If the infant is in respiratory distress, placing him on his abdomen is contraindicated. His head and the upper part of his body should be elevated.

In general the nursing care discussed in the section on prematurity applies to this infant since often he is a premature infant.

HYPOGLYCEMIA

Hypoglycemia occurs most commonly among male infants of low birth weight for their gestational age. Symptomatic hypoglycemia also occurs among infants of toxemic and diabetic mothers and in infants with erythroblastis fetalis. Symptoms of hypoglycemia may occur from a few hours to a week after birth. It may manifest itself by the presence of tremors, episodes of cyanosis, apathy, convulsions, apneic spells, weak cry, limpness, difficulty in feeding, or eye rolling. A blood glucose level of 20 to 30 mg. per 100 ml. usually accompanies the symptoms. Untreated symptomatic hypoglycemia is potentially serious because of its deterimental effects on the central nervous system.

Treatment consists of immediate intravenous infusion of 50% glucose for immediate relief of symptoms followed by a continuous infusion of 10% glucose until blood glucose levels have stabilized. Early formula feeding, if tolerated, is recommended. Therapy is usually necessary for a few days to several weeks, after which it should gradually be discontinued.

NEONATAL TETANY

Tetany in the newborn stems from a decrease in serum calcium associated with an increase in serum phosphate. It usually occurs during the first week of life. Transient hypoparathyroidism, diminished ability of the kidney to excrete phosphate, and a high phosphate load from undiluted cow's milk formula have all been considered predisposing factors in causing neonatal tetany. Symptoms most frequently encountered are irritability, muscular twitchings, tremors, convulsions, and laryngospasm. The important diagnostic criteria are

a reduction of the serum calcium concentration to 7.0 mg. per 100 ml. or less and a serum phosphate concentration above 8.0 mg. per 100 ml. A low serum magnesium concentration is frequently observed.

Symptoms respond dramatically to intravenous administration of 5 to 10 ml. of calcium gluconate in a 10% solution. It may be necessary to repeat the dose. Calcium should be given orally for approximately a week, preferably as calcium chloride. These newborns should be given a milk mixture with a high calcium-to-phosphorus ratio, that is, 3 or 4 gm. of calcium per gram of phosphorus.

FACIAL NERVE PARALYSIS

Paralysis of the facial nerve usually results from pressure over the facial nerve in utero, during labor, or from forceps during delivery. When the infant cries, there is movement on only one side with the mouth being drawn to that side. The eye does not close on the affected side. Prognosis is usually very good because the injury is secondary to pressure and not laceration of the facial nerve. Therefore recovery will occur within a few weeks. The exposed eye should be cared for.

Nursing care of the infant should be carried on as usual with special attention during feeding because sucking may be difficult for the infant. The physician will order therapy for the exposed eye.

Bell's palsy

Bell's palsy is rarely seen in infants, but it is included here because it is a form of facial nerve paralysis.

Isolated, acquired neuritis of the seventh cranial (facial) nerve can occur suddenly in childhood; it is similar to facial nerve palsy in the adult. The cause is unknown in most cases, but the weakness of the facial muscles frequently follow otitis media or respiratory infections.

True idiopathic Bell's palsy is rare in children younger than 2 years of age (Fig. 12-14). If facial palsy is diagnosed in this age group, diseases such as bulbar poliomyelitis, tumor of the brain stem, and viral damage of the facial nucleus should be considered.

The clinical signs of Bell's palsy are deletion

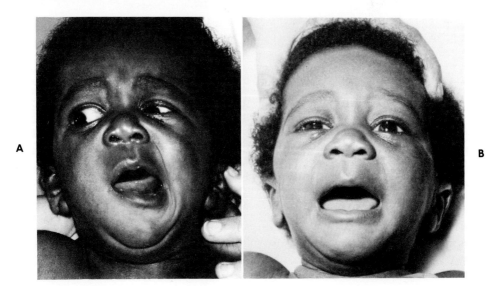

Fig. 12-14. Idiopathic Bell's palsy in 2-month-old child. **A,** Before treatment. **B,** Complete recovery after treatment with steroids.

of the nasolabial fold on the affected side and a pulling of the corner of the mouth to the opposite (nonaffected) side as well as inability to close the eyelid and wrinkle the forehead on the affected side.

The majority of children with idiopathic palsy make a good recovery within a few weeks to several months.

Treatment should consist of protecting the cornea by the use of an eye pad and instillation of methylcellulose drops. Administration of corticosteroids early in the disease is believed by some authors to speed recovery by reducing the edema surrounding the facial nerve. Surgical decompression of the facial nerve may be helpful but is rarely performed in children.

HEMORRHAGIC DISEASE OF THE NEWBORN

Hemorrhagic disease of the newborn is a self-limited bleeding disorder that usually occurs during the first week of life. The bleeding results from a deficiency of the coagulation factors dependent on vitamin K. Since most vitamin K in the body is synthesized by bacteria of the colon and the newborn infant has not yet developed a bacterial flora in his colon, his vitamin K level falls rapidly during the first few days after birth. This decreased vitamin K level interferes with an adequate production of prothrombin by the liver, which is the reason why all infants have relatively low levels of prothrombin during the first few days of life.

Clinical symptoms—bleeding from the skin, navel, mucous membranes, or viscera—may occur with or without trauma, usually between the second or third day of life. The most serious complications are intracranial hemorrhage and anemic shock.

Treatment consists of giving 1.0 mg. vitamin K_1 oxide by intramuscular injection to all newborns immediately after birth. If significant blood loss occurs, a blood transfusion is given to supply red blood cells and to correct the prothrombin deficiency.

The nursing care is that of the normal newborn with special care in handling the infant to avoid further trauma and resulting bleeding. The nurse should frequently observe the umbilical wound for evidence of bleeding and the stool for the presence of blood.

SUDDEN INFANT DEATH SYNDROME (CRIB DEATH)

Sudden unexpected death in a previously normal 2- to 4-month-old infant is common enough to constitute a major health problem. Although families at all socioeconomic levels have been affected, several studies pointed to an increased incidence in the lower social strata. Infants who are usually well nourished and free of any evidence of illness are found dead in their crib or carriage several hours after being fed.

Many studies have failed to reveal the cause of crib deaths. The most commonly proposed theories are (1) overwhelming infection with unknown viruses, (2) unknown errors of metabolism, and (3) disorders of neurologic mechanisms that might lead to laryngospasm or failure of cardiac conduction.

It is important to remember that most of these deaths are not caused by parental negligence. The parents should be supported emotionally to make them feel that they could not in any way have been responsible, by either commission or omission, for the infant's death. They should be told that there is nothing to suggest that greater care or concern on their part would in any way have prevented the event.

NEONATAL NARCOTIC ADDICTION

Narcotic addiction in this country has become common, and many narcotics users are women of child-bearing age. Some of the most common drugs incriminated in addiction are heroin, morphine, meperidine (Demerol), and barbiturates. A newborn infant of a habitual narcotic user is a potential addict whose addiction began in utero. Narcotic withdrawal symptoms will occur soon after delivery when the drug supply is cut off after the umbilical cord is ligated.

The clinical manifestations of neonatal addiction consist of restlessness, hyperirritable, hyperexcitability, sleeplessness, and a high-pitched cry. Excessive lacrimation and salivation, nasal stuffiness, and sweating are also observed. The infant eats well but fails to gain weight. In the absence of treatment the infant becomes seriously ill and dies of convulsions, respiratory distress, cyanosis, and apneic episodes.

The diagnosis is suspected when the mother has multiple needle punctures, cellulitis, thrombophlebitis, and withdrawal symptoms. Testing of blood and urine specimens for the sus-

pected narcotic is ordered soon after birth since the narcotic metabolites disappear rapidly.

Drugs such as paregoric, chlorpromazine, and phenobarbital have been used in the treatment of these infants. Pareneteral administration of fluids and calories may be needed in more severe cases. Long-term follow-up in a limited number of cases has shown those infants and children to be normal.

BRACHIAL PALSY

Brachial palsy is the result of injury to the nerve roots of the brachial plexus. A prolonged and difficult labor is associated with this condition. The paralysis may be of the entire arm, it may involve only the lower arm (Klumpke paralysis), or it may involve just the upper arm (Erb-Duchenne paralysis).

The Erb-Duchenne type of brachial palsy is the most common type of paralysis in the newborn. The arm cannot voluntarily be abducted from the shoulder or externally rotated, and the forearm cannot be supinated. The Moro reflex is absent on the affected side. The injury occurs when traction is exerted on the head during delivery of the shoulder.

The prognosis is excellent because most of the time the paralysis is caused by edema and hemorrhage about the nerve fibers. There should be a gradual return of function within a few months.

The treatment is conservative. The arm should be immobilized in a position of maximal relaxation. If the hand is paralyzed, padding should be placed in the fist. Massage and range-of-motion exercises are done daily to prevent contraction deformity. Surgical procedures on the nerve fibers may be considered when the infant is 6 to 12 months of age if function of the arm has not returned.

CEPHALOHEMATOMA

Cephalohematoma is a condition in which there is a subperiosteal hemorrhage under one cranial bone. This swelling does not manifest itself until several hours after birth because the periosteal bleeding is slow. It does not cross the suture lines. No treatment is necessary. The hematoma usually disappears within the first 6 weeks of life.

CAPUT SUCCEDANEUM

In caput succedaneum there is edema of the scalp. The edema may cross the suture lines and is located on the portion of the head that presented during delivery. No treatment is necessary. It disappears within a few days after birth.

INTRACRANIAL HEMORRHAGE

Intracranial hemorrhage may result from trauma during delivery. Extreme lethargy may be the first symptom the infant shows after birth. His actions are not like those of well infants. Other symptoms that may be seen are unusual irregularity of respirations, restlessness, either pallor or cyanosis, convulsive seizures, failure to suck well, a high-pitched cry, vomiting, and a tense or bulging fontanel. The nurse's responsibility is in making pertinent observations and in reporting them.

REFERENCES

Abramowicz, M., and Kass, E. H.: Pathogenesis and prognosis of prematurity, N. Engl. J. Med. **275:**878, 938, 1001, 1053, 1966.

Baird, D.: The epidemiology of prematurity, J. Pediatr. **65:**909, 1964.

Behramen, R.: The high-risk infant. In Shirkey, H. C.: Pediatric therapy, ed. 4, St. Louis, 1972, The C. V. Mosby Co.

Behrman, R. E., and Hsia, D. Y.-Y.: Summary of symposium on phototherapy for hyperbilirubinemia, J. Pediatr. **75:**718, 1969.

Bender, S.: Problems of prematurity, Practitioner **204:**366, March, 1970.

Brown, A. K.: Neonatal jaundice, Pediatr. Clin. North Am. **9:**575, 1962.

Callon, H.: The premature infant's nurse, Am. J. Nurs. **63:**104, February, 1963.

Caplan, G.: Patterns of parental response to the crisis of premature birth, Psychiatry **23:**365, 1960.

Chinn, R.: Infant gavage feeding, Am. J. Nurs. **71:**1964, October, 1971.

Committee on Fetus and Newborn: Standards and recommendations for hospital care of newborn infants, Evanston, Ill., 1971, American Academy of Pediatrics.

Cornblath, M.: Hypoglycemia in the newborn, Pediatr. Clin. North Am. **13:**905, 1966.

Crowley, M.: When a high risk infant is born, Am. J. Nurs. **75:**1696, October, 1975.

Farquhar, J. W.: The child of the diabetic woman, Arch. Dis. Child. **34:**76, 1959.

Ferguson, A. B.: Orthopedic surgery in infancy and childhood, ed. 4, Baltimore, 1975, The Williams & Wilkins Co.

Fishbein, J. F., Shadravan, I., and Hebert, L.: Idiopathic Bell palsy in a 2-month-old child, Am. J. Dis. Child. **128:**112, 1974.

Gluck, L.: Newborn special care. In Shirkey, H. C., editor: Pediatric therapy, ed. 5, St. Louis, 1975, The C. V. Mosby Co.

Heller, H.: Infant identification, Hospitals **44:**57, February, 1970.

Hervada, A. R., and Hartnett, E.: Specialized care for premature and high-risk infants, Hospitals **40:**54, October, 1966.

Hill, R. M., and Desmond, M. M.: Management of the narcotic withdrawal syndrome in the neonate, Pediatr. Clin. North Am. **10:**67, 1963.

Kitterman, J. A., et al.: Catheterization of umbilical vessels in the newborn infants, Pediatr. Clin. North Am. **17:**895, 1970.

Krumpe, M., and Kleinman, L.: Care of the infant with the respiratory distress syndrome, Nurs. Clin. North Am. **6:**25, March, 1971.

Leukens, J.: Hemolytic disease of the newborn. In Gellis, S. S., and Kagan, B. M., editors: Current pediatric therapy, ed. 6, Philadelphia, 1973, W. B. Saunders Co.

Lundeen, E. C., and Kunstadter, R. H.: Care of the premature infant, Philadelphia, 1958, J. B. Lippincott Co.

Neal, M. V., and Nave, C. M.: Ability of premature infants to maintain his own body temperature, Nurs. Res. **17:**396, September-October, 1968.

Nelson, N. M.: On the etiology of hyaline membrane disease, Pediatr. Clin. North Am. **17:**943, 1970.

Owens, C.: Parents' response to premature birth, Am. J. Nurs. **60:**1113, June, 1960.

Potter, E. L.: Pathology of the fetus and the infant. ed. 2, Chicago, 1961, Year Book Medical Publishers, Inc.

Review your knowledge of narcotic addiction in the newborn, J. Obstet. Gynecol. Neonatal Nurs. **2:**72, January/February, 1973.

Segal, S.: Neonatal intensive care, Pediatr. Clin. North Am. **13:**1149, 1966.

Segal, S.: Oxygen: Too much, too little, Nurs. Clin. North Am. **6:**39, 1971.

Silverberg, M.: Diseases of liver and biliary tract. In Shirkey, H. C., editor: Pediatric therapy, ed. 4, St. Louis, 1975, The C. V. Mosby Co.

Smith, C. A.: Diagnosis and treatment; use and misuse of oxygen in treatment of prematures, Pediatrics **33:**111, 1964.

Stern, L., and Denton, R. L.: Kernicterus in small premature infants, Pediatrics **35:**483, 1965.

Valdes-Dapena, M. A.: Sudden and unexpected death in infancy: A review of the world literature, 1954-1966, Pediatrics **39:**123, 1967.

Williams, S. L.: Phototherapy in hyperbilirubinemia, Am. J. Nurs. **71:**1397, July, 1971.

Wood, B. S. B.: Development of jaundice and anemia in the newborn, Nurs. Mirror, **136:**23, February 9, 1973.

Yates, S. A.: Stillbirth—what staff can do, Am. J. Nurs. **72:**1592, September, 1972.

Zahourek, R., et al.: Grieving and the loss of the newborn, Am. J. Nurs. **73:**836, May, 1973.

13

Nursing care of
THE CHILD WITH CONGENITAL DEFECTS

One of the major health problems of childhood is that of congenital malformations. As a cause of death it ranks second in infants under 1 year of age (Table 9-1). (Conditions classified as "certain diseases of early infancy" rank first.) Mortality from congenital malformations ranks second in children 1 year to 4 years old (Table 9-5), third in children 5 to 14 years old (Table 9-6), and seventh in young people 15 to 24 years old (Table 9-7). The severity of particular malformations is found to vary. Some are incompatible with life, whereas some can be totally corrected; others, even though treated, leave the child with a handicap.

In an effort to know more about the prevention and treatment of congenital malformations, many birth defect centers have been established by the National Institute of Neurological Diseases and Blindness as well as by the Pan-American Health Organization. Also there is an International Association for the Study of Congenital Malformations.

Although it is believed that congenital malformations may be due to genetic factors, chromosomal abnormalities, adverse environmental factors during intrauterine life, and/or the interplay of these factors, more needs to be known of specific factors causing defects. The roles of nutrition, certain drugs, excessive irradiation, and infections during the pregnancy of the mother are discussed in Chapter 2. By techniques used in experimental research, defects have been produced in animals, but this does not necessarily mean they can be reproduced in man in the same way.

From Table 13-1 it can be seen that deaths from congenital anomalies of the heart and circulatory system far surpass others in total numbers. Next, in consecutive order, rank deaths from malformations of the central nervous, respiratory, digestive, and musculoskeletal systems. Table 13-1 represents *mortality* figures from congenital defects. There is a high *inci-*

Table 13-1. Deaths under 1 year and infant mortality rates, United States, 1973*

Cause of death†	Number	Rate‡
Congenital anomalies (740-759)	8,953	285.4
Anencephalus (740)	784	25.0
Spina bifida (741)	445	14.2
Congenital hydrocephalus (742)	439	14.0
Other congenital anomalies of central nervous system and eye (743, 744)	338	10.8
Congenital anomalies of heart (746)	3,354	106.9
Other congenital anomalies of circulatory system (747)	642	20.5
Congenital anomalies of respiratory system (748)	573	18.3
Congenital anomalies of digestive system (749-751)	465	14.8
Congenital anomalies of genitourinary system (752, 753)	324	10.3
Congenital anomalies of musculoskeletal system (754-756)	305	9.5
Down's disease (759.3)	95	3.0
Other congenital syndromes affecting multiple systems (759.0-759.2, 759.4-759.9)	994	31.7
Other and unspecified congenital anomalies (745, 757, 758)	195	6.2

*Modified from Summary Report Final Mortality Statistics, Rockville, Md., 1973, Public Health Service, U.S. Department of Health, Education, and Welfare (Table 10).
†According to International classification of diseases, eighth revision, 1965.
‡Per 100,000 live births in specified group.

337

dence of some defects that do not cause death, such as clubfeet, polydactyly, and hypospadias.

COMMON PSYCHOLOGICAL FACTORS

The arrival of a new infant, especially a first one, should bring a great deal of happiness to parents; yet in some instances it proves to be an unhappy crisis in their lives. For months the parents have anticipated and carefully planned for the infant; perhaps older children in the family have been told about the expected arrival of another member and they have helped in the preparation for the newcomer. Then the momentous occasion comes, the infant is born, and the family is told that the infant has a defect—he is different from others. What this does to the mother, the father, and relatives depends on the particular people involved. The pediatric nurse can only speculate as to the possible effect of this news. She must remember that the abnormality that is a common condition to her—a cleft lip and palate, clubfoot, or spina bifida—is something new, maybe repulsive, and perhaps even gruesome to parents. It is advisable to let the parents see the infant as soon as the doctor has explained the condition to them so that the parents will not imagine the defect worse than it really is.

Solnit and Stark (1961) recommend that the mother be allowed a period of mourning for the well child she did not have—the infant who has been the object of her dreams. They further suggest for the mother both rest and participation in making realistic plans for the infant's care as a means of helping her in this critical time.

The mother may feel guilty, believing she caused her infant to have a defect. Her husband and his family may think something is odd about her ancestry. There may even be an estrangement between the mother and father because of this. Another possibility is that the mother may feel she has failed her husband and failed as a woman. Both parents may suffer from loss of self-esteem. They did not produce a ''normal'' infant. Perhaps neither husband nor wife wants any more children because of their fear of producing another child with a defect.

Feelings and attitudes toward the infant take many forms. The parents may be repelled by the defect. The mother may reject the infant and may either neglect him or hide her hostility by oversolicitude. On the other hand, the mother may accept the infant but be overly protective and attentive, to the detriment of her own physical and mental health, her husband's, and her children's. She may devote her entire attention to the infant and neglect the rest of the family's needs. Complete absorption with the infant's needs may indicate a feeling of guilt. The mother may be trying to expiate her feeling of sinfulness by zealous care of the infant. The mother may regard the birth of the infant as punishment for something she did wrong.

The mother and the father both need emotional support. The pediatric nurse may first meet the parents in a private doctor's office, in the outpatient department, or on the pediatric unit. The way the nurse greets and speaks to the parents helps or hinders the belief that they are ''worthy'' parents. Their self-esteem needs to be bolstered.

The nurse should remember that the way and manner in which she handles and accepts the infant will influence the parents. If they see the nurse is able to accept the deformed infant, the parents may hope there may be others in the community who can likewise accept their infant. Seeing the nurse talk to and cuddle the child with a defect is reassuring to his parents. In the hospital situation, nurses' prompt attention to the infant's physical needs may relieve some of the parents' tension.

The attitudes of siblings of the child may reflect those of the mother (loving, overprotective, rejecting). On the other hand, siblings may be hostile to the infant if the infant takes most of the mother's attention.

The nurse needs to let the mother understand she realizes it is harder to care for a child who has special physical needs than it is to care for a well child. The nurse should express interest in the amount of the mother's rest and sleep, in the mother's nutrition, and in her recreation or any activities she has in the community. The mother should be encouraged to maintain the same recreational interests she had before the child was born. If she does this, then for the sake of mental hygiene she should get away from the child at least once during each week. This is of paramount importance. The nurse should be able to suggest community resources, if necessary, that will allow the mother time away from the pressure of caring for the child. It is the only way to keep a sense of balance and maintain good mental hygiene. Staying with the afflicted child constantly may, in time, make the care of the child harder and more laborious for the mother. Also, the mother's fatigue and possible depression will affect her relationships with other members of the family.

The public health nurse who visits the home of the child with a congenital defect should remember that the mother needs her attention as a person just as much as, and perhaps more than, the infant does. Also, the nurse should be concerned with the adjustment of other members of the family to the infant with a defect. To the extent to which they are able they, too, should share in the care of the child, know him, and play with him.

During the preschool years of the child with a defect the parents should see that he plays with others and learns the beginning of cooperation, sharing, and participation. His attending a good nursery school and kindergarten, taught by well-prepared teachers, would be invaluable. This child lives in the same world other children do and must learn as a child to be able to get along with others. The teacher and parents can be mutually useful to each other.

During the school years, especially during the preadolescent and adolescent years when the respect of his peers is so important to him, the child should be aided in developing some particular skill in which he can excel: swimming, horseback riding, performing athletic stunts on the trapeze or ropes, ice-skating, roller-skating, etc. Feelings of self-confidence from this skill will carry over into other social areas.

Services available

The nurse is part of a health team in aiding parents to adjust to such an infant or child and to help initiate and implement a plan for his care and treatment.

The parents may wish to take the child to a private physician for treatment, or they may want to have the child evaluated at a crippled children's clinic.

Referral of the infant to a crippled children's clinic is usually made by a physician through the health department of the county in which the family resides. The program in most states is operated under the auspices of the state health department. Local crippled children's clinics are set up in various health districts in the state. Services are offered to children from birth to 21 years of age. The adolescent in his later teens may be directed by the clinic to a vocational rehabilitation center. This is usually a division of the state rehabilitation center, which is frequently under the jurisdiction of the state board of education.

Crippled childrens' services are intended not only for the child with an orthopedic defect but also for the child with certain other types of defects such as a congenital heart malformation. Eligibility of children with defects varies from state to state since the program is supported by matching state and federal funds.

Because many infants in rural areas are delivered by a midwife the *public health nurse* may be the first person (of medical personnel) to see the infant with a gross deformity. She has a responsibility to encourage and assist the parent in planning for medical evaluation and treatment of the child's problem. Also, it is her responsibility to help meet the recommendations made by a physician.

The *hospital nurse* may see the child with a defect in the neonatal period, in the outpatient department, or in the hospital unit when he is admitted for treatment. The child may have to have more than one hospital admission for the medical care of the condition. The nurse has the opportunity to help both the child and his family adjust to the child's condition, as well as to guide the parents in the promotion of the health of the child.

ORTHOPEDIC DEFECTS
Clubfeet
Nature of the condition

The word *talipes* is used in connection with certain foot deformities. *Talus* is a Latin word that means ankle, and *pes* means foot; therefore

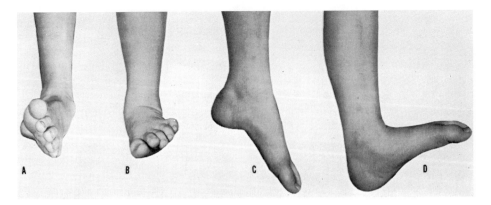

Fig. 13-1. Four cardinal positions of foot deformity. **A,** Varus; **B,** valgus; **C,** equinus; **D,** calcaneus. (From Raney, R. B., and Brashear, H. R.: Shands' handbook of orthopaedic surgery, ed. 8, St. Louis, 1971, The C. V. Mosby Co.)

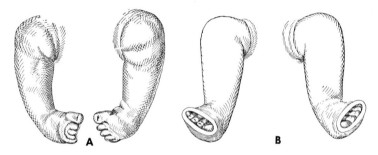

Fig. 13-2. Bilateral talipes equinovarus in infant. **A,** Before correction. **B,** Undergoing correction in plaster casts. (From Raney, R. B., and Brashear, H. R.: Shands' handbook of orthopaedic surgery, ed. 8, St. Louis, 1971, The C. V. Mosby Co.)

talipes refers to a deformity that causes the patient to walk on the ankle (Raney and Brashear, 1971). There are four cardinal positions in foot deformity: talipes varus (inversion), talipes valgus (eversion), talipes equinus (plantar flexion), and talipes calcaneus (dorsiflexion). Sometimes there are combinations of deformities, such as equinovarus (the most common type of clubfoot) and calcaneovalgus.

The sooner treatment is begun, the better. To obtain the best results this should be within the first 3 months of life (Raney and Brashear, 1971). The treatment includes not only correcting the deformity but also developing sufficient muscle tone in the affected limb so that the correction can be maintained. This entails supervision of the child until the growth of his foot is complete.

Exactly how the child's foot is treated depends on the age of the child, the extent of the deformity, and the doctor in charge.

Often the child's affected foot is put into a special shoe (clubfoot prewalker shoe) that is fastened to a steel bar. The unaffected foot is placed in a straight, laced shoe that is fastened to the bar in a neutral position. The affected foot is placed in a position optimum for correction of the deformity. (The bar has adjustable screws.) The steel bar is available in different lengths for infants and children of various ages.

Other doctors may manipulate the foot and place it in a series of plaster casts. These casts are changed at intervals during a period of 3 to 14 days until the correction has been reached; then a final cast is left on for 4 to 8 weeks

(Raney and Brashear, 1971). A night splint may be used to keep the foot in an overcorrected position for a number of months after that. Also, special exercises are taught to the mother to do for the child at home. Operative procedures may be used if the foot relapses into its former position.

Role of the nurse

Identification of defect. As the nursery nurse surveys the newborn infants, she notes that all of the infants hold their feet in a varus position (inversion). This is normal for newborn infants; however, if the nurse cannot easily turn the foot into the normal position or if the varus position is an extreme one, she should record this and call it to the doctor's attention as soon as possible. She should be able to identify the fact that one foot is different from the other. If there is the slightest question in her mind, she should discuss this with the doctor. Remembering that talipes equinovarus is the most common type of clubfoot may help her, as well as knowing that the condition is usually unilateral and is more common in boys than in girls. Also, the nurse should bear in mind that, if an infant has one defect, he may have others. Hydrocephalus (p. 419) and spina bifida (p. 387) are sometimes associated with clubfeet.

In her home visits the public health nurse should always look at the feet of the infants, even if she has actually called to see the grandmother in the home. Her relationships within the home should be such that the parents are proud to exhibit their children. Infants do not usually have on socks or stockings so that the nurse can notice the infant in his crib without obviously examining the child's feet. If she sees an infant or child with a foot in an abnormal position, she should talk with the mother about his receiving medical supervision. On the other hand, it should be remembered that many midwives still deliver infants in rural areas, and a child may never see a doctor or nurse until he starts to school and has to be immunized against certain communicable diseases.

The child health conference is another place where the nurse may see an infant with an untreated foot deformity. Before the doctors examine the infants the nurse has the opportunity to see and screen patients. When she sees something that the doctor should know about, she can either make a special note of it on a paper attached to the chart or she can tell the doctor verbally so that the doctor will be sure to examine the limb under question and advise the mother accordingly.

To summarize, the nurse has a responsibility for recognizing that one foot of a child is different from the other or that both feet are different from normal feet. She should either draw the doctor's attention to this or try to see that the mother gets the infant to a clinic or private doctor. The earlier treatment is begun, the better are the chances for a well-functioning foot in later childhood.

Cast care. If the infant lives some distance from the hospital and his doctor has decided upon frequent cast changes, the infant may be hospitalized for a few weeks. When the infant is returned from the cast room to the unit, the main areas of the nurse's concern are (1) drying of the cast, (2) circulation in the limb, and (3) care of the skin near the cast.

A fan or heat lamp should not be used on the wet cast because the outside of the cast will dry while the inside will remain wet. To have the cast dry evenly the infant's position needs changing. He can be turned from one side to the other and propped with a blanket, pillow, or folded pads.

Since an infant is small, a folded blanket or pillow can be used under both little legs to elevate them. If the circulation is good, the toes will be warm and pink. If there is swelling or coldness or if good color does not return immediately after the nurse presses the nailbed of one toe, the cast may be too tight. In watching the circulation the nurse needs to realize the infant cannot tell her that he cannot move his toes or that his toes feel numb. It is up to the nurse to be conscientious in her observation of the circulation. If the infant fusses as though he is in pain, this should be reported and a mild sedative ordered. Older infants are likely to be more uncomfortable than young infants. Any excess plaster on the toes or legs can be washed off with a little cold water or acetone.

Although there is padding under the cast, there is usually no stockinet used with a cast that is on an extremity for a short time. As a result, it will be necessary for the nurse to petal the edges of the cast with adhesive around the thigh and foot or the edges will crumble; also, the edge of the cast, especially on the thigh, might irritate the skin. A square piece of adhesive placed on the cast like a diamond holds well. Each petal should overlap the next. An applicator can be used to tuck the adhesive under the cast smoothly. Around the cast on the foot smaller pieces of adhesive should be used.

Two or three times a day special skin care should be given (in the morning, in the afternoon, and in the evening). The nurse can take a warm damp washcloth, pull back the skin on the thigh next to the cast, wash it well, and then wipe it. Next, using a little rubbing alcohol on her hand, the nurse should massage the skin well around the cast. The alcohol toughens the skin. Powder must not be used since it cakes. The toes of the child can be washed with a washcloth and wiped, but the only way to get between the toes is to use a cotton applicator. This can be moistened in the water and used to cleanse between the toes. To get under the edges of the cast near the toes with an applicator, again the nurse should pull the skin back with pressure of her thumb. The mother should not only be shown how to give cast and skin care but she should also do it under supervision of the nurse before she takes the infant home.

Meeting psychological needs. The psychological needs of the infant need consideration. Sometimes the parents, as well as nurses, are hesitant to pick up an infant with a cast or one with any special equipment. The infant needs to be held when he is fed and at other times be given affection in the many ways described in Chapter 9 in the discussion on promotion of health of the infant. Also, the infant needs sensory and motor stimulation. A toy could be fastened to his bed and other recreational diversion provided. The manner in which an infant is handled and cared for will influence him. The nurse could let the mother hold the infant while the bed is being made, or during visiting hours the nurse might pick up the infant a moment, talk to him, and hold him. After that she might ask if the mother or father would like to hold the infant.

Preparation for discharge. Before the infant is discharged the nurse needs to ascertain whether the mother understands when and where to return to see the infant's doctor. In addition, she should find out what the mother knows about the infant's care and supplement the mother's knowledge as necessary. Demonstration and a return demonstration of the infant's care should not be left until the day of discharge.

Many of these infants are cared for under crippled children's services. A referral to the public health nurse in the district where the child lives allows for continuity of care of the child. The hospital nurse should be explicit in her referral as to what instructions she has already given the parents.

Dislocation of the hip
Nature of the condition

Congenital hip dislocation or dysplasia is a common congenital orthopedic deformity. The incidence is high in Latin races; it is rare in blacks and is more common in girls than in boys. Unilateral dislocation is more common than bilateral dislocation.

Raney and Brashear (1971) define congenital dysplasia as "a malformation of the hip joint, with which a subluxation or dislocation of the hip is often associated at the time of birth or shortly thereafter. Three degrees of congenital dysplasia have been described: acetabular dysplasia, subluxation, and dislocation." In acetabular dysplasia the acetabulum is shallow. This phase can go into subluxation in which the head of the femur rides upward and outward although it is still in contact with the acetabulum. Complete dislocation occurs when the head of the femur is completely out of the acetabulum.

Unilateral hip dislocation

When the nurse is caring for the infant in the newborn nursery or sees him at home or in a child health conference, she should be alert to signs of dislocation of the hip. Prior to weight bearing, manifestations shown by young infants with unilateral dislocation include (1) prominence of one hip, (2) extra folds in the thigh near the gluteal region, and (3) unequal length of the thighs (Fig. 13-3). When the physician examines the infant, he places the child on his back, flexes the knees to 90 degrees, and tests for limited hip abduction by pressing against the knees. X-ray films are taken to confirm the diagnosis.

When the child with unilateral hip dislocation begins to walk, he limps because one leg is shorter. This may cause slowness in learning to walk. Older children may tire after exertion. There will be some lordosis and abdominal protrusion but not as much as when there is bilateral dislocation. In addition to this, particular signs for which the physician looks include (1) Trendelenburg's sign, (2) Ortolani's sign, and (3) telescoping, or "piston mobility." A positive Trendelenburg sign is elicited when the child stands with his weight on the affected hip and the pelvis is tilted downward on the normal side. In a normal situation the pelvis would tilt upward (Raney and Brashear, 1971). Ortolani's sign is a snap or click heard when the head of the femur rides over the acctabulum rim. Telescoping, or "piston mobility," is an up-and-down movement of the greater trochanter and head of the femur that is felt in the buttock

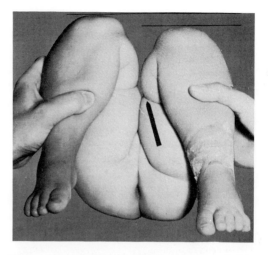

Fig. 13-3. Knee level test (Allis' sign) for unilateral congenital dislocation of the hip in a girl 2½ years of age. With infant supine on a hard surface, hips and knees are fully flexed. When the test is positive, knee on the dislocated side is lower. Note increased depth of the left thigh fold, which also suggests dislocation. (From Raney, R. B., and Brashear, H. R.: Shands' handbook of orthopaedic surgery, ed. 8, St. Louis, 1971, The C. V. Mosby Co.)

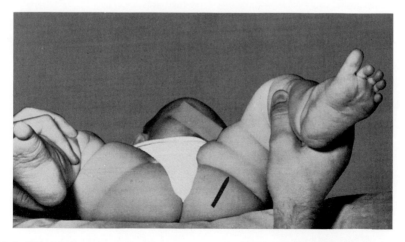

Fig. 13-4. Abduction test for unilateral dysplasia of the hip in an infant 8 months of age, who has subluxation on the left side. When the test is positive the thigh on the dysplastic side cannot be abducted so far as the thigh on the side with a normal hip. Note deepening of the proximal fold in the left thigh, which also suggests dysplasia. (From Raney, R. B., and Brashear, H. R.: Shands' handbook of orthopaedic surgery, ed. 8, St. Louis, 1971, The C. V. Mosby Co.)

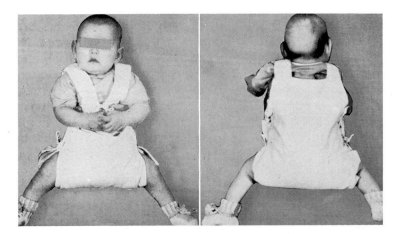

Fig. 13-5. Pillow splint (Frejka) used to maintain abduction of the hips. (Courtesy V. L. Hart; from Raney, R. B., and Brashear, H. R.: Shands' handbook of orthopaedic surgery, ed. 8, St. Louis, 1971, The C. V. Mosby Co.)

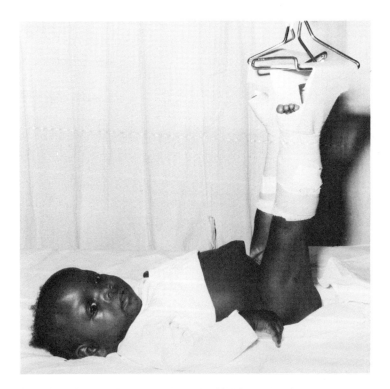

Fig. 13-6. Congenital bilateral dislocation of hips in child 9 months of age. Bryant traction is being applied prior to open surgical reduction of the hips. Note presence of umbilical hernia.

when the thigh is extended, pushed toward the patient's head, and then pulled distally.

Bilateral hip dislocation

The nurse can observe the following signs of bilateral hip dislocation in a young infant before the weight-bearing period: (1) wide perineum, (2) flat gluteal muscles, and (3) prominence of both hips. When the child with bilateral dislocation begins to walk, he shows a characteristic "duck waddle" gait. To get his balance such a child leans backward. This produces lordosis and a prominent abdomen (pot belly). In examining the child the physician tests for limited abduction of the hips and telescoping, or "piston mobility."

Treatment

The earlier the treatment is begun, the more favorable are the results.

When the condition is diagnosed early in infancy, the affected hip (or hips) may be placed in a position of increased abduction by use of a pillow splint (Fig. 13-5), or a special brace may be used.

In children between 1 and 3 years of age, often closed reduction of the hip is done after the femur has been pulled down by skeletal traction. A Steinmann pin or a Kirschner wire is used. If closed reduction cannot be accomplished easily, an open reduction is done. After the hip is reduced it is held in position by a hip spica cast with the legs of the child at 90 degrees of abduction in a frog-leg position. The length of time the cast is left on varies with the doctor and the development of the acetabulum. Usually this position is maintained for 6 to 9 months. During this period the cast may be changed about every 6 weeks. After 6 to 9 months the child's legs are repositioned in a 45-degree angle, and another cast is applied. After a few months in this position the child is admitted to the hospital, the cast is completely removed, and beginning exercises in physiotherapy are started. (This includes pool therapy.) The child is first allowed to move fully in his bed; then, when he can straighten his legs to a normal standing position, he may walk on them.

The treatment of children older than 3 years varies, but usually skeleton traction is done first and then open reduction of the hips; sometimes, however, a closed reduction may be done.

Role of the nurse

Identification. The nursery nurse is responsible for identifying and reporting to a doctor if there are asymmetrical folds in the thigh, if one thigh is shorter than the other, or if one hip is different (more prominent than the other). Often the nurse makes these observations while bathing or diapering an infant.

In her contacts with infants and toddlers in the home and in well-child conferences, the nurse should be on the lookout for a limp, a waddling gait, or anything that appears different from normal posture. In addition, she can make the same observations of the small infant that the nursery nurse does. It is essential for those in contact with children to be aware of anything that appears to be abnormal since the earlier treatment is begun, the better.

Aiding hospital adjustment of child. When a child is admitted to the hospital with a dislocated hip, special efforts should be made to help him adjust since he will be hospitalized for several weeks. Moreover, a child who is not happy does not eat well, and nutrition is extremely important to the growth of tissues and bones.

Information should be obtained from parents about whether the child drinks from a bottle or cup, what fluids he likes, and whether he is used to table food or junior pureed food. It is good to know, too, whether he is used to being fed or whether he feeds himself (see Chapter 11).

If the patient is a toddler, the nurse should ascertain from the parents whether he has been toilet trained. Soiling of the cast later can be more easily avoided if he has been toilet trained. If the child is toilet trained, when does he usually defecate and how often does he urinate? What words does he used to express his toilet needs? (Refer to Chapter 11 for further discussion of orienting a new child to the hospital.)

Traction care. When traction is applied, it is the nurse's responsibility to see that the weights hang free and are not resting on any part of the crib. The nurse should note whether the traction is in place and whether the child is up in bed sufficiently so that his foot is not resting against the end of the crib. The use of a waist or jacket restraint may be necessary to keep a young patient in the right position. The traction needs to be observed hourly.

The skin of the child will not break down easily if buttocks, back, and elbows are massaged briskly at least three times daily (morning, afternoon, and bedtime). These areas should be washed with soap before being massaged. Having a dry bed also helps to keep the skin in good condition. The child of 2 or 3 years should not be asked if he wishes to go to the toilet but offered the bedpan or urinal at the times the mother has said the child usually urinates and defecates. When any small child first wakes up (in the morning and after his nap), he needs to empty his bladder, so he should be given the bedpan then. After breakfast children frequently defecate, so they should be placed on the bedpan at that time. In general the preschool child does not go over a period of 2 hours without emptying his bladder.

Recreation is important as a tool to keep the child happy. The child in traction should be a daily customer of the "Play Lady."

Postoperative nursing. (For details of routine preoperative and postoperative care see pp. 296 and 298.)

After either a closed or an open reduction of the hip the nurse has the responsibility for proper care of the cast since a hip spica cast will be applied. The child is likely to be in a frog-leg position. (For discussion of circulation and skin care and cast care see p. 341, under care of a child with a clubfoot.) To that discussion may be added that pillows should support the child's cast as necessary. The child should be turned about every 4 hours when the cast is wet; after that he should be turned about every 2 hours.

The head of the bed should be elevated so that, if the child voids, urine (from a little girl) is less likely to soil the back of the cast. The children who are not toilet trained should have a diaper folded like a perineal pad and tucked under the edges of the cast around the perineum. Over this can be placed a large diaper pinned on each side as usual. The large diaper keeps the pad in place.

When the older child uses a bedpan, some waterproof material should be tucked under the edges of the cast around the perineum and perhaps a diaper over that to protect the sides of the cast. Special cast panties can be used for older children so they will not be unduly exposed.

Various ways to keep the child happy should be devised. For children who are immovable a toy that moves, such as a small car on wheels, is important. The child's crib may be turned so he sees other children. The crib can be taken into the playroom or moved next to a window. The small child can be lifted by the nurse and held in a chair (one without arms). Occupational therapy has been mentioned. Occasional parties relieve the monotony. Songs and music on a record player help. Picture books can be used. A play bag can be fastened to the bed so that he can drop his toys into it.

The 2-year-old can help to feed himself. He can also help in washing hands and face.

Preparation for discharge. Care of the child's cast, as well as means of protecting the cast, should be explained to the mother and demonstrated before the child leaves the hospital.

It is particularly important to discuss with the mother various means of making the child feel that he is one of the family. He is going to be in the cast for a period of months. There is no reason the child with a hip spica cannot be taken for rides in an automobile or be taken on a family picnic. At home he should be wherever the family usually are: the kitchen, living room, porch, or whatever room is used. He could be placed on the couch or on the floor in his cast. He should see other people so he will not have a difficult time in meeting new people later. His future social adjustment will then be easier. If left to himself, the child could very easily regress to a more infantile level. His psychological needs are the same as those of any other young child.

A referral to the public health nurse should be made. The hospital nurse should be very explicit in telling the former what her own suggestions to the mother have been.

Readmission and final discharge. When the child is readmitted and the last cast is removed, the nurse must remember that the child is not accustomed to sitting up. He should be propped up with pillows to a position where he is comfortable. Children move as much as they can, so each day he will be more active. His first weight bearing may be supervised by a physiotherapist. After the child becomes used to standing his pleasure in taking steps by himself is a joy to all.

The importance of keeping clinic appointments should be emphasized since these children have to be followed over a period of time to make sure there is no relapse.

Torticollis

Congenital torticollis is seen more frequently in girls than boys and is associated with difficult deliveries.

The sternocleidomastoid muscle is the main structure involved. It is contracted and shorter than the muscle on the opposite side of the neck. A mass may be felt in this muscle. The head is tilted toward the involved side, and the chin is turned toward the opposite shoulder. The shoulder on the affected side may become

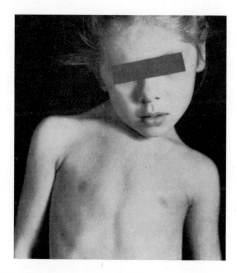

Fig. 13-7. Congenital torticollis in a 5-year-old girl. Note flexion of the head and neck to the right, pointing of the chin to the left, flattening of right side of the face, and high right shoulder. (From Raney, R. B., and Brashear, H. R.: Shands' handbook of orthopaedic surgery, ed. 8, St. Louis, 1971, The C. V. Mosby Co.)

elevated as the deformity progresses. Also there may be cervical dorsal scoliosis and asymmetry of the face (Fig. 13-7).

If the nurse in the newborn nursery cannot place the baby's head in a straight line with his body or if she feels a lump on one side of his neck, this should be reported at once. There are varying degrees of this disorder and the older the child becomes, the more difficult the problem is to treat.

In infancy gentle stretching to an overcorrected position, along with special exercises, may overcome this condition. In older children or in those with severe deformity, resection of the muscle is done and an overcorrected position maintained by plaster, brace, or traction. Exercises are also used.

(For nursing care of a child in traction see p. 345; for cast care see p. 341, under the discussion of congenital dislocated hip.)

Metatarsus varus

Metatarsus varus is a condition in which there is adduction of the forefoot at the tarsometatarsal joints. If untreated, the child walks in a clumsy manner. It is one of the causes of pigeon toe. Stretching exercises may be done, and special shoes may be prescribed. In severe cases application of a plaster cast may be necessary. After correction is attained special shoes may be necessary for a period of time.

Miscellaneous orthopedic abnormalities

There are other deformities that are deserving of a definition rather than a discussion so that the nurse will understand terminology she may read on a chart or terminology used verbally in relation to a particular deformity.

Polydactyly refers to supernumerary fingers and toes.

Syndactyly is a union of fingers or toes, usually the third and fourth fingers or the second and third toes.

Brachydactyly is abnormal shortness of the fingers and toes resulting from lack of one of the phalanges.

Split hand or **split foot,** described as "lobster claw," is manifested by a deep cleft in the anterior part of hand or foot. It is associated with polydactyly and syndactyly.

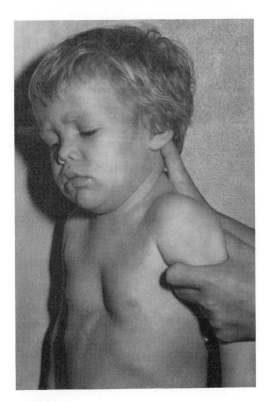

Fig. 13-8. Pectus excavatum in a 6-year-old boy.

Amelia is absence of an extremity or extremities.

Phocomelia is absence of a proximal portion of a limb or limbs.

Klippel-Feil syndrome is a condition in which there is a fusion of two or more of the cervical vertebrae; consequently the child has a short neck. In addition, there is absence or limitation of motion of the head, a low hairline, and often a mongoloid type of face. There are varying degrees of the deformity.

Arthrogryposis multiplex congenita (myodystrophia fetalis) is a congenital condition in which there is generalized fibrous ankylosis of the joints of the upper and lower extremities.

Pectus excavatum (funnel chest) is the indentation of the lower part of the sternum in most instances due to a short central tendon of the diaphragm (Fig. 13-8). The condition is usually congenital, and surgical improvement may be attempted for cosmetic reasons or if compression causes pulmonary embarrassment.

CARDIAC DEFECTS
The problem

Congenital malformations are one of the ten leading causes of death in infancy and in childhood (Tables 9-1, 9-5, 9-6, and 9-7). Among the commonest types of congenital defects is congenital heart disease. The fact that it accounts for at least half of all deaths caused by congenital defects in the first year of life helps the nurse to realize the importance of this condition. In addition, it is the commonest type of heart disease in childhood. The mortality of children with congenital heart disease is highest during the infancy period. In the first month of life about one third of infants born with this condition die. Although some of these infants have problems so complex that they cannot be saved at the present time, many of the infants with congenital heart conditions can be helped if their condition is diagnosed and treated early.

Fetal and postnatal circulation

To understand the nursing care of children with heart defects it is well for the nurse to review both fetal (Fig. 13-9) and postnatal (Fig. 13-10) circulation to understand the immediate circulatory readjustments that allow adequate blood flow through the lungs. A few of the salient points are reviewed in the following paragraphs.

Equally as important as the onset of breathing at birth are the immediate circulatory readjustments that allow adequate blood flow through the lungs. Prior to birth the source of oxygen supply to the fetus is the placenta. The lungs are mainly nonfunctional during fetal life; therefore it is not necessary for the fetal heart to pump much blood to the lungs. Blood returning from the placenta passes through the ductus venosus, mainly bypassing the liver. Then most of the blood entering the right atrium from the inferior vena cava is directed through the *foramen ovale* into the left atrium. Thus the well-oxygenated blood from the placenta enters the left side of the heart rather than the right side and is pumped into the aorta to flow mainly into the vessels of the head and forelimbs.

The blood entering the right atrium from the superior vena cava is directed through the tricuspid valve into the right ventricle. The blood is deoxygenated blood from the head region of the fetus. It is pumped by the right ventricle into the pulmonary artery, then through the *ductus arteriosus* into the descending aorta and through the two umbilical arteries into the

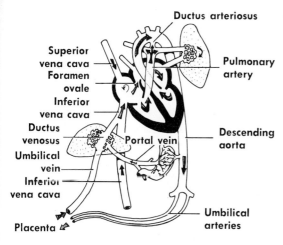

Fig. 13-9. Fetal circulation.

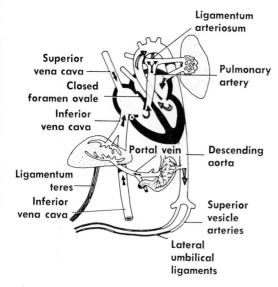

Fig. 13-10. Normal circulation.

placenta. Thus the deoxygenated blood becomes oxygenated (Fig. 13-9).

After birth changes in the circulation occur whereby the infant's source of oxygen is the lungs. When the umbilical cord is ligated, the lungs expand. This causes a great increase in the pulmonary blood flow. The foramen ovale, ductus arteriosus, and ductus venosus become functionally closed because they are no longer needed. In the majority of cases the ductus arteriosus closes by the eighth week of life and the foramen ovale by the end of the twelfth week. Consequently the heart pumps blood to

the lungs via the pulmonary artery and to the body via the aorta (Fig. 13-10).

An explanation of common types of congenital heart defects is included here before a discussion of nursing care relative to them (Fig. 13-11).

Incidence and etiology of cardiac defects

A functional circulatory system has been established by the fourth week of intrauterine life, while the architecture of the heart is complete by the eighth week. Occasionally the heart is malformed during fetal life; the defect is called a *congenital anomaly of the heart*. It is estimated that 1% of newborns have anomalies of the heart that are severe enough to produce symptoms.

Some of the more widely accepted etiological factors that produce congenital heart defects are (1) maternal infection due to rubella, Coxsackie virus B infection, and toxoplasmosis, (2) teratogenic effect of drugs and radiation, (3) heredity, that is, those caused by defects inherent in the genes, and (4) vitamin deficiency.

Diagnosis

The diagnosis can usually be established from the medical history, physical examination findings, electrocardiography, and roentgenograms. The history should include questions about the child's general activity, exercise tolerance, feeding behavior, and response to infections. The mother should be asked if the child had any cyanotic episodes, dyspnea with minimal exertion, and swelling of the face or extremities. The abnormal physical findings are variable and should be included in the description of a specific defect rather than making general statements about a child with congenital heart disease. The electrocardiogram measures the changes in the electrical potentials of the heart, thereby permitting recognition of the presence or absence of relative hypertrophy of the atria and ventricles. Roentgenograms of the chest with or without barium swallow permits the radiologist and pediatric cardiologist to evaluate the size of heart, the size of a particular chamber, the condition of the pulmonary vascular bed, and the size of pulmonary arteries and great vessels.

Table 13-2. Normal cardiovascular pressures and oxygen saturations in children

Location	Pressure (mm. Hg)	Oxygen saturation (percent)
Right atrium	3 (mean)	75
Right ventricle	30/3	75
Pulmonary artery	30/10	75
Left atrium	8 (mean)	95
Left ventricle	100/8	95
Peripheral artery	100/60	95

When doubt exists about the type and severity of the cardiac defect or there are indications for corrective cardiac surgery, a cardiac catheterization should be performed. The cardiac catheterization is performed under local anesthesia and heavy sedation. A small radiopaque catheter is introduced through a peripheral vein in the leg or arm and threaded into the heart. After the catheter is inside the heart, blood samples for oxygen saturation are obtained, systolic and diastolic pressures of each heart chamber are recorded, and selective angiocardiography and cineangiocardiography are performed. A patient may have all of these tests done or only selected ones, depending on what the pediatric cardiologist desires to obtain from the catheterization. The nurse should assure the parents that this is a diagnostic test and not a corrective surgical procedure. The procedure is not dangerous but is not without risk. After the catheterization the nurse should record vital signs frequently, observe for hemorrhage from the site of the cutdown, and watch for changes in the peripheral pulses and color in the extremity on which the procedure was performed. Any irregularities should be reported at once.

Types of cardiac defects

Basically there are three major types of congenital anomalies: (1) stenosis of the channel of blood flow in the heart or a closely allied major vessel, (2) left-to-right shunt, which is a defect that allows blood to flow directly from the left heart or aorta to the right heart or pulmonary artery, thus bypassing the systemic circulation, and (3) right-to-left shunt, a defect that allows blood to flow from the right heart or pulmonary artery directly into the left heart or aorta, thus

bypassing the lungs. The acyanotic type of congenital heart disease exists when there is no abnormal communication between the pulmonary and systemic circulations, or when a connection is present and the higher pressure forces the blood from the arterial (oxygenated) to the venous (deoxygenated) side of the circulation. Peripheral blood therefore has normal oxygen saturation. In the cyanotic type of cardiac defect there is a communication between the pulmonary and systemic circulations through which venous (unoxygenated) blood enters the systemic circulatory system. Cyanosis is present as a result.

A discussion of the most frequently occurring cardiac defects from each of the three major types will be presented in this section:

1. Acyanotic defects
    a. Obstruction of vessel
        (1) Pulmonary stenosis
        (2) Coarctation of aorta
    b. Left-to-right shunt
        (1) Patent ductus arteriosus
        (2) Interventricular septal defect
2. Cyanotic defects (right-to-left shunt)
    a. Tetralogy of Fallot
    b. Tricuspid atresia
    c. Transposition of great vessels

Acyanotic defects

Obstruction of vessel

Pulmonary stenosis. In pulmonary stenosis there is obstruction of the outflow of blood from the right ventricle due to a constrictive abnormality of the pulmonary valves or muscular ring inside the right ventricle (Fig. 13-11). The blood flow from the right ventricle into the lungs is greatly impeded, causing the right ventricular systolic pressure to rise to 75 to 100 mm. Hg instead of the normal 30 mm. Hg. The right side of the heart becomes dilated and hypertrophied at an early age. Before right heart failure occurs the stenotic area can be enlarged by surgical maneuvers so that the heart resumes normal function.

Coarctation of the aorta. Coarctation of the aorta is a short, localized narrowing of the aorta usually just beyond the origin of the left subclavian artery (Fig. 13-11). Coarctation may also occur at other sites such as in the thoracic or

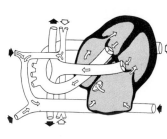

Coarctation of the aorta

Coarctation of the aorta is characterized by a narrowed aortic lumen. It exists as a preductal or postductal obstruction, depending on the position of the obstruction in relation to the ductus arteriosus. Coarctations exist with great variation in anatomical features. The lesion produces an obstruction to the flow of blood through the aorta causing an increased left ventricular pressure and work load.

Anomalous venous return

Oxygenated blood returning from the lungs is carried abnormally to the right heart by one or more pulmonary veins emptying directly, or indirectly through venous channels, into the right atrium. Partial anomalous return of the pulmonary veins to the right atrium functions the same as an atrial septal defect. In complete anomalous return of the pulmonary veins, an interatrial communication is necessary for survival.

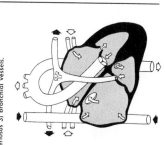

Subaortic stenosis

In many instances, the stenosis is valvular with thickening and fusion of the cusps. Subaortic stenosis is caused by a fibrous ring below the aortic valve in the outflow tract of the left ventricle. At times, both valvular and subaortic stenosis exist in combination. The obstruction presents on increased work load for the normal output of the left ventricular blood and results in left ventricular enlargement.

Tricuspid atresia

Tricuspid valvular atresia is characterized by a small right ventricle, large left ventricle and usually a diminished pulmonary circulation. Blood from the right atrium passes through an atrial septal defect into the left atrium, mixes with oxygenated blood returning from the lungs, flows into the left ventricle and is propelled into the systemic circulation. The lungs may receive blood through one of three routes: 1) a small ventricular septal defect 2) patent ductus arteriosus 3) bronchial vessels.

Truncus arteriosus

Truncus arteriosus is a retention of the embryologic bulbar trunk. It results from the failure of normal septation and division of this trunk into an aorta and pulmonary artery. This single arterial trunk overrides the ventricles and receives blood from them through a ventricular septal defect. The entire pulmonary and systemic circulation is supplied from this common arterial trunk.

Atrial septal defects

An atrial septal defect is an abnormal opening between the right and left atria. Basically, three types of abnormalities result from incorrect development of the atrial septum. An incompetent foramen ovale is the most common defect. The high ostium secundum defect results from abnormal development of the septum secundum. Improper development of the septum primum produces a basal opening known as an ostium primum defect, frequently involving the atrio-ventricular valves. In general, left to right shunting of blood occurs in all atrial septal defects.

Ventricular septal defects

A ventricular septal defect is an abnormal opening between the right and left ventricle. Ventricular septal defects vary in size and may occur in either the membranous or muscular portion of the ventricular septum. Due to higher pressure in the left ventricle, a shunting of blood from the left to right ventricle occurs during systole. If pulmonary vascular resistance produces pulmonary hypertension, the shunt of blood is then reversed from the right to the left ventricle, with cyanosis resulting.

Complete transposition of great vessels

This anomaly is an embryologic defect caused by a straight division of the bulbar trunk without normal spiraling. As a result, the aorta originates from the right ventricle, and the pulmonary artery from the left ventricle. An abnormal communication between the two circulations must be present to sustain life.

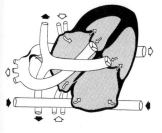

Patent ductus arteriosus

The patent ductus arteriosus is a vascular connection that, during fetal life, short circuits the pulmonary vascular bed and directs blood from the pulmonary artery to the aorta. Functional closure of the ductus normally occurs soon after birth. If the ductus remains patent after birth, the direction of blood flow in the ductus is reversed by the higher pressure in the aorta.

Tetralogy of Fallot

Tetralogy of Fallot is characterized by the combination of four defects: 1) pulmonary stenosis 2) ventricular septal defect 3) overriding aorta 4) hypertrophy of right ventricle. It is the most common defect causing cyanosis in patients surviving beyond two years of age. The severity of symptoms depends on the degree of pulmonary stenosis, the size of the ventricular septal defect, and the degree to which the aorta overrides the septal defect.

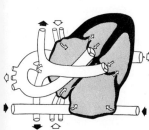

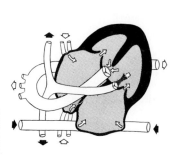
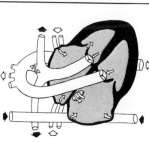
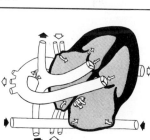

Fig. 13-11. Congenital abnormalities of the heart. (From Ross Clinical Education Aid, No. 7, Columbus, Ohio, Ross Laboratories, Publishers.)

abdominal aorta. The pulse is stronger and the blood pressure higher in those arteries proximal to the coarctation than in the more distal vessels. The diagnosis is made when one notes such a discrepancy between the two arms or between the upper and lower extremities. If symptoms are present, they may include headache, pain in the legs on exercise, and heart failure. The severity and site of the coarctation are established during cardiac catheterization by differential pressure determinations and angiocardiography. The optimal age for surgical excision of the coarctation is between 8 and 15 years. Surgery should be performed to assure normal life expectancy and to eliminate the threat of bacterial endocarditis.

Left-to-right shunt

Persistent patent ductus arteriosus. The ductus arteriosus normally closes shortly after birth. When the ductus remains open, blood under pressure from the aorta is shunted into the pulmonary artery (Fig. 13-11). As a result, oxygenated blood recirculates through the pulmonary circulation, causing an increase in the pulmonary blood flow and vascular resistance. There may be no symptoms, but, if present, they may include exertional dyspnea, repeated upper respiratory infections, and delayed growth and development. The presence of a continuous murmur in the second left intercostal space is pathognomonic of a patent ductus arteriosus. Roentgenograms and electrocardiography reveal cardiomegaly as well as right and left ventricular enlargement. Surgical treatment is simple: the patent ductus is ligated. The optimal age for the operation is between 18 months and 3 years. After the repair the heart becomes normal in size, and growth and development become normal.

Interventricular septal defect. Interventricular septal defect consists of an opening in the cardiovascular system between the right and left ventricles (Fig. 13-11). Because the systolic pressure in the left ventricle is normally about six times that in the right ventricle, a large amount of blood flows from the left to the right ventricle whenever an interventricular septal defect is present. As a result the right ventricle becomes dilated and hypertrophied. The defect varies greatly in size. In the large

defect, congestive heart failure, pulmonary hypertension, pneumonia, and retarded growth may be the accompanying symptoms. On the other hand, if the defect is small, then the child may not have any presenting symptoms. The major abnormal physical finding is the presence of a harsh pansystolic murmur heard loudest at the fourth left intercostal space. The chest roentgenograms and electrocardiogram help in confirming the diagnosis. The exact size of the defect is established at cardiac catheterization, which is always performed prior to scheduling surgery. Pulmonary artery banding, a palliative procedure, is performed in very young infants too small to be placed in the heart-lung machine but who have an established need for diminishing pulmonary blood flow. The treatment is by surgical closure of the defect, which involves the use of cardiopulmonary bypass by means of a heart-lung machine. The optimal age for surgery is between 5 and 15 years, providing that pulmonary hypertension is not present. Without surgery the prognosis is poor unless the septal defect is small.

Cyanotic defects (right-to-left shunt)

Tetralogy of Fallot. Tetralogy of Fallot is the most common type of cyanotic congenital heart disease. Pathologically, the four anomalies found in this defect are (1) pulmonary valvular stenosis, (2) interventricular septal defect, (3) right ventricular hypertrophy, and (4) dextroposition of the aorta (Fig. 13-11). Hemodynamically, when the right ventricle contracts, the outflow of blood is resisted by the pulmonary stenosis and blood is shunted across the ventricular septal defect into the aorta. This results in persistent arterial desaturation and cyanosis.

Cyanosis is the most outstanding clinical manifestation. Cyanosis is not usually present at birth unless there is a severe degree of pulmonary valvular stenosis. The cyanosis is most prominent in the mucous membranes of the lips and mouth and in the fingernails and toenails. It usually becomes apparent between 3 and 4 months of age and is often diagnosed during routine physical examination. Clubbing of the fingers and toes may be present by the age of 1 or 2 years. Dyspnea occurs on limited exertion. Characteristically children assume a *squatting* position for relief of dyspnea due to physical effort. *Paroxysmal dyspneic attacks* (anoxic "blue" spells) are a particular problem during the first 2 years of life. The infant becomes dyspneic and restless, cyanosis increases, and gasping respirations result. Episodes are frequently followed by sleep and weakness. The onset of the attacks are usually spontaneous, although they seem to be more common after feeding, crying, or bowel movement. The spells are associated with further reduction of already compromised pulmonary blood flow, which results in hypoxia and metabolic acidosis. The anoxic spells are treated with oxygen to relieve hypoxia, morphine for sedation, and sodium bicarbonate for correction of acidosis. Propranolol (a beta adrenergic inhibitor) is used to prevent the occurrence of the hypoxic spells in patients with uncontrollable recurrent severe spells. Growth and development may be delayed in patients with tetralogy of Fallot. Polycythemia and an elevated hematocrit value usually occur. A harsh, loud systolic murmur is heard most intensely along the left sternal border.

Roentgenograms of the chest reveal a *boot-shaped heart (coeur en sabot)* with decreased pulmonary vasculature. Electrocardiogram demonstrates the presence of right ventricular hypertrophy. Cardiac catheterization with angiocardiography establishes the severity of defect.

The medical management consists of preventing and controlling syncopal attacks with drugs, preventing infections, and the reduction of the hematocrit or hemoglobin levels by venesection.

In recent years tetralogy of Fallot has been treated relatively successfully by surgery. A palliative procedure in infancy or early childhood is performed by anastomosing the aorta and pulmonary artery (Potts procedure), thereby correcting the cyanosis by increasing the pulmonary blood flow, but thus does not correct the defects. In older children the shunt procedure most commonly used is the Blalock-Taussig operation, in which the subclavian or innominate artery is anastomosed to the pulmonary artery. These shunt procedures are performed so that complete repair can be postponed until the child is older (6 to 8 years) and has gained weight (40 pounds or more). The surgical treatment of choice for the vast majority of patients is by open heart repair with closure of the ventricular septal defect and relief of the pulmonic stenosis by means of a cardiopulmonary bypass. After complete repair the patients are asymptomatic and able to lead unrestricted lives.

Tricuspid atresia. In tricuspid atresia, a cyanotic type of cardiac defect, there is no opening between the right atrium and right ventricle (Fig. 13-11). The blood returning to the right atrium has to flow through an interatrial defect into the left atrium and left ventricle. A ventricular septal defect or patent ductus is usually present to permit blood to flow into the lungs; hence the pulmonary blood flow is diminished thereby producing cyanosis in early life. Most of these patients die within the first year of life unless a palliative shunt procedure is performed. The diagnosis is suspected on electrocardiogram by the presence of left axis deviation and hypertrophy. It can be confirmed by cardiac catheterization. There is no corrective procedure available at present, short of transplantation. Only palliative procedures aimed at increasing pulmonary blood flow in patients with severe hypoxia (Potts or Blalock-Taussig operation) are being performed.

Transposition of great vessels. In transposition of the great vessels the aorta arises from the right ventricle and the pulmonary artery from the left ventricle (Fig. 13-11). The pulmonary veins enter the left atrium, and the inferior and superior vena cava drain into the right atrium. The unoxygenated systemic venous blood enters the aorta, whereas the oxygenated pulmonary venous blood enters the lungs. To provide for oxygenated blood to enter the systemic circulation a patent ductus, ventricular septal defect, or atrial septal defect must exist; death results if there is no mixing of the blood through one or more of the defects. It is one of the most significant cardiac abnormalities encountered in the first month of life. It accounts for the most common cardiac cause of cyanosis and heart failure in the first 2 months of life. The majority of the infants have an increase in pulmonary blood flow, which results in a moderate to severe degree of pulmonary hypertension. The hemodynamic changes in the pulmonary system determine the clinical symptoms and prognosis.

The main clinical symptom is the presence of cyanosis in the first few days of life. The cyanosis is severe and progressive. Dyspnea, congestive heart failure, and failure to thrive become apparent during the first weeks of life. Examination of the heart reveals a loud systolic murmur.

The chest roentgenogram and electrocardiogram are useful in helping establish the diagnosis. Cardiac catheterization and angiocardiography are performed to establish the diagnosis.

The medical management in transposition of the great vessels is to give digitalis to relieve the symptoms of congestive heart failure, administer oxygen to relieve severe hypoxia, and correct metabolic acidosis by infusing sodium bicarbonate. If the cardiac catheterization demonstrates a small atrial defect, a larger communication may be created by performing a balloon atrial septostomy. The palliative procedure of creation of a larger atrial septal defect will result in improvement of the hypoxia and metabolic acidosis. Other palliative surgical procedures that may be indicated are pulmonary banding if there is severe pulmonary hypertension, aorta–to–pulmonary artery shunts to increase pulmonary artery blood flow, and ligation of the patent ductus arteriosus to decrease the pulmonary blood flow if a ventricular septal defect is present along with the ductus arteriosus. It is hoped that these temporary procedures will permit the child to grow and develop until he is 5 years of age, when complete corrective surgery may be performed. The results of the corrective surgical procedure for transposition of the great vessels are good as long as the child does not have pulmonary vascular obstruction.

The infant in cardiac distress

Heart failure. Heart failure is a common manifestation of congenital heart disease in infants. The majority of congenital cardiac malformations may cause heart failure during this time of life. Heart failure may be sudden in onset and result in sudden death before the condition is recognized. Dyspnea may be the first sign of heart failure and may be shown by mouth breathing and flaring of the alae nasi. Tachypnea with intercostal and usually subcostal retraction are the usual physical findings later in the course of the disease. Persistent tachycardia in the range of 180 to 200 beats per minute is common. Heart sounds may become poor, thereby making it very difficult for the examiner to count the rate. Cyanosis often accompanies heart failure as a result of pulmonary congestion. This type of cyanosis is usually less intense in the infant with a cardiac defect permitting a right-to-left shunt to occur.

Role of the nurse in the newborn nursery

Observation. Some infants with congenital heart disease, especially those with truncus arteriosus, tricuspid atresia, or transposition of the great vessels, may show cyanosis, respiratory distress, or heart failure as early as the postdelivery period. The particular responsibility of the nursery nurse is a vigilant alertness for symptoms and signs that might indicate cardiac distress or failure. These are not the same in infancy as in childhood and adulthood.

1. Cyanosis. Cyanosis will draw the nurse's attention to the infant, but not all cyanotic infants have congenital heart disease. Cyanosis may develop in an infant who has a tracheoesophageal fistula, congenital lobar emphysema, the respiratory syndrome of hyaline membrane disease, or tracheomalacia. It is important to describe the location of cyanosis. When an infant is admitted to the nursery, the nurse should inspect his entire body; she should do this also during bath time each day. The nurse needs to note whether the infant has cyanosis over his entire body, only the lower extremities, only the lips, or circumorally. Is the cyanosis deep or light in color? Does the body become more cyanotic when he is fed or when he cries? (If the infant's color improves with crying, he is overcoming some atelectasis.)

2. Behavior. Restlessness and irritability are associated with an infant in congestive heart failure. He is suffering from air hunger.

3. Tachycardia. The pulse of the infant in cardiac distress is consistently higher than that

of a normal infant. He has a decreased amount of oxygen, and the heart is trying to compensate by pumping harder.

4. Dyspnea. Dyspnea may be shown by chest retractions, mouth breathing, and flaring of the alae nasi.

5. Feeding. The infant may seem to tire easily in feeding and have choking spells. There is difficulty in feeding him.

6. Appearance of the skin. Because of generalized edema, the skin of the infant may seem to be thicker than the skin of a well infant. It is possible that this will not be seen until the end of the first week of life.

Symptoms the nurse observes vary with the severity of the particular defect of the infant; however, if any of the foregoing symptoms are seen, the nurse should record them on the nurses' notes and draw the attention of the physician to them.

Aiding with diagnostic measures. If the physician believes the infant may have heart disease, several diagnostic measures are done.

A complete blood count is taken. In children with a cyanotic type of heart disease, polycythemia is present. There is an elevated hematocrit value and an increased number of red blood cells. Because of this there is increased viscosity of the blood. For this reason the infant is more susceptible to cerebral thrombosis.

A cardiac series of x-ray films of the chest is taken. These films show the size and shape of the heart. An electrocardiogram is usually done at the bedside of the infant. It measures the electric potential generated from the heart muscle.

If the foregoing measures plus physical findings indicate that the infant may have a heart defect, a cardiac catheterization is done to determine the type of defect. A small tube is passed via a vein (usually in the arm or in the femoral region) into the heart. Samples of blood in vessels and intracardiac chambers are taken and studied; also, pressures in these same areas are measured. The infant is usually heavily sedated for this procedure.

An angiogram is often done as part of the cardiac catheterization. Some radiopaque substance is injected into a vessel or a specific chamber of the heart and then x-ray films are taken. Abnormal shunts and obstructions may be demonstrated in this way.

Understanding the plan of medical care. The plan of care varies with each particular infant. Usually, because of congestive heart failure, which produces respiratory embarrassment, the infant is (1) placed in oxygen, (2) digitalized, and (3) given morphine and diuretics. The infant is then reevaluated a little later as to the need for immediate surgery. If the infant does not respond to medical treatment, surgery is considered. The aim of operative procedures is to improve the circulation of the child. Palliative approaches are considered because open heart surgery using a heart pump oxygenator carries a high mortality in infancy, especially in those infants who weigh less than 20 pounds or have less than 1 square meter of body surface. In the near future new techniques will be devised in which the operative risk is less than at present.

Role of the nurse on the pediatric unit

The infant in the newborn nursery who has congenital heart disease may be transferred to the pediatric unit, or an infant may be admitted there who is older than the infant in the neonatal period of life. The nurse's main responsibility to infants who are in heart failure is centered around their rest and feeding, measures to relieve dyspnea, and an ever vigilant observation of the infants. The condition of an infant may change quickly.

Observation. In addition to observing any symptoms of cardiac distress, the nurse should note the nutritional status of the patient. The general appearance of the infant is often one of retarded growth and development. He may be thought younger than he really is.

Weighing. The infant should be weighed on admission and daily thereafter. It is important to know whether the infant is gaining, losing, or remaining stationary in his weight.

Feeding. Feeding the infant often presents difficulties because of increased dyspnea and choking spells. It is better to give him small feedings at frequent intervals (every 3 hours) than to have larger feedings every 4 hours.

The infant is usually receiving limited fluids. A formula is chosen that is high in calories but low in sodium content. (Patients in congestive heart failure usually have a restriction of sodium since that promotes retention of fluid in the tissues. In congestive heart failure there is impaired ability of the kidneys to excrete salt.) The infant's cereal should be selected in terms of salt content as well as the infant's age. The nurse should read the label on the cereal box carefully.

Because of the infant's dyspnea it may be wise to utilize most of the formula on the cereal and then to see if the infant will accept the remainder by cup feeding. Less effort is required to drink from a cup than to suck. Infants vary—some like milk from a cup and some do not. Other foods may be given that are appropriate to his age. If he has very severe dyspnea, feedings may have to be given by nasogastric tube.

How the infant takes his feedings by mouth and how dyspneic he becomes during feeding time should be included in the nurse's notes each time he is fed. The plan of feeding a particular infant has to be individualized.

Measures to relieve dyspnea. If the infant shows difficulty in breathing, he should be placed in Fowler's or semi-Fowler's position—whichever seems to give him the most comfort. This can be accomplished by putting the infant in an infant carrier seat (Fig. 11-8). Some older infants sit upright in tailor fashion with crossed legs. A knee-chest position may help other infants, but unless the child has had morphine or a sedative, he may be resistant to the latter position. A Croupette or oxygen tent may be prescribed for the infant; cool air often seems to help him. The effectiveness of the Croupette or oxygen tent can be judged by the rate of the infant's respirations. If they were 60 respirations per minute when he was out of the tent but dropped to 40 respirations per minute after he was in the tent for a short time, then obviously the oxygen and coolness aided him. Also, the infant should relax and be less restless in any oxygen tent.

It is a frightening experience to have difficulty in breathing. If possible, a member of the infant's family should be encouraged to say with him at least part of the day. The nurse needs to see the infant frequently, not only because of his physical condition but for emotional reasons as well. (See p. 293 for discussion of the care of a child in a Croupette.)

Rest. Rest is essential to lessen the work of the heart. It slows the metabolism so the infant will need less oxygen. Work should be so organized that the infant does not need to be constantly disturbed. The nurse needs to gather the supplies necessary in caring for the infant, execute the care with gentleness and dexterity, and then allow the infant to rest. If he is in a Croupette, the aid of another nurse or assistant nurse is helpful in maintaining the comfort of the infant while bed linen is changed. Perhaps the infant's mother will lend her assistance. Some infants need to rest between bath time and feeding time. An individual plan must be made for each infant.

The infant's needs should be either anticipated or met very promptly so that he will not need to cry to show he needs attention. Under the stress of crying, dyspnea is worse. During her contacts with the infant, the nurse needs to speak soothingly to him and to pat and caress him. Being held in the nurse's or mother's arms promotes relaxation. This should be done at least once on every nursing shift.

The child under 1 year of age usually has a morning and an afternoon nap. At the time the infant is admitted, information should be obtained about his habits and then an effort made to be consistent with his routine at home.

Often there is an order for morphine for the infant in congestive heart failure. Rest and relaxation are so important that this medication should be given freely, in accord with the prescribed dose and frequency.

Administration of medications. Digitalis or one of its derivatives is usually prescribed for the infant as well as morphine. A diuretic is prescribed as necessary for a particular infant. The amount of digoxin ordered is so small that the infant can often drink it from a paper medicine cup much more easily than he can take it by spoon or medicine dropper.

Understanding the plan for future care. If the infant is responding well to medical management, the physician may decide to delay surgical measures. In that case the infant may be sent home to be followed in a clinic or by a private physician until a later date when elective surgery may be done. Digoxin continues to be given to the infant. If the infant is not responding to medical management, the physician may recommend to the parents that palliative surgery be done.

In planning for the infant's home care, the nurse must make sure the mother knows how to give digoxin and how to care for her infant. The mother may be afraid of the infant or be anxious lest she harm him. If at all possible, the mother should care for the infant under the nurse's supervision before the infant is discharged. If this is the mother's first child, it may be well to refer this infant to the care of a public health nurse. Besides doing further teaching about home care, the public health nurse can give emotional support to the mother.

The infant with a congenital heart defect with medical management needs careful medical supervision by a physician, through the outpatient department of a hospital, or in a special heart clinic under the auspices of the crippled children's services. If the infant is not responding to medical measures, operative procedures may be planned immediately. (For responsibilities of the nurse during a hospitalization of the infant or child for surgery, refer to p. 417.)

The child admitted for study
Role of the nurse

Although the pediatric nurse may care for infants with congenital heart disease who are in heart failure, she may also come in contact with infants and children who have been referred to the hospital for diagnosis and evaluation. They may not be acutely ill; indeed, some may be ambulatory.

Aiding the child's adjustment. Every effort should be made to help orient the mother and the child and to help make this hospitalization a pleasant one, even if there are a few painful events. The relationship of both the child and his mother to the nurse plays an important part in the child's next hospitalization. In her contacts with the parents and the child the nurse should remember that, in all likelihood, the child will be readmitted later for another evaluation and/or surgery. The experiences both he and his mother have in the current hospitaliza-tion will influence his ability to adjust to later admissions.

Daily care. Many of these infants and children are receiving ordinary routine care. Older children are permitted to ambulate. On the other hand, each child's care should be individualized. The infant of 4 months may do better on feedings every 3 hours than every 4 hours. The child with coarctation of the aorta may have such hypertension that bed rest is more suitable than ambulation. Recreation should be provided according to the needs of the particular child.

Assisting with diagnostic measures. There are various laboratory tests and examinations with which the nurse assists. (Refer to p. 355 for common diagnostic measures.) The child should receive an explanation of what is going to be done in accordance with his age and ability to understand. When x-ray examinations are scheduled, the 3- or 4-year-old child can be told, "This is a special camera to take a picture of your chest," and for cardiac catheterization, "A tiny tube is going to be placed in your arm that will go to your heart. You may be asleep or very sleepy then because the medicine you get makes you want to sleep."

Explanations do not help the toddler or infant, but an unhurried manner and matter-of-fact behavior assumed by the personnel can aid him in meeting painful situations. Comforting the child after an unpleasant procedure such as a venipuncture is important in restoring the child's emotional equilibrium.

Understanding plans for elective surgery. After diagnostic tests are done and the child's particular condition has been evaluated and diagnosed, plans are made for future care. Opinions vary as to the exact age at which each type of defect should be corrected. A brief explanation is given here concerning the kinds of correction done for the common types of congenital heart conditions. (For the role of the nurse when surgery is performed refer to p. 417.)

Palliative procedures

Palliative procedures for infants with certain types of heart defects are performed via closed heart surgery. These operations alleviate distressing symptoms; later the child may return to have definitive surgery. As mentioned earlier, open heart surgery using a pump oxygenator carries a high mortality in infants under 1 year.

Listed here are common cardiac defects, together with the particular types of palliative operative procedure that may be done.

1. Tetralogy of Fallot. Various shunting procedures may be done to improve the circulation. Few children with tetralogy of Fallot progress throughout early childhood under medical management. In the Blalock-Taussig operation (frequently done) the blood is shunted from the subclavian artery to the right pulmonary artery. In the Potts-Smith procedure the shunt is between the descending aorta and the left pulmonary artery. In the Glenn procedure the blood is shunted from the superior vena cava to the right pulmonary artery.

2. Ventricular septal defect. The main pulmonary artery is banded to reduce pulmonary arterial pressure and blood flow.

3. Transposition of the great vessels. The Blalock-Hanlon procedure is frequently performed. This is the creation of an atrial septal defect. This is often preceded by an attempted atrial balloon septostomy. In this procedure a catheter is introduced into the heart via the femoral vein. It has a small deflated balloon at its tip, which is pushed through the foramen ovale, inflated, and pulled back. This creates a septal defect to improve the circulation.

Definitive surgery

1. Patent ductus arteriosus. An infant with this condition should have it corrected during infancy, whether or not the child shows symptoms. The surgical procedures consist of multiple ligation of the ductus or, preferably, a division of the ductus. These procedures have a very low mortality risk. This is done via closed heart surgery. Complications that may occur if the condition is not treated include congestive heart failure, bacterial endocarditis, aneurysm formation, and pulmonary hypertension.

2. Coarctation of the aorta. The coorrection of this defect is done in the early school years (9 to 12 years of age) by closed heart surgery. A resection of the constricted segment of the aorta is done, and there is an anastomosis of the cut ends.

The following operations are done by open heart surgery using a pump oxygenator:

3. Aortic stenosis. There is a total correction of the defect.

4. Pulmonary stenosis. There is a total correction of the stenosed segment as well as correction of other defects seen in direct visualization of the heart.

5. Tetralogy of Fallot, atrial septal defect, ventricular septal defect, and transposition of the great vessels. As discussed earlier, the child with these defects may have had palliative surgery performed in infancy but have definitive surgery with a total correction of defects when he reaches school age. Few children with tetralogy of Fallot progress throughout early childhood without surgical intervention. (See Chapter 15 for nursing care of the child with cardiac surgery.)

Planning for interim home care

Until the child reaches the age at which the surgeon will operate, plans for home care need to be made. Instructions to the mother should include those pertaining to medications, nutrition, and prevention of respiratory infection.

When the child goes home, the mother should have exact directions as to any medications the child is to receive. The doctor will specify the type of diet (often high in protein, calories, and vitamins) to give the infant or child. The nurse may discuss mealtime and any previous problems the mother had and perhaps suggest ideas for a pleasant mealtime so the child will take food. Nutrition helps to build the child's resistance to infection. Midmorning nourishment (a custard, milkshake, etc.) and something to eat after the child's afternoon nap are acceptable to the child and easier than taking a lot of food in the three meals of the family.

Playing outdoors in good weather and observing regular nap and bedtime hours may help to prevent infection, increase the appetite, and keep the child in as nearly optimum condition as possible. The child sets his own limits in physical exertion. Members of the family or visitors who have colds should stay away from him. Immunizations should be given as usual. Periodic visits to the dentist (if the child is over

2 years) should be begun or continued as the case may be.

Perhaps it would be best if special privileges are not given to the cardiac child, since they may confuse him. (Refer to p. 338 for discussion of psychological factors in the care of the handicapped child.) The family routine should be as nearly normal as possible. However, the nurse should be understanding if the parents are oversolicitous of the child. She should be understanding, too, of how a father might feel toward an undersized and underdeveloped child if he himself is a strong person.

Here again the nurse needs to help the parents to see the importance of meeting their own emotional and social needs so they can maintain a more objective view of the total situation. If the mother stays with the child all the time, never going out socially or taking an opportunity to be away for even a few hours during the week, her relationships with the other children and her husband may suffer. Also, she and the handicapped child will not enjoy each other as much.

If the mother of an infant would feel more secure if a public health nurse visited him, a referral should be made. Of course, if there is any question as to the adequacy of the child's home care, a referral should be made.

GASTROINTESTINAL DEFECTS
Cleft lip

The nurse in the delivery room first sees the infant with a cleft lip, then the nurse in the newborn nursery, and finally the nurse on a pediatric unit. In areas where midwives still deliver many infants the public health nurse may see the infant in a home visit. Seeing an infant born with a cleft lip is a shock to everyone. No one who is present either in a delivery room or in the home expects an infant with an obvious defect to emerge from the mother—neither the nursing personnel, the doctors, nor the mother. It is important that the nurse maintain her composure and be careful of her facial expression.

Nature of the condition

A cleft lip is one of the common congenital anomalies. It can be either bilateral or unilateral

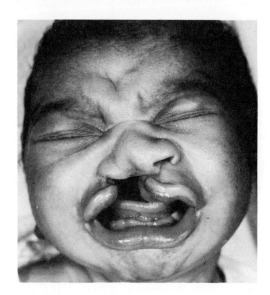

Fig. 13-12. Unilateral complete cleft lip with complete cleft palate and alveolar ridge defect.

(Figs. 13-12 and 13-13). The condition occurs most often on the left side of the mouth. Boys are affected more frequently than girls.

Doctors vary in the time they choose for operation to close the cleft. Some may do it within the first hours of life, whereas others wait until the infant weighs 10 pounds or is about 3 months old. Very early operations are often motivated by the parent-child relationship. Some surgeons like to make sure first that the infant has no other medical problem, is gaining weight, and is healthy. Because of eruption of deciduous teeth and because the bony structures are harder to manipulate as the infant gets older, the operation should be done, if possible, not later than the fourth month. Nutrition of the infant and his own adjustment are to be considered. If the infant is not caressed and fondled, he does not thrive. If parents are repulsed by the infant, they are unlikely to give the loving care he needs. On the other hand, if the mother is oversolicitous, she may hold the infant all the time, centering her attention on him. This is not good for the infant, the mother, or the father. Only that parent who emotionally is quite mature seems able to be objective.

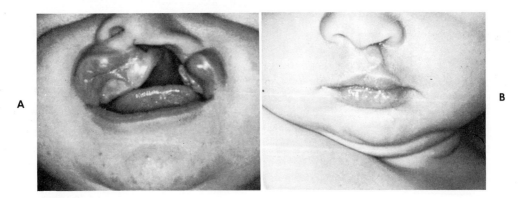

Fig. 13-13. A, Unilateral complete cleft lip with complete cleft palate and alveolar ridge defect. **B,** Same infant after repair of the cleft lip. (From Martin, L. W.: Pediatric surgery—general. In Shirkey, H. C., editor: Pediatric therapy, ed. 5, St. Louis, 1975, The C. V. Mosby Co.)

Nursing care in neonatal period

Observations in the newborn nursery. The nursery nurse needs to look at the infant carefully as she admits him to the nursery. If an infant has one deformity, he may have others. The nurse should be particularly sure to look inside the infant's mouth to see if there is also a cleft palate, since a cleft lip and palate are often associated. (For general nursing care of the infant in the newborn nursery, refer to Chapter 4.)

Introduction to parents. It is well for the parents to see the infant as soon as possible after the doctor has told them about the deformity, since the imagination of both parents may make the deformity seem worse than it is. The longer the delay in seeing the infant, the greater may be the effort required of the parents to look at their deformed child.

When the nurse takes the infant to the mother, the nurse might hold the infant in her arms for the mother to see instead of just handing the infant to the mother. The mother may not wish to hold the infant at first. If the mother looks at the infant and touches him, the nurse might place the infant on the mother's bed; otherwise, she should place him back in his crib and leave the mother and infant together so they can get acquainted just as any new mother and infant need to.

If the mother asks the nurse the cause of the deformity, the nurse should answer truthfully that the cause is not known. Actually, the doctor has probably already told the parents that it was nothing either of them did that caused the cleft. This is important, since one parent may blame the other. Knowledge that the cause of the cleft is not known may alleviate guilt feelings of the parents, but the fact still remains that their child is different from others. (For further discussion of psychological factors, refer to p. 338.)

Feeding. Feeding the infant with a cleft lip presents a problem to the nurse. She has several alternatives. Spoon feeding has been found very successful and can be used whether the infant has a unilateral or a bilateral cleft; likewise, cup feeding can be used. If the infant has a unilateral cleft, a special nipple with a rubber flap can be used on the formula bottle so the infant can suck from the bottle. Another method to use with the infant who has a unilateral cleft is for the nurse to elevate his head and shoulders on a pillow; then with one hand she can hold a regular baby bottle with the nipple in the infant's mouth and with the other hand press the cleft together by placing an index finger on one cheek and thumb on the other. The nipple should be directed to the good side of the infant's mouth.

When the infant has a bilateral cleft, the nurse can use an Asepto syringe with a rubber tube at the end that extends for an inch beyond the syringe. The infant can be held in her arms when being fed.

Sometimes a bottle that has large holes in the

nipple is used, but milk comes rapidly from such a bottle and the infant could easily choke on it.

Whatever method the nurse uses, she should burp the infant before feeding, several times during the feeding, and again at the end of the feeding. The infant with a cleft lip swallows more air in feeding than a normal infant. Burping will help prevent regurgitation of formula.

Preparation for discharge. If this is the mother's first child, she may need a considerable amount of information about the care of an infant besides the knowledge of feeding technique (p. 174). Also, the mother needs to practice feeding the infant under supervision. This will give her more self-confidence. Prior to her leaving the hospital, plans are usually started for the surgical treatment of the infant. The parents may wish to have a private doctor care for the infant, or they may want to have the infant referred to a local crippled children's clinic.

If there are other children at home, they need to be told that the new infant's mouth has a cleft and that he will need an operation when he is a little bigger. The children need some preparation before they see the infant.

It is nice if a public health nurse can see both the mother and the infant before the mother leaves the hospital. As was mentioned in the discussion of psychological factors, the mother needs emotional support, especially in going home and facing neighbors, friends, and relatives. The public health nurse should have very specific written information from the hospital nurse as to what instructions have been given to the mother and what plans for the infant have been made.

In all contacts with the mother and/or the father of the infant with a cleft lip, both the hospital nurse and public health nurse should remember that the way she handles and fondles the infant is going to influence the parents' own attitude to the infant. Both parents also need acceptance by the nurse. It is normal for the mother to grieve for the well infant she did not have, and it takes her a little time to accept her responsibility for this handicapped infant. Being involved in definite plans for the infant's welfare and future helps the mother to adjust to the situation.

Preoperative nursing care

Emotional support of parents. When the infant is admitted for operation, the pediatric nurse should be gracious in her greeting to the parents. If the nurse holds the infant gently and fondles or talks with the infant, the parents may be more at ease. The parents may have ambivalent feelings about their infant's operation. They want the defect corrected, but they may feel hesitant and anxious about subjecting him to the procedure. Letting parents share in the care of the infant before operation in some way, such as undressing him or holding the infant for the physician's examination on admission, sometimes helps in relieving tension. (For emotional support of parents at the time of the operation, refer to p. 417.)

Prevention of infection. The infant should be assigned to a room with children who do not have any infections or draining wounds. A "clean" nursery is ideal.

Nurses or personnel with any respiratory infection should not care for the infant or be around him. The infant's position needs changing at least every 2 hours in the daytime and every 4 hours at night. Change of position includes rocking the infant, holding him, or propping him on alternate sides. As infants and children turn in their sleep and move around, the night nurse needs to make frequent rounds to see that they are adequately covered.

Feeding. The infant should be fed preoperatively in the same manner in which he will be fed postoperatively. This gives him a chance to get used to the method of feeding. Usually an Asepto syringe is used with a rubber tip extending 1 inch beyond the end of the syringe. This is safe and convenient. The infant can be held in the nurse's arms as usual during the feeding.

Immediate preoperative care. Refer to p. 296 for immediate preoperative care.

Postoperative nursing care

Refer to p. 297 for details of general postoperative care of infants and children. Specifics in the care of an infant with repair of a cleft lip (cheiloplasty) are given here.

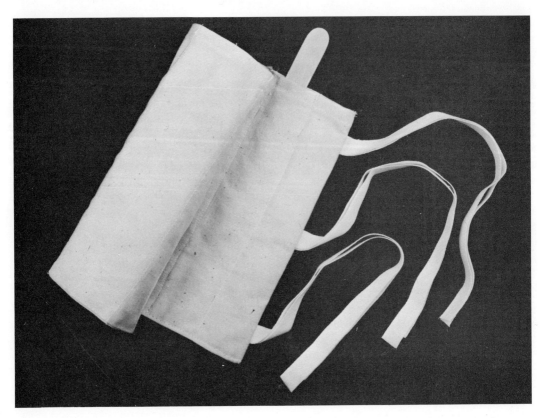

Fig. 13-14. Elbow restraint. (Courtesy The Children's Memorial Hospital, Chicago, Ill.)

Preventing injury. Before this infant is awake from the anesthesia the recovery room nurse should apply elbow restraints (Fig. 13-14). They should be placed over the infant's long-sleeved undershirt. The middle tie should be fastened first and then the others. The undershirt should be brought as a cuff over the restraint at the wrist and pinned with a small pin. The top of the restraint should be pinned also. If the infant is very young, the tongue blades that fit into the grooves of the restraint may need to be cut shorter so they will fit comfortably. The tongue blade should be as large as the distance from the inner aspect of the infant's wrist to the axilla. The elbow restraint keeps the infant from putting his fingers in his mouth or touching his lip.

When the infant is returned to his own room, the nurse on the unit should make sure the elbow restraints are in place. These restraints must be kept on at all times. A 4-month-old infant can be very active and it is safest to have another person hold the infant's arms while the infant is being bathed. Undue chances of injury should not be taken. On the other hand, both arms should be released (one at a time) and exercised several times during the day. A good time to do this is after each feeding of the infant.

Avoiding strain. The Logan bow, used by some doctors, helps to prevent strain on the lip. If the adhesive holding the bow in place becomes damp, it can be changed. One person will have to hold the cheeks of the infant with thumb and finger to avoid strain, while another person places fresh adhesive on the Logan bow and then reapplies it.

Crying is a strain; therefore its causes should be eliminated as far as possible. Every effort should be made to anticipate the infant's needs and to keep him comfortable and content. Phenobarbital is often ordered for these patients. It should be given frequently enough to keep the infant from having discomfort from his

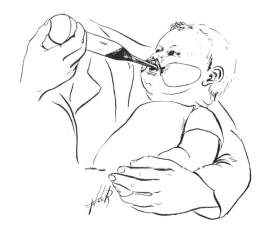

Fig. 13-15. Nurse feeding an infant with Asepto syringe with rubber tip (infant whose cleft lip has been repaired). Logan clamp over repaired lip helps to prevent strain on the suture line. Note that the nurse has one of the infant's arms behind her and is holding the other with her hand.

operation and consequent restlessness. If the infant does cry, the nurse should investigate the possible cause promptly and try to alleviate whatever is distressing the infant.

Maintaining nutrition. Usually the infant returns from the operating room with an intravenous infusion. This is discontinued as soon as oral fluids are retained and the intake of the infant is adequate. Glucose water can be offered orally. The infant can be fed by means of an Asepto syringe with a rubber tip just as he was the day previous to operation (Fig. 13-15). The rubber tip of the syringe should be directed toward the unaffected side of the mouth. Frequent burping is still essential, but the nurse should seat the infant upright in her lap and rub his back to do this rather than put him over her shoulder. Insofar as possible the same nurse on each tour of dtudy should feet the infant every day so she and the infant do not have to go through a period of adjustment each time.

Care of the sutures. The sutures need special care to keep them clean and to prevent the formation of any crusts over them. After each feeding the nurse can take a sterile applicator with a cotton tip, dip it into saline solution (or any solution ordered by the physician) and very gently cleanse the suture line. She should use as many applicators as necessary. If the nurse

steadies the infant's head with one hand and talks to him while she is cleansing the suture line, the infant does not seem to object to this treatment. Sometimes there are dried secretions in the nose. These need attention, since the presence of dried nasal secretions interferes with breathing and eating. Sutures are usually removed about 10 days after the operation. Dissecting scissors and forceps are used to do this.

Nursing-parent relationship. The mother may need time to adjust to her infant. The birth of the infant and his operation have constituted a big even in the mother's life. The sight of the sutures and elbow restraints on the infant might make her hesitant to touch and hold him. If the infant has not been at home before this hospitalization and has remained in the hospital since his birth, the mother needs to become acquainted with him. Having some supervision while she holds the infant may help the mother to feel more secure.

The nurse should remember that the parent's ego needs boosting. She should praise efforts the mother makes in helping her with the care of the infant. If the mother is staying with the infant, the nurse can also urge the mother to take adequate time for her meals as well as encourage her to go outside the hospital every day for at least a short time. Evidence that the nurse is concerned with her needs also may help the mother's self-confidence. If a good relationship is established between the nurse and the parent, the parent will be benefitted.

Preparation for discharge. Actually the care that this infant should receive to keep him well is essentially the same as for any normal infant (p. 174). By the time the infant is ready to go home usually he can be bottle-fed, but the nurse needs to check this point with the particular doctor of the infant as some physicians postpone bottle-feeding until later. The mother should not be overwhelmed with instructions. How much the mother needs to learn about the general care of the infant depends on what previous knowledge and experience she has had in the care of infants. The mother is usually pleased with the results of the operation and is happy to receive any suggestion about the infant's care. Before discharging the infant, it would be well to let the mother care for the infant under the nurse's supervision. If the nurse believes the mother needs help and supervision, a referral can be made to a public health nurse.

Cleft palate
Nature of the condition

The infant with a cleft lip may or may not have an associated cleft palate. There are varying degrees of severity of the cleft palate. A child may have a complete cleft or only a partial cleft. The care of the child with a cleft palate involves the plastic surgeon, the orthodontist, and the speech therapist.

In 1943 the American Academy of Cleft Palate Prosthesis was formed. Later, in 1949, the association was reorganized and the name changed to the American Association for Cleft Palate Rehabilitation. There are state programs for the child with a cleft palate under the direction of state services for crippled children in the state department of health, in universities, and in large medical centers. A list of the locations of these programs can be obtained from the Membership Directory, American Association for Cleft Palate Rehabilitation. The first objective of this organization is the encouragement of scientific research into the causes and nature of cleft palate and cleft lip (Olin, 1960).

A child with an unrepaired cleft palate may be the object of ridicule by classmates and acquaintances because of his nasal speech. He may be so embarrassed and self-conscious that his social and emotional development suffers. The speech impediment may make a difference in his parents' and his siblings' attitudes toward him. His speech may hinder him from attaining vocational goals he sets for himself. From lack of adequate attention and care for the child born with a cleft palate the community and country may be the loser.

Planning for surgical procedures

Doctors vary as to the age they consider optimum for repair of the palate. In general the trend is to wait until the child is 18 to 24 months old because of the growth of anatomical structures involved. The chief reason for operation is the child's speech. Any eating difficulties could be eliminated by the use of a special prosthesis that fits over the cleft palate.

Nursing care in the newborn nursery

Observation. When the newborn infant is brought from the delivery room to the nursery, it is possible that no one has yet discovered he has a cleft palate. The doctor may not examine the infant carefully until later. The nurse should always look into the mouth of every infant that she receives into the nursery.

In one instance a mother brought her new infant to the outpatient department of a hospital soon after she had been discharged from the hospital. She complained that the new infant was hard to feed and acted like his older brother, who had a cleft palate. Did the new infant have one? On examination it was found that he did.

Introduction to the mother. The same comments made about introducing the infant with a cleft lip to his mother are true of the infant with a cleft palate, except that this defect is not obvious to one just looking at the infant.

Feeding. If the infant has only a cleft palate, he may be fed by a regular nipple and bottle if he is fed slowly, burped often, and held with the upper part of his body elevated. Breastfeeding may be done if care is taken of the infant's position during feeding. When he burps, some milk may come back through his nose if there is a cleft in the roof of his mouth.

If the infant has a bilateral cleft lip and palate, he may be spoon fed, cup fed, or fed with an Asepto syringe with a rubber tip or by a bottling having a special nipple.

Other general factors in his care are the same as those of any well newborn infant (Chapter 4).

Preoperative teaching. Besides use of care in feeding, the mother should be advised to be sure to teach the infant to drink from a cup before he is readmitted for a repair of the palate. After his operation he is not going to be able to suck from a bottle so it is easier if he has already learned to drink from a cup. As mentioned in Chapter 5, an infant usually tries to hold his own bottle at about 8 months of age. When this occurs, the mother should try substituting a cup for the bottle. To make the toddler's adjustment to the hospital easier the mother might have a babysitter or a relative care for the child for short periods of time so that he becomes used to being with people other than his parents and is less dependent on their constant presence.

Hospital admission for surgery

Preoperative nursing care. The adjustment of the toddler to the hospital is the main problem. The toddler is old enough to know that the hospital unit is an unfamiliar place and that there are new and strange people around him. If the mother can remain with him, it will help him to accept his new environment.

The toddler can either walk or be taken to the playroom in a stroller. Play is a pleasant diversion for him and helps the time to pass more quickly. The role of the "Play Lady" on a pediatric unit is an important one.

If there are other mothers in the playroom with their sick, handicapped children, the mother of the child with a cleft palate may feel less alone in her own tragedy.

Elbow splints should be placed on the child for a short time so he can get used to them. This may help him to fuss less after his operation when he sees and feels them on him. It is helpful to the parents as well as the infant if he is sedated before he leaves the hospital unit to go to the operating room. (Refer to pp. 415 and 417 for a discussion of psychological factors in surgical operations and emotional support of the parents.)

Postoperative nursing care. The main objectives of the nursing care postoperatively are to prevent injury or infection to the suture line, to prevent strain on the wound, and to give adequate fluids.

To prevent injury to the sutures, elbow splints should be placed on the child's arms immediately so he will not put his fingers in his mouth. When he is completely out of the anesthesia, they can be removed when the nurse or mother is with the child and can supervise him. Although he may be given toys to play with, this also must be done under supervision to see that he does not put them in his mouth if his elbow splints are off.

To prevent strain on the sutures the child should be kept comfortable and content to prevent crying. Possibly he needs a sedative for discomfort the first few days postoperatively

and certainly something at bedtime. Physical comfort helps to prevent crying, but fear of new surroundings and anxiety due to separation from his mother may cause crying; therefore it is advantageous for the child's physical condition as well as his emotional status to have the mother or some familiar adult present. If the child is doing well postoperatively, he may be allowed to go to the playroom. This is a happy occasion for him. Also, a good afternoon nap may heighten the child's tolerance of frustration and any physical discomfort.

The physician leaves explicit orders about his diet. Usually the child is on a liquid diet for 2 weeks and then a soft diet is allowed. If the fluids offered are ones that the child enjoys, he is more likely to take them. He should be fed by spoon or cup; a straw, drinking tube, or bottle should not be used. Also, if fluids are presented to him in a little glass (fruit glass) or even poured from a large glass into a glass medicine cup, the toddler is usually more willing to take the fluids. To get the toddler to take enough fluids may be difficult. The nurse needs to offer fluids frequently and use ingenuity in getting the child to swallow them. Sometimes the toddler likes to have a variety of fluids brought to him at the same time and to rotate between them. The nurse needs to be persistent. Some water should be given after other fluids are taken. It is helpful if the head nurse specifies on the treatment sheet or Kardex the amount of fluids to be given on each shift. That sets a definite goal. If the child becomes dehydrated, then, of course, an intravenous infusion has to be given.

In planning for the discharge of the child the nurse should be sure the mother understands what diet the child is permitted and when the child is to return to the clinic or private physician's office.

Related follow-up care

Although the object of the operation is to enable the child to speak better, a referral to a speech clinician is often made. The pattern of speech of the parents is going to influence the small child's speech. Depending on the child, he may need considerable help with speech patterns or he may need very little help. The problem is an individual one. The speech clinician

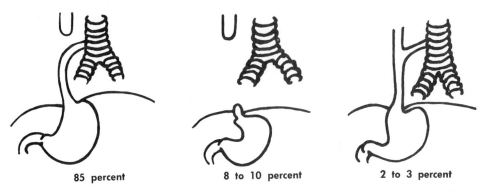

Fig. 13-16. Diagrams to illustrate the most common types of esophageal atresia with or without fistula. These comprise 95% to 98% of atresias of the esophagus and of tracheoesophageal fistulas. (From Coryllos, E.: Surgical emergencies in respiratory difficulties of newborn infants. In Abramson, H., editor: Resucitation of the newborn infant, ed. 3, St. Louis, 1973, The C. V. Mosby Co.)

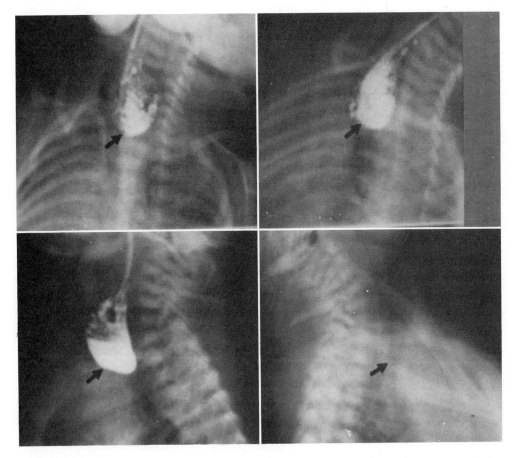

Fig. 13-17. Chest x-ray films in esophageal atresia. The contrast medium is seen filling a blind pouch in the upper portion of the esophagus. None has entered the lower esophagus, stomach, or trachea.

may need to see the child at intervals throughout the preschool period.

An orthodontist should see the child by 5 or 6 years of age when permanent teeth begin to erupt, since any broken alignment of teeth influences the speech of the child. Some orthodontists prefer to see the child earlier.

Atresia of esophagus and tracheoesophageal fistula
Nature of the condition

Congenital esophageal atresia and tracheoesophageal fistula are discussed in this book in some detail, not because of their frequency but because of the importance of the nursing care in the management of these patients.

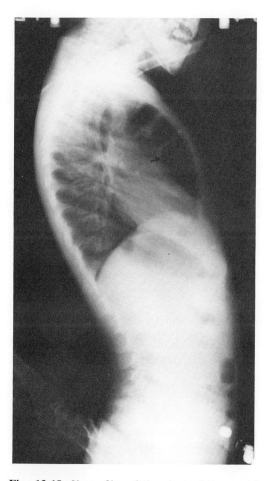

Fig. 13-18. X-ray film of the chest of 7-year-old child with a colon transplant for the treatment of esophageal atresia. Note air in the colon (arrow).

An illustration and descriptions of each type of esophageal atresia are included. Note that the commonest type is the one in which there is a blind upper esophagus while the lower esophagus communicates with both the stomach and the trachea.

The condition can be corrected by surgery, but what is done depends on the infant's condition and what is found at the time of operation. The upper and lower parts of the esophagus are usually anastomosed together and the fistula closed. A gastrostomy is done for the purpose of feeding during the immediate postoperative period.

Observation in the newborn nursery

It is the nursery nurse who may well be the first person to call the doctor's attention to an infant with this condition. That an infant has been cyanotic in the delivery room but was better after suctioning may not sound significant to the nursery nurse as the delivery room nurse gives her the report on the infant's condition when he is transferred to the nursery. Many normal newborns need suctioning at first; however, any infant who has experienced distress in the delivery room does need careful watching.

An infant with tracheoesophageal fistula is likely to have several recurrent episodes of cyanosis and excessive salivation. The nurse may have to aspirate repeatedly. If the infant is on his abdomen, she may find a large amount of mucus on the sheet. When the nurse gives the infant his first feeding, some 12 hours after birth, he may choke, cough, and become blue. His respirations will be very labored. If the nurse does not stop instantly and suction the infant or even hold him upside down for a moment, there is danger of asphyxiation. Since the esophagus ends in a blind pouch, the feeding will spill over into the trachea as soon as the pouch is filled. At best, this may cause a pneumonitis. It is fortunate that the first feeding of the infant is water or glucose solution. The doctor should be called at once. Until he comes, careful observation of the infant is essential. Not only may secretions from the nasopharynx go into his trachea but, if the infant cries, air via the fistula is pushed into the stomach and distends it. This also may cause increased respiratory embarrassment.

In anticipation of the doctor's arrival the nurse can get a new French catheter (No. 10-12) for the doctor to use. If the infant has an esophageal atresia, the catheter cannot be passed into the stomach. The physician will try to pass the tube through the nose and down the esophagus. (A soft catheter might just curl up in the pouch, so a new one that is relatively stiff should be used.) X-ray studies are made for several reasons. One is to learn the length of the upper esophageal segment and whether there is a fistula. Another is to determine the presence or absence of air in the stomach. Lack of air in the stomach shows there is no fistula. Also, a chest x-ray study aids in determining whether there is pneumonitis or any cardiac pathology. As already stated, an infant with one defect often has others. Cardiovascular and gastrointestinal anomalies such as imperforate anus are frequently associated with atresia of the esophagus.

Preoperative nursing care

Prior to operation the nurse is concerned with close observation of the infant for color and signs of respiratory distress, the positioning of the infant, and care of the intravenous infusion and the Isolette.

The Isolette is used with high humidity to control the temperature of the infant and to aid in liquefying bronchial secretions. The infant with this condition is often a premature infant. Constant vigilance by the nurse is necessary. She must be alert to the color, signs of respiratory distress, and general behavior of the infant. When awake, a well infant is active. Is this infant quiet and listless or is he responsive and active? The nurse must have a bulb syringe and other means of suctioning the infant on hand at all times so she can use it when necessary. She must bear in mind that the infant could aspirate secretions from the blind pouch and that gastric juices could be forced via the fistula into the tracheobronchial tube. Sometimes a catheter is placed in the esophagus and suction applied to prevent aspiration of saliva.

The infant is placed in a position so that the upper part of his body is elevated, and he is turned on alternate sides frequently. Positioning is so important that it should be discussed with the physician. There are two problems to consider: during the operation, the left side of the infant is in a dependent position; therefore would it be best to have the infant for shorter periods on his left side prior to operation? If his left side is up, it facilitates drainage to the trachea. On the other hand, pneumonitis of the right lobe is common, and the suggestion is made that some physicians desire the infant to be placed longer on his left side so that his right side will be uppermost for longer periods of time.

Postoperative nursing care

In the postoperative period a nurse should be with the patient at all times. The infant will still be in an Isolette or a Croupette with high humidity. For the first 24 hours, at least, parenteral fluid administration will continue.

Besides alertness in observations of his general condition, the nurse's main concern will be the feeding and the prevention of pneumonitis.

In order to avoid pneumonitis and/or atelectasis, positioning the infant is important. Beside turning the infant on alternate sides, the infant's head and chest should be elevated (Benson, 1964). Frequent suctioning is necessary. Endotracheal suctioning is done sometimes by the nurse and sometimes by the physician. Usually the physician wishes the infant to be fed by gastrostomy tube during the first week and sometimes longer. A small amount of glucose water is begun first at frequent intervals, then dilute feedings, and finally formula. Half-strength skim milk is sometimes used before formula. When he is fed, the infant should be held in a semierect sitting position. Since there is danger of aspiration of formula and/or mucus, care needs to be exercised. The stomach is first aspirated through the gastrostomy tube with an Asepto syringe, then the formula is allowed to run in by gravity alone. If the formula goes in too quickly, it may fill the stomach, back up into the esophagus, and spill into the trachea.

The esophagus has been likened to a funnel.

The upper part of the esophagus (the former blind pouch) is the wide top of the funnel, and the lower segment is the bottom. If the infant is fed too fast, the funnel will overflow, and the feeding will be aspirated. At the slightest sign of increase in respiration, the nurse should stop feeding. Sometimes the infant is fed by drip method through the gastrostomy tube instead of by the Asepto syringe.

When feedings are begun orally, a medicine dropper with a rubber tip or an Asepto syringe with a rubber tube at the end of it should be used. The nurse should feed very slowly. Again, the infant needs to be propped in a fairly erect position when fed.

A film by portable x-ray equipment is usually taken between the third and fifth days, before oral feedings are begun, to see if there is any leakage around the anastomosis. If there is a recurrent fistula, the infant may choke and cough as he did before the operation.

These infants may be in the hospital for some time. They need to hear the nurse talk to them and feel her touch them gently. Stroking of their heads and backs often seems to soothe them. When the infant is allowed in a crib and out of the Croupette or Isolette, he needs to be held and mothered. The infant must feel the will to live. Just what this physical experience of operation, difficult respiration, and uncomfortable suctioning was to him is difficult for nurses to know, but, if the infant shows no interest in his surroundings when he is getting better physically, mothering him becomes particularly important.

Preparation for discharge

The mother of the infant with a tracheo-esophageal fistula has not had the opportunity of handling and knowing her little one before he became a patient. Her first sight of him may come after he has been placed in an incubator; then the infant is operated on, and she may see him next with even more strange-looking equipment. The equipment alone may frighten her. The fact that the infant has to be constantly attended by a nurse impresses her. Add to this the fact that the infant has at least one defect. By the time the infant is well enough to be in a regular crib or bassinet, the mother may well be afraid to touch him. By this time perhaps she rejects him. She may be physically tired from the process of birth. The infant's birth has brought nothing but sorrow, anxiety, and expense. Like some other mothers who have given birth to infants with defects, she may think she has failed as a woman even though the doctor has assured her that the cause of this developmental defect is not known.

An effort should be made to explain to the mother and to the father any equipment being used. Whenever the mother does visit the infant, the head nurse or team leader should talk to her and make her feel welcome, beside giving the mother any news she can about the infant. Just as with other infants having defects, the way the nurse treats and handles or talks about the infant influences the parents.

As a step in getting to know her infant better, the mother should be encouraged to visit the infant whenever she wishes. The mother might assist the nurse by handing her articles she needs, such as a sheet or blanket. When the infant is well enough to be taken from the incubator, the mother might hold him in her arms as a positive step in realizing that this is her infant and that she soon will be caring for him at home. When the infant is finally sucking from a bottle, she can feed him.

Before the actual discharge of the infant the mother should spend at least 1 day at the hospital taking full care of the infant under the supervision of the nurse. What the nurse teaches the mother about the infant's care will be guided by what the mother already knows from caring for other children.

Imperforate anus
Nature of the condition

The defect of imperforate anus represents an arrest or abnormality of embryonic development. There are several ways in which an imperforate anus has been classified. Ladd and Gross (1937) described four types: type I, in which there is stenosis of the anus; type II, in which there is a thin membrane over the anus; type III (the commonest), in which the rectal pouch ends blindly some distance above the perineal skin; and type IV, in which there is an anal canal, but the rectum ends in a blind

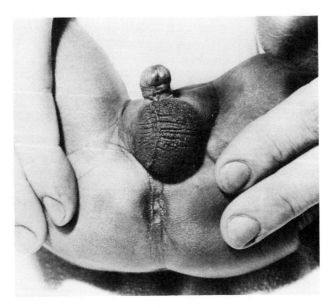

Fig. 13-19. Imperforate anus in 1-hour-old infant. Note the presence of first degree hypospadius and right undescended testicle.

pouch. Another method of classification (Swenson, 1969) is according to location—whether the lesions are high or low. In males the lesion is usually high, often with a fistula to the urinary tract. In females the lesion is likely to be low. There may be a fistula to the perineum or posterior vaginal wall. Stenosis of the anus is treated by manual dilatation. Other types are corrected by definitive surgery unless the infant is immature or has other serious anomalies. In that case a temporary colostomy is done. Fistulas are repaired at the time of the definitive surgical procedure.

Care is taken to avoid constipation so there will not be fecal impactions. Children who have low lesions are usually able to attain normal function without the aid of suppositories or enemas.

Preoperative nursing care

In the care of the newborn infant the nurse should be alert to observe and record the passage of meconium, whether this is in the delivery room or newborn nursery. If the infant passes no meconium within an 8-hour period after delivery, it should be reported to the physician. The fact that a rectal thermometer can be inserted is *not* necessarily an indication that

the infant has a patent anus and rectum. It is possible that the infant has an anal canal present, but the rectum ends in a blind pouch; however, taking a rectal temperature does furnish the nurse with an opportunity to see if there is an anal opening or if there is just a dimple or depression. To reiterate, observation and recording of stools of the newborn is a vital matter. If fecal material is not passed and the infant is fed, signs of intestinal obstruction will develop, such as abdominal distention and vomiting. Respirations may become shallow and rapid as the abdominal distention progresses.

A urine specimen is collected in infants because, if there is a fistula between the bladder or urethra and rectum, fecal material may be seen under a microscope.

Frequency of voiding is one index to the infant's need for parenteral fluids and should be met with accuracy. The infant's diaper should be observed hourly.

The nurse may assist the physician as he evaluates the infant for other anomalies and has various diagnostic tests done.

The mother should be given an opportunity to see and hold the infant before he is taken to the operating room. If the mother questions the nurse as to the cause of the defect, the nurse can truthfully answer that the cause is not known.

In summary, the main concerns of the nurse in the preoperative care are (1) observations (frequency of urination, passage of meconium, distention, and vomiting), (2) assisting with diagnostic measures, (3) emotional support of the parents, and (4) prevention of aspiration of vomitus. It is a wise rule in the nursery never to leave a newborn on his back. He should be propped on alternate sides or placed on his abdomen.

Postoperative nursing care

(For a discussion of general postoperative care see p. 297.) If a colostomy is done, there are several ways in which care may be given. A gauze dressing may be used over this, or one of several types of disposable stoma bags may be used. If a bag is used, the skin around the stoma should be carefully cleansed first and possibly karaya gum or benzoin applied to the skin around the stoma. The bag can then be applied so that stool will not touch the skin. If only a gauze dressing is used, each time the infant has a defecation (usually after he is fed), the skin around the colostomy should be washed and dried carefully to prevent excoriation. The dressing can be held in place by Montgomery straps or a roller bandage. The dressing should be checked at least every 4 hours to see if it needs changing. Daily baths given in a manner similar to that for any healthy infant will aid in keeping the skin in good condition.

Some physicians prefer gauze on small infants because of the tendencies of the skin and reaction to adhesive substances needed to hold the bag in place. Parents sometimes prefer gauze to a bag. The infant over 6 months will poke and pull at dressings of any kind. Putting on a one-piece overall in the daytime and a one-piece sleeper at night may solve the problem.

If the infant does *not* have a colostomy but an anus is constructed, the main nursing concerns are preventing infection of the operative area, watching for distention, describing the character of the stools, and giving the feedings as prescribed.

An axillary temperature is taken, not rectal. There must be meticulous cleansing of the perineal area after each defecation. Irrigations with warm water are frequently used. In cleansing, care must be taken to avoid hurting or dislodging the sutures. These sutures are usually removed a week or 10 days postoperatively. No dressing is used. The infant may be placed on a sterile pad, or his legs may be placed in Bryant's traction. To prevent infection antibiotics may also be prescribed. A Foley catheter is commonly used because of loss of bladder tone after this type of surgery. It should be connected to straight drainage. Irrigation is seldom necessary.

Until bowel function returns, as exhibited by bowel movements, decompression of the gastrointestinal tract is accomplished by a nasogastric tube or a temporary gastrostomy. When the former is removed, clear fluids are given by mouth (glucose water) and then a formula. The nurse can hold the infant in her arms to feed him.

Preparation for discharge

Since this infant, like the infant with tracheoesophageal fistula, is one whom the mother does not know well, the comments made on p. 369 about caring for the infant before discharge are true in this case also. If the baby has a colostomy, the mother needs to see how care is given and to give the care herself, under supervision, before the infant is discharged. She needs reassurance that the red mass seen on the abdomen does not pain the infant.

If definitive surgery has been done, the physician may give the mother specific directions relative to the infant's care at home.

The nurse should ascertain whether the mother understands the doctor's directions in regard to care of the anus, to diet, and to use of stool softener and/or enemas. Exact information should also go on the public health nurse's referral. Constipation and fecal impactions may be prevented by following directions.

Megacolon (Hirschsprung's disease)
Nature of the condition

Hirschsprung's disease is another name for megacolon; it is also known as aganglionic disease of the intestinal tract. In this condition there is an absence of ganglion cells in a segment of the intestine. Since there are no peristaltic waves in the affected segment to carry the feces along, chronic constipation results. In time the abdomen of the child becomes protuberant since the bowel just above the affected segment becomes very distended with feces. It could cause acute intestinal obstruction in a very young infant.

In appearance the child is pale and thin, even though he has marked abdominal distention. His nutritional status is poor. His extremities may look emaciated. Often he is fretful and irritable.

When the physician does the physical examination of the infant and does a rectal examination, it is unlikely that any fecal material will be on his glove since the obstruction is high in the intestine.

A barium enema is a helpful means of diag-

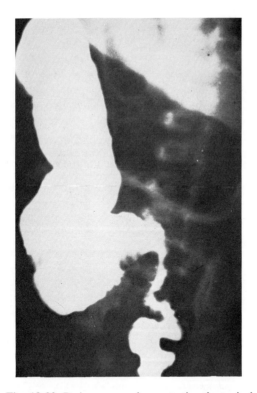

Fig. 13-20. Barium enema demonstrating the typical narrow distal rectal segment and sudden proximal dilatation of Hirschsprung's disease. (From Martin, L. W.: Pediatric surgery—general. In Shirkey, H. C., editor: Pediatric therapy, ed. 5, St. Louis, 1975, The C. V. Mosby Co.)

nosing megacolon, as is a rectal biopsy. The biopsy is to look for ganglion cells.

Because of the poor nutritional status of the infant, a temporary colostomy is usually performed. When the infant is older, is in good condition, and weighs about 30 pounds, definitive surgery is done and the affected segment is excised. An anastomosis is done between the ends of the intestines involved.

Preoperative nursing care

Other than making pertinent observations and giving such medications as vitamins and stool softeners, the main responsibilities of the nurse are in relation to giving of enemas prior to operation, trying to get the child to eat (low-residue diet), mothering him, and providing suitable recreation for him.

When giving enemas, the nurse should be sure to use saline solution, never tap water. Tap water enemas can result in water intoxication with resulting convulsions, shock, and death. Enemas should be given gently. If the solution is not expelled, it should be siphoned back. Often an oil enema is given for retention the evening before a saline enema is administered.

Sometimes a year-old-infant, if he is placed in a high chair to eat, becomes more interested in food and more willing to eat, but the anorexia of these children makes mealtime a problem.

The nurse might try holding the infant in her lap when she feeds him. Any suitable food the year-old infant can pick up in his fingers should be given. The infant should be allowed to try to feed himself. (For discussion of feeding infants and children, refer to pp. 176 and 202.) If the child is 15 or 18 months old and still is drinking from a bottle, it is not a good time to change his habits unless he readily accepts a cup. That the child take and retain fluids is more important than the manner in which he gets the fluid.

Some toddlers with this disease are more fussy and irritable than others. The fussy, forlorn toddler may derive comfort from being rocked. Another may like a push-and-pull toy, a nest of boxes, or other suitable play equipment. Time spent in the playroom with a recreation director or the "Play Lady" usually provides a happier day. If the mother can be present for at least part of each day, there is less separation anxiety.

Postoperative nursing care

For general measures in postoperative care see p. 297; for care of a child with a colostomy see p. 371. If definitive surgery has been done, the nurse's responsibilities are in the areas of taking care of the nasogastric suction, taking care of the Foley catheter, monitoring parenteral fluids, and making observations relative to abdominal distention and the passage of flatus and/or stools. (For detailed discussion of the care of the child with parenteral fluids, see p. 301.)

As soon as evidence of peristalsis is present, gastric suction is discontinued and oral fluids are begun. The child should be offered fluids without milk first, in whatever method he took fluids previous to the operation. Actually more oral fluids are usually taken by infants by bottle than by cup. Sweetened fluids like glucose water are usually more acceptable than plain water. When this is retained, fluid with milk can be given, and then either a low-residue or a regular diet for age is given.

If the child has severe distention and liquid stools, an enema may be ordered. A barium enema is usually ordered postoperatively to see especially if the colon can empty itself.

Usually by the fourth or fifth postoperative day the child is allowed to be up and around. He enjoys sitting in an infant tender, high chair, or play pen and playing with suitable toys. A short walk to the playroom and back may entertain him, or he may like to have his bed pulled close to the window so he can look out.

Preparation for discharge

Young infant. If the infant has a colostomy done in the neonatal period, the nurse should remember that the mother does not know the infant well. The nurse should help them to become better acquainted before the infant goes home. (See comments under discussion of the infant with tracheoesophageal fistula.) Whether the infant is in the neonatal period of life or later in infancy, the mother should see the colostomy and should watch the nurse caring for it after the

infant has a defecation. She should be reassured that the red mass on the abdomen does not hurt the infant and is not painful. It may take the mother some time to get used to seeing the colostomy before she can take care of it herself, but before the child is discharged the mother should be caring for it under supervision.

It is well to refer this infant to a public health nurse. The mother needs emotional support in caring for the infant and in accepting the fact that this infant is temporarily different from others. Later, when the baby weighs about 30 pounds and is between 1 and 2 years of age, he will return for further operation.

Toddler or young child. The mother of the child who has had a colostomy and now has had definitive surgery may feel a sense of relief. The nurse should be sure that the mother understands the importance of returning to the doctor's office or the outpatient clinic when designated. Directions as to diet should be clear and simple. If a low-residue diet is ordered for an indefinite period, the mother should be told explicitly what foods to avoid, as well as what foods the child can have. As cultural patterns of eating vary, the nurse needs to find out what

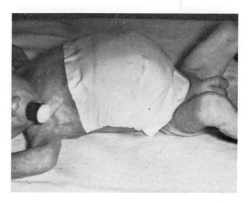

Fig. 13-21. Photograph of a 6-week-old infant immediately following the establishment of a colostomy for Hirschprung's disease. Because of the poor nutritional state, only colostomy was performed and definitive surgery was deferred until the infant was 1 year of age. (From Martin, L. W.: Pediatric surgery—general. In Shirkey, H. C., editor: Pediatric therapy, ed. 5, St. Louis, 1975, The C. V. Mosby Co.)

foods are frequently eaten at home and then see what parts of the usual family meal the child can eat.

The nurse who sees the child in the doctor's office or the outpatient clinic will probably note that the child has gained weight and has an improved physical appearance and that the distention has gradually decreased. Some patients always have some distention, especially if the colon was greatly dilated before operation.

The mother must be cautioned not to interfere in any way with the child's bowel movements in the toilet-training period. Let her observe when the child usually has a defecation and place him on the toilet chair at that time. She should be matter-of-fact and not scold if there are accidents. Toilet training is as much social development as it is motor development. (For a discussion of toilet training see p. 207.)

Pyloric stenosis
Nature of the condition

Pyloric stenosis is a congenital anomaly that the nursery nurse does not see since symptoms of the condition do not manifest themselves usually until the second or third week of life. The parents proudly take home the infant, who is usually their firstborn. He seems like a healthy infant, but then he begins to vomit. The first reaction of the mother (or the grandparents) may well be that the mother has not given the infant the right care or fed him properly.

If the physician to whom the parents take the infant believes that the infant has pyloric stenosis, he will refer him to the hospital, where the pediatric nurse sees the infant.

Pyloric stenosis is a condition in which there is a hypertrophy and hyperplasia of the pyloric musculature. As a result the lumen of the pyloric canal is obstructed, impeding emptying. The condition is congenital in origin. It usually occurs in the firstborn infants and males. Common manifestations of this condition, besides vomiting, include peristaltic waves, constipation, loss of weight, and a tumor mass the size of an olive at the pylorus. The tumor felt is the increased size of the circular musculature.

Treatment

As a rule the treatment is surgical after electrolyte imbalance (potassium, sodium, and chloride), fluid losses, and anemia (if present) have been corrected. Thiamine chloride, ascorbic acid, and vitamin K are usually given parenterally before operation. It is important that the infant be in good condition before surgery is undertaken. A cutdown intravenous is usually done. The infant is on nothing by mouth and receives nutrition parenterally.

Preoperatively the stomach may be lavaged and the tube left in the stomach during operation to relieve postoperative vomiting through removal of stomach secretions and swallowed air (Vaughn and McKay, 1975). A pyloromyotomy is done (Fredet-Ramstedt method). The circular muscle of the pylorus is split, allowing the stomach mucosa to project up through it so there is a larger opening for the passage of food. Postoperatively, glucose water is tried. If tolerated, a small amount of formula is given at frequent intervals. Gradually the amount of formula is increased and also the length of time between feedings is increased to normal intervals of either 3 or 4 hours. (Often a small infant is fed every 3 hours and a larger one every 4 hours.) The infant can be discharged about a week after his operation.

Preoperative nursing care

When the infant is admitted with the tentative diagnosis of pyloric stenosis, the nurse should see that he is assigned to a room where there are only infants with "clean" conditions, that is, where there is no infant with a condition that is infectious or contagious. The infant with pyloric stenosis is still in the neonatal period of life and has little resistance to any infection; moreover, as a preoperative patient, he must be protected by every effort against an infection.

In her care of this infant the responsibilities of the nurse are (1) accurate daily weighing of the infant, (2) prevention of infection, (3) monitoring of intravenous fluids, (4) skin care, and (5) accurate observations. The number and character of stools should be recorded as well as frequency of voiding. The latter is one measure of the state of dehydration. Other signs are poor tissue turgor, sunken eyes, depressed fontanel, dryness of mucous membranes, retracted abdomen, and grayish pallor. Vomiting, if present, should be noted but, if the infant is not given anything by mouth preoperatively, he is not likely to vomit. In projectile vomiting, which is characteristic of an infant with this condition, vomitus is not seen on the sheet of the bed, but at some distance from the crib. It is not bile stained. If there are any specks of blood in the vomitus, it may be from a ruptured blood vessel. In bathing or diapering the infant the nurse should watch for gastric peristaltic waves. They move counterclockwise across the upper abdomen.

In prevention of infection and/or pulmonary complications, the infant's position needs frequent changing. He should be turned on alternate sides. If he has an intravenous infusion in an ankle, the nurse must be careful not to let the infant lie directly on it. This would interfere with the flow of fluids. While the infant's bed is being made, the mother might hold the infant for a brief period. This constitutes a change of position.

The nurse needs to feel the infant's feet to see if he needs more covering. Sometimes a small blanket or diaper wrapped around his feet helps to keep the infant warm and comfortable.

Wiping the infant's lips with a wet cloth and moistening his tongue may help the baby if he is receiving nothing by mouth; also, the infant may enjoy sucking a pacifier.

(Refer to p. 301 for nursing responsibilities relative to an intravenous infusion.)

Accuracy in weighing is important, since it may reveal a lack of expected weight gain since birth and also as a basis for knowing whether the infant gains or loses weight after being admitted. In addition, the weight of the infant is important in estimating parenteral fluids and medication needs.

The nurse may be called upon to assist the doctor when he draws blood. Blood is needed not only for a complete blood count but also for a study of electrolyte balance and carbon dioxide content of the blood (or carbon dioxide combining power). If the infant has done a great deal of vomiting prior to admission, he may be in metabolic alkalosis. Later, in looking at the laboratory report, the nurse should note if the carbon dioxide content of the blood or the carbon dioxide combining power is elevated. Infant values are a little different from those for children or adults. In alkalosis the sodium is high because the hydrochloric acid in gastric

juice is lost in vomiting, and chlorides are low. Alkalosis may precipitate tetany, so calcium is given. If the infant is in severe alkalosis, his respirations may be reduced in rate and depth and he may have periods of apnea. An understanding of the laboratory report helps the nurse to see the reason why certain drugs and solutions are given parenterally.

When the doctor is examining the infant on admission, he may ask the nurse to get him a bottle of glucose water. He feeds it to the infant to see if the infant vomits it or has peristaltic waves after taking some fluid. The doctor will let the nurse feel the tumor (thickened pyloric muscle) if she asks him. It is about the size of an olive.

When a barium swallow is ordered, oral fluids (if being given) are withheld after midnight. The nurse may or may not accompany the infant to the x-ray department. The mixture of barium is put in a nursing bottle and the infant sucks it through the bottle. The object is to obtain a picture of the esophagus, both the exclude a stricture and to outline the pyloric canal. In pyloric stenosis the pyloric canal is long and narrow.

For general measures in preoperative care and immediate postoperative care see pp. 296 and 297.

Postoperative nursing care

The main responsibilities of the nurse in the postoperative period are (1) monitoring parenteral fluids until they are discontinued, (2) giving oral feedings to the infant, (3) continuing observation for vomiting, stools, and general condition of infant, and (4) educating the mother about the infant's care.

The cutdown intravenous infusion that was started on admission is usually continued after the operation until it has been ascertained that the infant is retaining oral feedings and is doing well. For particular points in care of an infant with intravenous therapy see p. 301.

In general, glucose water is offered first to the infant; then, as stated under treatment, small amounts of formula are given frequently. Gradually the amount of formula is increased as is the length of intervals between feedings until the infant is back on a normal schedule.

How he takes the feeding and whether he

retains it should be recorded. A little vomiting is not significant. Some regurgitation of the feeding is not unusual; however, any regurgitation or vomiting should be recorded and reported.

Preparation for discharge

Of all congenital anomalies, this condition may be the least traumatic for the infant and mother. After operation the infant should do well.

As the infant who has pyloric stenosis is usually the first child and a boy (consider the father's pride in him), the mother may need considerable help in planning the infant's care. The infant was home probably just 1 or 2 weeks before hospital admission. Also, it is advisable before the infant is discharged to inquire about the mother's health; often is has been less than 6 weeks since the infant's birth.

Perhaps the first specific step toward helping the mother when the infant goes home is to permit frequent visiting while the infant is in the hospital so she will not feel she is taking home a new infant. Let the mother continue her acquaintance with her infant. Even in the period of preoperative care the mother can sit with the infant, talk to him, pat his hand, and under supervision hold the infant. During the postoperative period of care, the mother might be helpful to the nurse in handing her articles and she might hold the infant at times. Under supervision she can feed the infant when he is back on his usual feeding schedule.

It is important to try to bring the father also into the care of the infant since it may be his first child and positive attitudes to the infant are important. The father may resent the infant because he is taking so much of the mother's time and before the infant's arrival the mother's attention had been centered on him. This requires an adjustment for the father, and he needs to feel important to the infant. Nurses in the hospital can plan to help meet this need of the new father by letting him participate in the infant's care. Bottle-feeding technique (p. 68) can be explained to the father so that he, too, can hold the infant and give him a feeding. Also, explanation should be given to the father that the infant requires affection and must be held,

talked to, and soothed. The infant's physical status demands it, and he eats better, sleeps better, and acts happier if he receives affection. Both parents may be hesitant to touch the infant after his operation.

If the mother does not know how to make the formula, a demonstration of this should be given to her. Also, the nurse should explain that this infant should receive immunizations just as any others do. (See Chapter 9 for further discussion of teaching relative to promotion of health of an infant.)

A public health referral may be helpful. Even one home visit by the public health nurse may make the mother feel more secure.

Omphalocele
Nature of the condition

Omphalocele is a herniation, or protrusion, of the abdominal contents into the base of the umbilical cord or through a defect in the skin of the anterior abdominal wall (Fig. 13-22). The herniation is usually covered with a delicate membrane of peritoneum. The omphalocele may be small or may be large enough to contain the liver and intestines. The diagnosis is made by inspection.

Treatment

Immediate surgical repair, before infection takes place or the tissues have become dry or the sac has ruptured, has been considered essential for survival. Replacement of the viscera in the abdomen and closure of the abdominal wall is the procedure of choice. A Silastic bag is sutured around the sac to form a pouch over the exposed abdominal contents. The bag is suspended from the top of the incubator (Fig. 13-23). Every few days pressure is exerted from the top of the pouch, thus forcing the abdominal viscera gradually back into the abdominal cavity. The defect is then sutured closed. Respiratory distress and failure frequently result because of the marked abdominal distention preventing the diaphragm from functioning normally and the chest from expanding.

Large omphaloceles that cannot be closed surgically may be "tanned" by using 2% aqueous solution of thimerosol (Merthiolate).

The mortality rate remains high, even with

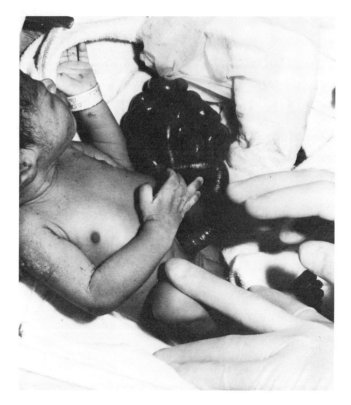

Fig. 13-22. Omphalocele in a newborn infant before surgical treatment. Note intestines lying on a sterile sheet.

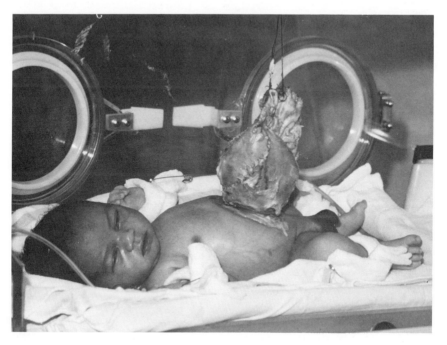

Fig. 13-23. Newborn with an omphalocele. A Silastic bag is sutured around the omphalocele to protect the exposed abdominal contents. The bag is attached to top of Isolette.

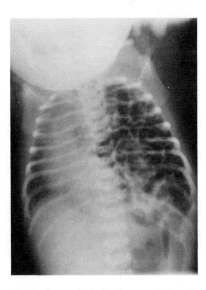

Fig. 13-24. Congenital diaphragmatic hernia. Note coils of air-filled small bowel in the left hemithorax. Operative correction was successfully performed 1 hour after birth.

newer surgical techniques, because of the seriousness of this defect and other associated anomalies that are also present.

Diaphragmatic hernia
Nature of the condition

Diaphragmatic hernia is a congenital defect in the diaphragm that permits the herniation of the abdominal contents into the thoracic cavity (Fig. 13-24). The lesion is most common on the left side. The lesion may range from a slight to an extensive protrusion of the liver, spleen, stomach, and intestines into the thoracic cavity.

Diagnosis

The symptoms of a severe lesion are respiratory distress, including cyanosis and dyspnea beginning from birth. In less severe states the symptoms may appear later during the neonatal period or even later and may include vomiting, severe colicky pain, dyspnea, and discomfort after eating. When the bowel fills with gas the bowel sounds may be heard on auscultation of the chest. The diagnosis is confirmed by roentgenograms of the chest. The films demonstrate the presence of air-filled bowel in the

chest, shift of the heart to the opposite side, and other organs in the thoracic cavity.

Treatment

Surgical repair is immediately indicated. Until the child can be brought to surgery he should receive oxygen as required to relieve cyanosis and positive pressure ventilation if needed to help expand the lungs. Gastric suction is used to remove secretions from the stomach. The newborn infant should be positioned with his head and thorax higher than the abdomen and feet to facilitate the downward displacement of abdominal organs. He may be placed on the affected side so that the unaffected lung can expand fully. The operation consists in replacing the abdominal viscera in the abdominal cavity followed by repair of the defect. Difficulty in restoring the viscera in their proper place may occur since the development of the abdominal cavity may be incomplete.

Nursing care

Gastric suctioning, correct positioning of the infant, and control of body heat are important nursing care procedures preoperatively. During the postoperative period gastric suction should be continued, intravenous fluids should be given until infant is fed orally, and blood transfusions are administered if the child develops anemia. Gavage feedings are preferable on the second and third day after surgery to prevent him from swallowing air. (For general measures in postoperative care see p. 297.)

Umbilical hernia

An umbilical hernia results from an imperfect closure or weakness of the umbilical ring. A portion of the intestine or omentum will usually be present in the hernia. This defect occurs in all races but is most common in blacks. The hernia is diagnosed by the presence of a bulge under the skin at the navel (Fig. 13-25). The hernia becomes most pronounced when the child cries, coughs, or strains. They can be easily reduced by applying pressure on the hernia sac. Most of the defects are small; however, some as large as a grapefruit have been reported.

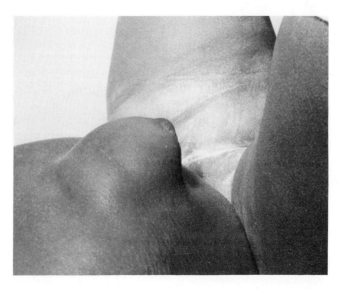

Fig. 13-25. Large umbilical hernia in a 1-year-old girl. Child is in traction for the management of congenital hip dislocation.

Treatment

The majority of umbilical hernias will disappear spontaneously by 6 years of age. "Strapping" or "binding" the hernia will not prevent its increase in size nor will it cause it to resolve at a faster rate. The "strapping" procedure may cause excoriation of the skin if it is not cared for carefully and frequently. Surgery is advised if the umbilical hernia is still present at 6 years of age, causes symptoms, strangulates, or continues to enlarge.

GENITOURINARY TRACT DEFECTS
Obstructive conditions

The nurse may encounter a child in the hospital who was admitted for pyelonephritis (p. 414); then, after diagnostic procedures such as an intravenous pyelogram have been performed, learned that the child has an obstruction to the normal flow of urine. If there is an obstruction anywhere along the genitourinary tract, there is a pooling of stasis of urine behind the obstruction. This is conducive to bacterial growth. Pus cells are seen in a microscopic urine examination. Such a child is referred to the hospital because of an infection; however, all children with pyelonephritis do not have a congenital anomaly causing an obstruction. Because some do, an intravenous pyelogram is usually done.

In addition to those with infection, children often may be admitted to the hospital because of some irregularity or interference with the flow of urine or with signs of renal insufficiency. These conditions could be caused by the presence of congenital anomalies.

The mother may say the child constantly dribbles, voids very little, or has difficulty in starting to void. The child's bladder may be distended or may look like an abdominal tumor.

In renal insufficiency, tests for renal function are not normal. Urine is increased in volume with low specific gravity; pyuria, casts, and red blood cells may be present; and blood pressure is elevated.

Common congenital anomalies that could cause an obstruction include strictures of the urethra or ureter, bladder neck obstructions, aberrant renal vessels, kinked ureters, and unilateral cysts.

Bladder neck obstruction is a condition that results from congenital hypertrophy of valvelike folds of the bladder neck or posterior urethra. History of a poor stream, hesitancy, and dribbling may suggest the condition. The presence of residual urine and superimposed infection is the rule. Since the lesion causes obstruction to the normal flow of urine, it usually leads to enlargement of the bladder, hydronephrosis, and progressive loss of urine function. Diagnosis is made by obtaining an excretory urogram, voiding cystourethrogram, and cystoscopy. Instrumental dilatation is of some therapeutic value; however, the Y-V plasty enlargement of the bladder neck or posterior urethra is more commonly employed since the operation offers an accurate and effective repair under visual control.

Hydronephrosis, a condition in which there is dilatation of the renal pelvis and calyces, is due to some obstruction of the drainage mechanism. There is a mass in the kidney region, in addition to the manifestations of obstruction already discussed.

In addition to general nursing care of any child admitted with a genitourinary condition, special emphasis should be placed on accurately recording the oral intake and the urine. If the child is still in the diaper stage, a double check should be placed in the urine output column if the diaper is saturated with urine and just one check if the diaper is wet. If diapers are changed every 2 hours in the daytime and every 3 to 4 hours at night (when the infant is awakened for fluids and feedings), a meaningful record can be kept.

The nurse participates in diagnostic measurements for these children by aiding in renal functions tests, intravenous pyelograms, and retrograde pyelograms.

The obstructive conditions named previously are amenable to surgery. General preoperative and postoperative nursing care is given. (Refer to p. 415 for a discussion of psychological factors involved in the care of a surgical child. Care of a Foley catheter is discussed on p. 299.)

Other anomalies of the genitourinary tract

1. There may be *absence of a kidney* or a *small malformed kidney.* If the other kidney functions well, the malformed kidney is removed (a nephrectomy). A small kidney has a poor blood supply and is more susceptible to infection.

2. Another malformation is that termed *horseshoe kidney.* In this condition both kidneys are fused together in the shape of a horse-

shoe. This may be compatible with life, but there is often an associated anomaly that requires operative intervention.

3. In *polycystic disease* of the kidney there are many minute cysts in the cortex and medulla of the kidney. There is considerable abdominal enlargement. This is not the same as multiple cysts of the kidney. Usually both kidneys are involved. On x-ray examination an elongation of the renal pelvis and major calyces is seen. This causes the roentgenogram of the kidney to appear as a "spider pelvis." If the condition is very severe, the infant may die shortly after birth. Hypertension, nephritis, a urinary tract infection, renal insufficiency, and/or congestive heart failure may occur.

4. *Hypospadias* is a common anomaly of the genitourinary tract. In this condition the meatus opens on the ventral surface of the penis. Other anomalies often occur with it, such as undescended testicles and ventral bowing of the penis (chordee).

Usually a two-stage procedure is done for this condition. If a chordee is present, that is corrected first and the child readmitted at a later date for further operative procedures. After operation the penis is swollen and tender. It is difficult to keep the child flat in bed. A slightly elevated headrest allows him to eat better and be more content. A cradle over the operative site will keep the bedclothes from touching a sore area. Since the child will be readmitted for the final stage of the operation, his adjustment to the hospital as well as his parents' adjustment is particularly important. The child usually has this operation done prior to school age so that when he enters school, he will be the same as other boys. (For a discussion of psychological factors affecting a child and his parents in a surgical condition, refer to p. 415.)

5. *Phimosis* means a tight foreskin of the penis that will not retract over the glans penis. There are various techniques by which a circumcision may be done. Many parents ask to have a circumcision done prior to taking the infant home from the hospital after his birth. Some parents have this done for religious reasons.

In some nurseries the infants are given a sugar nipple to suck while this is done. No anesthesia is used for infants. After the circumcision the nurse needs to watch closely for any bleeding. Often a strip of petrolatum gauze is placed around the penis after the operation.

6. *Undescended testicles (cryptorchism)* is a condition in which one or both testicles fail to descend into the scrotum. In fetal life the testes are in the abdomen, but they should descend into the scrotum in the eighth month of fetal life.

There are varying opinions as to the optimum age for surgery, but it is generally thought advisable to operate between the fourth and fifth birthdays. There are several reasons for this. The undescended testicle may be inadequate in its spermatogenic function, but it can secrete testosterone. If testes remain in the inguinal canal, they are more likely to be injured. Also, neoplasms develop more frequently in undescended than in normally located testes.

If the operation is done before the child starts school, a considerable amount of embarrassment is avoided (because of the appearance of the scrotum). No growing boy wants to look different from others. The body image of the child suffers when he has either unilateral or bilateral undescended testicles. The name of the operation is orchidopexy.

7. *Inguinal hernia* is usually of the indirect type and results from the presence of a congenital diverticulum of peritoneum that passes through the abdominal inguinal ring and into the inguinal canal. This is due to failure of the processus vaginalis to obliterate after the descent of the testis in the male and after fixation of the ovary in the female. The size of the hernia will vary, depending upon the size of the sac extending through the external inguinal ring or into the scrotum (Fig. 13-26). The hernia will become apparent when the intraabdominal pressure increases enough to force a viscous or peritoneal fluid into the hernial sac. It is 10 times more common in the male than in the female and is the most common of all hernias.

An inguinal hernia does not produce symptoms in an infant until the hernia sac becomes filled with partially obstructed bowel. The child may become irritable and fretful, refuse his feedings, or become constipated. Partial bowel obstruction will result in strangulation of the bowel and gangrene if the hernia sac is not

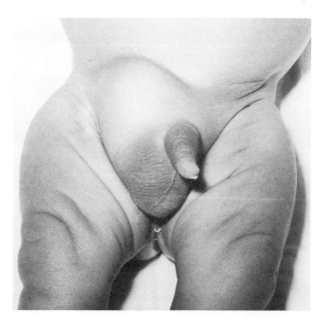

Fig. 13-26. Ten-month-old boy with a large right inguinal hernia that extends partially into the scrotum.

emptied and the defect repaired. Incarceration of the hernia is diagnosed by the presence of a mass that is irreducible and firm below the external inguinal ring. It may occur at any age but is most common during the first 3 months of life.

All inguinal hernias should be surgically corrected early in life because of the high risk of complications. When incarceration occurs, reduction of the hernia should be attempted by placing the child in the Trendelenburg position, applying ice packs to the inguinal region, and administering a sedative. Spontaneous reduction can occur. If the hernia remains incarcerated and strangulated, immediate operation is indicated.

Postoperatively collodion may be applied over the sutures to protect them from contamination. As soon as the infant tolerates water feedings, the preoperative formula and diet are resumed. The child is frequently discharged the day of the operation.

8. *Hydrocele* is a condition that is usually due to delayed closure of communication between the tunica vaginalis and the peritoneal cavity. Fluid collects in the scrotum. Sometimes the fluid is absorbed in the infant's first year of life, but, if there is a change and the hydrocele becomes even larger, communication is still open. This can be corrected by surgery. Often there is an inguinal hernia with this condition. General preoperative and postoperative nursing care is given to the infant or child.

9. *Exstrophy of the bladder* is a rare condition occurring once in every 30,000 to 50,000 births, so that only a brief description will be given. In this anomaly the bladder and the urethra are open and their lining forms part of the body surface. There is a constant seepage of urine, and the skin can easily be excoriated. In surgery for this condition the ureters may be transplanted to the colon; then in a later operation the penis is reconstructed in males and the anterior vaginal wall in females. The abdominal wall is repaired.

10. *Pseudohermaphroditism* is a congenital malformation in which the appearance of the external genitalia is ambiguous. Some children may have masculine-appearing genitalia and yet in exploratory operation be found to have nor-

mal female reproductive systems. These children have plastic operations on the external genitalia and are then raised as females.

Other children may appear from their external genitalia to be girls and yet are found to have testes. The uterus and tubes are absent. There may even be development of the breasts. Because of amenorrhea and because of a mass found in the groin (testes), this condition is discovered. The male pseudohermaphrodite is raised as a female since he is already oriented to a female role. At puberty an orchidectomy may be done.

11. *Hermaphroditism* is not as common as pseudohermaphroditism. The child possesses gonads of both sexes. From the external genitalia it is difficult to know whether the child is male or female. Sometimes the child may have the normal genitalia of one sex and the gonads of the opposite sex. In many instances the male gonad is removed; thus for practical purposes the child is a female.

NEUROLOGICAL DEFECTS

There are several neurological defects of infants that the nurse in the newborn nursery may see if the affected infant has been delivered in the hospital; if not, the public health nurse may see the infant at home or in a child health conference. Some of these abnormalities such as spina bifida with a meningocele are apparent at birth; others such as the Arnold-Chiari malformation may give no symptoms until the infant is older. Birth of an infant with a defect is a shock to the parents. (See p. 338 for discussion of psychological aspects of the care of infants with congenital defects and also for a discussion of the etiology and incidence of congenital malformations.)

Attention is called to the importance of the nurse's observation of the infant when he is admitted to the newborn nursery. It is of some significance for the nurse to know that over half of all infants with congenital defects have some involvement of the central nervous system.

Microcephaly

Microcephaly is a condition in which the head is unusually small. There has been an arrest in the development of the brain. This may be apparent to the nurse in looking at the infant. Besides the smallness of the head, she sometimes sees that the skull is narrow and the forehead slopes back. The nose and maxilla appear prominent. If microcephaly is not severe, the nurse's attention may not be drawn to the head; however, as part of any newborn nursery routine, either the nurse or the doctor should measure the head. This is true in the child health conference as well. Charting the measurements on a graph (p. 165) allows one to see whether the circumference of the head is unusually small in comparison to the average.

If the public health nurse sees the infant in a child health conference or at home, she may notice that his development is delayed. The microcephalic child represents one type of child with mental retardation for whom the parents might care at home while he is small. Whether he is ever institutionalized depends somewhat on the child's social adjustment and whether there is a member of the family who can supervise him when he gets older.

Cranium bifidum
Nature of the condition

Cranial bifidum occultum is a fusion defect of the cranium. When the nurse looks at the infant, she might not notice anything abnormal about the infant's head since there is skin overlying the brain; however, when she washes the infant's head, she can feel a soft spot where she expected to find the skull. The commonest site in which this occurs is the occipital region, with the parietal and frontal regions next in frequency. No treatment is needed in this condition.

Where a herniated sac is protruding from the fusion defect, it is called an *encephalocele*. The sac may contain only meninges and fluid (a *cranial meningocele*), or it may contain neural tissue and a portion of the ventricle (an *encephalocystocele*) or herniated nervous tissue with a portion of the cerebral ventricle plus fluid (an *encephalocystomeningocele*). As it is often difficult to ascertain preoperatively how much nervous tissue is in the herniated sac, the term *encephalocele* is commonly used for all types. If the sac contains brain tissue as well as meninges, there are often associated abnor-

malities. The brain may be malformed. Such conditions as microcephaly and hydrocephalus might be present.

In general, surgery is performed within the first weeks of life for several reasons. If the membrane over the sac is very thin, there is danger of its rupturing. Also, the child-parent relationship needs consideration as well as each parent's own adjustment to the realization that the infant not only has a defect but has one that is very unsightly. In the operation the meninges or nervous tissue is pushed back and the sac excised.

Role of the nurse

When parents first see the infant, it may be kinder to cover or lay a sterile towel over the herniated sac. Let them see the infant's face; then remove the towel if they prefer it. If parents know that an operation will be performed before the infant leaves the hospital, they may not wish to see the sac. Sometimes imagination may make the condition seem worse than it is so that it may be best if the parents do see the defect.

In caring for the patients the nurse needs to be sure that nothing presses against the herniated sac, since the sac is thin and may rupture. This could result in meningitis. The nurse needs to turn the infant frequently and carefully. She should prop him well on his side so that he does not roll back against the herniated sac. Both before and after the operation, she should watch for signs of increased pressure such as vomiting, tense or bulging fontanel, irritability, lethargy, seizures, and/or signs of mental retardation such as slowness in general development. The infant can be picked up for feedings if the nurse is careful. If she feels unsure of herself, the infant can remain in bed during feedings. The infant can be burped by the nurse holding him over her shoulder or seating him in her lap, supporting him with her hands.

Craniosynostosis (craniostenosis)
Nature of the condition

Craniosynostosis is a condition in which there is premature fusion of one or more of the cranial bones, either at birth or soon afterward.

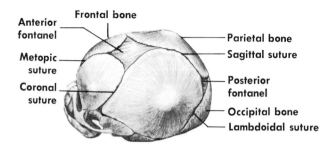

Fig. 13-27. Sutures of fetal skull.

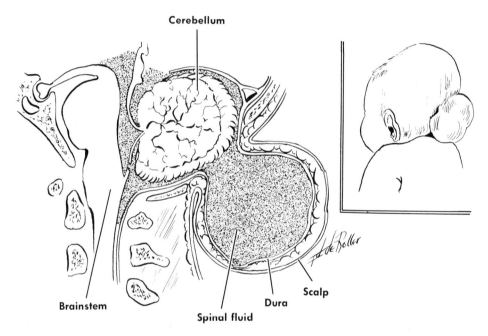

Fig. 13-28. An encephalocele may contain brain tissue along with cerebrospinal fluid.

Ordinarily there is a fibrous union between the cranial bones by the age of 5 or 6 months but no solid bony union until considerably later (Matson, 1961). When premature fusion occurs, deformities of the skull result, but of particular importance is the effect on the central nervous system, since cerebral compression may result. Skull x-ray examinations confirm the diagnosis of craniosynostosis. Its cause is unknown, although there is a familial incidence in one type called craniofacial dysostosis (Crouzon's syndrome). The condition is found more frequently in males than females.

The type of cranial deformity depends on the suture or sutures involved. The sagittal suture is the most frequently involved. When it closes prematurely, a long narrow head results, since lateral growth is limited. This condition is called *scaphocephaly*. There is a narrowing of the fontanels, or they are obliterated. The coronal suture is the next most frequently involved. When it is closed, this condition is called *brachycephaly*. The skull appears wide, since the anteroposterior growth is limited. In this type, signs of increased pressure are more commonly seen as well as anomalies of other parts of the body such as a cleft palate and syndactyly of hands and feet. In *trigonocephaly* there is a premature fusion of the metopic suture. The child with metopic synostosis has a

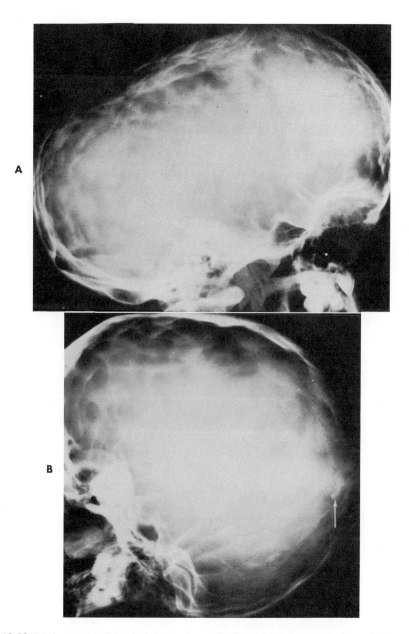

Fig. 13-29. Various type of craniostenosis. **A** and **B,** Sagittal craniostenosis. Lateral views of skull show scaphocephalic head deformity and abnormally prominent digital markings. **C,** Crouzon's disease. Grotesque face and syndactyly of both hands are apparent in this patient. In profile the exophthalmos, beak nose, and underdeveloped maxillae are also apparent. **D** and **E,** Trigono-cephaly. This 4-month-old boy was studied because of keel-shaped forehead, **D,** noted on routine examination. Skull x-ray film, **E,** revealed only a forelateral anterior fossa. (From Neurology in pediatrics by Patrick F. Bray. Copyright © 1969 Year Book Medical Publishers, Inc. Used by permission.) *Continued.*

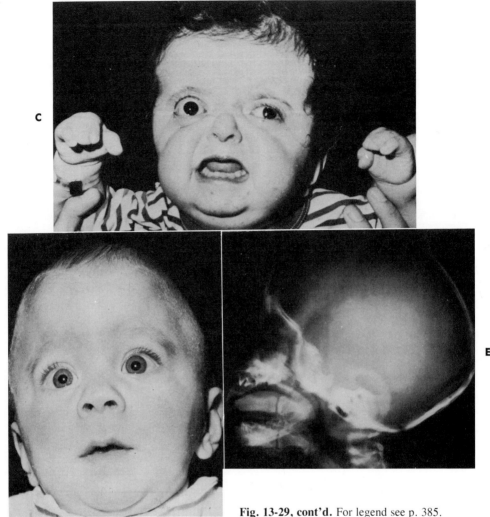

Fig. 13-29, cont'd. For legend see p. 385.

noticeable keel in midforehead. When there is a fusion of several or all sutures, the name *oxycephaly* is given to the condition. In oxycephaly the skull appears pointed, since it expands in the direction of the anterior fontanel, hence the name *turricephaly* is sometimes used. In another type, craniosynostosis may be associated with similar premature closure of sutures of the facial bones, producing unusual facial characteristics such as beak nose, small maxilla, and prominent forehead. In this case the name *craniofacial dysostosis* (Crouzon's syndrome) is applied. In *Apert's syndrome* (acrocephalosyndactyly) there is premature closure of the coronal suture plus anomalies involving fingers and toes or syndactylism. The head has a pointed appearance.

Surgical treatment

Surgery is performed as early as possible since cerebral compression and hence brain damage may result. In addition, early surgery aids the cosmetic results. In surgical treatment the affected suture is opened wide, and measures are taken to avoid closure of it.

Role of the nurse

The public health nurse may see an infant with an odd-shaped head at home or in a child health conference. A grossly deformed head suggests the possibility of craniosynostosis.

One that has generalized asymmetry may be caused by positioning of an infant who cannot move around himself. For example, if a parent leaves a young infant flat on his back all the time, the back of the infant's head may be flat. A head with a prominent occiput may be normal, but, if it is associated with delayed development and rapid head growth, hydrocephalus may be developing. A localized bulging could be indicative of one of several abnormal conditions such as encephalocele. In any event a head that is shaped differently from the usual head needs medical evaluation. This may be accomplished by having the mother take the infant for a general physical examination.

The nurse in the hospital will see the infant who is admitted for surgery. She should be alert to note the infant's ability to respond in accord with his age. Also, in some types of craniosynostosis, signs of increased pressure are present, such as unusual drowsiness, vomiting, and twitching or weakness on one side of his face in sucking the bottle.

After the operative procedure the head of the bed is elevated as for any patient who has had a craniotomy. The infant could be placed on an infant seat and elevated to the desired position. There is a tendency for the child to lose blood following the repair of a craniosynostosis. Any signs of increased pressure or staining of the patient's dressing should be noted. The general condition of the infant needs watching closely since shock from the operation may occur. The infant needs to be turned frequently during his postoperative period to avoid skin necrosis near the operative site. The infant's head should be handled gently because it is the operative area. Glucose water is given when the infant recovers from anesthesia, and if retained, his usual feedings are resumed.

Congenital dermal sinus

In congenital dermal sinus there is a dimple in the spine, usually in the lumbo-sacral region, although it could be anywhere along the spine. Often this dimple or pore has a hair or a port-wine mark near it. It comes from an incomplete closure of the neural tube in embryonic life. The sinus needs to be completely excised since it could become infected.

Spina bifida occulta

Spina bifida occulta is a defect of one or more vertebrae. Since the defect is covered by skin and since it produces no symptoms in an infant, the nurse may not realized anything is abnormal. Sometimes, though, there is a tuft of hair, a dimple, a pigmented area, or a subcutaneous lipoma. Often this condition is not recognized except by accident when part of the spine is being x-rayed.

In some instances there may be motor weaknesses of the lower extremities or even incontinence. However, it is more common for the child to have no symptoms.

Spina bifida with meningocele or meningomyelocele
Nature of the condition

In addition to the defect in the vertebral arches there is sometimes a cystic mass. If the herniated mass contains meninges and fluid but

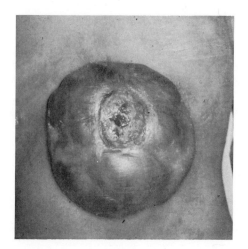

Fig. 13-30. Large meningomyelocele in the lumbo-sacral region in a 19-day-old boy. The apex of the mass consisted of neural tissue, not covered by epithelium, and in this region there was an escape of cerebrospinal fluid. Only moderate neurological deficit was present, with preservation of bladder and bowel function. The lesion was repaired, using a pedicled skin graft. Eighteen days later hydrocephalus was treated, using a ventriculoatrial shunt. This patient continues to do well 10 years after operation. (From Correll, J. W.: Pediatric neurosurgery. In Shirkey, H. C., editor: Pediatric therapy, ed. 5, St. Louis, 1975, The C. V. Mosby Co.)

no neural tissue, it is called *spinal meningocele.* If there is also a portion of the spinal cord and even nerve roots, it is *spinal meningomyelocele.* The nature of the neurological damage that is associated with this depends on the extent and location of the neurological deficit. The neurological deficit can include motor, sensory, and sphincter dysfunction. There may be flaccid or spastic paralysis of the legs and incontinence of urine and feces. Reflexes may be absent since the sensation below the involved area may be impaired or lost. Deformity of the feet is common. There may be rectal prolapse.

These spina bifida defects occur most commonly in the lumbar region, but they may be located in the sacral, thoracic, or cervical region.

Treatment

Unless there are symptoms from associated diseases, such as lipomas or dermoid cysts, *spina bifida occulta* does not require any treatment. Occasionally, as previously mentioned, there may be some motor weakness of the lower extremities or even incontinence. A plastic repair is done for the *meningocele,* or *spina bifida cystica* as it is sometimes called. The meninges are pushed back within the spinal canal and the sac is excised. Plastic repair is also done for the infant with a meningomyelocele.

In recent years there has been considerable impetus to perform this procedure as an emergency procedure on the day of birth. Evidence is increasing that, the earlier the procedure is performed, the less the neurological deficit will be. It has also been noted that chances of infection are less when these procedures are performed on the newborn infant.

Even if the infant with meningomyelocele has had surgery, he may need medical supervision for years depending on the extent of other deformities or weaknesses in the musculoskeletal system. He may have paralysis from the waist down (paraplegia). The aim of medical and nursing care is to make him as independent as possible.

Role of the nurse

If the infant has been admitted to the newborn nursery, he may be transferred to the pediatric unit or he may be discharged from the newborn nursery with instructions that he be brought back at a later date for admission to the pediatric unit in a hospital. As already stated, operative procedures may be done in the newborn period. A discussion of the nursing care of the infant with a meningomyelocele is given in some detail here because of the frequency of this type of neurological defect.

Hospital admission. The same psychological factors exist concerning this infant as have been discussed earlier in this chapter relative to the care of any infant with a congenital defect. Whether the infant is admitted to the pediatric ward or the newborn nursery, the manner of the nurse toward the infant, the nurse's acceptance of him as shown by her facial expression and her method of handling the infant, is most important to the mother. Also, the mother needs to know that she, too, is accepted and not considered abnormal because she had an abnormal infant. The nurse's behavior to the parents is equally as important as her manner toward the infant. After the doctor has told the mother about her infant's abnormality, the nurse in the newborn nursery who takes the infant to the mother's bedside will have to be careful that her feelings of dismay concerning the infant are not apparent to the mother. The nurse should be cognizant of the fact that until there is an evaluation by the pediatrician and the neurologist, the extent of neurological damage is not known. For instance, the infant may have a meningocele, not a meningomyelocele.

Nursing observations

Description of tumor mass. On admission of the child the nurse should note and record the kind and the condition of the skin overlying the tumor mass on the spinal column. Is the skin thin and transparent? Is it normal appearing? Is the skin in good condition? If there is any redness or if the tissue appears to be ulcerating, this should be recorded. The nurse should examine the mass to see if there are signs of leakage of fluid. If there are, it should be reported immediately.

Motor activity. The nurse should note whether the infant moves both of his legs when stimulated, just one leg, or neither of them. Do the legs appear to be either spastic or flaccid? If the infant has a cervical meningomyelocele, the nurse should see whether he moves both of his upper extremities; these may be involved in the neurological deficit.

Alertness and general development. The nurse should note the responsiveness and general behavior of the infant. Is his motor, social, and adaptive behavior in keeping with his age? Sometimes there is mental retardation when the infant has meningomyelocele. Presence of bulging or full fontanel should be recorded, together with any signs of lethargy or irritability, as this may signify intracranial pressure due to a developing hydrocephalus.

Presence of other abnormalities. When one abnormality is present, there is often another; the nurse should look for those especially associated with spina bifida, cleft palate, clubfeet, syndactylism, and prolapsed rectum. Congenital dislocation of the hip may be present in an infant who has meningomyelocele.

Constant dribbling of urine and feces. Throughout the day the nurse can note whether there is constantly a wet diaper and whether the infant has a normal defecation or the stool is passed in small pieces. Dribbling of urine and feces often causes redness of the anal and perineal area.

Behavior of parents toward baby. Noting and recording the behavior of the parents toward the infant at time of admission is a help to all personnel when they approach the parents during their care of the infant. Parents may need special help in accepting the handicapped infant. The social worker may play an important role in the total care of this infant.

Measuring the head. The nurse should not wait for the doctor to order measurement of the infant's head. She should do this on admission and daily thereafter. Even though hydrocephalus may not be apparent on admission, this condition may develop.

Care of the tumor mass. The cystic tumor must be observed closely for any evidence of leakage of fluid, as this could lead to meningitis. If there is a dressing over the mass or if skin covering the mass is ulcerated, the nurse should be careful to avoid contamination of the tumor mass by feces and urine. That, too, could lead to infection. Unless the skin is transparent, it should be gently washed daily with an antiseptic solution. The physician may suggest saline soaks alternating with gauze dressing impregnated with a bland ointment until epithelization should occur.

Positioning. The infant's position needs changing frequently. He may be placed on his abdomen or on either side. He should not be on his back or have anything pressing against the tumor mass, since that could cause rupture of the herniated sac with a possible resulting meningitis. Additional pressure against it could cause unconsciousness. The meningocele communicates with the subarachnoid space, so pressure on this leads to increased intracranial pressure. When the infant is on his side, he should be propped in position by means of a rolled towel, pad, or a small blanket placed behind his shoulders and upper part of his back. Another rolled pad should be placed against the buttocks, avoiding, of course, any pressure on the tumor mass, wherever it may be located—cervical, lumbar, or sacral region.

If the infant's legs are weak or paralyzed, they need to be supported comfortably when on his side. The infant may be placed in Sims' position with the upper leg resting on a folded blanket or small pillow.

Feeding. When the nurse is feeding the infant, he may be held just as any infant is but, of course, care should be exercised not to have pressure against the tumor mass.

The infant's diet is the same as that for any infant of his age. Both his appetite and the vigor with which he sucks should be noted. Difficulty or unusual slowness in sucking should be recorded. This behavior is often associated with mental retardation and/or brain damage.

Bathing. Some variation in the usual procedure of infant bathing has to be made, since the infant cannot be on his back. Of course the nurse may find it convenient and easy to sponge and wipe him on one entire side of his body, turn him, and then do the other side. If the tumor mass is covered by normal skin, the infant may be put in the tub.

The perineum and diaper area should have meticulous care if the infant is constantly dribbling urine and fecus. In addition to perineal and anal care at bath time, this area should be cleansed carefully at least every 4 hours (before each feeding). The use of a bland ointment may prevent excoriation of the skin.

Exercise. If the infant has weakness or paralysis of an extremity or extremities (as is expected with a meningomyelocele), passive exercises should be done. A physiotherapist or physician may give special directions; otherwise, the nurse may put the affected extremities through general range-of-motion exercises. A shortened or tightened heel cord can thus be avoided.

Meeting emotional needs. The head nurse should be careful in her assignment of an infant with this condition. The infant with an obvious abnormality may be one whom some nurses do not wish to handle; consequently the infant may receive less attention than others. He needs affection just as much as other infants do. Also, the nurse who is unable to be objective in handling an infant with this condition communicates her feelings to the infant by the way she handles him.

Assisting with diagnostic measures. In addition to the physical examination of the infant, x-ray studies of the spine, a myelogram, and possibly a lumbar puncture (spinal tap) are done. An intravenous pyelogram is usually done on the infant who constantly dribbles urine. There may be urogenital abnormalities. The nurse may assist the neurologist in his muscle and sensory examination of the infant; likewise, she may assist the orthopedic surgeon as he evaluates othropedic conditions.

Immediate preoperative nursing care. For general preoperative care of the patient refer to p. 296, and for psychological aspects relative to the nurse's responsibility to the parents refer to p. 415.

Postoperative nursing care. For general care during the immediate postoperative period refer to p. 297. When the infant is returned to the unit from the recovery room, there is usually an intravenous infusion running in his ankle or arm. (Refer to p. 301 for nursing care of an intravenous infusion.) If the doctor has ordered fluids as tolerated, the nurse can offer the infant glucose water orally. When he retains glucose water, half-strength formula may be tried and then full-strength formula.

The infant's position should be changed every 2 hours. Gentle and careful handling is essential since the infant's back is sensitive and painful. When lifted, the infant sometimes holds himself rigid. Because of this, during the first 48 hours the infant might be more comfortable if left in bed for his feedings. The head of the crib can be elevated. In this period the infant does enjoy being stroked or patted and having the nurse talk softly and pleasantly to him.

It is still necessary to watch for signs of hydrocephalus. Head circumference should be measured daily. Signs of increased intracranial pressure should be observed, especially a bulging fontanel, irritability, lethargy or drowsiness, and prominence of scalp veins.

Paralyzed or weak extremities should receive the same care as preoperatively; likewise, there should be special care to the diaper area of the infant who constantly dribbles urine.

The dressing on the infant's back should be protected from infection by urine and feces. Soiling of the dressing should be reported to the surgeon. The diaper may be placed between the infant's legs, but if the operative site is low on the patient's back, the diaper cannot be pinned in place. It must be folded away from the dressing. Leaving the crib elevated slightly will help to avoid contamination of the dressing by urine. Since many infants defecate after a feeding, the nurse should see whether the diaper needs changing after she feeds him. If he does not defecate then, the diaper needs to be checked hourly so there will be less likelihood of the dressing becoming soiled. A soiled dressing should be called to the doctor's attention at once.

Preparation for discharge. The mother should be shown the operative site of the infant before she takes him home. She may be afraid to handle the infant after his operation. She should not only be allowed time to watch the nurse bathe, dress, and feed the infant before he is discharged but she should also participate in his care. She needs to become acquainted or reacquainted with the infant, as the case may be. Feeding him, under supervision of the nurse, after she has held the infant once or twice may help her to feel she is important to the infant. It may be well to have the mother care for the infant throughout one entire day before she takes him home. Also, the mother should be instructed to take the infant to a doctor or a well child clinic periodically for guidance in nutrition, for immunizations, and to see if he is growing and developing in the expected manner.

The infant who had a *simple meningocele* needs the same care that any infant does; however, the infant with a *meningomyelocele* who has neurological defects such as sphincter disturbances and paralysis or weakness of one or both extremities needs special care all his life. If there are other associated anomalies, such as clubfeet, they too will need attention. Depending on the particular associated anomalies and the neurological deficit, the mother needs definite direction in regard to further medical attention for the child. It is very much the nurse's responsibility to make sure the mother understands to what clinic she will return and on what date. If the infant has loss of sphincter control, the mother needs instruction about skin care. If he has weakness of either or both lower extremities, she needs a demonstration of how to position the child for comfort when he is in his crib or baby carriage, and she should be shown exercises for his feet to prevent foot drop.

If the infant is discharged without an operative procedure on the cystic tumor mass, the nurse needs to discuss with the physician what he wishes to be used in care of the skin with cystic tumor. If the tumor does not have a thin transparent skin, the physician may prescribe washing with an antiseptic solution. The nurse does not have the prerogative to suggest treatment, even an ointment, for this. Parents may be reluctant to touch this mass and may neglect it completely. It could become infected. The mother and/or father should care for the tumor mass under supervision at the hospital before taking the infant home. The nurse's presence as she cares for the infant gives the mother a certain sense of security.

The child should be referred to the public health nurse for home visiting. The public health nurse not only gives the mother guidance in the care of the infant but is someone who can give emotional support to her and who accepts both the parents and the child, even though the child is different.

Follow-up care of the infant with meningomyelocele. Each infant has individual prob-

lems, so it is impossible to say exactly what care will need to be given in each instance. Extensive orthopedic care is often required for muscular weakness of legs and other deformities of the lower extremities. If there is congenital hip dislocation, this may or may not be corrected, depending on the strength of the hip musculature. Orthopedic operative procedures, casts, or other orthopedic appliances may need to be used in an effort to finally have the child walking—with leg braces and crutches, if necessary—so that he does not have to be physically dependent and helpless.

Specific teaching needs to be given to the parents and child regarding the use of various appliances. The hospital nurse, the nurse in the outpatient department, and the public health nurse should make every effort to be consistent with each other. Communication between them is essential.

The child who is a paraplegic may lack sphincter control and be incontinent. Training in bowel control requires patience and persistence. Just as a mother watches to see when her infant usually has a defecation and then places him on the toilet at that time, the same has to be done for this child. The child has to make an effort to defecate and to gradually become aware of the smallest kind of sensation that may tell him he is going to defecate. Often these children need a mild cathartic or stool softener to stimulate peristalsis; also, their diet must be well balanced with sufficient roughage. Whenever the child is successful in using the toilet, he should be praised; praise is more conducive than scolding in the development of bowel control. Sometimes, too, a ureteroileostomy is done, since the loss of sphincter control on urination represents a social and physical problem both to the child and to his parents. Care in regard to the ureteroileostomy bag needs to be given. The bag is worn all 24 hours.

Also, the nurse can interpret to the parents the handicapped child's needs for social interaction with others. Other children should be invited to his home. This handicapped child, like a normal child, needs to learn to share, to participate in activities, and to enjoy being with others.

The public health nurse has a special obligation in her home visits to the child to teach both the child and his parents ways in which the child can help himself. This makes his care easier for the parents and gives the child a sense of achievement. Particularly does the nurse need to emphasize the special need these handicapped children have for knowing that others love them. If the parents reject the child's handicap, the child may feel he is not liked as a person. He does not necessarily relate the parental rejection to his handicap.

As parents may resent and reject the child, the nurse should make every effort to further good relationships between the child and his family. Repeated clinic visits and hospitalizations are not only an expense but an inconvenience. Also, braces and special shoes are an added expense. Later, special arrangements may need to be made about school. In addition, the child requires more physical care than a well child, especially in regard to special exercises, care of braces, loss of sphincter control, and general handling.

At all times the nurse must remember that her acceptance of both the parents and the handicapped child is important for the future happiness of the child. A child with a handicap should be helped toward as much physical independence as possible, toward education in accordance with the level of his mental ability, and then toward vocational preparation. Throughout his childhood he needs to feel wanted and secure. He needs help, as does any normal child, in developing a set of values and philosophy of life.

The mental hygiene of the parents has to be considered in order that they can give to the child the support that he needs. Religion may prove a bulwark in a storm. The nurse should see whether the family is known to the local pastor in the church of the parents' faith.

DEFECTS OF THE EYE
Strabismus (squint, walleye, cross-eye)

Strabismus is a condition in which the eyes cannot be used at the same time for looking at an object. Strabismus may be congenital, and it is familial in 50% of cases. During the first month of life it may be difficult to tell whether true strabismus is present because of delay in developing conjugate following movements until the third month of life. The patient should be referred to an ophthalmologist for evalua-

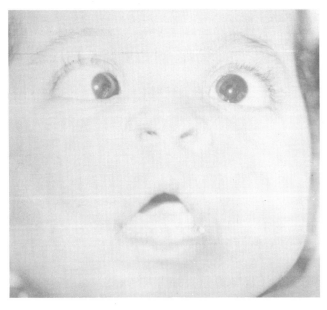

Fig. 13-31. Strabismus in child 9 months of age diagnosed in well child clinic. Ophthalmological consultation was recommended.

tion if the condition persists after 3 months of age (Fig. 13-31).

Classification

Paralytic strabismus is due to paralysis of a muscle. The eyes remain straight except when they are moved in the direction of the paralyzed muscle. Double vision may be present. In non-paralytic strabismus, which is the common type, all the muscles are capable of rotating the eyeball as they should, but they do not work together. Monocular strabismus involves one eye, while the other eye is always being used. Alternating strabismus is a condition in which either eye may be used for fixation while the other eye deviates.

Treatment

The treatment goal of modern ophthalmology is to obtain a pair of eyes that not only appear cosmetically straight but also function together in binocular single vision. Such a functional result is not frequently obtained in a child with strabismus; on the other hand, satisfactory cosmetic cures are frequently attained. Since even an infant may develop amblyopia, the child should be examined by an ophthalmologist as soon as strabismus is suspected. The medical management consists of prescription glasses, miotics, and orthoptics. The surgical treatment begins where the medical treatment ends. The correction of the deformity by surgery is considered when maximum improvement by glasses, miotics, and training has been attained, usually not before 3 or 4 years of age. If surgery is to be performed, it should be carried out before the child goes to school for psychological reasons. Otherwise, the child may be ridiculed and is likely to develop emotional disturbances.

REFERENCES
General

Altemus, L. A., and Ferguson, A.: Comparative incidence of birth defects in Negro and white children, Pediatrics **30:**86, 1965.

International Conference on Birth Defects, Fourth International Medical Congress, Amsterdam, 1974, Excerpta Medica.

Marden, P. M., et al.: Congenital anomalies in the newborn infant including minor variations, J. Pediatr. **64:**357, 1964.

Workany, J., and Fraser, F. C.: Congenital malformations. Vaughn, V., III, and McKay, R. J., editors: In Nelson's textbook of pediatrics, ed. 10, Philadelphia, 1974, W. B. Saunders, Co.

Psychological factors

Drotiar, D., et al.: The adaptation of parents to the birth of an infant with a congenital malformation, Pediatrics **56:**710, November, 1975.

Mercer, R. T.: One mother's use of negative feedback in coping with her defective infant, Maternal Child Nurs. J., **2:**29, Spring, 1973.

Owens, C.: Parents' reactions to defective babies, Am. J. Nurs. **64:**83, November, 1964.

Solnit, A., and Stark, M.: Mourning and birth of a defective child, Psychoanal. Study Child **16:**523, 1961.

Tisza, V., and Gumpertz, E.: The parents' reaction to birth and early care of children with cleft palate, Pediatrics **30:**86, 1962.

Orthopedic defects

Duthrie, R., and Ferguson, A.: Orthopedic surgery, ed. 7, Baltimore, 1973, The Williams & Wilkins Co.

Ferguson, A.: Orthopedic surgery in infancy and childhood, ed. 3, Baltimore, 1968, The Williams & Wilkins Company.

Ford, H. A.: Nursing a spina bifida child in a general hospital, Nurs. Times **66:**293, March 5, 1970.

Lane, P. A.: Home care of a toddler in a spica cast: what it's really like? Am. J. Nurs. **71:**2141, November, 1971.

Larson, C. B., and Gould, M.: Orthopedic Nursing, ed. 8, St. Louis, 1974, The C. V. Mosby Co.

Raney, R. B., and Brashear, H. R., Jr.: Shand's Handbook of Orthopaedic Surgery, ed. 8, St. Louis, 1971, The C. V. Mosby Co.

Shands, A., et al.: Pediatric orthopaedics. In Shirkey, H. C., editor: Pediatric therapy, ed. 5, St. Louis, 1975, The C. V. Mosby Co.

Stanisavijevic, S.: Diagnosis and treatment of congenital hip pathology in the newborn, Baltimore, 1974, The Williams & Wilkins Company.

Cardiac defects

Altemus, L., and Ferguson, A.: Comparative incidence of birth defects in Negro and white children, Pediatrics **36:**56, 1965.

Altschuler, A., Complete transposition of the great arteries, Am. J. Nurs. **71:**96, January, 1971.

Barnes, C. M.: Working with parents of children undergoing heart surgery, Nurs. Clin. North Am. **4:**11, March, 1969.

Benson, C. D., et al., editors: Pediatric surgery, ed. 2, Chicago, 1969, Year Book Medical Publishers, Inc.

Betson, C., et al. Cardiac surgery in neonates; a chance for life, Am. J. Nurs. **69:**69, January, 1969.

Danilowicz, D., Rudolph, A. M., and Hoffman, J. I. E.: Delayed closure of the ductus arteriosus in premature infants, Pediatrics **37:**74, 1966.

Edwards, J. E., Carey, L. S., Neufeld, H. M., and Lester, R. G.: Congenital heart disease, Philadelphia, 1965, W. B. Saunders, Co.

Glaser, H., et al.: Emotional implications of congenital heart disease in children, Pediatrics **33:**367, March, 1964.

Gould, S. E., editor: Pathology of the heart and blood vessels, ed. 3, Springfield, Ill., 1968, Charles C Thomas, Publisher.

Hall, D.: Coarctation of the aorta, Nurs. Clin. North Am. **2:**529, 1967.

Joseph, M.: Severe congenital heart disease in the neonate, Nurs. Mirror **131:**32, August 28, 1970.

Lambert, E. C., Canent, R. V., and Hohn, A.: Congenital cardiac anomalies of the newborn, Pediatrics **37:**343, 1966.

Nadas, A., and Fyler, D.: Pediatric cardiology, ed. 3, Philadelphia, 1972, W. B. Saunders Company.

Nora, J. J., and Meger, T. C.: Familial nature of congenital heart diseases, Pediatrics **37:**329, 1966.

Oestreich, P.: Children's reactions to cardiac catheterization—play interviews and interpretation, Nurs. Clin. North Am. **4:**3, March, 1969.

Stephenson, H. E., Jr.: Cardiac arrest and resuscitation, ed. 4, St. Louis, 1974, The C. V. Mosby Co.

Swenson, O.: Pediatric surgery, ed. 3, New York, 1969, Appleton-Century-Crofts.

Talner, N. S.: Congestive heart failure in the infant, Pediatr. Clin. North Am. **18:**1011, November, 1971.

Tesler, M., and Hargrove, C.: Cardiac catheterization: preparing the child, Am. J. Nurs. **73:**80, January, 1973.

Vaughn, V. C., III, and McKay, R. J., editors: Nelson's textbook of pediatrics, ed. 10, Philadelphia, 1975, W. B. Saunders Co.

Gastrointestinal defects

Atkinson, H. C.: Care of child with cleft lip and palate, Am. J. Nurs. **67:**1889, September, 1967.

Barbero, G.: Congenital hypertrophic pyloric stenosis. In Vaughn, V. C., III, and McKay, R. J., editors: Nelson's textbook of pediatrics, ed. 10, Philadelphia, 1975, W. B. Saunders Co.

Benson, C. D., et al., editors: Pediatric surgery, ed. 2, Chicago, 1969, Year Book Medical Publishers, Inc.

Davis, A. R.: Billy had a tracheo-esophageal fistula, Am. J. Nurs. **70:**326, February, 1970.

Gibbs, J. M.: Cleft palate babies: one mother's experience, Nurs. Care **6:**19, January, 1973.

Ladd, W., and Gross, R.: Congenital malformation of the anus and rectum, Am. J. Surg. **23:**167, 1937.

Martin, L.: Pediatric surgery—general. In Shirkey, H. C., editor: Pediatric therapy, ed. 5, St. Louis, 1975, The C. V. Mosby Co.

McDermott, M.: The child with the cleft lip and palate, Am. J. Nurs. **65:**122, April, 1965.

Nix, T. E., and Young, C. J.: Congenital umbilical anomalies, Arch. Dematol. **90:**160, 1965.

Olin, W.: Cleft lip and palate rehabilitation, Springfield, Ill., 1960, Charles C Thomas, Publisher.

Smith, R. M.: Anesthesia for infants and children, ed. 3, St. Louis, 1968, The C. V. Mosby Co.

Swenson, O., editor: Pediatric surgery, ed. 3, New York, 1969, Appleton-Century-Crofts.

Vaughn, V. C., III, and McKay, R. J., editors: Nelson's textbook of pediatrics, ed. 10, Philadelphia, 1975, W. B. Saunders Co.

Genitourinary tract defects

Holt, J. L.: A long term study of a child treated for hypospadias, Nurs. Clin. North Am. **4:**27, March, 1969.

King, L.: Pediatric urology. In Swenson, O., editor: Pediatric surgery, ed. 3, New York, 1969, Appleton-Century-Crofts.

Shirkey, H., editor: Pediatric therapy, ed. 5, St. Louis, 1975, The C. V. Mosby Co.

Williams, D. I.: Pediatric urology, New York, 1968, Appleton-Century-Crofts.

Neurological defects

Bierbauer, E.: Tips for parents of a neurologically handicapped child, Am. J. Nurs. **72:**1872, October, 1972.

Bray, P. F.: Neurology in pediatrics, Chicago, 1969, Year Book Medical Publishers, Inc.

Farmer, T., editor: Pediatric neurology, ed. 2, New York, 1975, Harper & Row, Publishers.

Ford, H. A.: Nursing a spina bifida child in a general hospital, Nurs. Times **66:**293, March 5, 1970.

Hermann, J., Pallister, P. E., and Opitz, J. M.: Craniosynostosis and craniosynostosis syndromes, Rocky Mt. Med. J. **66:**45, May, 1969.

Kapke, K. A.: Spina bifida, mother child relationship, Nurs. Forum **9:**310, 1970.

Matson, D.: Neurosurgery of infancy and childhood, Springfield, Ill., 1969, Charles C Thomas, Publisher.

Shillito, J., Jr., and Matson, D.: Craniosynostosis; a review of 519 surgical patients, Pediatrics **41:**829, 1968.

14

Nursing care of
THE CHILD WITH A LIMITED HOSPITALIZATION

MEDICAL CONDITIONS
Common psychological factors

When a child is brought into the hospital with an acute medical illness, neither the parents nor the child knew in advance that this would happen. With this in mind the nurse may be better able to understand the anxiety of the parents as well as that of the child. In addition to feeling physical discomfort, the child is suddenly faced with a strange environment and new people.

The parents' anxiety may be both for the physical condition of their child and the behavior of hospital personnel to the child as well as the adjustment of the child to the hospital. (Will strangers be kind to him?)

Since apprehension of the parents transmits itself to a child, the emotional state of the parents must be considered. Flexibility of visiting hours may be reassuring if parents are permitted to come and go from the hospital as they deem advisable and necessary.

Permitting the mother to help undress an infant or to hold him when the doctor examines him promotes a good relationship of nurse and mother. (If the mother believes that the nurse is pushing her aside and taking possession of the child, feelings of hostility may result. The mother should be allowed to share the care of the child.) Seeing the nurse do something to make the child more comfortable, such as positioning the child in a Croupette, aids the mother in understanding that medical personnel like children, are kind to them, and try to help them get better. This furthers a feeling of trust.

After the child's immediate needs have received attention, the nurse can ask the mother for information about phases of the child's care that will make the child's adjustment to the hospital easier. (Refer to p. 277 for adjustment of the child to the hospital.)

If the child is a toddler, it is particularly helpful to learn how he takes fluids (cup, glass, bottle). Knowing what fluids he likes is especially important in an acute respiratory illness. Asking the mother about the child's care shows the mother the nurse's sincere interest in the child and her acceptance of the mother.

The mother may believe the present illness of the child is a reflection of poor home care. The mother needs emotional support, and the nurse needs to communicate her feeling of empathy for the mother. The role of the nurse may largely be that of a good listener. Not only when the child is admitted should the nurse show her interest in the mother but also each day when the mother visits the child. If the mother stays with the child, on every tour of duty the nurse caring for the child should speak with her or both parents if they are present.

When a younger child is admitted, the nurse's attention is given to the mother (after the child's immediate needs are satisfied), since the behavior of the mother does influence the child. The mother tends to see the young child more as part of herself, whereas the child of school age is more an individual in his own right and can be dealt with more directly. The school-age child's fears center more around treatment. "What are you going to do to me?" is his thought. He reacts less to new people and strange sights than the infant or young child. He is more afraid of being hurt.

In helping the young child and infant adjust

to the hospital, nonverbal communication is the chief method. The way in which the nurse touches and handles the infant promotes tension or relaxation; the same holds for her tone of voice and her smile. Her promptness in meeting his needs for warmth, food, and general comfort will influence whether the child associates pleasantness and then affection for his nurse. The deftness with which the child is bathed, the techniques used in feeding, taking a temperature, and giving medication are all important to establishing a good relationship with the child and reducing fear in a strange place. The toddler, as he gets better, may enjoy swishing his hands in the bath basin and playing peekaboo or other games. Routines such as bathing need to be socialized. Meeting the young child's recreational needs helps his adjustment in convalescence. The nurse must remember that the infant and small child do not use the bell cord to summon a nurse. So seeing the nurse frequently, especially during the evening before he goes to sleep, aids in allaying fears. Singing to the young child or rocking him offsets possible loneliness.

The child should be assigned to the same nurse over a period of time on each tour of duty. This lessens the number of people to whom the child has to adjust and reduces emotional trauma to the child.

The presence of a familiar person—the child's mother or a relative—is comforting to the child unless, of course, the mother shows such apprehension and distress that she disturbs the child. This feeling communicates itself to the child.

The school-age child with an acute medical illness is different from the toddler or infant. As pointed out previously, the older child is afraid of being hurt. As new situations present themselves, he needs an explanation of what the doctor or nurse is going to do—having his temperature taken or blood pressure, being examined by the doctor, having a blood count taken, or going to the x-ray department. The presence of another child in his room often acts as an emotional support to the newly admitted child. As discussed in Chapter 11, knowledge of the routines and hospital day and understanding that a nurse is within call all 24 hours are impor-

tant to the child's adjustment. The effective use of pastel colors (for bedspreads and draw curtains) instead of white may lend a touch of warmth and make the room more attractive. Although the nurse is busy, she should make the most of the contacts she has with the child during bath time, giving medications, or helping to feed the child. She needs to let the child know she likes him. The nurse cannot pick up and cuddle the 8-year-old child as she does an infant, but she can call the child by his nickname, listen to what the child says, answer his call light quickly, smile at him, and talk to him. This means so much to the child! She can take the time to carefully explain treatments before they are given.

CASE ILLUSTRATION

A child overheard doctors talk about doing a spinal tap on him. He asked his nurse what that was. She told him he would have to lie on his side with his knees drawn up, that he would feel something cold on his back since one place was washed very clean. He would feel a needle prick, which would be medicine going into his back so that he would not hurt while the doctor drew out spinal fluid (which looks like water) from his back. After the treatment was done everyone commented on how cooperative the boy was. As his nurse put him back to bed the child said, ''Well, if you would just tell a guy what is going to happen, he wouldn't have to be afraid.''

If the child's mother does not stay with him, and often mothers do not with older children, the child needs to know when visiting hours are and when to expect to see his mother or parents again.

During convalescence, suitable recreational diversion is important. Time drags when there is nothing to do. Certain favorite games the child likes at home, as checkers, might be brought to him. Having his bed rolled out to a gaily decorated playroom is a nice change for the child. He usually sees other children there. An occupational therapist or the ''Play Lady'' can help find suitable diversion for him.

To be in acute discomfort is not pleasant, and it is important to keep the child's hospital stay from being essentially traumatic to him. Every effort should be made to help with this experience so that the child's attitude to illness, hospitals, and medical personnel is a positive one.

Respiratory conditions

Since the nursing care of older children with respiratory conditions is very similar to that of adults, the discussion here will be concerned chiefly with the nursing care problems of infants and young children. These are not the same as in older children.

Part of this difference is due to the anatomical and physiological structure of the young child; part is due to the manifestations of certain respiratory diseases in infancy (as pneumonia); and part is due to the fact that certain respiratory conditions are seen more commonly in young children than in older children (as laryngotracheobronchitis). In addition to this, some respiratory conditions in young children, such as aspiration pneumonia, might be prevented. The older child does not need the amount of surveillance that the infant and toddler need. Pertinent anticipatory teaching needs to be done by the nurse in her contacts with the mother or parents in the home, child health conferences, pediatric outpatient clinics, and hospital units.

Anatomical and physiological differences between adults and young children

When ill with a respiratory disease, the infant may have greater respiratory distress than the adult for several reasons. The lumen of his respiratory passages is smaller than an adult's, and, when edema is present due to inflammation, there is even less space. Also, the infant's trachea is smaller in proportion to his body than is the adult's, and the young infant has an ineffective cough reflex so his ability to remove obstructing exudate from the respiratory tract is limited.

Dyspnea is indicated by flaring of the alae nasi and by marked respiratory retraction: subcostal, substernal, suprasternal, supracostal, intercostal, or all of these. Other signs of respiratory distress in an infant include hoarseness, shallow respiration, tachycardia, increased respiratory rate, expiratory grunt, and restlessness. Restlessness may be an early sign of hypoxia.

A final point to consider in listing differences between the adult and the young child is the fact that the eustachian tube is both wider and straighter in the infant and young child than in an adult, so infection from the throat can travel quickly to the ear.

Nasopharyngitis and tonsillitis

One of the main problems in caring for an infant or toddler with pharyngitis or tonsillitis is related to his feeding. The infant's nose is small; if the mucous membranes are swollen and there are manifold nasal secretions, the child has trouble sucking a bottle or eating cereal and baby foods.

Some physicians prescribe nose drops prior to feeding, whereas others order oral decongestants. Suctioning each nostril with a rubber bulb syringe prior to feedings helps to clear the nose. (Refer to the technique in using nose drops and the use of a bulb syringe, p. 291.)

Steam inhalations or, preferably, cool moist vapor from inhalators will sometimes relieve the child. If it is a warm pleasant day, the sick toddler may profit from being outdoors for a short time.

Aspirin or acetaminophen (Tylenol) may be ordered for the young child. Antibiotics are avoided unless the infection is bacterial and seems serious.

Because an ear infection often accompanies any respiratory infection in young children, the mother (or nurse) should be told to let the physician know if the child is fretful, pulls at his ear, or gives any sign that his ear is painful. A sudden elevation of temperature could be due to an ear infection.

The child's appetite often decreases during an illness and he refuses solid food; however, ice cream, gelatin, custards, cream soups, and fluids should be offered. If the child has an elevated temperature, he usually accepts fluids well.

Rest (both in nap time and at night) is an important factor in aiding the child's resistance to infection. A tepid bath prior to nap time often helps the child relax and fall asleep more quickly. A warm room, in preference to a cold room, is often more comfortable for the young child while he sleeps; cold air may be irritating to the affected nasal, pharyngeal, or other mucous membranes. If the temperature of the child drops during his sleep, he may perspire. Damp clothing should not be left on the child but removed and dry clothing be substituted.

Acute bronchitis

Acute bronchitis is an inflammation of the bronchi. Often the trachea may be involved; the child may have tracheobronchitis. The disease is most frequently caused by viral agents, although such bacteria as the pneumococcus, the *Haemophilus influenzae* bacillus, and the *Staphylococcus* can cause it. Often the disease is preceded by an upper respiratory infection. Bronchitis is characterized by a persistent harsh and brassy cough. The cough may be so severe the the child vomits. When the cough is loosened, there is purulent sputum. Rales and rhonchi may be heard in the chest by the physician after the initial stages of the disease process. The fremitus caused by the secretions in the bronchi can be felt if the nurse places her hand over the infant's chest. The acute phase of the illness lasts about 5 or 6 days, although the child may continue to cough for another week or so.

The treatment consists of relieving the irritation and inflammatory process, diminishing the cough if too frequent or fatiguing, and decreasing the amount and thickness of the mucus in the bronchial tubes. Ampicillin is the antibiotic of choice when a bacterial infection is suspected or the organism has been isolated by culture. The child should be kept in a highly humidified atmosphere such as in a croup tent in the hospital or by the use of a cold water vaporizer at home. Potent cough suppressants should not be used in infants because it may suppress the cough reflex, thereby preventing clearance of the airway. When the cough is dry, irritating, and fatiguing, expectorants such as glycerol guiacolate may be used to thin and loosen the secretions. Antihistamines are never indicated because of their drying effect on the secretions.

Acute laryngotracheobronchitis (croup)

In actue laryngotracheobronchitis there is inflammation of the larynx, the trachea, and the bronchi. The etiology is usually viral but may be associated with *Haemophilus influenzae* type B and occurs more often in young children than in older ones. Sometimes the disease comes abruptly to the child, and sometimes it is preceded by an upper respiratory infection. The child is prostrated with high fever and severe dyspnea. Because of inflammation of the larynx and trachea, the child has a respiratory stridor or sometimes hoarseness. Since the bronchi are finally involved, there may also be difficulty on expiration. Retractions of the chest may be present because the effort to breathe is so great. The physician usually hears rhonchi and rales when he listens to the child's chest with a stethoscope. The child has a persistent cough, but the secretions are so tenacious, thick, and purulent that it is difficult for the child to bring them even to the back of his throat when he coughs. These secretions can cause emphysema (overdistention of the alveoli), respiratory obstruction, and even death.

Treatment of this condition is essentially twofold: treating the infection and maintaining an adequate airway. Throat and nasopharyngeal cultures should be obtained in all cases. Ampicillin is the antibiotic of choice because of its effectiveness against *Haemophilus influenzae*. If the child develops hypoxia secondary to the narrowing of the airway, very moist oxygen should be administered. In addition, cool aerosal mist is given by inhalation to help relieve the edema and inflammatory reaction of the mucosa of the larynx, trachea, and bronchi. Intermittent positive pressure breathing has proved to be of some benefit in the management of selected cases. A tracheotomy should be performed when the child continues to have increasing respiratory difficulty, fatigue, restlessness, and hypoxia despite these medical measures.

The nurse should be aware of the care of a tracheotomy in a small child. A tracheotomy set for a child contains an outer tube, with a plate that lies flat on the neck, and an inner curved tube. The outer tube remains in position the entire time. The inner cannula should be removed and cleaned frequently, and the trachea should be suctioned often as well. When the inner cannula is removed, it should be cleaned and replaced immediately because of the danger of outer tube becoming clogged with mucus due to its small size. Small children have died from such a closure when the nurse left the bedside for only 3 or 4 minutes.

Pneumonitis (pneumonia)

Classification and pathology. Formerly pneumonia was classified anatomically as lobar, in which a particular lobe or lobes are involved, lobular (bronchopneumonia), or interstitial. Bronchopneumonia is more common in young children than is lobar pneumonia because infection is more likely to be disseminated than localized.

In lobar pneumonia or bronchopneumonia the alveoli become edematous and filled with inflammatory cells, serum, red blood cells, and fibrin. The exudate found in the aveoli contains many bacteria of the kind causing the pneumonia. As the segments or lobes of the lungs become involved, there is a decrease in the amount of air entering the lungs, and the vital capacity decreases. These events are reflected in the child by intercostal retractions and flaring of the alae nasi.

The pathological findings in interstitial pneumonia are found in the interstitial spaces and bronchial mucous membrane of the lungs. The spaces and membranes become filled with cytoplasmic inclusion bodies, white cells, and exudate. Atelectasis, necrosis of the tracheobronchial epithelium, and emphysema may result.

With the use of antibiotics and chemotherapeutic agents, pneumonia is more likely to be classified according to its etiology. The main causes of pneumonia in a child are bacterial, viral, hypostatic, and aspiration. Of the bacterial group of pneumonias it is of some interest to know that the most common kind in infants and children is caused by the pneumococcus. Also, staphylococcal pneumonia has its greatest incidence in early infancy. The *Haemophilus influenzae* bacillus is not a frequent cause, but when it is the cause, meningitis may occur as a complication.

Prevention. Aspiration and hypostatic pneumonia can be avoided. If debilitated infants have their position changed frequently, hypostatic pneumonia might not occur. The young or weak infant is unable to turn himself from one side to the other without help. When the infant is turned on his side, a rolled pad or blanket should be placed at his back to hold him in position. In addition, rocking the infant and holding him for feedings are helpful.

Use of nose drops containing oil should be avoided since the oil could cause lipoid pneumonia. Zinc stearate powder or other powders used on an infant could be easily aspirated and should be used with care, if used at all. An older sibling in imitating his mother might shake a powder can over the infant and inadvertently let some of it go into the infant's mouth and nose. Also, a toddler or older infant might get hold of a powder can and put it in his mouth. If the can is open, this could be disastrous.

Various foreign objects (pins, nuts, popcorn, beads) may be picked up by the creeping infant or toddler and be aspirated. These can cause atelectasis, infection, or asphyxiation. Ingestion of kerosene can cause irritation of the respiratory tract. Children through 2 years of age still tend to put everything into their mouth, since the mouth remains an important sensory

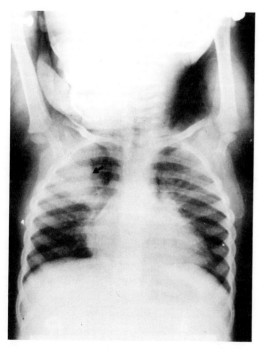

Fig. 14-1. Pneumococcal lobar pneumonia in a 5-year-old child. Note partial consolidation of right upper lobe.

organ. Anything potentially harmful must be kept away from them.

The aspiration of milk and food substances can cause pneumonia. When an infant is given his formula, his head and the upper part of his body should be elevated. After feeding he should be placed on his right side or his abdomen. If the infant is in a supine position and vomits or regurgitates milk, an aspiration pneumonia could result. Also, forcing a child or infant to eat may have disastrous results. The child could choke on the food and aspirate some. Popcorn and nuts should not be given to any children until they have their first permanent molar teeth. Since the small children cannot chew these foods, there is considerable danger of aspiration.

Child health conferences present a wonderful opportunity to teach mothers about the safety of young children and infants. The nurse in the hospital in her contacts with parents should be alert to opportunities for teaching as well as alert to the safety of the child.

Manifestations of pneumonia. In several ways the manifestations of pneumonia in young children differ from those in older children and adults. Pneumonia in young children is more disseminated than in older children. In older children pneumonia may be confined to a particular lobe or lobes (lobar pneumonia).

In addition to pneumonia being more disseminated, manifestations in the infant and toddler may be referable to the nervous and gastrointestinal systems. The infant may be brought to the emergency room of a hospital by his parents because he had a convulsion. Convulsions sometimes occur in infancy when the infant has a high elevation of temperature. On examination the infant may show signs of meningeal irritation, nuchal rigidity, hyperactive reflexes, and positive Kernig and Brudzinski signs. He may be in an opisthotonos position. The mother may say the infant vomited and has had loose stools for a few days. This is not uncommon. Loose stools are considered a *parenteral* diarrhea (secondary to the chief infection).

Another point of difference is that the infant does not expectorate if he has a cough. The cough reflex in infants is not always effective

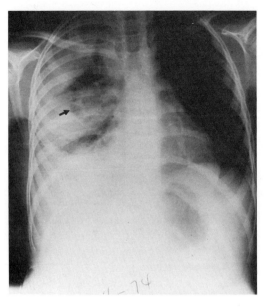

Fig. 14-2. Staphylococcal pneumonia in a 2-year-old child. Note the multiple air-containing cavities in the lung (end of arrow) characteristic of staphylococcal pneumonia.

enough to even bring secretions from the lungs to the back of the throat, but when this does happen the secretions are either swallowed or aspirated, depending to a large extent on the position of the infant. It is dangerous to leave an infant with pneumonitis in a supine position.

The infant may have greater respiratory distress than an older child (p. 397). The thoracic pain of which some adults complain is sometimes referred to the abdomen in a child. A young child does not complain verbally of pain, but if he lies with his legs drawn up or wants to stay on a particular side, it is usually indicative of pain.

The high white blood cell count (15,000 to 40,000) and high specific gravity of urine together with some hyaline casts and albumin are not dissimilar to laboratory data of an adult with bacterial pneumonia. In viral pneumonia the lymphocytic count is higher than the polymorphonuclear count. The reverse of this is true in bacterial pneumonia.

In a young infant or a very debilitated one sometimes it may be difficult for the doctor to find any abnormal sounds upon percussion and auscultation of the chest. Sometimes rales and rhonchi can be felt when a hand is placed over the infant's chest. X-ray examinations are helpful in making a diagnosis.

Complications. Otitis media, emphysema, and cardiac failure are less common complications since the advent of microbial therapy; however, pleural effusions still at times follow pneumonia. These may be purulent or nonpurulent. A serious complication is abdominal distention due to a paralytic ileus.

Home care. Some children with pneumonia may be treated at home if they have been seen by the doctor early in the course of the disease and there are no complications. The use of antimicrobial drugs has made this possible; however, usually many infants are hospitalized with pneumonia in the late winter and early spring. This is partly due to the severe dyspnea of the infant, the presence of diarrhea or other complications, and the problem of feeding when the infant is in acute respiratory distress.

Role of the nurse

The nursing actions involved in caring for a child with bronchitis, tracheobronchitis, and pneumonia vary in degree rather than in kind so they will be discussed together.

Observations. Because an infant's condition may change quickly, the nurse needs to watch the infant closely. Observations of an infant or child with pneumonia should be recorded at least once on every nursing shift. Anything about the infant that is different from what was previously recorded should be specifically noted. Care given and the infant's response to it should be recorded, in addition to the nurse's observation of his condition. Listed here are some of the significant factors to be watched for and included in written observations:

1. Quality of respirations (especially signs of dyspnea such as retractions, mouth breathing, flaring of the alae nasi, expiratory grunt, or inspiratory stridor)
2. Quality of the pulse (strong, weak, irregular, regular)
3. Color (pink, white, gray, blue)
4. Cough (dry, hard, loose, brassy)
5. Signs of spasticity or nuchal rigidity (best seen when handling infant during bath or feeding time)
6. Signs of dehydration (dryness of skin and mucous membrane, depressed fontanel, poor tissue turgor, sunken eyes)
7. Behavior (listless, restless, apathetic, irritable, active, playful)

Whether the infant has trouble in inspiration, expiration, or both should be noted carefully. In acute bronchiolitis there may be both expiratory and inspiratory distress. Death in this condition may come from exhaustion due to respiratory effort or from cardiac failure.

In describing the infant's color the nurse should observe the skin, mucous membrane, and fingernails of the infant. If crying improves the infant's color, this should be noted because the infant may have some atelectasis.

Behavior of a child gives a clue to the degree of his illness. The infant who makes no effort to move is indeed sick. Also, restlessness may indicate air hunger.

In judging whether the infant is dehydrated, the nurse should tell what she observes rather than give the interpretation of what significance she believes her observations may have. For example, dryness of the infant's lips may be from an elevation of temperature; on the other hand, there are other possible causes such as continuous loose stools.

Relieving dyspnea. Because of dyspnea the infant is usually more comfortable if the head of the crib is elevated. In a small crib it is easy to adjust the spring and mattress to whatever elevation is desired. In an Isolette the entire mattress can be elevated at one end. As the small infant cannot sit up, propping him up with pillows or pulling up the head of the bed of a large crib would result in the infant slumping into a U shape. This would make dyspnea even greater. The infant carrier or infant seat so frequently used by mothers to carry their infants might be used to advantage. The upper part of his body can be elevated as desired. The little seat can be held in place by straps as well as a pillow directly behind the seat.

Although an upright position helps to relieve dyspnea, cool moist air with or without oxygen usually does also. A Croupette is frequently ordered for the infant with dyspnea who has a respiratory infection. (For care of a child in a Croupette refer to p. 293). It is sufficient to point out here that, if the ice in the back of the Croupette is allowed to melt and the Croupette becomes warm, the respirations of the infant will increase, not decrease, and he will become more dyspneic.

Also, the crib should be made with cotton blankets because of the moisture of the Croupette. Stockings or cotton mittens can be used on the infant's hands to keep them warm. Because of poor circulation a diaper or small cotton blanket might be wrapped loosely around his feet and legs. The infant's clothes and covering become wet because of the moisture and should be changed every 3 hours when he has his formula.

Cough. Coughing is nature's way of removing obstructions from the airways. When the infant coughs, the nurse should seat him upright and place her hand over his chest to splint it as he coughs. Coughing accentuates any pleuritic pain. The cool moist air helps to liquefy the secretions so that the infant's cough should be looser after he has been in a Croupette for a time. If the infant's cough keeps him awake at night, the nurse should draw the physician's attention to this. A cough depressant may be ordered.

As noted previously, the infant does not expectorate, but if he breathes rather noisily, the nurse might try gently and carefully suctioning the infant either with an ear bulb syringe or a nasopharyngeal catheter. Sometimes a considerable amount of mucus is obtained and breathing is made easier.

Recording intake and output. Recording intake and output is another responsibility of the nurse. When fluids are given or offered, this should be written on the nurses' notes. If the infant is not taking enough fluids, an intravenous infusion may be started. All stools should be described, and if the diaper is wet when changed, this voiding is recorded. Some hospitals indicate that a diaper is very wet by placing two checks (✔✔) in the urine column of the nurses' notes instead of the usual one check (✔).

Nutrition. What is offered varies with the condition of the infant. If he is vomiting or has vomited, perhaps a parenteral fluid will be started. Glucose might be offered. If that is re-

tained, perhaps half-strength formula or skim milk may be ordered because of the low fat content. Liquids without milk that may be offered include weak tea and carbonated beverages. If there is no diarrhea, orange juice and other fruit juices may be offered. Sherbet and ice cream may be welcomed by a young child. A child who has fever but no gastric complications should be given foods that are high in carbohydrates, proteins, and vitamins. In fever the metabolic rate is increased. There is tissue destruction and fluids are lost.

Nutrition may well be a problem for the infant while he is acutely ill because of his dyspnea. Small feedings at frequent intervals usually are better than trying to get him to take a large amount at one time. A formula schedule of every 3 hours instead of every 4 hours helps. Offering small amounts of other fluids is better than urging the infant to take a lot. If the infant is very dyspneic, cup feeding should be tried. Sometimes, instead of a plastic cup, the small medicine cup might be used. Teaspooning fluids could be tried. If the infant is in an oxygen test or Croupette, he should be fed in the tent. (He might be taken out of the tent and held in the nurse's arms at other times for a short period.)

Skin care. The bath is important because the skin is an excretory organ. Also, the bath improves the infant's circulation. In place of having a bed bath an infant who is fussy and irritable might find it more pleasant to be soaped all over and placed gently in a basin of water to be rinsed. Afterward he can be placed on a cotton blanket and patted dry. This requires less handling and may be more soothing to him than a bed bath. However, if the infant's room is cold or drafty, this cannot be done without chilling the infant. In that case, bathing only the skin where surfaces are together would be better. Special attention should be given to the nose. If there are any dried secretions, the nostrils should be carefully cleansed with either a soft washcloth or a cotton applicator. While one nurse is bathing or holding the infant, another nurse should be making his bed. The infant's comfort and safety must be the first consideration in caring for him.

Daily bathing and changing the infant's position every 2 hours when he is awake are factors in maintaining good condition of the skin and preventing the skin from breaking down. (If the infant has diarrhea, see p. 408 for care of the skin.)

Rest. If the infant can be placed in a two-bed ward, rather than one having four or six beds, a great deal of disturbance to the infant will be eliminated.

How much rest the infant gets depends also on how comfortable the medical and nursing attention makes him in relieving dyspnea and in attending to his bodily needs. Part of his rest depends on the organization of work of the nurse. Whether she has assembled the equipment she needs before she begins to care for the infant or has to step out of the room for other supplies makes a difference to him. After gathering necessary materials the nurse should do whatever she plans and then let the infant rest until the next time she has specific care to give, such as offering fluids to the infant, changing his clothing, covering him, or turning him. The nurse can observe the infant's respiration and color and add ice to the Croupette without disturbing him.

Emotional support. The best emotional support might well be physical care, especially anything that relieves the infant's dyspnea. Prompt attention to bodily needs and general comfort helps to eliminate crying. (Crying only makes the infant more dyspneic.) To cry and not have prompt attention might lead to negative feelings, which in turn have an undesirable physiological effect. On the other hand, when the nurse is with the infant, she should talk to him pleasantly. It does not usually hurt the infant to be removed from the Croupette for a short time and held in the nurse's arms at least once on every tour of an 8-hour duty. Difficulty in breathing is frightening, and the infant needs reassurance. Every time the nurse comes to look at the infant she should smile and speak to him. As the infant cannot be interviewed, we do not know, but can only imagine, what he must feel like seeing no one in his room for long periods of time, especially when he is feeling uncomfortable. Certainly it is stressful.

If the infant is very little and is in an Isolette, the nurse can reach through the armhole and touch and stroke the infant. Nurses must not underestimate the feelings and intellect of any infant, however young.

Administration of medication. Penicillin is the drug of choice for pneumococcal pneumonia, but before a sensitivity report has been made, often penicillin in combination with another antibiotic or sulfa drug may be ordered. The medication can be given parenterally or intramuscularly. (See p. 290 for giving intramuscular injections.) Later the medication is usually ordered to be given orally. There should be distinct improvement of the infant's condition 12 to 24 hours after antimicrobial medication has been given. Medication is usually given for 7 to 10 days. This means that it is continued for several days after the temperature is normal.

Most strains of staphylococcal pneumonia are resistant to penicillin, sulfa drugs, streptomycin, and the tetracyclines. Methicillin and oxacillin seem to be effective against staphylococcal pneumonia at present.

Other antimicrobial drugs are ordered according to the sensitivity of the organism causing the pneumonia.

Although certain broad-spectrum drugs such as tetracycline have some influence against viral agents, infants and children with viral pneumonia tend to have a longer course of illness than children with a bacterial type of pneumonia. A medication for cough may be ordered if the cough interferes with the child's rest at night.

Temperature-reducing measures. Antipyretic medications may be ordered for an elevation of temperature. If a rectal suppository of aspirin is used, the nurse should not expect the temperature to drop as quickly as if aspirin by mouth is prescribed or Tempra syrup is given. The reason the infant's temperature is closely watched is that high elevation may cause a convulsion. If the Croupette is kept cool, the chances of a high elevation of temperature are less. (Various nursing measures used to reduce the infant's temperature are discussed on p. 292).

Convalescence. The nurse's description of behavior of the infant is significant to the doctor. When the infant begins to smile and be responsive socially, is active when awake, and is hungry, the nurse can be sure the infant is better. A well infant has a happy disposition; he sleeps and eats well.

It is at this point that the mother is likely to be most receptive to suggestions about the infant's care. Whatever advice the doctor gives should be carefully discussed with the mother to see that she understands it. Also, the nurse can inquire from the mother about periodic examinations of the infant, immunizations, and various measures that help to maintain the infant's health. The answers of the mother are the nurse's cue as to necessary and pertinent teaching.

It is important, too, that the nurse be cognizant of the mother's need of rest, relaxation, and recreation. The mother may feel fatigue from emotional anxiety, especially if she has remained in the hospital with the infant. Perhaps she should spend a day at home resting before the infant returns home. If the mother has learned to trust the nurses, she will be willing to leave the infant for 1 day while he is in the hospital.

Bronchiolitis

Bronchiolitis is a respiratory illness caused most frequently by the respiratory syncytial virus during the winter and spring months of the year. It is disease of early infancy; almost 90% of the children are less than 1 year, and 75% less than 6 months of age. The virus produces a generalized inflammation of the mucosa of the lower respiratory passages such as in the small bronchi, bronchioles, and pulmonary alveoli. As a result of the inflammation the lumen of the lower respiratory passages become narrowed and filled with thick, sticky mucus. Therefore air becomes trapped behind the partially obstructed passages, since it can enter during inspiration but cannot be expelled on expiration. The air remains trapped in the lungs each time the infant breathes, causing the chest to become overdistended.

Clinical symptoms. The symptoms of bronchiolitis will occur 5 to 7 days after an infection of the upper respiratory tract. Mild elevation of the temperature is usually present. The child is restless and anxious and also has a dry, hacking, nonproductive cough. The respirations are rapid and shallow and have a characteristic expiratory grunt. On auscultation of the chest diminished breath sounds, rales, and "wheezing" are found along with prolongation of the expiratory phase of respiration. Chest roentgenogram reveals overinflated lungs with patches of pneumonitis or atelectasis.

Prognosis. Bronchiolitis is a basically benign, self-limited viral respiratory infection. After 2 or 3 days of severe symptoms and signs of respiratory obstruction the child begins to breath easier and develops better air exchange. It is not unusual for mild symptoms to remain for 7 to 10 days. Deaths are uncommon.

Treatment. The primary aims of treatment are to improve the infant's air exchange and relieve hypoxia if present. Hydration and feeding should be maintained intravenously until the child is able to drink and eat without difficulty. Moist cool air in a Croupette or an ultrasonic nebulizer is usually used to provide maximum humidification of the atmosphere so that liquifaction of the secretions will result. Moist oxygen is administered whenever cyanosis is apparent. Antimicrobial therapy is reserved for infants with demonstrated bacterial complications or a concomitant bacterial infection and those that are dangerously ill. Corticosteroids have been used, but there is no strong scientific evidence available that they are beneficial in this disorder. Nursing care is similar to care of a child with pneumonia.

Bronchiectasis

Bronchiectasis is included in this chapter because of convenience. Since it is a chronic disease, rightfully it should be discussed in the chapter on long-term illness (Chapter 16). Bronchiectasis is a progressive and chronic disease in which there is inflammation and dilatation of the bronchi. The condition is seen less frequently than formerly. This is partly due to the use of antibiotics in treating the respiratory diseases that may act as predisposing factors in bronchiectasis. In prevention, prompt attention to respiratory illnesses and protection from pertussis are essential in young children.

When a child with this condition is admitted to the hospital for treatment and/or evaluation of his condition, the nurse will see him. Her areas of chief concern are weighing him accurately, encouraging him to eat, carefully supervising his rest periods, giving antibiotics and possibly expectorants, and aiding in postural drainage and aerosol therapy. The latter should be given after postural drainage to be most effective.

As changing the child's position or turning him may induce coughing, the nurse should plan her care with a vew to disturbing him as little as possible.

If the affected area of the lung is localized, surgery may be performed and a portion of the lung excised. Otherwise, efforts are directed toward controlling infection and reducing secretions. A prophylactic antibiotic is sometimes prescribed by the physician in an effort to prevent further respiratory infections.

Gastroenteritis (diarrhea)
Nature of the condition

Diarrhea is a symptom of a variety of disorders. Causative agents include bacteria, viruses, fungi, parasites, and intestinal protozoa. Noninfectious diarrhea could be due to aganglionic megacolon, celiac disease, parenteral infection, or some inborn error of metabolism such as an intestinal deficiency of carbohydrate-splitting enzymes. In areas where there are low hygienic standards, diarrhea could be caused by contaminated milk, formula, or other infant foods.

Dysentery is a severe form of diarrhea with blood and pus appearing in the stools. Amebic dysentery is due to intestinal infestation with *Entamoeba histolytica.* Bacillary forms include those due to *Shigella* and *Salmonella* organisms.

The four main groups of *Shigella* are *Shigella dysenteriae, Shigella flexneri, Shigella boydii,* and *Shigella sonnei.*

Bacillary dysentery is reportable to the Department of Public Health. Pus and blood are seen in stools of patients with this infection, as well as in dysentery caused by amebae. This is not true of other types of gastroenteritis (diarrhea).

A stool specimen is sent to the laboratory for examination, or a rectal swab is taken. The infant may be moderately or severely dehydrated and have some degree of acidosis. If he is not vomiting and he has only mild diarrhea, he may be given oral electrolyte solution; otherwise, he receives nothing by mouth for 24 to 48 hours, and attention is given to improving the infant's circulation and restoring electrolyte imbalance through parenteral therapy. Dehydration is caused by loss of water and electrolytes in stools or urine, through skin and lungs, and perhaps by vomiting. (Vomiting does not always accompany diarrhea.) The amount of dehydration is judged by the doctor partly by weight loss and partly by the appearance of the infant. Elevation of the blood urea nitrogen is indicative of a moderate degree of dehydration. Blood chemistries can aid in judging the severity of the acid-base imbalance in selected instances but cannot tell the volume of water or amount of electrolytes lost. After correction of the dehydration and electrolyte imbalance, the treatment depends on the cause of the condition.

Lomotil may be ordered to allay restlessnes and tenesmus. Kalose or kaolin combined with pectin might be used to improve the consistency of the stool. Antibiotics are ordered in accordance with the specific organism found (on culturing of the stool or by rectal swabs). Antimicrobial drugs used include the sulfonamides, the tetracyclines, chloramphenicol, polymyxin B, neomycin, and others. Perhaps in a mild infection or in a viral diarrhea no antibiotic will be ordered.

When the infant's stool becomes normal, skim milk or a milk with low fat value is often offered. Glucose water, barley water, and/or weak tea is often given between milk feedings. Ripe bananas and scraped apple may be added to the diet and then the infant's usual formula, full strength. Gradually the infant resumes the usual diet for his age.

Role of the nurse

Isolation. When an infant with diarrhea is admitted to the hospital, he should be placed on isolation, preferably in a room by himself. Until the physician ascertains on examination of the infant and/or on bacteriological study of stool (or rectal swab) that pathogenic organisms are not present, other infants on the unit or ward must be protected.

Observations. Recording observations will help the physician to know the degree of the infant's illness as well as his progress.

Stools. In the newborn nursery the quick recognition, recording, and reporting of a diarrheal stool will tell the physician that there is a sick infant who needs his attenton. On the pediatric unit the description of the stool of a diarrheal infant helps the physician to know the progress of the infant.

NORMAL STOOLS. In order to understand what constitutes an abnormal stool it is essential that the nurse have an understanding of normal stools of infants. The first stool of a newborn infant is black or greenish black and is sticky. It is called meconium. Next it turns a greenish brown when the infant is fed milk, then a greenish yellow, and finally about the fourth or fifth day the stool is yellow in color and soft or salvelike in consistency. The frequency of stools in the newborn is related to the frequency with which he is fed. The number may vary from three to five or six daily. The breast-fed baby has a golden yellow stool, whereas the artificially fed infant has a stool of somewhat lighter yellow.

During the first 3 or 4 months of life, breast-fed infants average two to four stools daily, whereas artificially fed infants average one to two stools daily. The stools of the latter have more odor. Whitish curds and small amounts of mucus may appear in the normal stool of an infant. This is of no particular significance.

ABNORMAL STOOLS. The character of the stools varies with the severity of the infection. The frequency varies from two or three to more than 20. In consistency the stools may first be loose with considerable mucus, then become yellow greenish in color and semiliquid, and finally may be watery. Large amounts of mucus may be present. Pus and blood are seen with bacillary and amebic dysentery. In diarrhea of the newborn the stools are frequently watery and are passed explosively.

The nurse should describe each stool according to amount (large, medium, small), color (brown, yellow, greenish yellow, or green), consistency (soft, loose, liquid), and any ab-

normal constituents such as pus, blood, and any large amounts of mucus. If the stool has a foul odor, this too should be noted, as well as the passage of any flatus. Each time the nurse changes the diaper the stool should be recorded. If she waits, she may forget and not record accurately. The last diaper of the infant should be saved for the physician to see and the previous one discarded.

Behavior. Behavior of the infant needs describing. In the newborn nursery the infant may be fretful or listless before the onset of diarrheal stool. He may not nurse as well. On the pediatric unit the way the infant behaves on admission and on each 8-hour nursing shift thereafter should be described. Is he alert or drowsy? Does he draw up his legs and cry before passing a stool? This is significant. Is he fretful, irritable, lethargic, or does he respond playfully and cheerfully to social stimulation? Is he wide awake, anxious looking, or relaxed and peaceful? Does he accept feedings eagerly or slowly? Perhaps he is stuporous. Whatever his behavior is, it should be recorded. As the infant feels better, he will become more cheerful and playful.

Dehydration. Clinical signs of dehydration in an infant include poor tissue turgor (loss of normal elasticity of the skin), dryness of mucous membranes and skin, sunken eyes, and sunken fontanel. Loss of skin elasticity is due to loss of subcutaneous tissue. Skin may hang in folds. However, a plump infant may be dehydrated but not show signs of dehydration except for the sunken eyes. This, then, is perhaps the best criterion of dehydration. As the diarrhea improves and as fluids (parental and oral) are given to the infant, there should be fewer signs of dehydration, or at least the signs should be less obvious.

Distention, tenesmus, and signs of abdominal pain. These should be noted. A sharp cry, if accompanied by legs being drawn up on the abdomen, helps to indicate abdominal pain.

Skin condition. The condition of the perineal region should be noted especially since the acid from the diarrheal stool can cause excoriation of the skin. Also, as these infants are very thin, bony prominences such as ankles, occiput, and hips may become irritated and reddened due to pressure.

Accurate weighing. The infant should be weighed on admission, both before the intravenous is started and afterward, since daily weights will be taken and compared to the admission weight. As has been stated, parenteral fluid therapy partially depends on the weight of the infant. If the infant's weight remains stationary after parenteral fluids have been begun and the infant is on nothing by mouth, the amount of fluid in a 24-hour period is increased. The weight and the increase or decrease of weight act as one indication of the condition of the infant.

Assisting with parenteral therapy. If the infant appears acutely ill on admission, the nurse can anticipate the doctor's needs and assemble equipment for blood to be drawn for blood cultures, for hemoglobin and complete bood count, and for determination of the serum levels of potassium, sodium, and chloride, as well as for determination of the plasma carbon dioxide level. The physician needs to know what electrolytes are low in concentration in order to replace them.

Vacutainer tubes are needed, together with their special needles, a 5 ml. syringe, and a tourniquet. Laboratory technicians usually draw blood to perform a complete blood count, electrolyte level, blood gases, and special chemistries; they bring their own equipment.

Equipment for an intravenous infusion should also be assembled. (See p. 301 for a description of the nurse's duties in regard to intravenous therapy.) Since the peripheral veins are often collapsed in a severely dehydrated infant, a cutdown intravenous infusion may be done. The most easily accessible superficial veins in infants are located in the scalp, wrists, and ankles. The site of infusion should be changed every 72 hours. The intravenous route is necessary for rapid administration of fluids and for their continuous administration over prolonged periods of time. Fresh whole blood, plasma, protein hydrolysate solutions, or hypertonic solutions are also given intravenously. Solutions may be given by "push" or continuous drip. The desired rate of flow is usually slow in infants and may not be easy to maintain. One drop per minute amounts to 3 to 4 ml. per hour, or 75 to 100 ml. per day. Attention here is

called to the fact that the nurse not only has responsibility for monitoring the fluids but also for the comfort and safety of the infant receiving an intravenous drip.

The aims of parenteral fluid therapy are (1) the repair of existing deficits and associated alterations of hemostatic processes by the rapid repair of intravascular volume and the gradual repair of pH changes, potassium deficit, and disturbances of osmotic pressure; (2) the replacement of continuing abnormal losses as they occur; and (3) the maintenance of normal needs, that is, providing normal requirements when they cannot be met in the usual (oral) administration. Ideal parenteral fluid therapy would involve some method of exact measurement of accumulated deficits and current normal and abnormal losses, with concurrent replacement of these demonstrated requirements. In practice these needs are estimated through a combination of clinical information and laboratory data, which reflect certain changes in the composition of extracellular fluid. Dehydration, with or without acid-base disturbance, is fundamentally a state of depletion of water and sodium chloride. In addition, a significant deficit of potassium is usually present. If renal function is adequate, both acidotic and alkalotic states can be treated satisfactorily by the infusion of neutral fluids (2.5% glucose water and 0.45% normal saline solution) containing sodium chloride, glucose, and water. Isotonic solutions such as Darrow's solution, Ringer's lactate, and modified Butler's solution are commonly used. Nonpotassium-containing fluids should be administered until an adequate renal output has been demonstrated. Preexisting renal, cardiac, or pulmonary disease may decrease the child's normal tolerance for fluid and electrolytes.

Nutrition. Nutrition is an especially important aspect of the nursing care of the infant with diarrhea because food affects the digestive tract and thus the stools of the infant. As stated previously, if the diarrhea is severe, food is withheld for 24 to 48 hours and fluids are administered parenterally. However, if the diarrhea is mild, if dehydration is not severe, and if there are no signs of circulatory insufficiency, lethargy, vomiting, or gastric distention, an oral electrolyte solution may be ordered. Later, skim milk is often given; glucose water, barley water, and/or weak tea is often given between milk feedings. Gradually the infant resumes his usual diet.

Food ordered is in the nature of a medication, and the nurse must be sure to adhere exactly to whatever diet the doctor has prescribed for the infant. On the other hand, if the stools become loose and/or liquid with the addition of more food, the doctor should be notified. Obviously the nurse should not continue the same feeding. Usually the doctor wishes the infant to go back to the previous diet.

Recording intake and output

Stools. As mentioned previously, each stool should be described according to amount, color, consistency, and any abnormalities. As soon as the diaper is changed, the stool should be charted.

Urine. Each time the infant voids or the diaper is found damp or wet there should be a check (✔) on the appropriate column in the nurses' notes. If the infant is very dehydrated, the urine may be scanty and concentrated and contain albumin and casts.

Vomitus. The amount lost in any vomitus of the infant has to be estimated. The nurse can make a more accurate estimate of the amount of fluid lost in vomiting if she measures 1 ml. and then 15 ml. and pours each in a separate place on a clean sheet spread on a bed. She can then note how large an area of wet surface there is.

Fluids and food. Careful charting of the following factors is essential: what fluid and/or food is offered, the amount taken, how it is taken (eagerly, slowly, or refused), and whether the infant seems satisfied after his feeding. As he gets better, his appetite should improve to the point of his appearing ravenously hungry. Accurate descriptions of his behavior toward food are essential if the nurse is going to function as a contributing member of the health team.

Affection. The infant with severe diarrhea is in special need of being petted, stroked, held, and rocked. He is a sick infant, sometimes in pain; yet, in spite of his emotional needs, the nursing and medical personnel are more likely to fondle and play with a pretty, responsive infant who is convalescing. It is a well-recognized fact that doctors' and nurses' "pets" get along better than others. If the emaciated infant with diarrhea were to receive extra attention, then he too (other factors being equal) might gradually be more responsive and look more alluring.

In planning the nursing care of the infant with diarrhea the head nurse or team leader should write on the Kardex or nursing care plan, "Hold and/or rock this infant every 4 hours." These hours could coincide with his oral feedings. Even if he is receiving parenteral fluids, the infant can still be picked up and held if care is exercised. Emotions influence the physical state of the infant, and the infant was brought to the hospital for the purpose of getting him well.

Skin care. The acid stool of the infant with diarrhea tends to cause redness and excoriation of the buttocks and perineal region. If the skin in the diaper area is not excoriated on admission to the hospital, the careful cleansing of the area after each defecation, together with the use of a bland ointment rubbed gently over the perineal region, may prevent excoriation of the skin. If it is already present, compound tincture of benzoin or other special ointments may be prescribed by the physician. Cornstarch can be very effective in healing the excoriation. Sometimes the area is exposed and a heat lamp is used. (The light bulb should not be more than 25 watts, and it should be at least 1 foot away from the infant.)

Changing the infant's position frequently will aid in avoiding the development of pressure areas over bony prominences and in preventing hypostatic pneumonia. The infant should be turned on alternate sides and propped. If he is very weak, placing him on his abdomen should be avoided. If he is left on his back, there is always the danger of aspiration.

A daily warm bath helps to stimulate the circulation, especially if the nurse wipes the skin dry using slight pressure rather than just patting the infant dry with a towel.

Administration of medication. Sometimes antibiotics such as neomycin are given by mouth; others may be given intramuscularly. Although on p. 290 there is a discussion of the administration of medicines, attention is called here to the fact that the diarrheal infant is usually a very thin infant. An intramuscular needle not longer than 1 inch should be used. In some instances when the infant is very emaciated and small, a needle shorter than 1 inch in length would reach the muscle.

Preparation for discharge. Suggestions and teaching to the mother should not be delayed until the last day the child is in the hospital but should be given as soon as the infant is better. At that time the anxiety of the parents for their child is alleviated, and they are anxious to do all they can to keep him well. The nurse should let the mother hold, feed, and diaper the infant. The nurse can notice whether the mother's technique is acceptable and whether she washes her hands after diapering the infant, and the nurse can adapt her teaching accordingly. Of particular importance is finding out how the mother prepares the infant's formula at home and how she manages storage of milk and infant foods (especially in hot weather). Whether the mother takes her infant to the doctor or a well child clinic for periodic visits and for immunizations is important for the nurse to find out. For other factors related to keeping the infant well, which might be discussed with the mother, refer to promotion of health, Chapter 9.

It would be indeed a utopia if all infants under 1 year of age could be referred to the public health nurse, but this is often impractical since there are insufficient public health nurses; however, for any infant who has been gravely ill it seems worthwhile to refer the infant to the public health nurse with the understanding that, if she finds he is receiving good care at home and the mother seems to handle the situation adequately, the family will be dropped from the caseload.

Prevention. Diarrhea is a symptom, and its prevention depends on it cause.

1. Epidemic diarrhea of the newborn. This can be prevented by following recommendations of the Committee on Fetus and Newborn of the American Academy of Pediatrics. There should be scrupulous aseptic technique in handling infants in the delivery room and the nursery. From an epidemiological viewpoint, rooming-in is safer for the infant than care in a newborn nursery, since the infant will have contacts with fewer adults and other infants. Sterile supplies in the nursery need culturing at frequent intervals. The formula room should follow the recommendations outlined by the Academy, and samples of formula should go periodically to the bacteriological laboratory. Diapers should be separated from the rest of the nursery linen.

Health regulations of personnel in the maternity service should be enforced, especially in the nursery. In hospitals that permit a certain number of days of sick leave with pay there is less chance of infants getting an infection from a nurse. Those personnel with any type of infection should stay far away not only from the newborn infant but from other infants as well.

Prompt isolation of any newborn infant suspected of being ill would also help to prevent an outbreak of epidemic diarrhea of the newborn. Accurate charting by nursery personnel helps draw the doctor's attention to abnormalities of infants.

2. Bacterial and viral gastroenteritis. Infants should be kept away from adults or children who have infections. Measures that help to maintain the infant's resistance and general health include adequate diet, cleanliness, sufficient rest and sleep, exercise, appropriate clothing, affection, and outings in good weather. As stated previously, infants do not thrive without affection. Also, good personal hygiene of adults who are handling the infant is important, as well as care in preparing the formula and in the handling and storage of infant's foods.

3. Dysentery. Discovery of carriers and patients with dysentery is possibly the first step toward prevention. Bacillary dysentery is a reportable disease, but amebic dysentery is reportable in only certain areas of the United States. If a public health nurse is at all suspicious that certain patients have dysentery, she can ask for help from the sanitation section of the county public health department. There must be sanitary disposal of human feces, protection against or elimination of flies, and provision of a safe water supply. Examination of a stool can be done, but the specimen has to be a fresh one.

Any cross-connection between water supply and sewerage must be eliminated. If well water is used by a given family, it should be tested periodically for the number and kind of organisms.

Since contaminated food is also a source of infection, raw vegetables and fruits should be washed well before eating. Water for infants should be boiled. The infecting organism can be ingested with food contaminated by feces of infected animals. Improvement of personal hygiene helps to interrupt the hand-to-mouth transfer of organisms that occurs when moist objects soiled with discharges from the patient are touched. Care of food, flies, fingers, and feces as the four F's is one way to remember the factors in prevention of dysentery.

For protection against *Salmonella* dysentery, especially, there should be a thorough cooking of all food derived from animal sources. There should be proper refrigeration of prepared or leftover foods, especially in hot weather, with protection against insects and rodents. Also, an effort should be made to control *Salmonella* infections among domestic animals.

Pasteurization of milk, meat and poultry inspection, and strict sanitary supervision of preparation and serving of all food are helpful measures.

Both the hospital and the public health nurse should be particularly aware of their teaching function relative to the preparation of food and fluids for infants and young children, as well as the care of diapers and handwashing after changing the infant's diapers and before feeding him.

Enuresis

Enuresis is defined as "involuntary discharge of urine" but is largely limited to involuntarily wetting the bed at night at an age when control could reasonably be expected. Bladder control at night is usually gained by 3 years of age. The incidence is higher in the institutionalized and children in the lower socioeconomic groups. There is a familial incidence, and boys are afflicted more than girls. The social handicap attending enuresis is evident.

There are many theories to explain the etiology of enuresis. The most frequently accepted theory is that the causes of enuresis are psychological disturbances in the child and emotional conflicts in the home environment. The conflicts often present are too early and vigorous attempts at toilet training, hostile mother-child relationship, and an unstable home environment.

Before treatment is initiated it is imperative to determine that the enuresis is not due to organic disease beyond the child's control. Initially a complete urinalysis and urine culture should be ordered. If the results are negative, the instructions for simple measures of bladder control are given to the parents and child. These include restriction of fluids at bedtime, voluntary withholding of urine during the daytime to increase bladder capacity, drugs such as atropine derivatives to decrease irritability of bladder, and imipramine (Tofranil) to lessen depth of sleep. If the measures outlined are carried out diligently, positive results are frequently attained within 4 to 6 weeks. When there are serious manifestations of disturbed child-family relations, the assistance of a pediatric psychiatrist or psychologist is indicated.

Acute glomerulonephritis
Nature of the condition

Acute glomerulonephritis, or acute hemorrhagic nephritis as it may be called, is most often seen between the ages of 3 and 7 years, but it may occur at any age. The onset of the condition may be abrupt and severe, or it may be mild.

Nephritis in children differs from that in adults. Acute glomerulonephritis is the most common type of nephritis in children but the least common in adulthood. In adults, nephritis is usually associated with degenerative changes. In addition, children's kidneys have greater power for regeneration after injury than those of adults.

Histopathologically, the glomeruli are large and appear bloodless due to compression of capillary lumens by swelling of the endothelial cells and an increased number of mesangial cells. Electron microscopy has revealed the presence of antigen-antibody complex on the basement membrane of the glomeruli. Group A

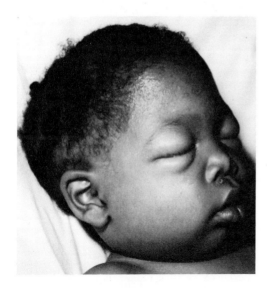

Fig. 14-3. Glomerulonephritis in a child 7 years of age. Note edema of eyelids and impetiginous lesion near right naris.

beta-hemolytic streptococci are associated most commonly with this condition. The antistreptolysin titer is high if the child has an active streptococcal infection. This is an autoimmune reaction. A nose and throat culture may demonstrate the presence of streptococcal infection. Often the child has had a respiratory infection for 3 to 4 weeks prior to the onset of symptoms.

The manifestation that is usually first noted by the mother is hematuria (blood in the urine). Other signs that are often present include some edema (especially puffiness of the eyes), albuminuria, hypertension, and azotemia (elevation of the nonprotein nitrogen constituents of the blood). Urinary changes may include decrease in the amount (oliguria), increase in specific gravity, and the presence of red blood cells, white blood cells, and casts. The abnormality shown by renal function tests varies in accord with the severity of the condition. An elevated blood urea nitrogen level is regarded as abnormal. It means urea cannot be cleared from the blood as quickly as is expected due to renal impairment. This test measures the function of the glomeruli to clear urea from the blood. The creatinine clearance test measures the rate at which the glomeruli clear creatinine from the blood. The rate would be diminished in an acute

renal condition. The Addis count also tests for active renal function. If renal function is impaired, the numbers of red and white cells and casts excreted in the urine in a 12 or 24 hour period are greatly reduced.

Headache, anorexia, and vomiting may be seen also; anemia often develops. Even though there may be no clinical evidence of heart involvement, abnormalities are often seen in repeated electrocardiograms. The heart may be enlarged.

The child is treated symptomatically. He usually remains in bed until his blood pressure has returned to normal. Penicillin is administered empirically or if the nose and throat culture is positive for beta-hemolytic streptococci. If the hypertension is mild, barbiturates may be ordered; if it is severe, other antihypertensive drugs are used, such as reserpine and hydralazine.

Within 2 weeks hematuria disappears and the temperature, blood pressure, and blood chemistry findings should become normal. Diuresis may occur for 2 to 4 days after admission. The child may lose several pounds, even though no edema can be seen. There may be some abnormal urinary findings for many months, even though the child is clinically well.

In general the prognosis in children is very good. Only 1% to 5% of children die in the acute phase. Possible complications are cardiac failure and hypertensive encephalopathy. Death from renal failure is rare.

Role of the nurse

Hospital preparation for the child. When the nurse is notified that a child with a tentative diagnosis of nephritis is about to be admitted, she should select a room that preferably has only two beds in it. Rest is the biggest single nursing factor that can help the child if he is hypertensive, so the fewer children there are in the room, the greater is the possibility of quiet. Two children can play games together, but if three or four are present, there is more excitement and hilarity. In addition, the larger the number of children in the room, the harder it is for the new child to adjust. Adjusting to one other child is easier. If possible, the bed next to the window should be for the new child, since personnel passing through the hall can be distracting.

In getting the child's unit ready, the nurse should obtain a urine specimen bottle and equipment to take blood pressure. If scales can be brought to the bedside, they too should be on hand. It will be necessary to keep a very accurate intake and output record; therefore, if there is a form for this in addition to the bedside notes, the forms should be placed in readiness for use. The necessity of this cannot be overstressed.

Observation. With the nature of the child's disease in mind the nurse needs to make pertinent observations on each 8-hour tour of duty. These observations include the following:

1. Behavior of the child—alert, active, listless, irritable. Listlessness and irritability could indicate a rising blood pressure. Development of severe anemia could make for apathy or indicate that the child has increasing heart involvement. Quietness alone might show fear of the hospital environment. If the child feels physically ill, his eyes are dull. A talkative, cheerful child feels well; an irritable, listless child does not.

2. Pulse. The rate should be recorded and a notation made on the nurses' notes as to whether the pulse is weak, full, of good quality, regular, or irregular.

3. Respiration. Beside the rate of the respiration, any sign of dyspnea (mouth breathing, noisy breathing, or orthopnea) should be noted.

4. Color. Has the child a rosy color? Pallor is associated with anemia and carditis. Cyanosis indicates circulatory insufficiency.

5. Edema. Puffiness around the eyes is sometimes seen. There may also be edema of the ankles. The child should lose weight in the hospital. If he gains weight, he is getting more edema.

6. Urine color. When the nurse takes the bedpan or urinal from the child, she should note the urine color. It may look like bright blood, be a dark reddish brown, or be yellow. Hematuria (if present) should lessen in a few days.

7. Appetite. The appetite of the child should be noted (and how much he takes). Food is important to recovery. If he eats poorly, the nurse can confer with the team leader in regard to possible approaches to the problem.

8. Untoward symptoms. Particular symptoms for which to watch, which might imply cardiac complications, are restlessness, orthopnea, and reluctance to lie flat. In hypertensive encephalopathy, symptoms for which to watch are marked hypertensive severe headache, irritability, and vomiting. Later, there may be visual disturbances, convulsions, and coma. Severe oliguria could be the first sign of renal failure. Complete anuria seldom occurs.

Fluid intake and output. Fluids are usually restricted for the first few days. If a child is overhydrated, it is more difficult to manage any hypertension. An accurate intake of all fluids should be kept, as well as an accurate account of urinary output. The nurse needs to point out to the child and his parents the importance of this record. The mother should be instructed to call the nurse to measure the urine if she (the mother) gives the bedpan to the child. If the child is 3 or 4 years of age, he may wish to be lifted onto a potty chair rather than use a bedpan. Small children sometimes push away a bedpan. Instruction is needed also in regard to the fluids the child takes.

Blood pressure. The child's blood pressure is taken at frequent intervals, especially when first admitted. Hypertension is treatable, and its adequate management can help prevent such complications as hypertensive encephalopathy, convulsions, and coma. Blood pressure should be measured with the child in a resting position. Any significant change in the blood pressure should be reported.

Weighing. The child needs to be weighed on admission and daily. This is best done prior to breakfast each day. In order for the weight to be accurate the child must wear the same amount of clothing each time. Also, the scales must be carefully balanced each time before he is weighed. Whether the child loses or gains weight is significant. Again, weight gain may be due to increased edema. The gain of 0.5 kg. is the equivalent of 500 ml. of fluid.

Skin care. A daily bath is important not only for comfort but also because the skin is an excretory organ and the kidneys are often impaired in their ability to excrete waste products. Since the child has to remain in bed, bony prominences (hips, ankles, knees, and elbows) need massaging at least three times daily (morning, afternoon, and evening). The back and buttocks should be bathed with soap and warm water and then massaged, at least in the morning and evening. Bedsores are easier to prevent than to heal.

Nutrition. Refer to p. 283 for a discussion of mealtime in the hospital. It is sufficient at this time to remind the nurse that her responsibility does not end when she gives a child a tray. Fixing the food so that the child can manage it readily and in other ways making mealtime pleasant is essential if the nurse is going to fulfill her obligation to the child. The aim of the nurse is to have the child eat food. Table salt is usually omitted from his tray. Fluids are restricted when there is severe hypertension.

Rest. As previously mentioned, rest is the biggest single factor in the child's recovery. As long as there is hypertension, the child remains in bed; however, being in bed is not the entire answer to rest. Placing the child in a two-bed unit rather than a larger one can reduce some external stimuli. Attention to the plan for the child's care during the 24-hour period might result in organization that would promote a quieter, more relaxed atmosphere.

If the mother or parents are present, what is their adjustment to their child's illness and hospitalization? If they are anxious and obviously apprehensive, this communicates itself to the child. This points up the necessity of considering the parents in the total plan of care.

The child's possible anxiety about himself and being in a hospital also needs consideration. The child's fears will depend somewhat on his age level as well as on his general adjustment at home. When one child's blood pressure was taken, the child inquired if that meant he had to have an operation. (For further discussion of psychological factors in a child's hospitalization, refer to the beginning of this chapter.)

Unless acutely ill and apathetic, the child may find it hard to stay in bed. A volunteer might read a story to him or play a game of checkers—some form of *quiet* recreation.

In the evening does the nurse bother to say "Goodnight" to the child and tell him that a nurse is there all night to care for him? In one hospital a night supervisor saw a child at 1 A.M. and again at 5:30 A.M. On the second visit the child said very sympathetically to the supervisor, "Didn't you sleep either?"

Other methods to aid rest include giving a complete bed bath rather than a self-help bath, seeing that conditions are such that the child can rest or sleep in rest hour and at night, giving attention to the appearance of the room, smooth organization of her own work, and not talking about the child's condition in his presence. As previously indicated, judgment is needed relative to the child's recreation. The color and decoration of the room can be depressing or cheerful.

The amount of activity allowed the child as his pressure drops near normal should be discussed with the physician. If the doctor says "bathroom privileges," does he mean unlimited or limited to three or four times a day? Is the child permitted to go to the playroom for occupational therapy, or should he remain in his room? Can he sit at a table for meals? When he is allowed to be ambulatory, how long should he be permitted to remain up at one time? In general, once the blood pressure has returned to normal, the child is allowed to be out of bed as much as he wishes.

Assisting with tests. The nurse assists with various tests that help to determine renal impairment. The child should have an explanation of what the test is and what it involves, according to his age and interest. The matter-of-fact behavior of the physician and nurse is somewhat reassuring to the child.

Usually a 24-hour urine collection is ordered, an Addis count, a blood urea nitrogent test, and a creatine or urea clearance test. (Refer to p. 311 for purpose of these tests.) A biopsy of renal tissue is sometimes done to obtain a culture of organisms, to clarify the diagnosis, and to assess the effect of drugs.

Administration of medication. Penicillin is usually given intramuscularly or orally. The first dose may be given intramuscularly and the other doses orally for 10 days. If there is a very elevated blood pressure, for example, a systolic pressure over 140 mm. Hg, antihypertensive and vasodilation drugs are ordered, such as reserpine and hydralazine hydrochloride (Apresoline). These are often given together. Reserpine allays anxiety as well as mildly reducing hypertension, whereas hydralazine is a stronger hypotensive agent.

Nursing care in complications. In cardiac failure, narcotics and digitalis may be ordered for the child. Because of dyspnea and to lessen the work of the heart the headrest is elevated.

In renal failure, which is rare, an indwelling catheter may be inserted and samplings of urine evaluated at frequent intervals. Careful attention is given to the electrolyte balance and the amount of fluid given. Intravenous therapy is frequent, and sometimes feedings through a nasogastric tube are given.

In hypertensive encephalopathy the nurse may be called upon to give anticonvulsant medications in addition to medications to reduce the blood pressure. If the child has convulsions, special care needs to be taken (p. 494). Spinal taps might be done to relieve pressure.

Preparation for discharge. When the child is ready to be sent home, the nurse should make sure that the parents understand when to bring him back to the pediatric clinic or to his own doctor. Instructions for the child's care at home, including the time when he can return to school, should be discussed with the physician. After the physician has talked to the parents the nurse should ascertain that the parents have understood the directions.

Pyelonephritis
Contacts of nurse with the child

Although the school nurse's attention may be called to this child because of pallor, failure to gain weight, and general apathy, the office nurse or hospital nurse is more likely to see this child, since pyelonephritis occurs more frequently in young children than in older ones.

Nature of the condition

Pyelonephritis is an acute infection of the renal pelvis and parenchyma. The most common feature that leads to the discovery of this disease is the presence of an increased number of white cells and bacteria on examination of the urine. Clinically it is usually not possible to localize infection specifically to the bladder (cystitis), renal pelvis (pyelitis), or renal parenchyma (pyelonephritis).

Infection of the urinary tract is very common in children. It occurs most frequently between 2 months and 2 years of age. Congenital malformations of the genitourinary tract are present in 50% to 75% of these patients. *Escherichia coli* is the organism responsible for the majority of these infections. Females in diapers have a higher incidence of genitourinary infections than males because of the relatively short urethra that is easily contaminated by stool. A congenital malformation of the genitourinary tract may obstruct the flow of urine, as in bladder neck obstruction (p. 379). Stasis of urine then occurs with resulting pyuria. This becomes a predisposing factor in the onset of pyelonephritis.

The clinical symptoms vary from no symptoms to acute illness with temperature of 105° F., chills, paleness, and toxicity. Symptoms related to the urinary tract may be that the child complains of dysuria, frequency, urgency, and back pain. In the very young child these symptoms are usually absent.

The diagnosis is established by the microscopic examination of the urine, looking specifically for increased numbers of white blood cells and bacteria. Urine obtained by "clean catch" method, bladder puncture, or catheterization is preferred for a urinalysis and urine culture. An intravenous pyelogram and a retrograde cystogram are performed to rule out any congenital malformation or malfunction of the urinary tract.

The aims of treatment are elimination of the infecting organism, removal of any obstruction to urine flow, and correction of any renal impairment. Specific antibiotic therapy is used after careful bacteriological culture and sensitivity test results are available. Ampicillin and sulfa drugs are the most commonly used drugs. If the child is critically ill, antibiotic therapy should be instituted immediately, before the culture reports are available from the laboratory. Surgical correction of the anomalies is carried out as soon as the child's general condition is stable. The urging of oral fluids or intravenous fluids are ordered to increase the urine flow. As the urine flow increases, the concentration of the urine decreases, thus improving kidney function.

Role of the nurse

If the child is not vomiting, fluids should be urged. If vomiting is persistent, intravenous therapy may become necessary. (For care of a child with an intravenous infusion see p. 301.) If the child has a high temperature, sponging him with tepid water and other measures to reduce the temperature may be used (p. 292).

In addition to providing measures of general comfort, the nurse will have to collect urine specimens. A girl should be well cleansed before collection of the specimen so there will be no vaginal secretion in the specimen. If possible, a midstream collection of urine from boys is desirable. In fact, several specimens may be necessary. As indicated previously, catheterization may be required for a sterile specimen of urine. Cultures of urine specimens aid in the diagnosis.

Renal function tests are often done to ascertain whether there is any renal impairment. Pyelonephritis, as stated, is not limited to a single part of the urinary tract. There is inflammation of the renal pelvis and renal parenchyma and sometimes inflammation of the ureters and bladder. These tests are usually done after the acute phase of the disease has subsided and the child is more comfortable. The nurse assists with such diagnostic measures as cystogram, intravenous pyelogram, cystoscopy, renal biopsy, and radiography. She needs to offer emotional support, especially to the young child, during these procedures. Parents as well as children need explanations of the procedures.

Antibiotics given depend on the susceptibility of the particular organism. If sulfa drugs are prescribed, plenty of fluids should be given since a good urinary flow should be present to prevent kidney damage.

Preparation for discharge. A medication is usually given to the child for a period of months after an acute attack of pyelonephritis in order to prevent a recurrence. If inadequately treated, chronic pyelonephritis may occur and eventually cause renal failure. Cardiac failure could result because of severe hypertension. The nurse must make sure that the parents understand where they can obtain the medication, how much the child should take, and how often it should be taken. Also, it is important that the parents understand when the child should return to see the physician in his office or in the pediatric outpatient department.

SURGICAL CONDITIONS
Common psychological factors

Psychological aspects of nursing care of children who have surgery performed are discussed here. Except for children having cardiac surgery, psychological aspects of infants having surgery for congenital defects have already been discussed in Chapter 13.

Home preparation. When the child is going to have an elective operation such as a tonsillectomy, parents have an opportunity to discuss the plans for it with the child and prepare him for the event. The office nurse is in a position to help parents with this problem. Children's books about hospitals are helpful to many children. They may like to look at the pictures in a book such as *Johnny Goes to the Hospital* or have the book read to them or both. The child might help to pack his suitcase to take to the hospital and decide what toy or play material he will take. The mother should tell the child whether she will be with him all the time or just part of the time. The parents could help the child play-act going to the hospital, the operating room, and home again.

The 2-year-old child is too young for any lengthy explanation, but he should be told the doctor is going to "fix" whatever area is involved: the clubfoot, the hernia, etc. His parents can show him the hospital building where he is going to be. If the parents are matter-of-fact in talking about it, this attitude is communicated to the child.

Preoperative nursing care. (See Chapter 11 for a discussion of general factors in the child's adjustment to the hospital.) It is sufficient here to emphasize the importance of introducing the child to others who are in his room or whom he sees in the playroom as well as the importance of explaining to the child any treatment before the nurse does it, no matter how routine it may seem to her.

The fact that parents may be apprehensive about the coming surgery on the child must not be forgotten. (This is particularly so when the operation is an emergency one.) Their tenseness may show in a refusal to let the nurse help undress the child, in an abrupt manner of speaking to hospital personnel, or in their facial expression. Their tenseness may be communicated to the child. The nurse should be patient and calm.

Some of the parents' apprehension can be allayed by the nurse's manner to the child and to them. If the nurse evidences her sincere interest and liking for the child, this helps the parents' adjustment.

Frequently, at least one parent remains with the child; but if one does not, the nurse should be sure to ask before they leave whether the child knows why he is in the hospital and also exactly what he has been told. What the nurse tells the child is based upon his previous knowledge. The nurse can furnish more specific details than parents: that medicine will be given the child before the operation to make him feel sleepy, that he will ride in an elevator to the operating room, that personnel there are doctors and nurses even though they are dressed differently with caps and masks, and that he will be asleep when the doctor takes out his tonsils or performs whatever operation is planned. If the child is going to the recovery room after his operation, he should be told this so he will know where he is on waking up. Of course, some explanation of the recovery room should be given to him.

Other explanations and preparation of the child by the nurse depend on what the operation is. If the child is going to have his tonsils removed, he should be told his throat will feel sore, as though he had a bad cold.

A child who is scheduled for cardiac surgery should be shown equipment that will be used following the operation. He should have some familiarity with a Croupette or oxygen tent, blood pressure apparatus, intravenous equipment, and a gauze dressing.

CASE ILLUSTRATION

A student in nursing inquired of a 7-year-old child why he was in the hospital. "The doctor is going to sew up a hole in my heart," the child replied. Then the nurse asked him if he would like to look at a book about another boy who went to a hospital, but not for heart surgery. The child took pleasure in recognizing familiar pictures—an otoscope, a stethoscope, a crib, a nurse with a syringe and needle in her hand. Then the nurse told the boy about his care after the operation. She showed him a Croupette, like one he would have. She introduced him to another child who had an intravenous running in his arm, just as he would have. The 7-year-old wanted to know if the intravenous hurt. The other boy replied in the negative. Then he replied, as an afterthought, "It just hurt when the doctor started it." The nurse and child talked about the fact that the child's diet the first day after the operation would probably be just fluids until he felt like eating more. The next day the nurse and the child reviewed their conversation of the previous day. Then the nurse put a dressing on a doll. She removed it with instruments the doctor would use to take off the child's dressing after the operation, she told him how the stitches would tickle when taken out, and then she taught the child to cough and deep-breathe.

The explanation the nurse gives to any child depends, of course, on how much the child can understand and what preparation he has had prior to his admission. Telling a child what is going to happen and giving the child time to think about it lessens the degree of adjustment the child has to make and prevents him from being startled. Perhaps sometime it will be possible to show children with elective surgery the recovery room before their own surgery; perhaps also the day will come when prior to surgery every anesthetist will visit the child he is to anesthetize, just as he does when an adult is the patient. In the operating room the child should be able to recognize the anesthetist as a familiar person, as a friend. Puppets can be used to explain preoperative medications, going to the operating room, etc.

Day of operation. If the operation is scheduled early in the morning (7 A.M. or 8 A.M.), it is wise for the child to have a bath the previous evening to avoid hurry the next morning and also to let him sleep longer. The child who has had his bath can have his pajamas changed and void first before the nurse gives him his preoperative medication. A bath would completely arouse him; consequently, it might take longer for the preoperative medication to take effect than it would otherwise. If the child does not go to the operating room until 9 A.M. or later, the nurse should plan to bathe him when the other children are having their breakfasts. If the nurse has this child void before she gives him the medication, she will not have to disturb him later. After the medication is given the mother may wish to hold the child in her lap if he is a young child. This is comforting to the child, and he may relax faster than if he is left in bed. The room should be darkened. If other children are in the room, perhaps they can go into the playroom so the child's room will be quiet. The medication will not take effect quickly if the child is distracted and constantly stimulated by noise and light. Perhaps someday studies will be done to determine what is appropriate soothing music that might be played during this time. Music can be conducive to relaxation.

When the operating room finally calls for the child, the young child should be transported in his crib rather than transferred to a stretcher. It is less disturbing. The older child should have been given an explanation in advance why it is easier for patients to be taken to the operating room on a stretcher than on a bed.

If the child is awake when he goes to the operating room, all personnel should make a special effort to be calm and matter-of-fact. Hurry and tension should be avoided, as tension is so easily communicated to children, particularly to young children.

The nurse assigned to the child should accompany him to the operating room and wait there until he is asleep. The child should be anesthetized in an anesthetizing room and then taken into the operating room after he is asleep. Seeing a lot of shiny instruments, as well as people who are masked and rubber gloved, is not conducive to relaxation; indeed, these sights may thoroughly frighten the child.

Emotional support of the parents. When the nurse returns to the unit, she should speak with the parents. She can tell them exactly how the child was when she left him. She should be truthful with the parents. They may imagine that the reaction of the child (if awake) to the operating room was far worse than it really was. The nurse can encourage the parents to take a walk outside the hospital or go shopping while waiting for the child to be returned to the unit. If they do not wish to leave the hospital, she could direct them to the coffee shop. They might like to know, too, where the hospital chapel is. Waiting for the outcome of an operation on a loved one is very difficult. Also, the nurse can explain she will call the operating room a little later and ask the condition of the child. It is reassuring to parents to know that their child's operation is partially finished and all is well.

The parents need emotional support during this difficult time. The operation may be as emotionally distressing to them as to the child, and possibly even more so. The parents may feel a certain amount of guilt. They have given their permission for the child to have an operation that possibly will cause him pain and discomfort. Also, the parents may wonder whether the child will survive the operation. If he cried and was upset when taken to the operating room, this too remains in the parents' memory while they wait for the child's return.

Postoperative nursing care. When the child is fully awake from the anesthesia, he should be given a medication either in the recovery room or on the unit. This is not just to allay pain but for psychological reasons. The child has had a difficult experience, and resting without discomfort will help to restore a certain emotional equilibrium. After sleeping he is more ready to face postoperative experiences.

The best supportive care in the immediate postoperative period is that which makes the child physically comfortable. It is hard to judge when a child is in pain unless he cries; but irritability, frequent changing of position, and restlessness point toward discomfort. Analgesic medications should be given freely during the first few days postoperatively. If a child feels comfortable, he is more likely to take fluids and eat; also, he can relax and sleep if he has no pain. After the first day, if the child is not nauseated, the nurse can ask the doctor to change the order for a subcutaneous or intramuscular analgesic medication to an oral one. This is more acceptable and less disturbing to the child.

General measures of comfort such as warmth, comfortable position, moistening of tongue and lips, washing face and hands with warm water, and letting a young child hold his favorite toy are all helpful. Anticipating his needs and relieving them may prevent discomfort. The older children need assurance that the operation is over. If the nurse frequently stops to look at the child, especially if his parents are not present, it is reassuring to him. Being a postoperative patient is a new experience, and the presence of a familiar person even for short intervals of time keeps him from a feeling of aloneness. The child may be somewhat bewildered that he does not feel like sitting up, playing, or doing anything.

The child's behavior is an index to how the child feels physically. The irritable fretful child is still sick. The quiet child may be having problems in adjusting to the hospital and his illness. The child who wants to sit up and who shows an interest in his surroundings and in play materials is feeling better. Gradually the child should be helped to increasing independence in washing, feeding, and entertaining himself.

In the days after his operation the nurse can encourage the older child to express his feelings about the operation. Sometimes the older child will talk about it; sometimes, like the preschool child, he can better express himself through creative play materials. Some of the older children may well express their feelings if asked to write a short story about a child who had an operation. Younger children like such creative materials as clay, dolls and doll equipment, toy hypodermic syringes, a stethoscope, crayons and paper, and the like. Their play helps them to assimilate this experience in their life. If the nurse watches the child in his use of these play materials, she may get a clue as to how he feels and what he thinks about his operation.

When the child feels well enough, pleasant experiences like eating in the playroom and diversional recreation should be provided. This, to some degree, helps to remove the unpleasantness of pain, fear, and discomfort and may leave a happier memory of the hospital with the child. As pointed out in Chapter 11, illness itself is not pleasant, but pleasant associations with the hospital may help the child to better make the hospitalization a positive experience rather than a negative one.

Tonsillectomy and adenoidectomy
Reasons for removal of tonsils and adenoids

Removal of tonsils and adenoids is not an emergency. It is not a routine operation and is recommended only after careful appraisal. The tonsils are lymphatic tissue and act as a mechanism against infection. When the child has an upper respiratory infection, the tonsils become hypertrophied and then reduce in size after the infection. In early school years tonsils are normally large, but all lymphatic tissue begins to decrease by the age of 12 years. The size of the tonsils alone is not a reason for removal, unless they are so large that they obstruct swallowing and breathing. Chronic infection and hypertrophy of the tonsils and adjacent tonsillar structures are an indication. Sometimes there is a persistent enlargement of cervical lymph nodes. Tonsillectomies are recommended for persistent carriers of diphtheria bacilli.

Mouth breathing, either day or night, is an indication for adenoidectomy, as are persistent rhinitis and alterations of the voice. There may be a nasal quality to the voice. Impaired hearing could result from hypertrophied adenoids with secondary chronic otitis media and recurring purulent drainage.

Psychological preparation of children

Refer to p. 415 for psychological aspects of care of these children. For additional emphasis, attention is drawn here to the importance of the nurse's asking the parents whether the child knows why he came to the hospital and exactly what he has been told. If the mother has not told the child why he is in the hospital and refuses to tell him, the nurse should report this to the physician *prior* to the time the mother or parents leave the hospital. It is essential for the child to trust his parents, and everything possible should be done to maintain that trust. It is difficult for some parents to explain to the child that he will have an operation, but if they do not, his confidence in them will be considerably lessened. The child must know about his operation and exactly when his parents will return to see him.

To whatever the mother has told the child about his operation, the nurse can add details about the routine in the particular hospital where he is. Sometimes the children have stories and games in the playroom and eat together there on the evening of admission. The day following the operation perhaps something special is planned, like having ice cream for breakfast. In any event, children should know what to expect: the routine, the preoperative medication, the method of going to the operating room, and whether they will wake in the recovery room or in the pediatric unit.

Preoperative nursing care

For details on preoperative care see p. 296, and for a discussion of the nurse's emotional support of the parent see p. 417.

Attention here is drawn to the fact that bleeding time, clotting time, and hemoglobin values are made preoperatively as a security measure. A very low hemoglobin level or prolonged bleeding and clotting time is an indication for delaying surgery.

Fluids should be urged the evening preceding the operation. Usually clear fluids can be given up to 6 hours prior to the operation. This means that if the child wakens during the night, he can be given fluids if it is more than 6 hours before his operation. Physicians' orders vary, and some may permit fluids to within 4 hours of operation. During the operation a good deal of blood is lost, so that adequate intake of fluids preoperatively is essential. If rectal anesthesia is given, the child should be weighed. The rectal anesthesia is given in the child's room. The room, of course, should be darkened and quiet.

Postoperative nursing care

At the close of the operation the child may be taken to the recovery room or returned to his room. If several children have been scheduled for tonsillectomies, possibly they could be placed in one room or in adjoining rooms in the pediatric unit. One nurse could be assigned to them. It is reassuring to the child if he can see at least one parent when he wakens from anesthesia; also, having the same nurse he had before his operation means less adjustment for the child and his parents.

When the child is still under the influence of anesthesia from his tonsillectomy and/or adenoidectomy, he should be placed on his abdomen with a pillow under his chest. His head should be turned to one side. The purpose of the prone position is to avoid aspiration. Lung abscess is a possible complication of a tonsillectomy. The nurse as well as the doctor has responsibility for prevention of it.

The nurse needs to be alert to any possible evidence of hemorrhage. Vomiting of bright blood is obvious, but constant swallowing is sometimes not noticed. The child may be restless. The pulse may start to increase in rapidity. Because of the possibility of hemorrhage the child needs watchful vigilance. An ice collar is often used around the child's neck when he has reacted from the anesthesia. How soon fluids can be given after the operation varies with different physicians, as does the diet that the child is allowed. Cold fluids the first 2 days (or ice cream) usually make the throat feel more comfortable than hot fluids.

As a rule, the child is discharged on the day after the operation.

Hydrocephalus
Nature of the condition

Hydrocephalus is a condition in which there is an excess of cerebrospinal fluid within the subarachnoid and ventricular spaces of the brain. It may be congenital or acquired. The cerebrospinal fluid is secreted by the choroid plexus. It flows from the lateral ventricle through the foramen of Monro to the third ventricle, through the aqueduct of Sylvius into the fourth ventricle, through the foramen of Magendie and the foramen of Luschka to the cisterna magna and the cisterna lateralis. Only a small part of the fluid enters the spinal subarachnoid space, whereas most of it circulates to the cerebral and cerebellar subarachnoid space. The spinal fluid is reabsorbed by the arachnoid villi. In hydrocephalus there is an obstruction of the circulation. Congenital malformations may be a cause, such as atresia (narrowing) of the aqueduct of Sylvius, atresia of the foramina of Luschka and Magendie (the Dandy-Walker deformity), or the Arnold-Chiari deformity. When hydrocephalus is associated with the Arnold-Chiari malformation, there

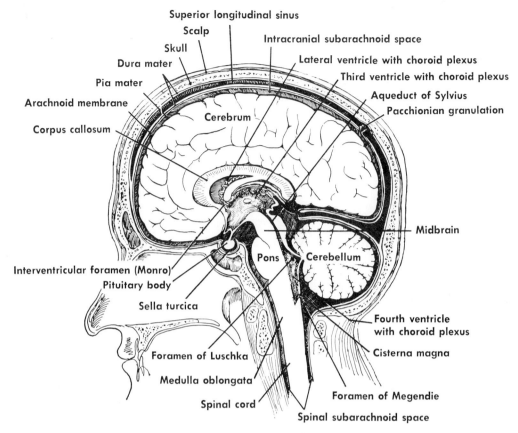

Fig. 14-4. Diagram of sagittal section of the head showing cerebrospinal fluid spaces and their relationship to the venous circulation and principal subdivisions of the brain and its coverings. (From Carini, E., and Owens, G.: Neurological and neurosurgical nursing, ed. 6, St. Louis, 1974, The C. V. Mosby Co.)

may be other malformations present, such as spinal meningocele.

The Arnold-Chiari malformation is an elongation of the cerebellum and the brainstem (medulla) with displacement through the foramen magnum into the cervical portion of the spinal canal. This might cause impaired drainage of the cerebrospinal fluid from the fourth ventricle, or such impairment of drainage could result from an associated anomaly as forking of the aqueduct of Sylvius or a malformed brainstem.

In addition to congenital malformations, hydrocephalus may also follow an infection such as meningitis or encephalitis, a subarachnoid hemorrhage, or a tumor in the brain. All these conditions cause an obstruction in the normal flow of the cerebrospinal fluid.

Hydrocephalus may be further classified as *communicating* or *noncommunicating*. Cerebrospinal fluid is secreted by the lateral ventricles. When hydrocephalus is present, there is an obstruction between the point of secretion and the point of absorption; however, the term *communicating hydrocephalus* indicates open communication between the ventricles and spinal subarachnoid spaces. In noncommunicating hydrocephalus there is an obstruction to this open communication.

In addition to measurement of the head, various diagnostic procedures are done such as radiological examination, lumbar puncture, pneumoencephalogram, a ventriculogram, and dye studies (p. 424).

Operative procedures

After a diagnosis has been made of progressive hydrocephalus and the point of obstruction has been located, operative procedures are done to avoid brain damage and/or increasing intracranial pressure. Severe mental retardation is only one complication of the increase in intracranial pressure. Weakness, spasticity, convulsions, and blindness could result, as well as loss of acquired motor achievements. Vomiting could interfere with the nutritional status of the child. At that point the child has to be tube fed. In untreated progressive hydrocephalus the child usually dies from intercurrent infection or inanition.

The most commonly used operation for correction of either communicating or noncommunicating hydrocephalus is devised to shunt the cerebrospinal fluid into the venous circulation—usually a ventriculo-auricular shunt. Less commonly the ventricular fluid may be shunted into the peritoneal or pleural cavities. In the past the fluid has also been shunted into other organs or spaces such as the gallbladder or into the ureter and hence into the urinary bladder.

Torkeldson's operation (anastomosis between the lateral ventricle and the cisterna magna) may be done if the obstruction is from a tumor or acquired lesion in the third or fourth ventricle or the aqueduct of Sylvius. This procedure is called a ventriculocisternostomy.

There are some disadvantages to every type of operation. In a subarachnoid ureterostomy (in which a ureter is anastomosed to the subarachnoid space) not only is one kidney sacrificed but hyponatremia and hypochloremia could occur from the loss of salt (in the cerebrospinal fluid) due to its excretion in the urine. In a ventriculo-auriculostomy, the one-way valve used (Spitz-Holter valve, Heyer-Pudenz valve, or Hakim valve) may cause a septicemia. Surgical revisions are necessary in the event of obstruction, of course, and are now frequently performed in anticipation of malfunction of tubing due to body growth. Shunting fluid to the peritoneal space may result later in adhesions, which obstruct the shunt.

If the procedure is done early and assuming there are no complications, intelligence of the child is frequently within normal limits. Unfortunately, many children are still seen late, and aside from accompanying cerebral defects, complications such as infection or shunt occlusions may result in a poor prognosis.

Preoperative nursing care

What are the main nursing responsibilities when the infant is admitted to the hospital or is born in the hospital?

Observation. As the nurse undresses the infant and takes his vital signs, she can note whether the fontanel is full, bulging, or pulsating, if the scalp is thin and shiny, if the scalp veins are prominent, and if the infant's developmental abilities are characteristic of his age. The infant may be either alert and responsive or irritable, drowsy, and lethargic. Fretfulness and irritability could denote head pain. Sometimes these infants are normal and intelligent, and

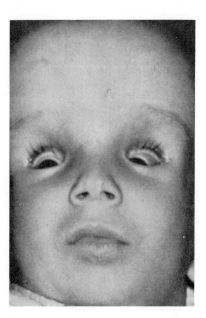

Fig. 14-5. Appearance of the eyes in an infant with hydrocephalus, showing the "setting sun" sign. (From Liebman, S. D., and Gellis, S. S.: The pediatrician's ophthalmology, St. Louis, 1966, The C. V. Mosby Co.)

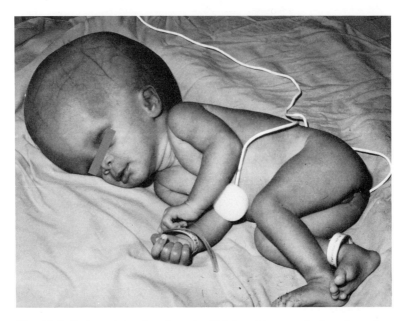

Fig. 14-6. Hydrocephalus in a 3-week-old infant. Note monitoring electrode.

sometimes they may be retarded. The nurse should particularly look at the eyes, as strabismus is common; also, the sclera is visible above the iris as the upper eyelids appear retracted. Other signs that the infant may evidence are a high-pitched shrill cry, retraction of the neck, extension and rigidity of the limbs, and widely separated sutures, with the head enlarged and out of proportion to the body. These help to denote increased intracranial pressure and should be recorded. Sometimes, as previously stated, there are other deformities.

Measuring the head. The circumference of the head should be measured on admission and daily thereafter to see if there is an increase in head size.

Nutrition. The infant should be on a diet for his age. The nurse can hold him in her lap to feed him as she does other infants. While feeding him, she should particularly note how the infant eats. If he has difficulty in eating and sucking or if he sucks slowly, this needs to be recorded because it may denote brain damage. Projectile vomiting after eating could be symptomatic of increased intracranial pressure.

Preventing skin decubitus. Because the scalp is thin the skin can easily break down. Also, the head is heavy, so the infant does not

move it as freely as a normal infant does, and he cannot hold it erect. The infant's head needs to be gently washed daily with soap and water. The palm of the nurse's hand, rather than her fingertips, should be used in bathing the head. In addition to that, the position of the infant needs to be changed every 2 hours. Holding the infant for feeding relieves pressure on the head. A soft infant pillow can be used under the head or, preferably, a square piece of foam rubber.

Affection. Even if the head of the infant is so heavy that the infant is cumbersome to lift and handle and even if he appears lethargic or severely retarded, the nurse must remember that he is conscious of her touch and the tone of her voice. Holding the infant when he is fed or otherwise cuddling him is important. Stroking him, handling him gently, and speaking soothingly all help. This infant must not be left in a crib with a minimum of handling. Specific explanations given by the head nurse to nursing aides about this infant's condition sometimes help to remove the general fear of an infant so different looking from others.

Assisting with diagnostic tests. The nurse may be called upon to take the infant to the x-ray department and to help the physician as he does a subdural tap, a ventricular tap, and/or a

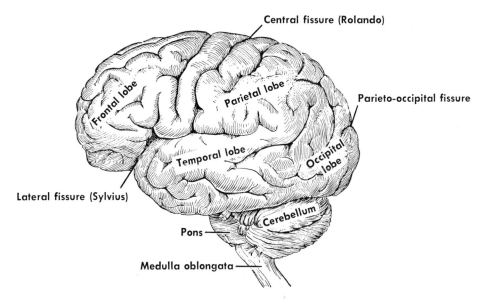

Fig. 14-7. Lateral view of a cerebral hemisphere (showing the lobes and principal tissues), the cerebellum, pons, and medulla oblongata. (From Carini, E., and Owens, G.: Neurological and neurosurgical nursing, ed. 6, St. Louis, 1974, The C. V. Mosby Co.)

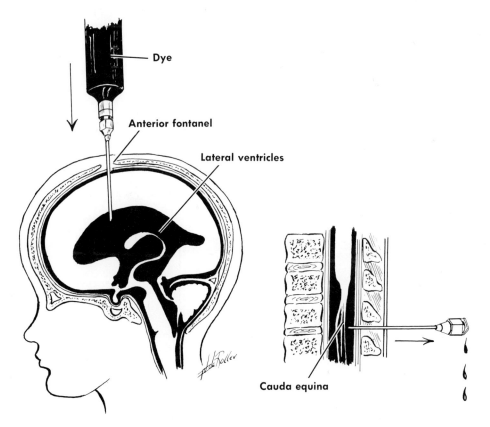

Fig. 14-8. When dye is inserted into the ventricle of an infant with communicating hydrocephalus, the dye can be recovered in the spinal fluid.

lumbar puncture. Special tests that verify the diagnosis and indicate the site of the obstruction include the following procedures.

Radiological examination. This shows head enlargement, wide sutures, thinning of the skull, and the particular location of occipital protuberance.

Bilateral subdural taps. Subdural taps are performed to rule out subdural hematoma or effusion.

Dye studies. For dye studies the nurse needs to get out equipment for a spinal tap plus two spinal needles. A spinal puncture needle is introduced through the coronal suture into the lateral ventricle. Another spinal needle is introduced into the lumbar space. The pressure is measured in both locations as an aid in seeing whether there is full communication between them. With the same needles in place, phenolsulfonphthalein or indigo carmine is introduced through the needle that is in the lateral ventricle. The length of time that it takes for the dye to appear in the spinal fluid in the lumbar space is noted. If there is full communication, the dye is seen within 15 minutes. If no dye appears in half an hour, there may be a complete block. Sometimes lumbar puncture is repeated after a few hours. The use of a dye is not entirely reliable, but the validity of the test is increased when spinal taps are repeated.

Collecting urine at definite times after the dye is injected is another method that aids in locating the obstruction. Twelve hours after the injection over one half of the dye should have been excreted.

Lumbar pneumoencephalogram. Again, spinal tap equipment needs to be obtained. A lumbar puncture is done, some fluid is withdrawn, and air is injected. If the hydrocephalus is of the communicating type, the air outlines the

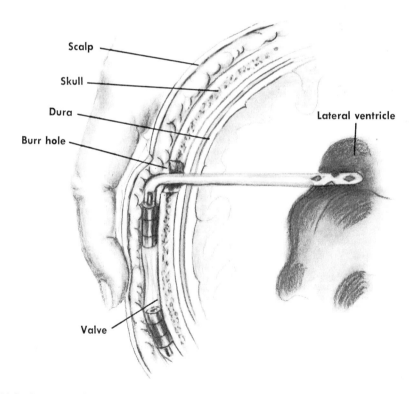

Fig. 14-9. One type of valve used in operations for children with hydrocephalus when fluid is shunted to enter the venous circulation, gallbladder, or other body cavity. Note the position of the index finger. This valve is pumped two or three times daily. Other types of valves do not have to be pumped.

ventricular system as seen by radiological examination. If the hydrocephalus is not communicating, a ventriculogram may be done. In this procedure air is injected into the ventricles directly.

Postoperative nursing care

See p. 298 for general postoperative nursing. Specific points in caring for the hydrocephalic child or infant include the following:

1. Leaving the head of the infant level with the body the first few days unless there are written orders by the surgeon to either elevate or lower the head. If the infant is allowed to sit up or is held with his head in an elevated position, too rapid a compression can cause vomiting and coma. On the other hand, the infant can be cuddled in the nurse's arms as long as he is held in a prone position.

2. Taking the temperature hourly if above 100° F. If it is above 100° F., this should be reported, since aspirin, Tempra syrup, or a tepid sponge may be ordered to reduce the temperature.

3. Giving specific antibiotics and other medications as ordered. An order for p.r.n. medication for pain may be requested from the doctor if there is none written and if the infant appears to be in discomfort.

4. Turning the infant on alternate sides every 2 hours—unless the physician wishes the infant turned only from his back to the unoperative side.

5. Caring for the intravenous infusion. (See p. 301 for nursing responsibilities.)

6. Offering the infant fluids and food. The nurse should offer glucose water. When this is retained, half-strength formula and then full-strength formula and the usual diet can be added. Glucose water should be offered even if the infant is receiving an intravenous infusion, since the infusion will be continued until it is apparent that the fluids will be retained and the infant is taking sufficient oral fluids.

7. Measuring the head daily. This should be done just as in the preoperative period.

8. Observing and recording any signs of increased pressure such as drowsiness, irritability, tense or bulging fontanel, lethargy, or projectile vomiting. These may signify that the shunt is blocked or that meningitis is developing. If blood pressure is being taken (and sometimes it is not in infants), the blood pressure would increase if there is an increase in cranial pressure.

9. Seeing that the dressing is in place. This is important since sometimes the dressing is not serving its purpose.

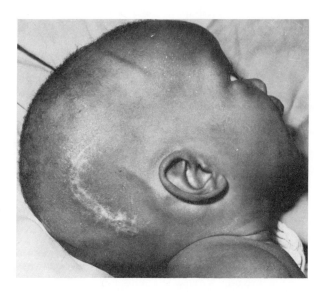

Fig. 14-10. Hydrocephalic infant with a ventriculoperitoneal shunt. Note the tubing under the skin of the scalp as it appears from the skull.

10. Pressing the valve. Depending on the type of valve used in a shunting procedure, the valve may need to be pressed at intervals. This is *not* necessary with all types of valves, so that information from the surgeon is needed about care of a particular infant.

Preparation for discharge

Before the child is discharged the nurse should make sure that the parents know the date the child should return to the private physician or the outpatient clinic. In addition, the mother should understand that if the child begins to vomit, seems lethargic, or becomes irritable, she should notify her physician at once or bring the child back to the clinic immediately.

Cardiac surgery

Refer to p. 350 for a discussion of types of common congenital heart defects and to p. 357 for possible surgical procedures. The use of a heart pump oxygenator has aided the progress of cardiac surgery for children and made possible the total correction of defects.

As explained in Chapter 13, infants under 1 year of age usually have cardiac surgery because they are in heart failure and are not responding well to medical measures or because, without surgical intervention, the defect would probably be fatal. These operations are sometimes in the nature of an emergency, and palliative surgery is done since, at present, open heart surgery using a pump oxygenator carries a high mortality risk for infants weighing under 20 pounds or having less than 1 square meter of body surface. Children with heart defects who have survived the first year of life with only medical supervision may have surgery in later childhood. There is a variation among surgeons as to what time they believe is best for elective heart surgery. Some preschool and school-age children are admitted for a total correction of defects for which they had palliative surgery in infancy.

When the pump oxygenator is used, the circulation of blood in the body continues, but, instead of going to the heart, the blood goes out the oxygenator by one route and returns by another to the systemic body circulation. The preferred site of return is the femoral artery.

Common congenital heart conditions that can be corrected in closed heart surgery (without the pump oxygenator) include patent ductus arteriosus and coarctation of the aorta. Palliative shunt procedures that relieve cyanosis and some respiratory embarrassment can be performed for an infant or young child with tetralogy of Fallot, ventricular septal defect, tricuspid atresia, and transposition of the great vessels. By means of open heart surgery with the pump oxygenator, a total correction of defects can be made for children with aortic stenosis and pulmonary stenosis. Children who may have had palliative surgery as infants for tetralogy of Fallot, transposition of the great vessels, or a ventricular septal defect return in later childhood for a total correction of defects (using the pump generator). (See p. 358 for further discussion of cardiac surgery.)

Hospital admission

For a detailed discussion of preparation of the child for hospitalization and a discussion of psychological factors involved in surgical procedures, refer to p. 415.

The child having elective cardiac surgery is usually admitted 2 or 3 days prior to the operation. This allows some time for the necessary laboratory work to be done such as complete blood count, hematocrit determination, typing and cross-matching of blood, and urinalysis. Also, further x-ray studies and electrocardiograms are often done.

The few days of hospitalization before the operation also give the child a chance to become better oriented and more familiar with the pediatric unit. The child should be given some explanation of his operation in terms of his age and ability to understand. "The doctor will fix your heart" might satisfy a 6-year-old child, but an older one might wish more particulars.

Equipment that might be used to aid the child postoperatively should be shown to him. A drawing that shows where the defect is might help. Children should be told they will probably be (or will be) in an oxygen tent or be wearing an oxygen mask when they awaken because it helps them to breathe better. They should be shown a tent and a mask. A Croupette should be set up so the young child can climb inside if he wishes. The nurse might hold a child's stuffed animal or doll inside the tent.

If the child has not seen blood pressure apparatus, this should be shown to him and his blood pressure should be taken. The child may like to squeeze the bulb. He should be told his blood pressure will be taken lots of times after his operation.

The child should be shown an intravenous setup, with an explanation that he will be fed by a tube in his arm to make him feel stronger.

Deep breathing and coughing can be practiced. The nurse can splint the sides of the child's chest with her hands just as she will do after the operation.

Preoperative nursing care

For a discussion of general preoperative nursing care, refer to p. 296. In addition, antibiotics are usually started prior to the operation.

Operative procedures

See p. 358 for a discussion of various common types of congenital heart defects and possible surgical procedures to relieve them.

Postoperative nursing care

Each hospital and/or surgeon may vary in particular procedures for the postoperative care of children with heart surgery. For example, after a Glenn procedure is done some surgeons do not wish any intramuscular medications or intravenous fluids or medications given above the waist of the child for 2 weeks after the operation. They wish to avoid the possibility of infection. Postoperative care in this section will be discussed in only a general way. Each hospital should have its own written policies, including details of care.

Equipment

1. Closed heart surgery. If the child is having closed heart surgery, an oxygen tent or a Croupette (whichever is used) should be set up in readiness for the child. An oxygen mask is frequently used for an older child. Suction with a nasopharyngeal catheter should be available and also a cardiac arrest tray, emergency drugs (vasopressors, vasodilators, and stimulants), a tracheotomy set, a drainage bottle for chest suction, a stethoscope, and a sphygmomanometer.

2. Open heart surgery. If open heart surgery is done, in addition to the preceding equipment, a hypothermia blanket should be placed on the bed ready for the child. It helps to regulate the temperature of the child by fluid circulating through it. Also, a monitor with four leads (one for each extremity) should be ready for use to measure the child's vital signs (blood pressure, electrocardiogram, pulse, and temperature). There are several kinds of monitors. The nurse reads and records information obtained from the monitor regarding the vital signs. When using the monitor for temperature elevation, it is important to secure the indwelling rectal thermometer to the patient with adhesive.

General care. There is often a special team of nurses to care for the child during the first 3 or 4 days after surgery, depending on the patient's progress and the procedure performed.

Position. When the patient is brought from the operating room, he should be placed on his side to prevent aspiration. The upper part of his body should be elevated. This is particularly important after a child has had the Glenn procedure done. This makes the work of the heart easier and breathing easier. When the child reacts from anesthesia, he should be turned every 1 to 2 hours unless otherwise ordered. At the time the nurse monitors the vital signs the child should be in a supine position.

Chest suction. The nurse assists the doctor in attaching the drainage bottle to the chest catheter. The tube from the child's chest should be attached to a bottle having a glass tube submerged in water. Certain points should be borne in mind when chest suction is used. The tubing must be long enough to allow the child to move. Excess slack should be coiled on the bed and not allowed to dangle. It should be free of kinks. The bottles should be in a special holder so they cannot tip or be inadvertently kicked over or be elevated. Bottles could be taped to the floor or tied to bed springs. The bottle must always be kept below the child's chest. (If the bottle is at chest level, negative pressure may suck water into the thoracic space. If above chest level, water goes in by gravity.) When it is necessary to change the water in the bottle, the tube should be clamped near the patient's chest with a hemostat before the water seal is broken. Drainage from the chest should be measured and recorded every hour. Blood replacement postoperatively is usually calculated according to the amount of chest drainage.

Chest catheters are usually removed when the drainage decreases, often by the third day.

Observations. The nurse should see that the child has an open airway. Noisy respirations may indicate need of suctioning.

The color of the child (watch the child's nail beds and earlobes) should be noted as well as the presence of bright blood in the drainage bottle or on the dressing. The nurse should watch for symptoms of hemorrhage and for shock. She should remember that a drop in blood pressure is not the first sign of these conditions. (See p. 297 for discussion of general postoperative nursing care.)

The nurse should be on the alert for any neurological symptoms such as twitching or paralysis. A cerebral accident may happen if the hematocrit level is high, as in tetralogy of Fallot. When the patient is conscious, the nurse should be on the alert to notice and report excessive irritability, irrational behavior, dizziness, and headaches.

It is important that all monitor attachments to the patient be checked periodically to ascertain whether they are in correct position and whether skin irritation exists. A patient could be allergic to the jelly used with equipment.

Vital signs. If the child is on a monitor, the nurse can read and record vital signs from the monitor. Temperature should be taken hourly or as ordered. Temperature readings are taken from an indwelling rectal thermometer. The temperature may be subnormal following surgery. Overheating or chilling the patient must both be avoided; neither one is good. Overheating increases the oxygen and metabolic demands for the body. As mentioned, a hypothermia blanket is used to control and regulate the temperature of the child who has had open heart surgery.

Occasionally it is desirable to measure the blood pressure by cuff, even though the child is on the monitor. The nurse should look at the patient's chart to ascertain what his blood pressure was prior to the operation for the sake of comparison. (Hypotension may result after open heart surgery for correction of tetralogy of Fallot because of a decrease in the cardiac output.) She should also be aware of what the normal blood pressure is in children of different ages.

If vital signs are not monitored, the pulse, blood pressure, and respiration should be taken every 15 minutes until stable. An apical pulse should be recorded, although a femoral, radial, and temporal pulse may be taken for comparison. Sometimes no radial pulse is felt following heart catheterization if the antecubital region is used. After shunts the radial pulse on the operative side might not be felt. The character of the pulse and respiration should be noted and recorded at intervals. The nurse should make sure that she has a blood pressure cuff of appropriate size for the infant and preschool child.

Croupette or oxygen tent. The tent needs to be maintained at the desired temperature and the oxygen checked at intervals to make certain the correct number of liters is flowing. An analysis of the oxygen content can be made about every 2 to 4 hours. The child should be kept dry. (For other responsibilities of the nurse in caring for a child in a Croupette, see p. 293).

The older child may have an oxygen mask instead of a tent. Care should be taken to see that it is in place and functioning properly.

Intake and output. An accurate record of fluid intake and output is essential because it influences the doctor in his decision regarding parenteral fluids. A Foley catheter is commonly used for patients who have been on the oxygenator to help evaluate renal function by measurement of hourly urine output and the occasional collection of a urine specimen. The 24-hour amount should be measured and recorded. If a child or infant does not have a Foley catheter, each time the infant or toddler voids, it should be recorded. The amount that the older child voids can be measured, then recorded.

During the time that nothing is taken by mouth, the child's lips and tongue may be dry. These can be moistened with water to keep the child comfortable.

(For care of intravenous fluids refer to p. 301.) During the immediate postoperative period, physicians guard against giving too much fluid, since they wish to avoid pulmonary congestion. When the infant is permitted oral fluids, glucose water is tried. If that is retained, a dilute formula or skim milk formula may be offered, and finally regular formula. A child is offered clear liquids, then liquids with milk, then soft diet, then the diet for his age. When trying to get toddlers or even 3-year-old children to take fluids, the nurse should be aware that sometimes they will accept fluids by bottle rather than by cup, glass, or straw. A variety of fluids is usually more interesting to drink than just one. A nurse must use her ingenuity and resourcefulness.

Laboratory and x-ray studies. From time to time during the first few days postoperatively, blood may be drawn in order to see if the child is in electrolyte balance. Also, chest x-ray studies with portable equipment are done, especially before and after chest tubes are removed. Electrocardiograms are done as necessary. The presence of "his" nurse and an explanation are important to a child.

Rest. Rest is necessary. Nursing procedures should be so organized as to permit as much rest as possible. Unnecessary handling should be avoided. An important adjunct to rest is emotional security. Tenseness and fear have a negative effect on respiration and circulation, whereas relaxation has a beneficial effect. When the infant becomes conscious, he should see the nurse and feel her hand patting him. Remember, he cannot interpret pain and discomfort. Sucking a pacifier might make him happy. A medication may be necessary. Presence of the parents or a familiar person helps. Sometimes holding a familiar toy helps a small child. The older child can be kept informed of progress and given encouragement. The infant, the preschool child, and the older child need all the emotional support they can get.

Prevention of respiratory complications. Frequent turning of the child is essential. The exact frequency during the first 24 hours may be specified by the physician. After the first day, unless the doctor indicates otherwise, the child should be turned at least every 2 hours. While he remains in bed, some elevation of the head of the bed is usually desirable.

The preschool and older child can be asked to breathe deeply, especially if a game is made of this procedure. When the child coughs, he can do it better if sitting upright and if the operative side is splinted by the nurse's hands. The oxygen mist liquefies the secretions so that they can be coughed up more readily. The small infant will not cooperate if asked to cough. For this reason more suctioning may be needed than for the older child. Suctioning sometimes starts the infant coughing. When he coughs, he too, should be elevated to a sitting position and supported. The affected side should be splinted in the same way as for the older child when he coughs.

Recreation. When the child is out of his tent and feels better, he becomes more active. The preschool child is not content to just hold a doll or stuffed animal. These children need mild recreation. A record player is useful. Also, a doctor's or nurse's kit often finds acceptance. Some of the small child's aggression, which cannot be communicated by language, is shown through his use of dolls and stuffed animals with material from the doctor's play kit. The temperature of the doll is taken. Hypodermics are injected forcibly. The doll may receive rough treatment. Other materials for self-expression, like clay or crayons, can be useful.

Exercise and ambulation. Usually within a week after the operation, or perhaps before this, the child is allowed out of bed. He should first sit on the side of the crib and dangle his legs. Some support should be under his feet. His pulse should be taken before and after dangling. The next day he is permitted to sit on a chair. After that, walking might be allowed for a limited time. The child's pulse should be taken before he gets out of bed, while he is up, and after he returns to bed. If the physician does not indicate how long the child should be out of bed, the nurse should limit the child to 15 minutes the first time he is up, then gradually increase the time each day.

The child who has had a ventriculotomy for total correction of tetralogy of Fallot is an exception to the preceding routine. Many surgeons tend to keep such a child on bed rest for at least 7 days. Explicit directions for the ambulation of this child need to be obtained from the physician.

Medication. Antibiotics are usually given preoperatively and postoperatively. If the child was on a digitalis preparation prior to the operation, it is often continued postoperatively. Medication for pain should be given as necessary. Sometimes in the first 24-hour period an analgesic may be given with intravenous fluids. When the child can retain fluids orally, the nurse may inquire if a medication for pain can be given orally.

Preparation for discharge

If the child is receiving a medication such as digoxin, the nurse should find out from the physician what dosage the child will have at home and then teach the mother how to give the medication. This is of particular importance in young children or infants who take digoxin in fluid form rather than a tablet.

The mother of the preschool child may need reassurance that the child does not need to be fed but can feed himself. Seeing the preschool child eating in the playroom with other children and helping himself is much more convincing to the mother than the best verbal advice.

General measures helpful for any preschool child's health such as eating, sleeping, and playing outdoors should be discussed with her. Regular hours for naps and bedtime are essential. Various factors in promotion of a child's health should be discussed with the mother. (Refer to Chapter 9 for discussion of the particular health problems encountered at different age levels.)

A definite plan should be made to teach the parents about the child's activities *before* he goes home. The doctor needs to be explicit as to what the school-age child can and cannot do. For example, can the child swim? Ride horseback? Ride his bicycle? Go coasting? Play baseball and football? Help with farm chores such as feeding animals or help with housework? Pick oranges? Exactly when can he return to school?

Children usually have less exertional fatigue and are more active after an operation. This is more of a problem with school-age children than with younger children, although the parents of the preschool child should be given explicit advice as to whether a child can ride a tricycle, swing, or climb on a jungle gym. If the child is permitted out of bed for only part of the day during the first month at home, the length of time out of bed should be specified.

Intussusception

The hospital nurse rather than the public health nurse is most likely to see the patient with intussusception. Intussusception represents an emergency condition. The office nurse should be familiar with the typical history of a patient with this condition so that, if the mother telephones, she will try to get in touch with the physician at once if he is not in the office.

Nature of the condition

Intussusception means the invagination of one portion of the intestine into another. In the majority of instances the child is under 1 year of age, is a boy, and is robust and healthy. The condition is rare in infants under 3 months and over 2 years of age (Vaughn and McKay, 1975). The infant who has been playing happily suddenly draws up his legs and cries as though in severe pain. This occurs at periodic intervals of 15 to 30 minutes. The child vomits. Fecal matter in the colon is evacuated. Later, vomitus is bile stained. After 12 hours blood usually appears in the stool, sometimes accompanied by mucus. The term *currant jelly stool* is used by some in describing the stools. The temperature of the child may rise to 104° to 106° F. With an increasing number of attacks the child grows weaker, becomes pale, and shows signs of shock. The abdomen may become distended and tender. As already stated, this is an emergency situation. After a period of 24 hours mortality from this condition rises sharply.

There are two possible treatments: one is to reduce the intussusception by hydrostatic pressure applied by enema and the other, more commonly used, is to open the abdomen and either reduce the intussusception or, if that is impossible, resect the bowel.

Hospital admission

When the infant is admitted to the hospital, the nurse needs to appreciate the parents' attitude to the situation. To have their child suddenly become ill, needing hospitalization and even an operation, may represent a catastrophe to them. A warm manner coupled with calmness on the part of the nurse may be helpful to the parents.

The nurse should take an axillary temperature of the infant, since the intussusception may protrude from the anus and look like a rectal prolapse. The infant's respirations may be grunting because of abdominal pain. They may be rapid and shallow if the infant is in shock. In addition to noting and recording the quality of respiration and any unusual appearance of his anus and rectum, the nurse should be alert to abdominal distention, the infant's color, the quality of pulse, and behavior. The infant may be restless and irritable or lethargic and unresponsive. Lying on his side with his knees drawn up may indicate pain. At all times the nurse must remember that the infant is sensitive to the way he is touched and handled, as well as to tones of voices.

Nursing care

The nurse should be ready to assist with intravenous fluids or even with blood transfusions. When the doctor feels the child's abdomen, he is looking for a palpable abdominal mass. Sometimes a barium enema is given as a diagnostic measure.

(For a discussion of the emotional support of parents during a child's operation turn to p. 417; for general measures of postoperative nursing care refer to p. 297.) The infant probably will be having an intravenous infusion. Possibly he will have a nasogastric tube. The nasogastric tube, if used, is attached to some type of suction apparatus. Until the infant can take oral fluids, his lips should be moistened and he might be offered a pacifier to suck. When the tube is removed, glucose water is tried orally. If the infant retains it, dilute formula is offered and then full-strength formula. The nurse needs to ask the surgeon for explicit written orders in regard to feeding the infant. The intravenous infusion will not be discontinued until the infant is retaining fluids orally and is doing well.

Particular postoperative nursing observations include watching for the passage of flatus and stool in addition to observing the general condition of the infant.

Appendicitis
Nature of the condition

Although appendicitis is more common among adults than children, it still represents the commonest cause of abdominal surgery in childhood. The nurse is most likely to see a child under 5 years of age with a perforated appendix, whereas the older child is more likely to have an uncomplicated appendectomy. The latter patient is discharged within 1 week.

A child of school age can better explain his symptoms and where he hurts. His pain is usually periumbilical at first and then located in the right lower quadrant. Typically, he complains of nausea, possibly vomiting, and his mother finds he has a low-grade fever. The doctor, on examination, finds tenderness in the right lower quadrant. A blood count usually shows leukocytosis. The child is referred to the hospital, and an emergency appendectomy is done. The child may ambulate the day following surgery and is home within a week.

The small child is different. He has less resistance to infection, the appendiceal wall is thinner and perforates more easily, the omentum is not sufficiently developed to adequately wall off the spread of infection, the course of the disease is faster, and the child cannot tell exactly where the pain is. It is harder for the physician to discover whether there is localized pain and tenderness, since it is difficult to get the child to relax when his abdomen is examined.

If the appendix has ruptured, a drain is placed in the appendiceal region during surgery, and the appendix is removed.

Preoperative nursing care

The nurse should note the posture of the child on admission to the hospital, since this may indicate pain. It is significant if the child has his legs drawn up toward his abdomen and is lying on his side. She should note also any irritability or restlessness and the character of his breathing. Grunting respirations and signs of dyspnea may be present in a child acutely ill with peritonitis as well as in a child with pneumonia. If there is fecal material on the thermometer when she withdraws it from the rectum, she should report this. Constipation can cause discomfort, pain, and even vomiting. If the doctor in doing a rectal examination finds fecal material in the rectum, he may order a low enema. The rectal tube should not be inserted more than 2 inches. This should be given gently and slowly. The enema can should not be placed higher than one foot above the child's hips.

Obtaining a clean urine specimen is important since, if there are urinary abnormalities, the child may have pyelonephritis.

In assisting the experienced physician with his examination of the child, the nurse may notice that he talks with the child first or examines the child's teddy bear and then feels some part of the child's anatomy that he is sure does not hurt. The abdomen (which is hurting) is the last part of the doctor's examination. The physician wants to win the child's confidence so that he will be relaxed when the abdomen is felt to see if there are local pain, tenderness, and spasm in the right lower quadrant. If the child is tense, it hinders his examination.

If the child has stools, the character of them should be noted and reported by the nurse. In gastroenteritis there could be pain and fever; however, diarrhea is a less common symptom than constipation in a child with appendicitis.

In looking at a report of blood work done, the nurse should be aware that a leukocyte count of 10,000 to 18,000 is expected in appendicitis; but if it is over 20,000 and the child appears acutely ill, the appendix may have already ruptured. If there is a luekopenia and the child appears acutely ill, he may have an overwhelming sepsis.

After the diagnosis of ruptured appendix or appendiceal abscess is established and prior to the operation, the nurse is usually called upon to help with nasogastric suction and intravenous fluids and to administer the prescribed antibiotics. Before the child has surgery he should be well hydrated and in electrolyte balance. If there has been much vomiting and the child has been unable to retain fluids, he may need considerable fluid replacement.

The doctor often orders that the child be placed in Fowler's position to let the abscess drain downward into the pelvic area and become more localized. In this position the back, buttocks, and bony prominences need massage several times daily for comfort and to avoid skin irritation. Children tend to slide down in bed so the child needs repositioning every 2 hours. Intramuscular medications given in the thigh may be less disturbing to the child than if given in the gluteal muscle. The child's lips may be moistened or wiped with a cool washcloth.

Postoperative nursing care

For immediate preoperative and postoperative care, see pp. 296 and 297, respectively. In addition to those nursing suggestions the nurse should ascertain whether the physician wishes the child placed in an oxygen tent postoperatively. The oxygen tent cools the child and reduces distention. Nasogastric suction is usually maintained for 48 hours after surgery or until there are visible signs of normal peristalsis. Any special equipment used should be explained to parents because the sight of it may make them even more fearful for their child.

The nurse should observe the child for restlessness and signs of pain. The children seldom complain of pain verbally so the nurse judges by the child's behavior whether he is in pain. If the child is uncomfortable, the nurse can request the physician to write a medication for pain if none has already been ordered. Morphine is frequently used for children with a perforated appendix.

Once the intravenous infusion and gastric suction are discontinued, the parents might like to hold the small child on their lap for a short time. If not, the child might like the nurse to rock him gently.

When the child is able to take fluids, water, clear broth, or a carbonated beverage should be tried. Liquids with milk can be started when clear fluids are retained, and then a soft diet can be given. (General postoperative care is discussed on p. 298.)

REFERENCES
Common psychological factors

Bakwin, H.: Psychic trauma of operations, J. Pediatr. **36:**262, 1950.

Bakwin, H., and Bakwin, D. M.: Behavior disorders in children, ed. 4, Philadelphia 1972, W. B. Saunders Co.

Dudley, N.: Linda goes to the hospital, New York, 1953, Concord-McConn.

Erickson, F.: Reaction to hospital experience, Nurs. Outlook **6:**501, Sept., 1958.

Gerst, H.: A child goes to the hospital, Springfield, Ill., 1965, Charles C Thomas, Publisher.

Kunzman, L.: Some factors influencing a young child's mastery of hospitalization, Nurs. Clin. North Am. **7**(1):13, March, 1972.

Levy, D. M.: Psychic trauma of operations in children, Am. J. Dis. Child **69:**7, 1945.

Roberts, M.: A doll goes to surgery, Am. J. Nurs. **63:**82, November, 1963.

Sever, J. A.: Johnny goes to the hospital, Boston, 1953, Houghton-Mifflin Co.

Shore, M., editor: Red is the color of hurting. Planning for Children in a Hospital. Washington, D.C., 1967, U.S. Department of Health, Education, and Welfare.

Smith, R. M.: Preparing children for anesthesia and surgery, Am. J. Dis. Child. **101:**650, 1961.

Sparks, L.: Humpty-Dumpty goes to the hospital, Can. Nurs **64:**34, March, 1968.

Medical conditions

Ballenger, J. J.: Diseases of the nose, throat, and ear, ed. 11, Philadelphia, 1969, Lea & Febiger.

Barnett, H.: Pediatrics, ed. 14, New York, 1968, Appleton-Century-Crofts.

Engle, M. A.: Treatment of the failing heart, Pediatr. Clin. North Am. **2:**247, 1964.

Fine, R. N., et al.: Hemodialysis in children, Am. J. Dis. Child. **119:**198, 1970.

French, R.: The nurse's guide to diagnostic procedures, ed. 3, New York, 1971, McGraw-Hill Book Co.

Gillis, S. S., and Kagan, B. M.: Current pediatric therapy, ed. 6, Philadelphia, 1973, W. B. Saunders Co.

Khan, A. J., and Pryles, C.: Urinary tract infection in children, Am. J. Nurs. **73:**1340, August, 1973.

McCrory, W. W., and Shibuya, M.: Long-term follow-up of acute glomeruli-nephritism children, N.Y. State J. Med. **68:**2416, 1968.

Shirkey, H., editor: Pediatric therapy, ed. 5, St. Louis, 1975, The C. V. Mosby Co.

Vaughan, V., III, and McKay, R. J., editors: Nelson's textbook of pediatrics, ed. 10, Philadephia, 1975, W. B. Saunders Co.

Surgical conditions

Achram, J.: Anesthesia for infants and children, Am. J. Nurs. **64:**107, August, 1967.

Barclay, L.: Blalock-Hanlon operation at eight days, Nurs. Mirror **131:**21, December, 1970.

Barnes C. M.: Working with parents of children undergoing heart surgery, Nurs. Clin. North Am. **4:**11, March, 1969.

Blake, F.: Open heart surgery in children; a study in nursing care, Washington D.C., 1964, U.S. Department of Health, Education, and Welfare.

Braney, M. L.: The child with hydrocephalus, Am. J. Nurs. **73:**828, May, 1973.

Cowley, C. M.: Repair of ventricular septal defect, Nurs. Mirror **39:**38 September, 1970.

Haggerty, R. J.: Diagnosis and treatment; tonsils and adenoids—a problem revisited, Pediatrics **41:**815, 1968.

Kingsley, H.: Children and anesthesia, Can. Nurse **63:**26, October, 1967.

Lloyd, P.: Postoperative nursing care following open heart surgery in children, Nurs. Clin. North Am. **5:**399, September, 1970.

Matson, D.: Neurosurgery of infancy and childhood, ed. 2, Springfield, Ill., 1969, Charles C Thomas, Publisher.

McCrory, W. W., and Shibuya, M.: Long term follow up of acute glomerulonephritis in children, N.Y. State J. Med. **69:**2416, 1969.

Mustard, W. M., et al., editors: Pediatric surgery, ed. 2, Chicago, 1969, Year Book Medical Publishers, Inc.

Shirkey, H. C., editor: Pediatric therapy, ed. 5, St. Louis, 1975, The C. V. Mosby Co.

Smith, R.: Anesthesia for infants and children, ed. 3, St. Louis, 1968, The C. V. Mosby Co.

Swenson, O.: Pediatric surgery, ed. 3, New York, 1969, Appleton-Century-Crofts.

Vaughan, V., III, and McKay, R. J., editors: Nelson's textbook of pediatrics, ed. 10, Philadelphia, 1975, W. B. Saunders Co.

15

Nursing care of
THE CHILD ACCIDENT VICTIM

COMMON PSYCHOLOGICAL FACTORS

The abruptness and suddenness of an accident with the consequent hospitalization or medical care at home is a difficult adjustment for both the parents and the child. It is a shock. If one or both of the parents believe they are responsible for the accident to the child, either directly or indirectly, the situation is distressing. Sometimes one parent may blame the other for the accident. A small child may think of himself as "bad" because of the burn he received and believe he is being punished for misbehaving. If the child has a head injury and is unconscious, the family may be in a state of acute anxiety.

The parents need a chance to discuss their feelings of surprise, grief, and guilt about the accident. They need a nurse who is willing to listen and let them talk, one who through empathy can give them sympathetic support. The nurse needs to be patient, to explain to the parents any procedures or treatments she is doing for the child, and to share the child's care with the parents if they so desire. The nurse's verbal as well as nonverbal communication to the parents is highly significant at this crucial time.

To avoid being judgmental of the parents, some nurses may need to discuss their feelings about the child's accident with someone who will help them to be objective—perhaps the head nurse or another staff nurse.

After any kind of accident the child needs reassurance. In a short space of time bewildering events have taken place. Verbal explanations are helpful, but a tone of voice, a smile, gentleness, and relief from discomfort may be more supportive emotionally. Even if a small child is too ill to play with a toy, the sight of play material or of cheerful pictures on a wall

may help him to feel less lost in space. Sleep and rest following an accident are essential in helping to restore emotional equilibrium.

Sometimes the services of a social worker and/or child psychiatrist are necessary in helping the parents and the child to recognize and to resolve their feelings about the accident.

BURNS

Burns constitute a common type of accident for children; yet most of these burns can be avoided if proper safety precautions are taken. The type and extent of burns vary somewhat with the age of the child. The infant and toddler are more likely to have burns from hot liquids (tea, coffee, water) spilled onto the head, neck, and upper extremities because they reach for things they cannot see and pull at the handles of pans, coffeepots, etc. The older child often has a more extensive burn since his clothing is ignited by fire from an unprotected fireplace, small open heater, or the like. Little girls' dresses catch on fire more readily than pants and shirts. Boys are more likely to be burned by inflammable liquids such as kerosene and gasoline (Boles, 1963). A toddler left in the bathtub alone may turn on the hot-water faucet and be scalded.

As a result of burns, the child may spend months in the hospital. The injury may be more than physical. Being burned is a difficult psychological experience for children (Long and Cope, 1961).

Role of the nurse
Prevention

Refer to p. 212 relative to the prevention of accidents in toddlers and preschool children. The public health nurse should develop a

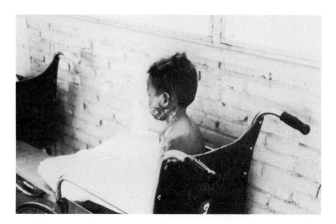

Fig. 15-1. Burned Vietnamese child. (Courtesy James Gerlock, M.D.)

safety-conscious eye. Both in home visits and in the child health conferences she can give mothers much needed education about safety precautions to take with both the inquisitive toddler and the older child. Posters, combined with a short talk in a child health conference, might prove highly profitable. The office nurse can often use posters and literature to good advantage.

In the elementary, junior, and senior high school, prevention of burns could be part of health and/or safety instruction. The school health nurse is in an excellent position to try to arouse teachers' interest in this subject and to act as a resource person. She might initiate plans for a school committee on health instruction to discuss this topic. Current statistics on the number of children receiving burns are always startling. Many of these would not have occurred had clothing and/or bedding been treated with flame-retardant chemicals! A new federal law, enacted in 1970, makes it mandatory that such cloth items be so treated after January 1, 1973. Studies are available on how many of the burns children received could have been prevented (Colebrook and Colebrook, 1956; Jensen, 1959). Local fire departments are usually ready to cooperate in a teaching project.

As both junior and senior high school students do considerable baby-sitting, it is essential for them to have information about the safety of small children.

Degree of burn

The degree or depth of a burn influences the metabolism of the patient. A first degree burn produces erythema and possibly mild blistering and peeling as in a sunburn. This may be painful. The superficial layers of the skin are affected. A second degree burn involves deeper damage to the skin and underlying tissue. In an extreme second degree burn, so much fluid may be lost from the intravascular compartment that the blood volume is reduced; in turn, this may produce hypovolemic shock. Renal flow is reduced. In a partial-thickness burn, there is usually a mottled, moist, and painful surface. Burns from hot liquid frequently produce a partial-thickness destruction of tissue. If there is an absence of sensation, then there may be a full-thickness destruction of skin or a third degree burn. A third degree burn involves muscle, nerve, and possibly even bone. Many children with severe burns have both second and third degree burns on their body. A white or charred surface of skin may be seen with a full-thickness or third degree burn.

Estimation of extent of burn

For a quick estimation of body burns in adults, Pulaski and Termison suggested the rule of nine. According to this rule, there is a division of body surface into areas representing 9% or multiples of 9%. The head and neck account for 9%, the anterior trunk 18%, the posterior trunk 18%, each lower extremity

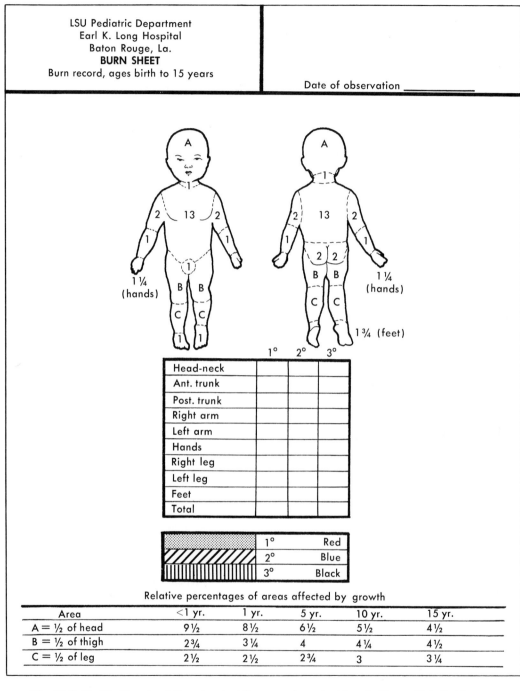

Relative percentages of areas affected by growth

Area	<1 yr.	1 yr.	5 yr.	10 yr.	15 yr.
A = ½ of head	9½	8½	6½	5½	4½
B = ½ of thigh	2¾	3¼	4	4¼	4½
C = ½ of leg	2½	2½	2¾	3	3¼

Fig. 15-2. Modified Lund and Browder chart for measuring extent (area) of burn. Note that the area of the skin burned is expressed as a percentage of the total body surface area. Because of marked difference in surface area of the head and lower extremities, the rule of nine used for adults does not apply to children. (Courtesy Louisiana State University Pediatric Department, Baton Rouge, Louisiana.)

18%, each upper extremity 9%, and the perineum 1%.

This rule of nine cannot be applied to young children since there is a relatively greater amount of surface area for the head and trunk and a lesser amount for lower extremities. MacMillan (1975) suggests approximate percentages of body surface to be used to evaluate the extent of body surface burned in a newborn, 3-year-old child, 6-year-old child, and 12-year-old child. Fig. 15-2 shows a modified Lund and Browder chart for measuring the area of burn in children.

Goals in treatment

Usually children who have burns are hospitalized if the burns cover more than 10% of the body surface. In the immediate or initial management, sedation is usually given to allay pain and apprehension. Intravenous fluids are begun to combat hypovolemic shock. Tetanus prophylaxis is given as well as appropriate antibiotic therapy. Blood is drawn for baseline laboratory determinations. Further treatment consists of maintenance of adequate body fluids, prevention of infection, and promotion of rapid healing without loss of function or scarring. Local treatment of burns varies. Because of possible psychic trauma from an extensive burn, attention is given to the child's mental hygiene. Every effort is made to lessen the trauma of the hospitalization as much as possible.

Initial care

All charred and smouldering clothing must be removed. *No ointment or grease should be placed on the burn.* The child can be wrapped in a clean sheet wrung out in cold water to bring him to the hospital. This helps to allay the child's pain and minimizes contamination of the burn. Although burns are painful, a third degree burn is less so since the nerve endings have been destroyed with the complete destruction of the skin.

Pain and apprehension can be allayed by sedation. Then care is directed toward the prevention and/or treatment of shock. Every effort is made to maintain an adequate circulation and thus prevent possible circulatory and/or renal failure. Shock occurs faster in infants and young children than in adults since the blood volume is smaller and there is relatively greater surface area in proportion to body weight.

When a child is burned, the rest of the body becomes dehydrated because plasmalike fluids go to the area of the burn and there is an enormous evaporative water loss from the burn surface. The hematocrit value is a good index of the degree of fluid loss; likewise, the urinary output is important. The kidneys try to conserve water. Consequently, in states of dehydration, urinary output reduces. A drop in blood pressure is actually a late sign of shock. A marked rise in the pulse rate is an earlier sign of shock as well as the pallor, coldness of skin, and behavior of the patient. Intravenous fluids help restore the blood volume and increase the renal function.

The infusion of intravenous fluids is begun immediately after blood has been drawn for blood chemistries, cross-matching, and typing. To the fluid may be added such vitamins as ascorbic acid, thiamine, and riboflavin. On the day of the burn injury about one half of the fluids for the 24 hours is given in the first 8 hours from the time of burning. One quarter of the fluid is given in each of the next two 8-hour periods. On the second day the child receives about one half the amount of fluids calculated for the first 24 hours. By the third day there is usually a diuresis. At this point the child needs calories and fluids low in sodium content. Intravenous fluids are discontinued when the child begins to take and retain oral fluids. A good guide to the need for fluids is the child's urinary output. (A Foley catheter is used if the child has a major burn: 12% of the body surface up to 8 years and 18% from 8 to 18 years.)

As part of the initial care, the child is given protection against tetanus; he may also be given an antibiotic. If the burn involves the perioral region, if there is singeing of nasal hairs, if the child is coughing up sooty material, or if the burn was obtained in a small enclosed area, then the burn is treated expectantly as a respiratory burn. The child is placed in a Croupette with high humidity and 40% oxygen. If this burn is seen within the first 12 hours, pharmacological doses of cortisone may be given in the intravenous fluids in order to minimize the risk of bronchospasm and edema. After 12 hours, administration of cortisone increases the risk of sepsis since the wound is likely to be contaminated and growth of bacteria present would be encouraged. A tracheotomy is only performed if there is frank respiratory distress relieved only by an airway, if there is considerable edema of respiratory passages, or if such obstructing edema is anticipated.

Local treatment of burn

Whether the child is taken to the operating room to have the burned area debrided or whether there is gentle cleansing of the burn in the emergency room depends on the physician. Also, what is placed on the burn after it is cleansed may vary with different physicians.

Any one of a variety of topical antibacterial agents may be used on second and third degree burns to prevent wound sepsis. Many types of bacteria cause sepsis, but the predominant ones are streptococci, staphylococci, and *Pseudomonas aeruginosa*. Silver nitrate solution (0.5%), gentamicin (Garamycin), and mafenide (Sulfamylon) are sometimes used, but silver sulfadiazine is more commonly used today. There are some advantages and disadvantages to each topical medication.

Silver nitrate solution stains everything it touches, but sheets or articles contacted can be treated with an organic iodine solution (such as Wescodyne or Betadine) before the black stain develops and then rinsed in water. This will prevent the stain. More important than staining is the fact that the use of silver nitrate solution changes the electrolyte balance, so that blood needs to be drawn at least every 8 hours to ascertain the electrolyte balance. Particularly sodium and chloride, and to a lesser extent potassium, are dialyzed out of the body into the silver nitrate–saturated dressings. At the same time the body absorbs water from the dressings and may become overhydrated. This is of particular importance in the first 3 to 5 days of treatment. When silver nitrate solution is used, the dressings on the child must be kept wet and changed two to three times daily. If left longer, the silver becomes more concentrated. These dressings make it hard for the child to ambulate. One more disadvantage to the silver nitrate is

that it does not penetrate the wound unless the burn is clean or debrided.

Gentamicin has the advantage of penetrating the wound. It is applied by mesh gauze impregnated with this ointment, or it can be used directly from the tube onto the surface with the gloved hand or a tongue blade. A disadvantage is that its use may allow for an overgrowth of resistant organisms such as *Pseudomonas* that are not susceptible to gentamicin. A further disadvantage is that it causes a delay of several days in the time of separation of the burn eschar and thus may delay time of full healing or grafting. It is available as a cream and an ointment.

Mafenide (Sulfamylon) also penetrates the burn and inhibits the growth of bacteria. Mafenide is painful to apply, and the child may need an analgesic before it is used. When this ointment is used, crusts form over the burn and the time the eschar separates is delayed. The eschar may have to be excised for skin grafts to be applied. Mafenide ointment must be washed off daily, preferably in a whirlpool bath. If the ointment is not washed off, drug-resistant organisms can grow between the dried, crusted drug on the body surface and the wound. The child is not to be left in water (bathtub, whirlpool) for more than 15 minutes because the water will dialyze considerable quantities of salt from the child. In addition, mafenide, a potent carbonic anhydrase inhibitor, may change the acid-base balance, which could result in metabolic acidosis. The nurse should be alert for rapid respirations (polypnea) and changes in mental state, both of which may herald acid-base disequilibrium.

Silver sulfadiazine ointment contains 1% silver sulfadiazine in a water-miscible base. Used experimentally for some time, now it is widely used by many in preference to other topical applications. It appears to have few disadvantages. It does not influence the acid-base balance as do 1% silver nitrate solution and mafenide. True, some cases of leukopenia have been reported following the use of this drug. The ointment is soothing to the child, and its application does not cause pain. The ointment does stain sheets, but these stains can be washed out.

Before silver sulfadiazine is applied, the skin should be washed very gently with Ivory or a nonallergenic soap. The nurse wears sterile gloves in washing the skin. She washes the skin with her gloved hands. (Gauze sponges would cause pain and are not necessary; the gloved hand is adequate.)

The ointment is applied also with a gloved hand to a thickness of 3 to 5 mm. It should be applied as often as necessary to maintain this thickness.

Twice a day the child is placed in a Hubbard tank or tub to wash off the ointment and the body surface. The area under the moist exudate is a good medium for proliferation of bacteria. Following the bath, ointment is reapplied.

The child is placed in bed on clean sheets with a cradle to keep the upper bedclothes from touching his skin. External heat needs to be applied to keep the child warm. The temperature of the room itself needs to be warm enough so the child is comfortable. If he is cold, the child shivers and his temperature begins to rise.

Following the bath the child is usually thirsty. His mouth feels dry. If he can take oral fluids, fluids that contain electrolytes or fluids to which electrolytes can be added are valuable.

In summary, maintenance of adequate body fluids, prevention of infection, and promotion of rapid healing without loss of function or scarring are the goals of treatment. The child with an extensive burn and prolonged hospitalization may well have psychic trauma. Psychiatric assistance may be needed for him, If so, frequent communication between the psychiatrist and those who care for the child is essential so that the latter will know best how to help him.

Nursing care
Initial care

In the initial period of hospitalization the nurse's main functions include helping to assess the patient's condition, trying to allay his fears and anxiety, obtaining necessary equipment, assisting with drawing of the blood, monitoring the intravenous fluids, and recording the urinary output.

When the child is admitted to the emergency room, the nurse should first take the vital signs. While taking them, she can observe any restlessness or signs of dyspnea. Respiratory distress may be present if the child has been burned on the neck and upper chest. This is also true of the child who has been exposed to intense heat or smoke, since this may cause edema of the mucous membrane of the respiratory passages. Wheezing and hoarseness help to indicate dyspnea. Restlessness is a primary sign of air hunger in both children and adults, and restlessness may also be seen in dehydration. Restlessness should not be mistaken for uncooperativeness, pain, or fright. Other important observations include the general color, responsiveness, and behavior of the child.

If there is respiratory difficulty, the nurse should bring a tracheotomy set to the room. Other materials to be assembled include intravenous equipment (cutdown instruments for an infant or child with extensive burn injury) and a Foley catheter if the patient has a major burn. Masks, gowns, gloves, and sterile sheets are usually in each emergency room.

The child must be weighed and measured, since this is helpful in estimating the fluid requirement. Clothing should be removed to see the extent of the burn. If it is necessary to cut the clothing, this should be done at the garment seams.

The nurse should keep in mind that the chief aim of treatment in the initial stage is prevention and/or treatment of shock. As stated previously, more fluids are administered intravenously on the first day than on later days. Until the child's vital signs are stable, he should not be moved from the emergency room.

Vital signs, medications given, urinary output, and all other pertinent observations should be recorded on the child's nursing care record. If a Foley catheter is inserted, the hourly output of urine is noted; if no Foley catheter is used, the amount that the child voids should be recorded. If the patient is an infant, a check (✔) can be made when the diaper is wet. The nurse can note the condition of the diaper hourly.

Daily care

Aims. In order to plan the nursing care the nurse needs to be aware of the general goals of medical treatment of a burned child. Prevention and/or treatment of shock was the primary aim in the initial period of the child's illness. After that, minimizing or preventing infection and promoting rapid healing without loss of function or scarring are the next goals. Septicemia is the biggest single cause of death of burned children now that shock is better controlled. Skin grafting is done as early as possible to minimize scarring and to prevent further loss of proteins, electrolytes, and fluids. To this end, getting the skin ready for grafting (by whatever method has been selected by the physician) is vital.

To accomplish these goals close teamwork of the physician, social worker, physiotherapist, dietician, and nurse is essential. The particular role of the nurse is outlined here.

Care of intravenous infusion. See p. 301 for a description of the nursing responsibilities relative to care of intravenous infusion. The nurse on the unit needs to continue the record of the nurse in the emergency room in regard to the intravenous infusion.

Prevention of infection. Sometimes a child is placed in a room by himself on reverse isolation. The patient is considered clean. On the other hand, there is a trend now not to place the child in isolation since infection probably comes from the child himself. The area of the burn is contaminated and infection may result from this. Under eschar formed, pathological organisms may grow. Topical medications or ointments do not necessarily prevent this growth.

Personnel caring for the child need to be free of any infection so they will not give the child any infection. Personnel wear gowns in caring for the child in order to protect their own clothing. Sterile gloves are used in applying a topical medication and in bathing the child in a tub.

An unpleasant odor from the dressing or discoloration of the dressing should be reported since it may well mean that infection is present. If the urine is greenish, it may denote that *Pseudomonas* is present.

Exercise. The child's position needs changing frequently to prevent hypostatic pneumonia and to minimize scarring and contracture. Often the child can turn himself with less pain than when turned by a nurse. If he is on a Stryker frame, he needs turning every hour or so. Exercise helps prevent contractures as well as respiratory infection.

Whenever possible, the child should ambulate. If the child gets into the tub daily for soaks, he should be encouraged to walk to the tub and back again. While he is in the tub, floating toys might be used so the child will become interested in playing and forget to be afraid to move his limbs. As the bathroom is very warm, he becomes thirsty and willingly takes fluids offered while he is in the tub.

Before getting back into bed again the small child may like to be covered with a sterile sheet and rocked for a while. It is comforting to him.

While he is sitting on the nurse's lap or when he is again in bed, the nurse can sometimes get the child to play again with her—in a way that involves his moving his arms and thus exercising them.

Preventing contractures. Exercising in the tub and ambulating help to prevent contractures. Using a footboard, keeping the body in good alignment, and encouraging range-of-motion exercises assist also. An extremity that is burned is usually wrapped and placed in a functional position. The dressing is removed when the child is placed in a tub. If the child's interest can be diverted from himself and guided into playing toys, he exercises his arms himself. Although these measures are helpful, the early and complete coverage of burned areas with skin grafts is essential if contractures are to be prevented.

Nutrition. During the fiirst 24 to 48 hours, oral fluids are not given to a child with extensive burns. He often vomits and there is danger of aspiration. In addition, oral feedings sometimes cause gastric and abdominal distention since a paralytic ileus is common.

After the first few days, fruit juice and fluids are given, and then a diet adequate to meet his health needs is given. Nutrition is important for healing to take place and for new tissue to grow. Crawford and Antoon (1973) point out there is a protein and calorie deficit. There is an increased evaporized heat loss from the skin. Because of the burn, the thermoregulatory function of the skin is lost. Fruit juice, eggnogs, custards, and ice cream should be offered between meals and at bedtime. (For discussion of mealtime see p. 283.) The nurse needs to return to the child's bedside frequently to offer fluids if the child takes only a small amount at a time.

Fluid intake and output. After oral fluids are begun, conscientious recording of fluids taken is important to see whether he is getting an adequate amount and also to see if desirable fluids are accepted.

If the child is extensively burned, he usually has a Foley catheter inserted, even though the catheter may be a means of introducing infection. When this is used, the amount of urine excreted is measured hourly during the first critical days. If the infant voids less than 10 ml. per hour or the child less than 20 ml., the physician should be notified.

Children less extensively burned who do not have a Foley catheter should be offered a bedpan immediately on waking in the morning and then approximately every 2 hours thereafter. The child's mother can usually tell the nurse what is the child's rhythm of urination. Sometimes it is easier to use an emesis basin into which the child can void, in preference to a bedpan, if there are burns of the thighs and buttocks or if sitting on a bedpan causes discomfort. A piece of rubber covered with a pad can be placed under the emesis basin when the child voids. The child can use the basin either when he is on his back or when he is on his abdomen. As it is likely to be the older child who is extensively burned rather than a toddler, bedwetting is not usually a problem; if, however, it is a toddler who is extensively burned, every time his diaper is changed a check should be placed on the nursing record under urine output so that everyone will know the child has voided.

Pertinent observations. In order to tell the condition of the child the nurse on every tour of duty should note the child's behavior (restlessness, listlessness, irritability, responsiveness) and observe the color of the child, any coldness of extremities, dyspnea, increase of stridor, or gross changes in the temperature, pulse, respiration, and blood pressure. Cold extremities, shivering, and cyanosis of lips and extremities indicate poor peripheral circulation. Continued thirst and restlessness may indicate inadequate hydration. A steady rise in temperature, pulse, and respiration coupled with vomiting, increasing restlessness, or prostration

may be a forerunner of the development of toxicity. Significant changes in vital signs and/or the behavior of the child need to be recorded and reported to the physician.

Mental hygiene. If a child is in a room by himself, it is lonely for the child and may further add to his emotional distress about the accident and his bewilderment in being in new surroundings. Having a special nurse all during the 24-hour period may be comforting if the nurse remembers the child's needs as a person. The nurse must be careful in what she communicates to the child nonverbally by her facial expression when she looks at an exposed area of the burn. The manner in which she changes the wet dressings, turns the child, etc. tells the child something about her. The dexterity with which the nurse cares for a patient can either lessen pain or increase it.

In every way possible the nurse should let the child see that she likes him. The psychic disturbance of a burned child may be very great. The child may regard the burn as a punishment and believe he did something that is wrong. He may think of himself as being an unworthy person. The young child often suffers separation anxiety, and even the older child may be unable to understand why his parents, who are all-powerful, cannot stay with him constantly.

As the child begins to feel better physically, suitable recreation should be provided. The older child needs to continue his school studies.

Recreation does not have to be only in the playroom at a certain hour, but at any time the nurse is with the child as she cares for him. As stated in Chapter 11, every nurse should have a repertoire of stories and games not requiring equipment that she can use as necessary.

If the child is not reasonably happy, he will not eat well and this affects the healing of the skin. Adequate sleep and rest are important considerations in maintaining emotional stability.

The child with an extensive burn and prolonged hospitalization may well have psychic trauma. Psychiatric assistance may be needed for him. If so, there need to be open channels of communication between the psychiatrist and those caring for the child.

Skin grafting

As soon as there begins to be a line of demarcation between the viable and the devitalized skin, the burned area may be debrided and skin grafts applied. If the child is severely burned, there may have to be multiple debridements and skin graftings. There is a trend to avoid early grafting of full-thickness burn areas. The grafts, except those for very small areas, are *split-thickness* grafts. The nurse plays an important role by promoting good nutrition both before and after skin grafting. Whole blood or plasma may be given to the child if his hematocrit or hemoglobin level is below normal or if the total protein of the blood serum is low. Some physicians believe that for skin grafts to take well the total serum proteins should be at least normal. There must be immobilization of the part that is grafted in order for the graft to take well. This is usually accomplished by pressure dressings for the first few days. Later, when the skin graft is exposed, nothing should brush against it. If the burn site is extensive, multiple skin grafts may have to be done.

Thighs are often used as donor sites, although skin from any unburned area could be used. Skin grafts from another person may be used if there is a large burn surface that needs covering as soon as possible because of the condition of the patient; however, such grafts always slough after a few weeks and the area has to receive other grafts.

The donor sites are usually covered with medicated gauze and then a pressure dressing. The pressure dressing helps to control any bleeding and is removed after a few days, and the area is exposed to heal. If the nurse sees that the dressing is soiled or wet, she should call this to the physician's attention so he can change the dressing or have the nurse change it.

FOREIGN BODIES
Gastrointestinal tract
The problem

Through 2 years of age the creeping infant and toddler tend to put everything into their mouths. The mouth is a sensory organ by which the toddler can tell if an object is soft, hard, smooth, sweet tasting, etc. Anything that can harm the child should be kept out of his reach.

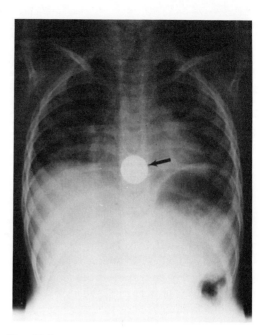

Fig. 15-3. Foreign body (coin) lodged in distal portion of esophagus. Coin was removed at esophagoscopy.

Even some 3-year-old children continue to put things in their mouths. Safety pins should be closed when not in use.

The incidence of swallowing foreign bodies is greatest in children from 1 to 4 years of age (Gross, 1953). Coins, pins (either safety pins or straight pins), and small toy parts are among the commonest objects that children have swallowed.

Manifestations

It is possible that the mother of a child may find an object in the child's stool without being aware the child had swallowed anything. On the other hand, the child may show difficulty in swallowing and have spells of choking. He could have dyspnea and hoarseness. Dyspnea results when there is compression in the trachea caused by the passage or lodging of a hard object in the esophagus.

Treatment

The child should remain on his usual diet. Cathartics and laxatives should be avoided, since rapid peristalsis increases the danger of perforation if the object is sharp.

The majority of foreign objects pass into the stomach and through the intestines; however, the progress of the foreign object is carefully watched by means of roentgenograms. All stools of the child should be carefully saved and examined to see if the object is passed. If the object lodges in the esophagus, it is removed by an esophagoscope. If the object is sharp or if it fails to progress after a period of time, surgical measures are usually employed since there is danger of irritation, ulceration, and possibly perforation. Some foreign objects in the duodenum can be removed by passing a magnet down the esophagus on the end of a Levin tube.

Respiratory tract

When a small child aspirates a foreign body, he may cough, wheeze, and choke. The mother may take the child to a physician because of a persistent cough or wheeze and discover the child has a foreign body in the bronchi. Dyspnea, hoarseness, and cyanosis can occur. Symptoms depend somewhat on the degree of obstruction that exists. A foreign body could cause asphyxia or atelectasis. It could also cause an inflammatory reaction.

Diagnostic measures include a roentgenogram of the chest, physical signs heard by the physician on examination of the chest with a stethoscope, and visualization of the object by laryngoscopy.

Foreign bodies in the respiratory tract are removed by a bronchoscope or other means as soon as possible. After a foreign body has been removed the child is usually placed in a Croupette or similar tent in which high humidity can be given. The nurse should watch the child's respirations carefully prior to surgery and after surgery. It is wise to have a tracheotomy tray on hand in the child's room for an emergency, also oxygen. After the removal of the object there may be edema of the respiratory passages so the child may be quite dyspneic.

Other organs

Nose

A toddler may insert small objects such as beans, buttons, pieces of crayon, seeds, or pebbles into the nose. The object frequently becomes lodged and, if it remains for a time, may produce a chronic blood-tinged mucopurulent discharge. The discharge is usually unilateral, which should draw attention of the parents to the fact that a foreign body may be present in the child's nostril. If the object is a pea or bean it may swell and cause respiratory obstruction or wheezing.

It is recommended that the child be brought to a physician for removal of the object. Some times forcible blowing of the nose with the other nostril closed may dislodge the foreign body.

Ear

Small children may insert beans, peas, pieces of paper and crayons, pills, or pebbles into the external canal of the ear. If the foreign body remains lodged for a while it may produce irritation and infection of the ear canal.

A physician should remove the object from the ear. The foreign body may be removed with alligator forceps under direct vision or by irrigation of the ear canal if organic material such as a pea or bean is present.

Vagina

Pencils, crayons, pins, or paper clips may be inserted into the vagina. If the foreign body remains lodged, a mucopurulent vaginal discharge will result. Diagnosis is confirmed by a KUB roentgenogram of the abdomen and rectal examination. Removal of the object by a urologist or gynecologist is recommended.

INGESTION OF POISONS

Role of the nurse

The public health nurse needs to know the gravity of the situation in regard to poisoning of children, both for the purpose of teaching prevention and for application of general home nursing. The hospital nurse may see some children brought to the hospital as a result of poisoning. Some of these children may be acutely ill or even in a coma. Others, who have ingested only a small amount or a less toxic poison, may be seen in the emergency room, where treatment is given, and then be allowed to go home. The nurse's reaction to the accident and her behavior to the parents are an important element in the care of the child. (Refer to the discussion of psychological aspects of accidents, p. 434.)

Prevention

Poisoning is especially common from 1 to 4 years of age. (For general information about prevention of accidents see p. 000.) It is sufficient here to emphasize again the importance of keeping potentially harmful drugs or solutions out of the toddler's reach. This includes cleaning fluids, lye, insecticides, rodenticides, aspirin, bleaches, and hydrocarbons such as kerosene. The tops of the cans should be screwed on tightly or fastened securely, as the case might be. Each drug or chemical should be kept in its own bottle or container. Medicines left from an illness of the child or adults in the family should be discarded. When medicines are administered to children during an illness, they should be called "medicine"—not "candy." Children need to be taught that medicines are meant to be taken when a person is ill but that, if a well person takes medicines, the medicine could make him sick. Preschool children who wish to "play doctor" can be given some candy such as peppermints to be used as medicine.

Potential hazards of certain drugs and compounds

1. *Boric acid solution,* whether used as an antiseptic in eye irrigations or for wet dressings, is a dangerous drug. In the home, plain soap and water is a better and safer disinfectant. The ingestion of less than a teaspoonful orally may prove fatal. Boric acid can also produce toxic symptoms if it is absorbed through the skin or used in the eyes. Renal failure can develop, as well as gastrointestinal symptoms and convulsions, as a result of ingestion. There is no specific antidote for boric acid, and treatment is symptomatic.

2. *Lye* may be ingested by the crawling baby or toddler who puts everything in his mouth. Stricture of the esophagus can result, as lye is caustic. The child may have to have repeated dilations over a period of months or may have to have surgery performed. Drano, which contains lye, should not be within the toddler's reach.

3. *Cationic detergents* such as Zephiran, Diaparene, and Ceepryn chloride should never be left on a bedside table of a child in the hospital or be left anywhere within reach of the young child. He need only take 1 to 3 gm. for the solution to be fatal. Death can occur within a few hours.

4. *Sodium hypochlorite,* contained in many bleaching solutions such as Clorox, could be fatal if 15 to 30 ml. were taken orally by children. There is pulmonary irritation and possibly edema of pharynx and larynx. Sodium hypochlorite is an acid and, as such, acts as a corrosive to the mucous membranes.

5. *Gasoline* or *kerosene,* if ingested, might cause pneumonitis or bronchitis. It is absorbed quickly. Even if the mother did not know a child had taken kerosene, she might smell it on the child's breath or hear the child coughing. The child also might develop an elevated temperature and be very drowsy.

6. *Insecticides* that are chlorinated (DDT, Aldrin, and Endrin) are very toxic, especially Aldrin. These substances can be absorbed through the skin. The symptoms that appear are usually related to the central nervous system. Respiratory failure may result. The use of substances such as sprays is a hazard to children.

Thiocyanate insecticides are also readily absorbed through the skin. They can cause dyspnea, convulsions, cyanosis, and respiratory failure. If children's hands become contaminated with these substances, their hands should thoroughly washed.

7. *Rodenticides* are substances, often containing thallium, that are used to kill rodents. Peanuts and grains coated with thallium salts look attractive, and a child may put them into his mouth. Alopecia is a late symptom, which may not be seen until several weeks after the ingestion of thallium. Immediate symptoms may be referable to the gastrointestinal system, whereas other symptoms such as paralysis or ataxia may be referred to the central nervous system.

8. *Aspirin* is such a common offender in poisoning of children that the symptoms of aspirin poisoning are given here. Respirations become deeper and faster. There is hyperventilation and consequently respiratory alkalosis; however, it

is the metabolic acidosis that may develop that is the most serious. Ketonuria may be present; there may be an elevated temperature. The child may have been poisoning by eating baby aspirin, believing it to be candy, or the mother may have given aspirin to a child during his illness without his physician's advice about the dosage.

Salicylate levels in the urine and blood should be obtained. A serum salicylate level of over 40 mg. per 100 ml. is considered toxic. Administration of syrup of ipecac or gastric lavage is employed only in the child who has ingested the aspirin 2 hours or less before the treatment is begun. Glucose solution, sodium bicarbonate, and electrolytes are drugs used frequently in the management of these children. These drugs will accelerate the removal of salicylate from the body. Vitamin K oxide is given to prevent bleeding since the salicylates produce a dicumerol-like effect. Exchange transfusion, peritoneal dialysis, or hemodialysis has been used to effect external removal of salicylates in children with life-threatening salicylism.

9. *Ferrous sulfate,* if taken as prescribed by a doctor, might not cause difficulties, but sometimes there is carelessness in taking this drug, since many people believe it to be harmless. It can cause vomiting, corrosion of the gastrointestinal tract, circulatory collapse, and hepatic damage.

In home visits the nurse needs to emphasize that no medicines should be taken unless they are specifically ordered by the physician.

Treatment

In general the treatment for ingestion of poisons is to remove the unabsorbed poison from the stomach as quickly as possible, unless the poison is a strong acid, alkali, or corrosive substance. This may be accomplished by placing a finger or a spoon handle as far down a child's throat as is possible in an effort to gag him and produce vomiting. It has been suggested that syrup of ipecac be used as an emetic, in doses of 10 to 15 ml., and repeated in 15 to 30 minutes if vomiting has not occurred (Arena, 1975). A small amount of mustard in water, or salt in lukewarm water, could be tried; however, time is important and, if the child does not vomit at once, it is better to get him to a hospital or private doctor's office immediately.

Every public health nurse should know the nearest poison control center. (A directory of these centers can be obtained from the National Clearing House for Poison Control Centers, Public Health Service, Division of Accident Prevention, U.S. Department of Health, Education, and Welfare.)

If substances containing strong alkalis have been ingested, dilute vinegar or fruit juices should be given; after acid poisoning, milk of magnesia can be used. Milk and raw egg whites act as precipitants for certain metals. Starch is an antidote for iodine.

If kerosene or gasoline has been ingested, *no* attempt should be made to have the child vomit, since aspiration may lead to bronchitis or pneumonitis. Vegetable or mineral oil should be given, since this slows the absorption of kerosene or gasoline.

When corrosives have been taken, such as lye or Clorox, no emetics should be given nor should vomiting be induced. Weak vinegar, fruit juices, plus water or milk should be given. Olive oil applied to the burned area of the mouth in lye poisoning may relieve pain.

When the child is taken to the hospital, a lavage is done unless the child has swallowed a corrosive. There is a difference of opinion as to whether a lavage should be performed on the child who has swallowed kerosene.

During a lavage, the head of the bed or table should be lowered. The nurse should inquire if the doctor wishes to have the washings sent to the laboratory for identification of the poison.

A specific antidote for the poison may be given, if there is one. Other treatment depends on the poison taken and the condition of the patient.

Lists of common poisons and their symptoms and treatment can be found in Shirkey's *Pediatric Therapy* and in *Nelson's Textbook of Pediatrics.* A list of counterdoses for home use is published by the American Druggist and can often be obtained at neighboring drugstores.

LEAD POISONING

The danger of chronic lead poisoning lies in the fact that brain encephalopathy can occur.

Since there are now regulations prohibiting use of lead in paints, the source of lead poisoning is likely to be from inhaling the fumes of an old storage battery or eating flakes of paint peeling from a fence or wall. This is more commonly seen among groups of a low socioeconomic level. It is associated sometimes with a child who has pica: an abnormal or perverted appetite for foreign materials such as dirt, ashes, or grass. Pica, when present, is usually observed in children during the first 3 years of life.

If a child develops acute lead poisoning, the symptoms that result may refer to the gastrointestinal, circulatory, or central nervous system. On admission to the hospital, some of the outstanding manifestations are vomiting, abdominal pain, irritability, muscular incoordination, hypertension, weakness, and convulsions. Hematological abnormalities are low hemoglobin level, decreased red blood cell count, and hypochromic microcytic red blood cells on the blood smear. The cerebrospinal fluid results usually reveal an elevated white cell count, increased protein, and an elevated pressure.

In acute lead poisoning there is a trace of lead in the urine, an increased density at the ends of long bones (shown by x-ray film), a blue lead line along the gums, and an excessive concentration in the blood and cerebrospinal fluid. In collecting a urine specimen, care must be taken to ensure that there are no lead contaminants in the receptacle used for collection. Coproporphyrin levels in the urine may be used in confirming the diagnosis and in screening children.

Early diagnosis and treatment are essential in preventing sequelae. Gastric lavage may be done in addition to giving the patient magnesium sulfate. Dimercaprol (BAL) together with edathamil (calcium disodium edetate) may be prescribed in order to remove lead from the system by causing mobilization of the lead in the bloodstream and its excretion through the kidneys.

If convulsive seizures are present, medications such as paraldehyde or sodium phenobarbital may be given. The nursing care in that instance would be the same as for any child having a convulsion (p. 494.) During the period when the child has hypertension and convulsions, all possible stimuli should be kept at a minimum. The child is handled as little as possible; however, he should be turned and propped on his side frequently enough to prevent the development of pneumonia.

During the child's convalescence, careful observation and evaluation for signs of mental retardation or emotional disturbances should be included in the plan of management.

FRACTURES
The problem

Fractures are more common in the child of school age than in the preschool child and infant. The school and the camp nurse may see a child with a fracture before the physician sees him. The nurse in the newborn nursery may encounter a newborn infant with a fracture, and the nurse on the pediatric unit may care for a

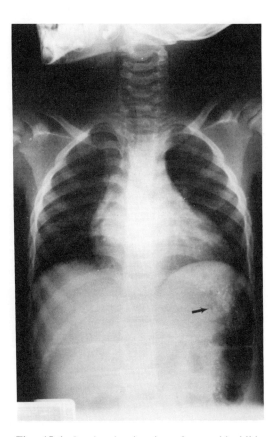

Fig. 15-4. Lead poisoning in a 3-year-old child. Note lead-containing paint flakes (end of arrow) in intestine that child ingested from paint peeling off wall in his home.

child who needs to be observed a few days after the application of a cast to a fractured bone or a child who is in traction after the reduction of a fracture. Many children are treated for fractures in a private physician's office or in the accident room of the hospital and then go home.

Definitions

A *simple* fracture is a break in the continuity of the bone. A *compound* fracture occurs when there is a communication between the bone and the outside. Fractures not due to trauma may occur in children with certain diseases such as osteomyelitis and tumors and with cysts of the bone. These are called *pathological* fractures. A *greenstick* fracture is one in which the convex side of a bone breaks but the concave side bends. If a bone is broken into three or more fragments, it is called a *comminuted* fracture. Terms such as *transverse, oblique,* and *spiral* allude to the direction or angle of the break.

Manifestations of a break

Loss of motion, pain, crepitus, swelling, and deformity of the part affected are all manifestations of a break. The injured extremity may be shorter or look different from the opposite extremity. In transferring the child with a fracture to a hospital, the affected part should be splinted to avoid further injury unless it is the elbow or the clavicle that is injured. In those cases the arm on the affected side should be placed in a sling. If the child has one injury, the nurse should look to see if there are abrasions, bleeding, or injuries in any other parts of the body. The child may suffer shock from the fracture so he should be kept warm.

Treatment

The aims of treating a child who has a fracture are to reduce the fracture, to maintain the reduction of the fracture, and to restore the function of the part injured. The earlier the fracture is reduced, the less swelling there is. Usually most of the fractures in children can be treated by closed reduction. Proper alignment in positioning is important; however, exact apposition or end-to-end contact of bone fragments is not essential to children. There can be some overlapping of bones, as children are still in the growing process. The reduction is most frequently maintained by a cast but sometimes by traction. Open reduction is rare in children. If it is done, the fracture is held in place by a nail, screws, or plate.

Children's fractures tend to heal more rapidly than adult fractures. Also, there is seldom any permanent limitation of motion of the injured part after prolonged immobilization. Physical therapy is not as necessary in treating children after fractures as it is in an adult.

Motion is not urged when children have fractures of the elbow. Pain will limit the child's motion of the part. When the child no longer has protective spasms, he will use the arm.

Fracture of clavicle

The clavicle is the most frequently fractured bone in children. In the newborn such a fracture could result from a difficult delivery. The neonate should be observed to determine if his arms move. If he has a fractured clavicle, he may appear to have a pseudoparalysis of the arm.

An older child may complain of pain in the shoulder and refuse to use the arm on the affected side. In order to relax the sternocleidomastoid muscle he may have his head tilted toward the affected side and his face away from it. One shoulder is lower than the other, and he will not raise his arm above shoulder level.

The child may be taken to the operating room and the fracture reduced under general anesthesia. A figure-of-eight pressure dressing or a plaster of Paris bandage may be applied to hold the reduced fracture in place.

After the clavicle is reduced the nurse needs to observe the circulation of the arm frequently. She should note the swelling, temperature of the fingers (extreme cold or heat), and any loss of motion of fingers. In judging the circulation of the fingers she should press against one of the fingernails on the affected side. With pressure the nail should blanch, but color should return immediately.

The child's position should be changed often enough to keep him comfortable. The injured part should be elevated on a pillow. Ice applied to swollen tissue sometimes helps to relieve pain. (Special skin care to the child with a cast,

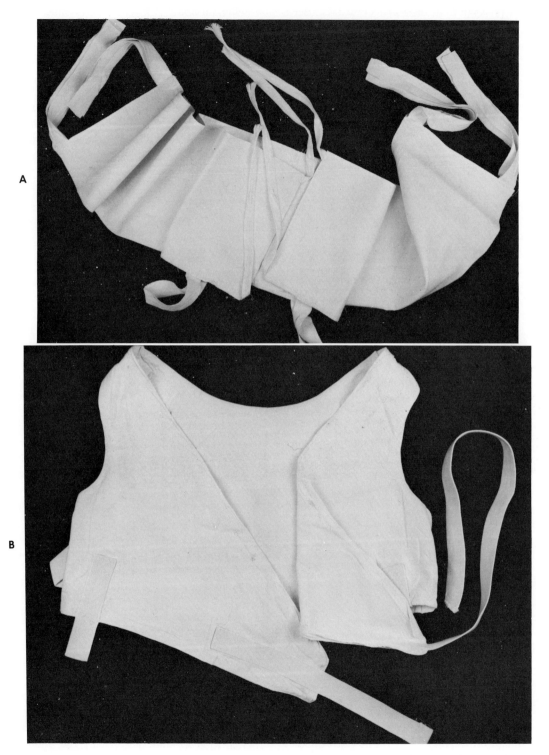

Fig. 15-5. A, Hibbs restraint. **B,** Waist restraint. The Hibbs and waist restraints can be used interchangeably for patients in Bryant's traction. (Courtesy The Children's Memorial Hospital, Chicago.)

as well as cast care, is described on p. 341.)

Medications for discomfort may or may not be necessary after the reduction. When making the child comfortable for the night, it is helpful if a sedative is given in order to ensure him a good night's rest. To break an arm and suddenly be hospitalized may be emotionally disturbing to the child. Sleep helps him to gain emotional stability. Of course, if he is in pain, he cannot sleep and should be given a medication.

Supracondylar fracture

The child with the supracondylar fracture is hospitalized for a few days to make sure the circulation is all right, since there is real danger of venous occlusion. The radial pulse of the affected arm should be checked at least hourly while there is still any swelling present. If no pulse can be felt, the physician needs to be notified at once. He removes the cast and extends the arm.

Other measures of nursing care are the same as those outlined for the child with a fractured clavicle.

Fracture of femur

The child who has a fractured femur and is under 3 years of age or less than 30 pounds in weight is often placed in Bryant's traction. An older child is placed in Russell's traction (skin traction) or skeletal traction with a Kirschner wire. Traction is used when there is a displacement of fragments of the bones. After several weeks the child is taken out of traction and a plaster of Paris cast applied.

Bryant's traction. When the child is in Bryant's traction, the nurse must make sure the circulation in both legs is good. (The uninjured leg is placed at a right angle to the body, as is the injured leg.) The legs should be rewrapped twice daily. When rewrapping them, the nurse should note if the adhesive has slipped on either of the legs. The child's position should be such that his buttocks are off the bed (or Bradford frame if that is used). A waist restraint or binder should be utilized to keep the child in position. Weights should hang clear and not be resting against the end of the crib. The weights should be placed in a canvas bag or secured firmly so there is no danger of their falling.

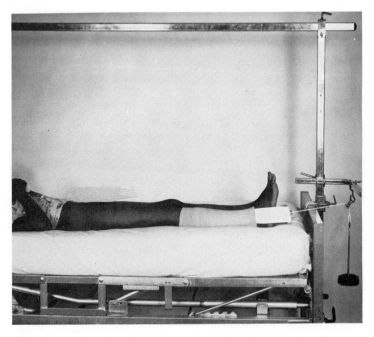

Fig. 15-6. Buck's extension, used to exert traction in the long axis of the lower limb with knee and hip in neutral position. (From Raney, R. B., and Brashear, H. R.: Shands' handbook of orthopaedic surgery, ed. 8, St. Louis, 1971, The C. V. Mosby Co.)

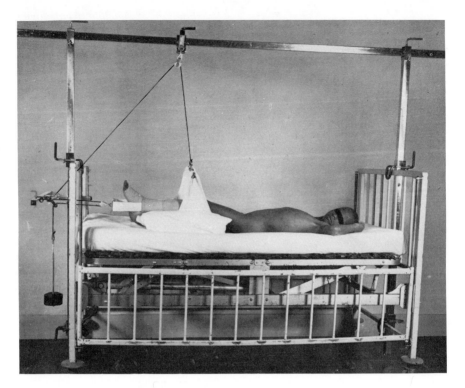

Fig. 15-7. Russell's traction, applied for a fracture of the left femoral shaft in a girl 5 years of age. This rope-and-pulley arrangement results in a traction force acting on the long axis of the femur that is approximately twice as great as the force that suspends the knee. This type of skin traction is especially useful for children over the age of 3 years and for adolescents. (From Raney, R. B., and Brashear, H. R.: Shands' handbook of orthopaedic surgery, ed. 8, St. Louis, 1971, The C. V. Mosby Co.)

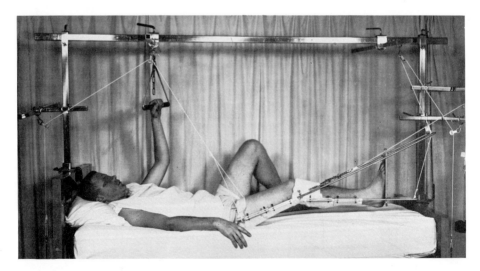

Fig. 15-8. Balanced skeletal traction. Traction in the long axis of the right thigh is applied by means of a Kirschner wire through the proximal portion of the tibia. The limb is supported by a Thomas splint beneath the thigh and a Pearson attachment beneath the leg. An additional attachment prevents foot drop. Weights apply countertraction to the upper end of the Thomas splint and suspend its lower end. By using his left limbs as shown, the patient can shift the position of his hips, without changing the amount of the traction. (From Raney, R. B., and Brashear, H. R.: Shands' handbook of orthopaedic surgery, ed. 8, St. Louis, 1971, The C. V. Mosby Co.)

The child is usually comfortable but needs diversional activity. Normally a child is active, and it is hard for him to be in bed for several weeks.

Russell's traction. If the child is in Russell's traction, again the nurse should make sure that the child's body is in alignment so the traction is serviceable. She should also see that the child has not slipped down in bed so his food is against the end of the bed and the traction is not effective. The foot of the affected leg is to be kept at a right angle to prevent development of foot drop. A special footplate is sometimes used for this. The uninjured leg should receive range of motion exercise at least daily.

An orthopedic bedpan, which is flat on one end, should be used for the child in traction. It is easier for the nurse to slip it under the child and causes the child less discomfort while he is using it than an ordinary bedpan. The child in traction is unable to wear pajamas, but every effort should be made to avoid undue exposure. A cloth **T** binder or loin cloth for this type of patient should be part of the linen supply of every pediatric unit. Special skin care to the child's back, elbows, and bony prominences should be done three to four times daily (morning, afternoon, evening before bedtime). At these times, also, drawsheets can be tightened and crumbs brushed from the sheet.

Since he will be in the hospital for several weeks, provision should be made for the child of school age to continue his school studies.

Compound fracture

A compound fracture is one in which the skin is broken and there is communication to the outside. When this kind of break occurs, the child is given prophylaxis against tetanus. The wound is carefully cleansed. The fracture is reduced and the position is often maintained by traction. The wound may or may not be sutured in accord with the physician's evaluation of it. If it is a badly contaminated wound, it may be left open rather than closed by suture in order to prevent the possibility of gas gangrene. Chemotherapy is usually ordered.

HEAD INJURY

It is of particular importance that the school nurse and camp nurse realize that any child who has had any type of trauma or injury to his head, particularly if there was a loss of consciousness, should be seen by a physician. A child can receive brain damage without having a fractured skull. The extent of brain injury does not necessarily show up immediately; therefore medical supervision is necessary for a period of time.

Minor head injury

If a child falls out of a tree, falls from playground apparatus, or falls off a horse, he may be stunned. He should be seen by a physician, but he might not be hospitalized.

If the child is at school when this happens and the school nurse is present, she should notice whether the pupils of his eyes are equal, whether he can move all extremities, and what degree of alertness he shows; if the child is at camp, the same is true. In addition, the nurse should look to see if he is hurt anywhere else. Vital signs such as temperature, pulse, blood pressure, and respiration should be taken. This establishes a baseline to see if there is any variation later. The physician may wish to examine the child at camp before having any x-ray films taken, or he may suggest that the child be brought to his office or a hospital. If the physician examines the child and decides not to hospitalize him, he may request that the child be awakened several times the first night to make sure he is sleeping and not slipping into a coma. Vomiting, increasing drowsiness, inequality of pupils, or persistent headache of the child should be reported at once to the physician.

When a child seems to be alert, acts as usual, and has a normal appetite, the amount of physical activity he is allowed is increased.

Severe closed head injury

Immediate care. When a child is injured in an automobile accident or otherwise is rendered unconscious by a closed head injury, attention should be given to establishing a sufficient airway for the child; next, the child should be so positioned that he cannot aspirate secretions. For the person in a comatose state the gag, swallowing, and cough reflexes are absent.

Hospitalization and nursing care. When the pediatric nurse is notified that a child is being admitted who has a head injury or was in an automobile accident, she should select a room for him, if possible, that has both oxygen and suction. If there is none, then a means of suction and oxygen should be made available for the child. Also, a padded tongue depressor should be at the bedside, as the child with a head injury sometimes has convulsions. For this reason, plus the fact that the child may be comatose, side rails should be fastened on one side of the bed. The side rail on the other side can be put in position after the child has been placed in bed.

When the child is admitted, the nurse should see if he has any dyspnea and position him to avoid aspiration of secretions, as noted earlier. Next she should take the vital signs immediately. Since the signs will be taken frequently (half-hourly or hourly) until they are stable, it is well if the nurse graphs his vital signs in a small supplementary chart. Any change in the pulse, respiration, blood pressure, or temperature can be readily recognized if graphed. A steady rise of blood pressure and/or diminishing of pulse and respiration may indicate increasing intracranial pressure and should be reported. Also, a persistent hyperthermia is serious.

Observations. Accurate and frequent observations of the child are essential in relation to his eyes, motor activity, and state of consciousness. The nurse should *not* record, "child is conscious." She should tell what the child says, whether he knows his name, whether he can follow a suggestion as "squeeze my hand," or if the child asks where he is and calls for his mother. All of this is important to record, as is also his general behavior, restlessness, or drowsiness. Besides this, the equality and appearance of the pupils of the eyes should be noted. They may be large and dilated or of pinpoint type; the pupils may be unequal or equal in size.

Whether the child can move all of his extremities should be noted also. The spontaneous activity of an infant should be recorded. If one extremity seems weaker than the other or if the child moves one hand or leg more freely than the other, this should be noted on the chart, together with any observation of spasticity. Important to know also is whether the child is able to void if he is conscious. Daily observations should include a comment about the hydration status of the child, that is, whether he shows any signs of dehydration. In addition, any marked changes in the child's vital signs should be reported.

Emotional support. The child with a head injury needs reassurance in his new surroundings. True, any hospitalized child does, but this child was hurt suddenly. He may not know what happened to him and to others who were with him. If possible, one of the family should remain with the child.

If he is alone, without one of his family, the head nurse should be able to secure a volunteer to sit with the child. Crying makes a headache worse and elevates blood pressure, so every effort should be made to help the child in his adjustment to the hospital.

Convulsive seizures. For care of a child during a convulsion see p. 494. Anticonvulsive medication may be prescribed, such as sodium phenobarbital or diazepam (Valium).

Oxygen therapy. Oxygen therapy may be used, as it is important that an impaired brain have sufficient oxygen. Restlessness may be a sign of air hunger. Oxygen may be prescribed by the physician in an effort to prevent brain damage due to anoxia.

Fluid intake and output. Fluids may be taken by mouth if the child is conscious; if he is not, intravenous fluid therapy may be started. If the child remains comatose, fluids and nutrition may be given by a nasopharyngeal tube. All fluids given (either orally, by gavage, or intravenously) should be recorded, as well as the approximate amount in any vomitus. An accurate record of his urinary output should also be kept. If the child is unconscious, he may be placed on constant bladder drainage.

Administration of medication. For restlessness, aspirin is frequently ordered. This may be given by gavage, by rectum, or by mouth, depending upon the patient and his condition. Paraldehyde, phenobarbital, or small amounts of codeine may be given for extreme restlessness. Narcotics are avoided, as the brain function is already depressed. Chemotherapy may be ordered if the child had a fractured skull or if the child is on constant bladder drainage. Restlessness is better controlled by medication than by restraining the child, since a child fights restraints and this would send his blood pressure even higher.

Temperature-reducing measures. Since the child's temperature is very often elevated, various measures to reduce temperature may be utilized (see p. 292). A tepid sponge bath may be prescribed and/or antipyretic medications as aspirin. A cool oxygen tent may help. Offering cool oral fluids is valuable if the child can take fluids orally. After those measures have been employed the temperature should continue to be taken every half hour because it is possible for the temperature to drop suddenly, especially in a young child.

Personal hygiene. If the patient is comatose, in addition to the general nursing measures for comfort, special attention should be paid to skin care and to oral hygiene. Secretions around the nares should be carefully cleansed. Special skin care should be given frequently to the back, buttocks, and bony prominences. Hair should be combed twice daily. If the patient has long hair, it may be best to part the hair and braid it. Attention should be given to the patient's bowel hygiene. When the brain is injured, the metabolism of the child is slowed. Constipation should be avoided. If the child fails to have a stool daily, the nurse should call this to the physician's attention.

Convalescence. When vital signs are stable, the activity of the child is *gradually* increased. Children with head injuries are ambulated as early as possible. As usual, the pulse should be taken before and after ambulation to see if there is much variation. If the child vomits or has a severe headache following ambulation, this should be reported to the physician. It is difficult to say how long a child may be hospitalized with a head injury. It depends on the child and the extent of the injury.

Fracture of skull

The nursing responsibilities for a child with a fractured skull are the same as for a child with a closed head injury, except that the nurse should watch for any bleeding from the nose or ear or evidence of hemorrhage in other areas such as the orbit and the periorbital tissues. These manifestations are associated with basal fractures. Hematomas may be associated with linear frac-

tures. Chemotherapy is usually prescribed prophylactically for children with basilar skull fractures.

Depressed fractures are sometimes seen in the newborn baby as a result of a difficult delivery. Older children may have a depressed fracture as a result of an automobile accident. A burr hole is made in normal bone, and the depressed bone is then elevated into position.

Open head injury

In open head injuries, prophylaxis against tetanus is given, as well as chemotherapy. The head is shaved around the injured area and the wound carefully cleansed. Local scalp wounds are usually sutured. If the wound is deep, the same principles of treatment hold true as for a compound fracture of other bones. (See p. 451.)

As there is danger of meningitis from an open skull wound, in addition to nursing care described under closed head injuries, the nurse should be alert to the presence of any rigidity or spasticity of the child's neck or body and also to undue irritability or drowsiness. A careful record of the fluid intake and urinary output should be kept.

Subdural hematoma

A subdural hematoma is a collection or accumulation of blood in the subdural spaces. This condition is due to direct trauma to the head. Older children can tell of a fall or injury, but sometimes parents of an infant do not give a history of an infant's injury. Trauma during the birth process is a possibility. The condition is not common in the newborn period of life but is seen most frequently in the middle months of the first year of life of the infant. The incidence decreases with the age of the infant. After the second year of life it is not seen unless older children suffer head injury in various types of accidents.

The nurse should be alert to symptoms of increased intracranial pressure secondary to the enlarging hematoma. Irritability, drowsiness, projectile vomiting, tense or bulging fontanels, and convulsions are all signs of increased pressure. A tight and glossy scalp is sometimes seen. There may be a separation of cranial sutures. If the nurse sees an infant with these symptoms in her home visits or in her other contacts with infants, she should urge the parents to take the infant to a physician for medical care.

When an infant is admitted to the hospital with a tentative diagnosis of subdural hematoma, the nurse should carefully observe him, since after a subdural tap is done, signs of increased intracranial pressure usually decrease in severity and then sometimes increase again before another tap is done.

When helping the physician in his examination of the infant, the nurse may see the physician pay particular attention to the eyes of the infant. This is because retinal hemorrhage ultimately develops in most of the affected children. It may not be present initially. During the physician's examination, the nurse will notice also that the infant's reflexes are hyperactive.

If the blood pressure and vital signs are ordered, the nurse should be quick to report an increasing blood pressure together with slow and irregular respirations. There is a widening difference between the blood pressure and pulse. This denotes increased intracranial pressure due to hemorrhage.

As stated, a subdural tap is done (via the anterior fontanel) as a diagnostic procedure. If a large amount of fluid is removed, there will be a decrease in the increased intracranial pressure, thereby making the procedure therapeutic as well as diagnostic. The same equipment needed for a lumbar puncture is used for this procedure. The head must be held securely during the procedure to prevent damage to the brain. If fluid is obtained from the subdural hematoma, it is usually brownish red in color (old blood).

Usually taps are repeated daily for almost 2 weeks. If the amount of fluid decreases each time a tap is done, the infant may convalesce

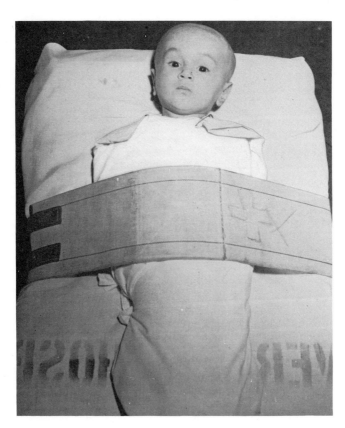

Fig. 15-9. Body restraint for subdural puncture. (From DeSanctis, A. G., and Varga, C.: Handbook of pediatric medical emergencies, ed. 3, St. Louis, 1963, The C. V. Mosby Co.)

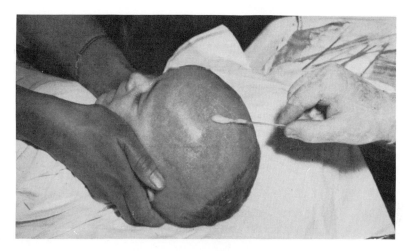

Fig. 15-10. Preparation for subdural puncture, including proper immobilization of the head. (From DeSanctis, A. G., and Varga, C.: Handbook of pediatric medical emergencies, ed. 3, St. Louis, 1963, The C. V. Mosby Co.)

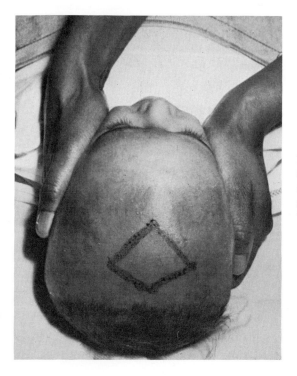

Fig. 15-11. Outline of margins of the anterior fontanel as a guide for subdural puncture. (From DeSanctis, A. G., and Varga, C.: Handbook of pediatric medical emergencies, ed. 3, St. Louis, 1963, The C. V. Mosby Co.)

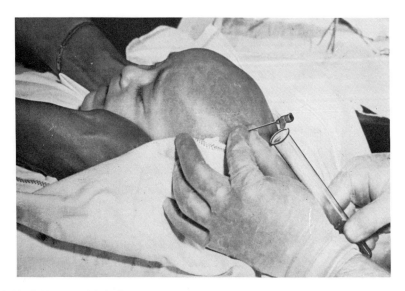

Fig. 15-12. Collection of fluid from subdural hematoma. (From DeSanctis, A. G., and Varga, C.: Handbook of pediatric medical emergencies, ed. 3, St. Louis, 1963, The C. V. Mosby Co.)

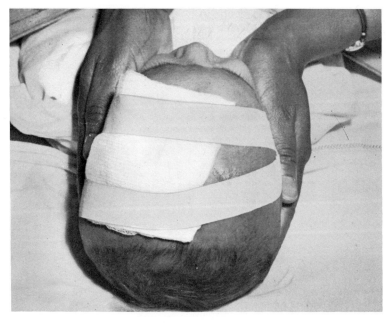

Fig. 15-13. Dressing in place after subdural puncture. (From DeSanctis, A. G., and Varga, C.: Handbook of pediatric medical emergencies, ed. 3, St. Louis, 1963, The C. V. Mosby Co.)

without further treatment. On the other hand, more drastic measures may need to be done if conservative measures fail. A craniotomy may be performed, with removal of the clot and as much of the membrane around the clot as possible.

Treatment is essential to the infant, since his brain grows rapidly and needs room for expansion. The prognosis for this condition is good if atrophy of the brain has not already taken place prior to operation or other treatment.

BATTERED CHILD SYNDROME

The battered child syndrome is an extreme form of a whole spectrum of nonaccidental injury and deprivation of children. The battered child is characteristically one who has suffered serious injury from intentional physical trauma by his parents or parent surrogates. The abuse may vary from neglect to such physical trauma that the child may die. The physical injuries may vary from mild bruising to fractures of the long bones and ribs to subdural hematoma with or without a skull fracture.

Incidence

Battering of children is one of the most serious concerns facing society. No one really knows the true incidence of the battered child syndrome. Kempe (1971) reports that the annual number of cases in the United States is estimated to be 30,000 to 50,000.

Authorities in this field agree that the true frequency is higher than is being reported. Kempe has estimated that at least 700 children are killed every year in this country by their parents or parent surrogates. Thousands more are permanently injured either physically or mentally. The majority of the battered children are under the age of 3 years because their age makes them defenseless against severe forms of punishment.

Clues in diagnosing child abuse

The battered child syndrome should be suspected when a child is brought into a doctor's office or hospital emergency room if (1) the child has an unexplained injury, (2) the child has dehydration and/or malnutrition without an obvious cause, (3) there are physical findings of

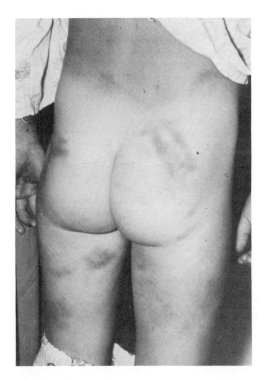

Fig. 15-14. Eight-year-old boy with multiple bruises caused by many beatings with a belt.

overall poor physical care, (4) the child shows an unusual fear of people and surroundings, (5) the child "takes over" care for the parents, (6) the parents see the child as "bad" or "different" in emotional makeup, (7) the child is dressed inappropriately for the injury, (8) there are multiple old and new bruises and skin injuries, (9) there are old and healing fractures, and (10) injuries are found during the examination that are not mentioned in the history.

Parents should be suspected of battering their child when they bring their child to a doctor's office or hospital emergency room and the evaluation reveals (1) a marked discrepancy between the history and the actual injury, (2) a history of repeated injuries, (3) that the parents are reluctant to give information or refuse to give consent for studies, (4) that the parents are hospital and doctor "shopping" for medical and emergency care, (5) that the parents have unrealistic expectations for the child, (6) contradictory histories between parents, (7) a delay in seeking medical care for the injury, (8) overreaction or underreaction to the injury, (9) a

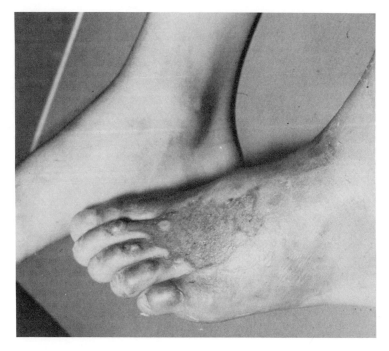

Fig. 15-15. Burn of foot caused by holding child's foot under hot running water from faucet.

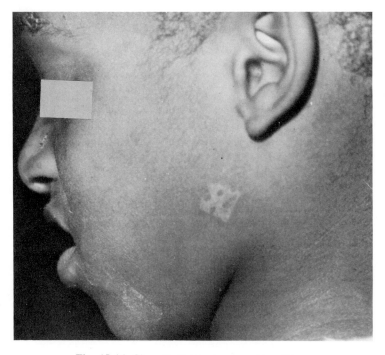

Fig. 15-16. Cigarette lighter burn on side of face.

disturbed parent-child relationship, and (10) familial discord or financial stress.

Whenever there is a suspicion of child abuse, protective services should be provided to the child immediately. Hospitalization of the child is usually required since most of the injuries will need constant medical attention. During the hospitalization a complete blood coagulation workup is performed to rule out a bleeding disorder, total body roentgenograms are taken to search for old and healing fractures, and a psychological evaluation is done to establish if any emotional trauma is evident in the child. After the workup is completed, the findings obtained from the medical history, physical examination, and laboratory examinations are assembled and correlated to establish whether the battered child syndrome is possible or not. If the diagnosis is established or suspected, the case is reported to the appropriate agency in the community dealing with child abuse and neglect for further evaluation of the home environment.

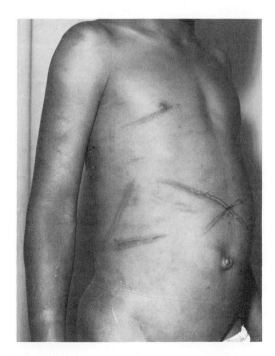

Fig. 15-17. "Cross mark" laceration of child's abdomen made with a knife as a means of "cutting the devil out of him."

Characteristics of abusive parents

Parents who physically abuse their children come from all walks of life and all socioeconomic levels. The type of child rearing that these parents practice has a high demand for the child to perform to gratify the parents. They frequently use severe punishment to ensure the child's proper behavior. Many of them have been emotionally deprived and abused as children. Abusive parents were raised in a family in which they were expected to perform well at all costs, as well as never having their emotional needs adequately considered or met. They learned to satisfy their parent's expectations and desires to avoid severe punishment. Many of these parents have no basic, firm cushion of self-esteem or awareness of being loved. They are in constant need of reassurance from their spouse, friends, and relatives. Any minor indication by relatives or spouse of a poor performance on their part may produce a crisis of unmet needs. In such a crisis, they repeat what they have learned during their childhood and turn to their child for nurturing and reassurance.

It is frequently very difficult for these parents to seek help. The greater the amount of aggression and abuse to which the parents were exposed in childhood, the more difficult it will be for them to seek help and the more severe is the abuse. The abusive parent who is unable to turn to his spouse for help will become inevitably frustrated and will often turn to the child for emotional support. The parent-child relationship becomes out of balance, and battering is more likely to occur.

In-depth observation and evaluation of the parents' attitude toward their children must be obtained. Usually each child has a special meaning to his parents. One child may be perceived as entirely gratifying and comforting to the parents. This child usually has learned to please his parents and how to avoid displeasing them very early in life. Such a child becomes overly controlled and submissive and therefore is rarely physically abused. Abusive parents frequently state that the child has thwarted their desires, interfered with their life, or just been a troublemaker for the family. They view the infant or child as older than his chronological age and as having greater physical ability and intellectual development than he actually has. A typical parent statement reflecting their feelings is "I never can do anything for myself because Sara is always sick" or "Joey is a miserable child, even when I am being nice to him." Persistent crying by an infant despite parental efforts to comfort or care for the child's needs may be interpreted by the parents as criticism of their efforts and evidence of their parenting inadequacy.

When battering occurs there is usually a crisis in the family. One element of the crisis may be that the child soiled his pants, has broken something, or has been disobedient. The child taxed the parents' tolerance to the breaking point. The other element of the crisis is some event producing lower esteem and desperate need for reassurance on the part of the parent. One common precipitant is the withdrawal or leaving of a spouse. Another example is an unwanted pregnancy, because the mother may be overburdened by the tasks of caring for her children. This is frequently the product of a disturbed sexual relationship between husband and wife.

Generally in order for a parent to abuse a child three things have to occur. These three components usually occur in some kind of sequence and are almost always seen in one or both parents. The three components are (1) the potential for abuse, (2) a very special kind of child, and (3) a crisis. *The potential for abuse* may exist if the parents were abused or neglected by their own parents, cannot turn to people when in need of help, have a poor marital relationship, and have unrealistic expectations of the child. A *very special kind of child* is one who is "different" in physical and emotional makeup than the other children in the family or is one who is constantly overdemanding and irritable as compared to the other child who is "good" and happy. An example of a *crisis* is present when there is no food, money, or job for the breadwinner. The crisis is usually a precipitating factor to battering and not an etiological factor.

Treatment of parents

In dealing with cases of child abuse, the objective should be to help both the parent and the child. The destructive pattern of behavior should be interrupted, as well as dealing with the emotional conflicts that have produced the behavior in both individuals. Some of the parents may have to be separated from their child to prevent further injury, whereas others may be allowed to continue caring for the child while they undergo some form of psychiatric therapy. It must be stressed that the parent is not actually guilty because his aggressive acts are based upon unreality. Therefore punishment to mobilize guilt is doomed to failure.

The parents will become very dependent on the therapist early during the treatment. These patients tend to wear one out emotionally; they are challenging and often almost ask to be rejected. The growth of dependency is accomplished by discussing alternative ways of problem solving, relieving frustration, and coping with children. The visits are mostly devoted to listening, understanding, and uncritical approval, with focus on the parents' needs rather than on the child's. Therefore, if the parents' basic needs are met, the child will be safe and the parents will become loving and giving to their children. In a few child protection centers where therapy of this kind is being offered, 80% of the children are back with their parents within 8 to 12 months of initiation of treatment.

Prognosis

The prognosis is dependent upon the length of time that battering occurs. Ten-year followup studies reveal that 40% of the children were emotionally disturbed, 50% had I.Q.'s below 80, and 60% had some failure in physical growth. Only 10% of the battered children in this sample fell within normal limits on measures of emotional, intellectual, and physical growth. If the children survive, they have a 90% chance of developmental retardation. In general, battered children possess a 6% to 10% chance of mortality.

Treatment of child

The nurse is one of the most important persons involved in the team approach to care for the abused child. Case finding and listening to the plea for help from battering parents can be accomplished when the nurse is able to recognize the symptoms that are predisposing to the battering. These symptoms may be recognized in the prenatal clinic prior to the birth of the child, in a pediatric office, in a health unit clinic, or in the pediatric ward of a hospital. Some frequent statements by these mothers are that of frustration at their crying infant, extreme distress over behavior of a child, and how difficult it is to care for this child. In most cases one parent or the other has made a plea for help that was not heard. The nurse should be very sensitive about a parent who brings a child to the physician for "no reason at all." The nurse should talk with the parent and obtain valuable information concerning (1) how the mother is facing the responsibilities of her marriage, home, and newborn infant, (2) what her stresses are and how she handles them, (3) how the new mother views her child and how she feels when cleaning the child when he is soiled with urine or feces, and (4) the amount of anxiety that a crying infant brings on, especially when the parents are alone with the infant.

When interviewing these parents it is safe and helpful to express a sympathetic understanding that the parent has been trying very hard to do well in the face of unusual difficulties and that the circumstances have created overwhelming problems. It is important to focus on the parents' problem and needs and to avoid centering attention on the child and his injuries. A promise to help get things organized will frequently bring a sigh of relief from the parents. Parents are in constant fear of punitive actions being taken against them if they reveal any information about themselves and the negative feelings they have about their children.

The nurse is an ideal person to evaluate and teach child-rearing practices to the parents. Parents need to feel a warmth of emotional support from the nurse. It is important to talk to the mother about feeding the child, discipline, and growth and development. Abusive parents, because of the idiosyncrasies of their own personalities, focus on particular phases of the child's growth and development and become distressed by the child's failure to perform adequately at such periods. The hardest time to cope with children is the first months of life because they are most demanding and the least rewarding to the parent. For some of these parents the stage of toilet training is when most of the

difficulties occur, whereas for others it is when the child begins to talk or walk. Persistent crying of an infant despite parental efforts to comfort or care for the child's needs is the most common precipitant to abusive behavior by a parent. The parent interprets the crying as criticism of their efforts and evidence of their inadequacy.

Abusive parents have an inadequate art of mothering or parenting. Lack of parenting in the abusive parents is because they were reared in a home where their emotional needs were never considered or met and they had to orient themselves toward parental satisfaction to avoid severe punishment. Many of the abusive parents were abused, severely punished, criticized, and expected to perform well to gratify parental needs during very early childhood. The nurse may give such parents assistance by working side by side with them to teach mothering abilities. She must encourage the mother to express her feelings about her role as a woman, wife, and mother. It becomes very trying and exhausting to work with this kind of mother. If the mother becomes very angry and upset, the nurse must continue to feel very sympathetic and understanding. Gradually, as the art of mothering improves, the marital relationship improves and the mother will begin to get a sense of pleasure and satisfaction from her child. As the feeling of acceptance and attention occurs, the parent in turn is better able to minister to needs of the child.

An accomplishment from the nurse's efforts has resulted if the mother states "my child is interesting and lots of fun."

Prevention

After a child has been diagnosed as being a battered child there are three possible solutions to prevent recurrence of battering:

1. The child is temporarily placed in a relative's home or foster home while the parents obtain professional counseling, and the child is returned home when safe.
2. The child is returned home with the parents under protective services by the juvenile court or department of family services; the parents would also be expected to get professional counseling.
3. The child could be placed for adoption

since the home would never be safe for his return.

The greatest reason for prevention of recurrence of battering is to help the child grow up without physical abuse so that when he becomes a parent he will not be a battering parent. Preventing the abuse will interrupt the generation-to-generation cycle of the battered child syndrome.

The establishment of child protection centers to help coordinate the multidisciplinary agencies has proved to be effective in many communities. The personnel employed by the center are social workers, pediatric nurses, psychologists, psychiatrists, lawyers, and police officers. The objectives of a child protection center are (1) to improve methods of early diagnosis of child abuse, (2) to develop treatment programs for the child and parents, (3) to improve community attitudes toward handling children and family, (4) to develop coordinated community services, (5) to improve professionals' attitudes toward child abuse cases, (6) to develop evaluation and training programs, and (7) to do research. Child protection centers that have been in operation for some time have shown that there are (1) a decrease in the death rate due to child abuse, (2) a decrease in recurrence rate of child abuse, (3) an increase in the number of early reports of child abuse, and (4) an improvement in communication between agencies.

Mothers Anonymous and Parents Anonymous are self-help groups that have developed in the larger cities of the United States. These groups attempt to provide a place and an atmosphere in which abusive parents can share their feelings with other parents who have also been destructive toward their own children. The abusive parent becomes dependent upon someone in the group. This friend can give support, love, and affection and can be sensitive to needs of the parent that have never been understood or met before. The friend is always available during a time when a crisis occurs in the home.

In most cities day care centers are available where battering parents can place their children while they do something for themselves or be alone for awhile. These centers should be able to help parents interact with their children and develop support from each other. We must al-ways remember that most battering parents love their children most of the time.

In larger cities crisis nurseries are becoming available to battering parents to provide a place for them to bring their children when they are on the verge of battering them because of a fear of losing control or of a situation that is too stressful. After a period of cooling off, the parent returns to pick his child up and returns home in much better shape to care for his needs.

Abusive parents who are severely disturbed should be managed by a mental health clinic team, family counseling service, or private psychiatrist or psychologist. The hospital medical and nursing staff should provide the parents with the treatment resources available in the community. The arrangements to see a professional person should be made by the parents before discharge of the child.

All states have laws that make child abuse a criminal offense and require physicians and nurses to report it to the proper agency. Most of the laws contain a section that provides full protection to the person reporting the abuse. Many states have laws establishing protective social services that will provide protection of the child and treatment for the parents. Nurses may be required to testify in court about abuse cases; therefore accurate and detailed notes are important in helping to recall observations. Termination of parental rights may become necessary for the good and safety of the child. However, only a few states provide laws that allow termination of parental rights. In states without this law, children are left in foster care until they become of adult age.

REFERENCES
Common psychological factors

Bakwin, H., and Bakwin, R.: Behavior disorders in children, ed. 9, Philadelphia, 1972, W. B. Saunders Co.

Barnes, C.: Support of a mother in the care of a child with esophageal lye burns, Nurs. Clin. North Am. **4**:53, March, 1969.

Bowden, M., and Feller, I.: Family reaction to severe burn, Am. J. Nurs. **73**:317, February, 1973.

Brooks, M.: What play in the hospital? Nurs. Clin. North Am. **5**:431, September, 1970.

Hyde, N.: Play therapy—thr troubled child's self-encounter, Am. J. Nurs. **71**:1366, July, 1971.

Kjaer, G.: Psychiatric aspects of thermal burns, Northwest Med. **68**:537, June, 1969.

Long, R., and Cope, O.: Emotional problems of burned children, N. Engl. J. Med. **264**:1121, 1961.

McFarland, R., and Moore, R.: Childhood accidents and injuries. In Talbot, N., et al., editors: Behavioral science in pediatric medicine, Philadelphia, 1971, W. B. Saunders Co.

Vigliano, A., et al.: Psychiatric sequelae of old burns in children and their parents, Am. J. Orthopsychiatr. **34:**753, 1964.

Burns

Antoon, A. Y., Volpe, J. J., and Crawford, J. D.: Burn encephalopathy in children, Pediatrics **50:**609, 1972.

Artz, C., and Moncrief, J.: The treatment of burns, ed. 2, Philadelphia, 1969, W. B. Saunders Co.

Bleck, E. E.: Causes of burns in children, J.A.M.A. **158:**100, 1955.

Boles, E. T., Jr.: Burn management in children, South. Med. J. **56:**1089, 1963.

Caudle, P. R. K., and Potter, J.: Characteristics of burned children and the after effects of the injury, Br. J. Plast. Surg. **23:**63, 1970.

Claudia, S.: TLC and Sulfamylon for burned children, Am. J. Nurs. **69:**755, April, 1969.

Colebrook, L., and Colebrook, V.: The prevention of burning accidents, Br. Med. J. **1:**4980, 1956.

Crawford, J., and Antoon, A. Y.: Burns. In Kagan, B., and Gellis, S., editors: Current pediatric therapy, ed. 6, Philadelphia, 1973, W. B. Saunders Co.

Haynes, B. W., Jr.: Management of burns in children, J. Trauma **5:**267, March, 1965.

Jacoby, F. G.: Nursing care of the patient with burns, ed. 2, St. Louis, 1976, The C. V. Mosby Co.

Jensen, G. D.: Prevention implications of a study of 100 children treated for serious burns, Pediatrics **24:**623, 1959.

Lund, C. L., and Browder, N. C.: The estimation of areas of burns, Surg. Gynecol. Obstet. **79:**352, 1944.

Margolius, F.: Burned children, infection, and nursing care, Nurs. Clin. North Am. **5:**131, 1970.

MacMillan, B.: Management of burns in children. In Shirkey, H. C., editor: Pediatric therapy, ed. 5, St. Louis, 1975, The C. V. Mosby Co.

McGregor, I. A.: Fundamental techniques of plastic surgery and their surgical application, ed. 5, Baltimore, 1972, The Williams & Wilkins Co.

Polk, H., and Stone, H. H., editors: Contemporary burn management, Boston, 1971, Little, Brown & Company.

Quinlan, E.: Dietary treatment in burns, Can. Nurse **61:**375, 1965.

Smith, E. I.: Acute management of thermal burns in children, Surg. Clin. North Am. **50**(4):805, 1970.

Waller, J., and Manheimer, D.: Nonfatal burns of children in a well-defined urban population, J. Pediatr. **65:**863, 1964.

Wood, M., Henry, H. A., and Price, W. R.: Silver nitrate treatment of burns, Am. J. Nurs. **66:**518, 1966.

Foreign bodies, ingestion of poisons, and lead poisoning

Arena, J.: Poisoning and its treatment. In Shirkey, H. C., editor: Pediatric therapy, ed. 5, St. Louis, 1975, The C. V. Mosby Co.

Byers, R. K.: Lead poisoning: review of literature and report on 45 cases, Pediatrics **23:**585, 1959.

Cachia, E. A., and Fenech, F. F.: Kerosene poisoning in children, Arch. Dis. Child. **39:**502, 1964.

Covey, T. J.: Ferrous sulfate poisoning, J. Pediatr. **64:**218, 1964.

Etteldorf, J. N., et al.: Intermittent peritoneal dialysis using 5% albumin in the treatment of salicylate intoxication in children, J. Pediatr. **58:**226, 1961.

Fowler, R. S., et al.: Accidental digitalis intoxication in children, J. Pediatr. **64:**188, 1964.

Gross, R.: The surgery of infancy and childhood, Philadelphia, 1953, W. B. Saunders Co., p. 246.

Jensen, G. D., and Wilson, W. W.: Preventive implications of a study of 100 poisonings in children, Pediatrics **25:**490, 1960.

Kopito, L., et al.: Chronic plumbism in children. Diagnosis by hair analysis, J.A.M.A. **209:**243, 1969.

Pickering, D.: Salicylate poisoning; the diagnosis when its possibility is denied by the parents, Acta Pediatr. **53:**501, 1964.

Reed, A. J.: Lead poisoning—silent epidemic and social crime, Am. J. Nurs. **72:**2180, December, 1972.

Segar, W. E., et al.: Peritoneal dialysis in infants and small children, Pediatrics **27:**603, 1961.

Shirkey, H. C., editor: Pediatric therapy, ed. 5, St. Louis, 1975, The C. V. Mosby Co.

Skellenger, W.: Treatment of poisoning in children, Am. J. Nurs. **65:**108, Nov., 1965.

Vaughn, V. C., III, and McKay, R. J., editors: Nelson's textbook of pediatrics, ed. 10, Philadelphia, 1975, W. B. Saunders Co.

Verhulst, H., and Crotty, J.: Childhood poisoning accidents, J.A.M.A. **203:**145, 1968.

Fractures

Blount, W. D.: Fractures in children, Baltimore, 1955, The Williams & Wilkins Co.

Drain, C. B.: The athletic knee injury, Am. J. Nurs. **71:**536, March, 1971.

Hilt, N. E., and Schmitt, E. W., Jr.: Pediatric orthopedic nursing, St. Louis, 1975, The C. V. Mosby Co.

Larson, C. B., and Gould, M.: Orthopedic nursing, ed. 8, St. Louis, 1974, The C. V. Mosby Co.

McFarland, R. A.: The epidemiology of motor vehicle accidents, J.A.M.A. **180:**289, 1962.

Raney, R. B., and Brashear, H. R.: Shands' handbook of orthopaedic surgery, ed. 8, St. Louis, 1971, The C. V. Mosby Co.

Reeves, K.: Children's reactions to head injuries, Am. J. Nurs. **70:**108, January, 1970.

Swenson, O.: Pediatric surgery, ed. 3, New York, 1969, Appleton-Century-Crofts.

Head injury

Brandesky, G.: Severe head injuries in children; treatment and long-range outlook, Clin. Pediatr. **4:**141, 1965.

Carini, E., and Owens, G.: Neurological and neurosurgical nursing, ed. 6, St. Louis, 1974, The C. V. Mosby Co.

Matson, D.: Neurosurgery of infancy and childhood, ed. 2, Springfield, Ill., 1969, Charles C Thomas, Publisher.

McFarland, R. A.: The epidemiology of motor vehicle accidents, J.A.M.A. **180**:289, 1962.

Reeves, K.: Children's reactions to head injuries, Am. J. Nurs. **70**:108, January, 1970.

Young, J.: Recognition, significance and recording of the signs of increased intracranial pressure, Nurs. Clin. North Am. **4**(2):223, June, 1969.

Battered child syndrome

Bullard, D. M., et al.: Failure to thrive in the neglected child, Am. J. Orthopsychiatr. **37**:680, 1967.

Clark, J., and Sawyer, J.: I solemnly swear—a nurse testifies to child neglect, Nurs. Outlook **68**:35, April, 1968.

Committee on Infant and Preschool Child, American Academy of Pediatrics: Maltreatment of children: the battered child syndrome, Pediatrics **50**:160, July, 1972.

Fontana, V.: The maltreated child, the maltreatment syndrome in children, Springfield, Ill., 1964, Charles C Thomas, Publisher.

Hall, M.: The right to live, Nurs. Outlook **15**:63, August, 1967.

Helfer, R., and Kempe, C. H., editors: The battered child, Chicago, 1968, University of Chicago Press.

Holter, J. C., and Friedman, S. B.: Principles of management in child abuse cases, Amer. J. Orthopsychiatr. **38**:127, 1968.

Hopkins,: The nurse and the abused child, Nurs. Clin. North Am. **5**:589, December, 1970.

Jacobziner, H.: Rescuing the battered child, Am. J. Nurs. **64**:92, June, 1964.

Kempe, H., et al.: The battered child syndrome, J.A.M.A. **181**:17, 1962.

Kempe, C. H.: Paediatric implications of the battered baby syndrome, Arch. Dis. Child. **46**(245):28, 1971.

Klein, M., and Stern, L.: Low birth weight and the battered child syndrome, Am. J. Dis. Child. **122**:15, July, 1971.

Paulsen, M.: Legal protections against child abuse, Children **13**:42, March-April, 1966.

Pollock, C.: Early case finding as a means of prevention of child abuse. In Helfer, R., and Kempe, C. H., editors: The battered child, Chicago, 1968, University of Chicago Press.

Shydro, J.: Child abuse, Nursing '72 **2**:37, December, 1972.

Symposium on Child Abuse (Rochester, N. Y., October 19, 1971), Denver, 1972, The American Humane Association, Children's Division.

16

Nursing care of
THE CHILD WITH PROLONGED
MEDICAL SUPERVISION

COMMON PSYCHOLOGICAL FACTORS

The child who has an illness with which he has to live, such as rheumatic carditis, diabetes, or cystic fibrosis, has problems relating not only to himself but to his family as well. Most of the conditions discussed in this chapter stay with the child throughout his life. During this time, he may have acute episodes of the disease in which he is hospitalized more than once. These acute episodes are discouraging to both parents and child. A discussion of the child with nephrosis is included because of his repeated hospitalizations in early childhood, although in later childhood he may be free of the condition.

First, let us consider the possible effects of a chronic condition on the child. If the child has diabetes or rheumatic carditis that is under control, he does not look different from other children; but he knows that he is not the same, that there is something unusual. During the period from 10 to 15 years of age, this is especially hard since he longs to identify with his peer group and to be just like them. This is the height of the gang age—the age in which each sex enjoys primarily the companionship of members of their own sex. In addition during the adolescent period, the healthy teenager is concerned about his body. Indeed, he may feel lonely or different from others and wonder if he has been adopted. At the same time he is striving for independence and dislikes what seem like arbitrary rules and regulations. When a patient has a chronic health problem, there are certain rules in which it is essential that he conform, lest he have an acute episode of the illness and have to return to the hospital. For example, even if a diabetic teenager is on an unrestricted diet (p. 471), he still has to test his urine and give himself insulin. It is normal for this diabetic child or for the child with rheumatic fever who has to take an oral antibiotic for an indefinite period to feel rebellious at times. As the young person progresses from elementary school to junior and then senior high school, it is important for him to take increasing responsibility for maintaining his health, especially during the teenage period. This reduces possible nagging from parents, although it does not mean that the parents do not supervise this son or daughter.

To what extent the child with a chronic condition thinks he is different from others is determined first by how well he feels physically, second by the philosophy of his family toward his condition, and third by the way those unrelated to him behave toward him.

The school nurse and the public health nurse who sees him at home are in a vital position to aid the child. If they know his treatment and his limitations, they can emphasize the child's need of being given responsibility and treated exactly like other children with no special privileges. The less attention drawn to him, the more relaxed the child can be. To be in school the same as others and to enjoy the same activities insofar as his condition permits is very important to a child. Where there is a question about an activity—bicycle riding, participation in scout activities, roller skating, dancing, and more competitive athletics—then the doctor should be contacted for advice.

465

In maintaining and promoting his health, the public health nurse (or school health nurse) has a responsibility to see that he keeps hospital clinic appointments or appointments with his own doctor. When a child is feeling well, often he and his family do not realize the importance of medical follow-up examinations; nor do they understand the importance, for example, of having the child with cystic fibrosis continue with breathing and postural exercises, or having the child with rheumatic carditis continue to take an oral antibiotic.

When the child is hospitalized and remains there for 2 or 3 weeks, a month, or even longer, he misses contacts with other children, he misses school and home, he is bored, and, if he does not feel acutely ill, it is very trying to stay in bed. Besides this, children may well regard frequent physical examinations as invasions of privacy. They both resent and fear being repeatedly stuck with a needle, whether it is by a doctor or nurse. If the family cannot visit the hospital more than weekly, the child may feel rejected and forgotten. The so-called "good" child who makes no trouble may be close to despair.

What can be done to avoid or offset negative factors? After all, the child's attitude toward readmissions is influenced by his experiences on former admissions. Cheerful surroundings, recreational diversions, attractive meals, school (if he is well enough), and the presence of other children his age make hospitalization easier to bear. Special birthday or other parties give the child something to anticipate and to discuss afterward. Parents should be encouraged to send postcards and suggest to the child's friends at home that they do likewise. Seeing the charge nurse on each shift, if only for a few minutes, helps to give the child a sense of protection and a feeling that someone cares about him.

The child who has cystic fibrosis or nephrosis is often a young child, who may find separation from parents even harder than do children of school age. Visiting privileges should be planned to meet the needs of the individual child.

For the child who is at home and unable to attend school, the public health nurse might be instrumental in getting a visiting teacher for the child. She might also see if the family is known to the local church of the family's faith. She could contact the scout office to see if the child at home could participate in any kind of scout activity or if a scout leader or older scout could visit the child weekly for diversional purposes. Possibly there would be a circulatory library from which books could be secured for him.

The child who is in bed at home might like a plant that he can water daily and watch grow or want to put a sweet potato in a glass with water and in time see the vine grow from it. Goldfish, a canary, or a pet of some kind—perhaps a kitten—may provide fun. Other games or play materials should be in accordance with the child's age and interests. The public health nurse's visit in itself is a diversion for him. Other children should be invited to the home to play or visit with the child if his social and emotional development is not going to be neglected. Perhaps he could be placed on a couch or cot in the living room or room where others in the family spend most of their time. In this way the child might feel more as if he is part of the family.

On the other hand, what do repeated episodes of hospitalization or a long hospitalization mean to the family of the child? In those diseases in which there is a familial tendency (diabetes, rheumatic fever, cystic fibrosis), there may be renewed guilt feelings each time the child is returned to the hospital. Because of this the family may be oversolicitous, or they may feel they cannot do enough for the child. Also, the parents may be depressed and discouraged. They have tried to follow the physician's advice and yet here the child is once more in the hospital.

If there are other children in the family, should the mother neglect them and remain with the sick child in the hospital? If the hospital is some distance away from home, there may be a problem of transportation. In addition, there is the cost of hospitalization. Even if some of the child's expences are paid by an agency such as crippled children's service, the parent is usually expected to pay something toward hospitalization costs.

From distress to depression to discouragement the parents may finally come to a feeling of hostility toward the child. There may be a change in the child-parent relationship and possibly in the relationship of other siblings toward the child who is a special expense and who takes so much of the mother's attention, especially if she stays with the sick child during his hospitalization.

To try to maintain desirable family relationships is important. Services of a medical worker are of great importance when caring for any child who has a chronic disease or a condition that requires repeated hospitalizations.

Parents as well as the child need emotional support. In the hospital and clinic this can be given by all members of the medical team, but at home it is the public health nurse who can be of special assistance. The mother may receive help from talking with neighbors, but the nurse is in a better position to understand the possible ambivalence of the mother's and the father's feelings toward the child. The mother needs to feel that the nurse accepts and likes her, especially if the child's condition is one with a familial tendency. The nurse can encourage the mother to express herself and yet, at the same time, point out that at least the mother does have the privilege of loving and caring for a child. In the Bible, Jesus said, "Let the little children come unto me, for of such is the Kingdom of Heaven."

It is helpful to the mental hygiene of parents if they, like parents of children with congenital abnormalities (p. 338), have at least one outside interest, something that gives them pleasure outside of the home. Even the brief separation of a few hours helps them to keep the situation in better perspective. The mother who is at home for the entire day may be more depressed than the father who has his work.

In conclusion, if a child has a condition requiring prolonged medical supervision, not only does the child but also the child's family have to live with this condition and make friends with it. For the entire family to try to continue living just as they would ordinarily is important for each member. The focus of attention should not be the limitations of the disease. The emphasis should be on what the child can do rather than on what he cannot do. If the affected child can acquire a special skill in keeping with his condition, this will bolster self-confidence.

ALLERGY

An allergic condition represents the hypersensitivity of the body to certain substances. These substances serve as antigens in the body and produce symptoms of allergic reactions. Infantile eczema, rhinitis, hay fever, and asthma are examples of allergies.

Causes of allergies include genetic factors, foods, inhalants, pollens, emotions, and physical factors. Common foods to which an allergic young child may be sensitive are wheat, cow's milk, citrus fruits, eggs, chocolate, and fish. House dust is an inhalant to which an allergic child is often hypersensitive. Common pollens come from trees, grasses, and ragweed. Materials containing wool may be irritating to the skin. The dander from household pets may cause an allergic reaction.

Measures for control
Environmental control

Through elimination and avoidance of specific agents, if that is possible, the symptoms of an allergy may be abated. When a child has any history of allergy, measures for general environmental control of allergens should be instituted. Neither stuffed animals and toys nor pets should be permitted. Particular attention should be paid to the child's bedroom. It should be damp-dusted daily. Rugs, upholstered furniture, venetian blinds and drapes should be taken from the room. It should be furnished with the bare necessities only—a bed, a dresser, and a wooden chair. If possible, the clothes of the child should be kept in another room and he should dress and undress in a room other than his bedroom. Cotton blankets should be substituted for woolen ones. The mattress should have a plastic covering on it and a foam rubber pillow be substituted for a feather pillow. The door to the bedroom should be kept shut and also, during the daytime, the windows. An air conditioner in the summertime is helpful. In selecting clothing for the child, wool should be avoided. Food such as chocolate, citrus fruits, wheat, and eggs should be omitted from the diet.

Drugs

Antihistamines are the group of drugs most commonly used to produce symptomatic relief from an allergy. The antihistaminic drugs block the action of free histamine on the tissues, thus relieving the symptoms of hay fever, allergic rhinitis, and urticaria. They are less effective in the relief of asthma.

Epinephrine (Adrenalin) given subcutaneously is the most important adrenergic drug used in the management of atopy and anaphylactic reactions. It is highly and rapidly effective in relieving asthma, urticaria, and anaphylactic reactions to insert stings, drugs, and injected allergens. Isoproterenol (Isuprel) is another drug of the group. It is used chiefly by inhalation and sublingual administration in the management of asthmatic patients.

Corticosteroids are used to inhibit a wide variety of immediate and delayed allergic reactions by stimulation of the secretion of endogenous adrenal hormones. They are usually used in patients who have severe and chronic manifestations of allergic disease. When they are used, they should be used with care because of their many undesirable side effects.

Drugs are used for the quickest relief of allergic disease. Symptomatic drug treatment is not curative in allergic disease, and recurrence of symptoms must be expected when the drug being administered is stopped.

Desensitization

If the child is not relieved by the preceding measures, skin testing is done to see what the child is allergic to, and steps are taken to desensitize the child accordingly with extracts of the appropriate antigens.

Manifestations of allergy

Infantile eczema

Infantile eczema is uncommon in breast-fed infants. Sometimes the condition is due to contact irritants. It is frequently associated with a dry skin and is most often seen on the extremities and exposed surfaces, including the scalp. Through scratching, the skin becomes excoriated. Weeping of involved areas and sometimes bleeding may be seen. There may be a secondary infection.

When the skin is weeping or shows raw areas, soaks with various solutions such as Burow's solution or saline solution may be used. Later, starch baths or Alpha-Keri added to the bath water may allay itching. Coal tar preparations and other ointments may be used when the infection and/or weeping has been cleared. Corticosteroid ointment or Vioform ointment is sometimes used. Antihistamines are usually prescribed for the itching.

Because of the susceptibility of the infant with eczema to infections, especially respiratory ones, he is not hospitalized if it is at all possible to treat him as a private patient or to treat him in a pediatric clinic of a hospital outpatient department. The infant whom the hospital nurse sees in the pediatric unit has a severe case of eczema.

In planning the daily care of the infant the nurse should bear in mind that this infant has all the needs of any normal infant, plus needs for the special care of his skin. The infant needs affection and cuddling even more than the well infant, but because his physical appearance is not appealing, it is likely that he will receive less of it than other infants. He needs exercise and sensory stimulation. Food is important, and he does not like to be kept waiting when he is hungry. He may have even less power to cope with frustration than other infants. Emotional factors are sometimes involved in any form of allergy.

In cleansing the infant, soap is not used, but water or oil. The skin should be treated with whatever is recommended: compresses, special baths, or ointments. The nurse needs to be conscientious in giving special skin care, since ointments and compresses help to allay the intensity of the itching. An infant's arms need to be restrained by elbow cuffs so that he cannot scratch himself. Certainly once on every tour of duty the nurse should remove the infant's restraints in order to let him exercise, but of course she should watch to make sure that he does not scratch himself. Fingernails should be cut short. Recreational diversion helps to distract the infant's attention from himself.

Fluids should be offered these infants frequently, since the skin often is very dry. The infants may be on a regular diet for age if the formula is *not* made with cow's milk. Evaporated milk and a Sobee or Nutramigen formula are usually prescribed. Citrus fruits, eggs, and foods containing wheat are usually omitted from the diet. When the infant is being fed, he can be wrapped in a sheet and held in the nurse's arms. This can be one of his exercise periods.

The nurse needs to have patience with the eczema infant, who is irritable and fussy because he is in discomfort. Sometimes a medication is prescribed to allay the itching.

Before the child is discharged it is important that the parents understand special directions for the child's diet; also, the general environmental control should be explained to them. The infant's need for play and warmth of affection should receive emphasis.

Many children over 2 or 3 years of age sometimes seem to outgrow the eczema and to build up resistance and tolerance to the factors responsible for it; however, some continue to show some symptoms or allergic manifestations such as hay fever and asthma.

Asthma

Asthma is a common condition in which there are usually wheezing respiration and paroxysms of coughing. The child often has a feeling of tightness in his chest and may complain of not being able to breathe. The anxiety produced by the latter may lead to a vicious cycle of increased breathing, calling into play auxiliary muscles of respiration (the neck accessories and nasal alae), increased hyperinflation, and great inefficiency in breathing. The child may sweat profusely, sit upright, and appear pale and even cyanotic.

The primary problem is one of diffuse airway obstruction, partly due to bronchiolar and bronchial smooth muscle spasm, mucosal edema, varying degrees of inflammatory reaction, and/or retained thick secretions. The increased airway resistance and decrease in usable lung space (due to hyperinflation) lead to increased breathing effort and changes in the pattern of breathing. The child with chronic or recurrent asthma frequently suffers a variable but persistent state of airway obstruction.

In childhood, most asthma is on an allergic basis, although it may sometimes occur only during periods of respiratory infection. Seldom is an emotional factor paramount. Emotional tensions in the home are often a natural result of repeated and frightening attacks. In infancy, asthma often is the result of an infectious process compromising already tiny air passages.

The allergic nature of asthma is confirmed by a family history of allergic disorders, seasonal or environmental changes in symptoms, and positive reactions to common inhalant allergens, such as tree or grass pollens, ragweed, house dust, or molds.

Vigorous physical exertion (such as swimming, basketball, or even laughing loudly at television) may so alter the breathing pattern as to induce some degree of transient bronchospasm and wheezing. This has too often led to unnecessary and unfortunate restriction of a child's activity and resulted in friction in the home.

Management of the child with asthma centers chiefly around providing environmental control to allow minimal indoor exposure to common allergens (such as feathers, animal dander, wool, molds, house dust, and occasional foods) and irritants (tobacco smoke, strong odors, too dry air). Keeping bedroom windows closed in the daytime or providing an air conditioner in the bedroom is helpful in controlling outdoor pollen. If significant, hyposensitization to suspected common pollen and mold allergens, as well as house dust, is usually desirable. Medication should always be considered supplemental to environmental controls rather than as a substitute. Acute episodes are usually managed initially with epinephrine, with long-term therapy usually built around oral ephedrine. Aerosol medication can often be substituted for an injection for treating the acute episode in the home, but the nurse must be certain that the patient does not substitute the short-acting aerosol bronchodilator for long-acting oral preparations. This can and may lead to severe dependency on the aerosol unit. Corticosteroids are usually reserved for treatment of hospitalized patients whose condition is severe or for addition to the already stated regimen in patients with chronic and severe asthmatic states, which produce either physical handicapping or considerable absence from school.

DIABETES MELLITUS

The office nurse may see the child with diabetes before he is acutely ill, since the child's mother may complain because he is underweight, or the diabetes may be discovered when a routine urinalysis is done because the child is ill with a respiratory or other infection. On the other hand, the infant or young child may be brought into the hospital in a diabetic coma before it has been discovered that he has diabetes.

The onset of diabetes is rapid. The disorder may be precipitated by an acute infection, a physical injury, a severe emotional disturbance, or some other stressful situation. That diabetes may be inherited is not necessarily known to all parents; consequently, even if a close relative has diabetes, parents do not always watch for the disease in their child.

The school nurse's attention may be drawn to the child because he is losing weight and seems easily fatigued. Of course, the school nurse may be informed that there is a diabetic child in a certain school. In that situation the nurse has a chance to help the school personnel develop a better understanding of the illness and a chance to help the child and his family learn to live with this condition without feeling unduly handicapped.

Nature of the condition

Diabetes mellitus is a metabolic disturbance in which there is insufficient production of insulin. This interferes with the metabolism of carbohydrates, fats, proteins, and minerals. The relationship of this disease to endocrine glands other than the pancreas is not completely understood. Diabetes is inherited, probably as a recessive trait.

The nurse needs to review the anatomy and physiology of the pancreas in order to have an appreciation of what happens when the pancreas is not functioning normally.

Hyperglycemia (excessive sugar in the blood) and glycosuria (sugar in the urine) are associated with abnormal carbohydrate metabolism. Since glucose is not used by the peripheral tissues, hyperglycemia results. Glycosuria occurs when hyperglycemia exceeds the renal threshold. Through the resulting polyuria there is excessive loss of electrolytes and water.

Ketonuria and ketonemia are associated with abnormal fat metabolism. When there is impaired storage of glycogen in the liver due to insufficiency of insulin, fat combustion is substituted for carbohydrate. The breakdown of fats causes the formation of ketone bodies. These ketones are discharged into the blood. Ketonuria occurs when the peripheral tissues are unable to oxidize ketone bodies as rapidly as they are formed and when the number of ketones in the blood exceeds the ability of the kidney to excrete them and the ability of peripheral tissues to oxidize them. Accumulation of ketone bodies causes increased polyuria so there are further disturbances in the electrolyte and acid-base balance. The presence of acetone in the urine shows that there is an excessive formation of ketones. This is serious. The accumulations of ketone bodies in the blood, impaired renal function, the loss of a fixed base, and dehydration are factors in the development of acidosis. The child can go from diabetic acidosis to coma and death.

The disease is diagnosed by finding sugar in the blood and urine. Normally, there is no sugar in the urine. If the blood sugar level is higher than 200 mg. per 100 ml. or if a fasting blood sugar level is higher than normal, diabetes is suspected. A glucose tolerance test may be done if there is a question.

If acidosis is present, the carbon dioxide content of the blood or the carbon dioxide combining power is lowered. The pH is acid. Sometimes there is an elevated nonprotein nitrogen. In the urine, acetone is present, and occasionally albumin and casts.

In treating the child with diabetes the aim is not only to control the metabolic aspects of the disease but to promote normal growth and development and to have the child phychologically adjusted. Growth is stunted in uncontrolled diabetes. Administration of insulin is essential because it restores the normal metabolism.

There is a difference of opinion as to the diet of the child. One type of diet is a prescribed diet, which is measured. Exchange lists of food are available.* Insulin is essential to renal metabolism of glucose. Fasting blood sugar should be within a normal range in the treated child. The other plan is to permit a nonrestricted diet in which the child eats according to his appetite and in accord with food requirements of nondiabetic children. The amount of insulin should be enough to avoid ketonuria but to permit some glycosuria. Advocates of this regimen believe that there are fewer reactions with this program and less psychological stress. They believe that hyperglycemia without ketosis is not harmful.

Advocates of the prescribed diet believe that hyperglycemia and glycosuria are harmful and are factors in the development of degenerative diseases of the kidneys, eyes, and cardiovascular system.

Special problems of diabetes in childhood

There are differences to be considered between the child with diabetes and the adult with diabetes. Familiarity with these differences helps the nurse's understanding, and in consequence she may be of greater assistance in getting the child to the physician sooner than she might otherwise.

The onset of diabetes in children is more rapid than that in adults. In contrast to the obesity seen in adults, diabetic children are thin. They fail to grow and thrive. In uncontrolled diabetes, growth is stunted. Symptoms of polydipsia (excessive thirst), polyphagia (excessive appetite), and polyuria (excessive urine) are seen in children just as in adults. However, in a child the polyuria may result in bedwetting after the child has been toilet trained. Secondary skin infections are common around the genital area in small children. Hair on the body of young children has an unusually soft texture.

Intercurrent infection and disease such as mumps, measles, and respiratory infections increase the problem of controlling diabetes. When ill, children need more insulin. Illness, especially hospitalization, may mean emotional stress and that, too, affects the need for insulin. Other factors affecting this need are exercise

and growth. When the child is active, he needs less insulin; with increased growth he needs more.

The diet has to be one that meets the growth needs of the child in various stages of his childhood and adolescence. In addition, children are more active than adults and have a more rapid basal metabolism. Caloric requirements are more crucial in children than in adults. Exercise and activity of children are variable; for example, on Saturdays the schoolchild is more active than on weekdays. It is easier to adjust the insulin of the child than the food.

Psychological adjustments may be hard for an adult but may be even more so for a child, especially at the time the adolescent body changes are occurring and he is concerned about his "normalcy." In the adolescent period there may be increased rebellion against restrictions in diet, testing of urine, taking insulin, etc. If the child cannot eat what the family eats, this is hard for him. He feels different from others. If he is eating the school lunch and cannot have what is allowed others, this marks him as different. He may feel inferior, which could lead him to be either an unduly withdrawn child or an aggressive troublemaker. Taking his lunch to school may cause less stress to the diabetic child.

The child with this disorder needs chances to succeed and the encouragement that accompanies a specific skill in order to build up feelings of confidence. Although any child needs companionship and supervision to help in learning to share, participate, and cooperate, the diabetic child especially needs to know he is one with others and is accepted and liked.

The attitude of the family toward the child is also a factor that influences the child to a great extent. (For further discussion of psychological factors in long-term illness see p. 465.)

Role of the nurse

Nurse in the child health conference. In taking the history of the child when he is first admitted to the conference, the nurse should ask if any relative has had diabetes. If the reply is positive, the nurse should call this to the physician's attention. She should compare the present weight of the infant with the birth weight

---

*The American Dietetic Association, 620 N. Michigan Ave., Chicago, Ill.

and watch to see if there is a steady, normal increase in weight and height at successive visits. Variation from expected levels should be reported to the physician.

School health nurse. A teacher may draw the school nurse's attention to a child who is very thin but has an unusually large appetite at lunchtime. Also, the teacher might notice the unusual frequence with which a particular child needs to go to the bathroom. The nurse should be alert to any such behavior of the child and refer the child for medical attention. Such a child may have diabetes.

If a child attending school is known to be diabetic, the nurse should make friends with both the child and his family to evaluate health instruction needed and to interpret the child's needs to the school.

Hospital nurse. A diabetic child may be admitted for regulation of his insulin and diet, or the nurse may see the child brought into the hospital in diabetic acidosis or coma.

Observations. If the child is in a *precomatose* condition when he is admitted, typical manifestations that the nurse should note and record include flushed cheeks, cherry red lips, acetone breath, hyperpnea, nausea, and vomiting, and possibly body pain, especially abdominal pain. If the child is *in coma,* there may be Kussmaul breathing (severe hyperpnea), rigid abdomen, soft eyeballs, and sunken eyes, in addition to the acetone breath and cherry red lips. Symptoms of dehydration are often present. Sometimes the respirations are grunting in character. The pulse is weak and rapid, and the blood pressure may be subnormal.

When the child is being adjusted to insulin, it is essential to watch for symptoms of insulin shock or reaction. These symptoms are variable. There is a change in the behavior of the child. He may suddenly become irritable and restless, or if playing with toys, he may become quiet and pale. An older child may complain of sudden hunger. There is a definite change in his behavior, no matter which direction the behavior takes. There should be orange juice on hand, which can be given the child in an emergency, or if this happens just prior to a meal, the tray or part of it can be served immediately. As soon as the child has taken food, he feels,

looks, and acts better. At all times the nurse assigned to the child should know the result of the last urine test, relative to both sugar and acetone. If the patient is not receiving enough insulin, he may show signs of diabetic acidosis. Precomatose symptoms have already been discussed.

The condition of the skin of the child should be carefully noted to see if there are any abrasions, bruises, or signs of infection. Skin infections are common in diabetic children. They heal slowly.

Skin care. The child needs a daily soap-and-water bath. If he is ill and in bed, special care needs to be given to elbows, ankles, and bony prominences several times a day. His position needs frequent changing while he is in bed.

Assisting with tests. The nurse may need to assist the doctor or laboratory technician while he takes blood for blood chemistries. The presence of the nurse when blood is drawn is particularly helpful to small children.

Collecting specimens of urine at certain intervals for testing for sugar and acetone is also part of the nurse's responsibility. Labeling each specimen correctly and sending it to the proper laboratory call for conscientiousness and exactness on the nurse's part.

Testing the urine. The child's urine is tested at various times in accord with the illness of the child and directions of the physician. Frequent testing is done during an illness, but when the child seems stabilized, possibly testing twice a day for sugar and once a day for acetone is all that the physician may believe is necessary.

While stabilizing the child, often the physician requests that urine be collected and tested four times a day (before each meal and at bedtime). In the morning the first voided specimen should be discarded. After drinking water the child should void again and this sample tested. This sample may show no sugar, but the previous sample might. The first voided specimen is really a night specimen.

Clinitest tablets or Benedict's solution is used to test urine for sugar. Acetest tablets or acetone test powder can be used to test urine for acetone. If the child is on a restricted diet, the hope is that no sugar will show in the urine; but if he is on a nonrestricted diet, it is acceptable to have a little sugar spilling in the urine all the time. The child is less likely to have insulin shock or be "shocky." However, no matter which diet the child has, the presence of a positive acetone test is very serious. If the acetone test is positive, the physician should be notified, since ketosis could be occurring. Additional insulin is given immediately. Blood chemistries may be done and further action taken in terms of the results of the blood chemistries.

Administering insulin. Insulin, as stated previously, is essential to normal glucose metabolism. Prior to its first use in 1922, life expectancy was very short. Now, there are various types of insulin available, differing mostly in the rapidity with which they work. Often the physician orders a combination of a slow-acting and a quick-acting insulin to be used. Infants and preschool children are more likely to be given a modified insulin rather than a long-acting type. The unmodified, regular insulin is the most rapid-acting insulin. NPH insulin has its greatest effect 7 to 11 hours after injection and generally has an effect for 20 to 24 hours. Protamine zinc insulin and lente insulin have maximal effect about 12 to 18 hours after injection and last for 24 hours. Globin insulin has maximal effects about 8 hours after injection and lasts about 18 hours. Often a maintenance dose of a long-acting insulin is ordered, and the regular insulin is adjusted according to urine tests. When the child is stabilized after the initial attack of diabetes, he may not need insulin for a few weeks; then he shows glycosuria and needs it. As he grows older, more insulin is required. Sometimes the adolescent and his family believe the diabetes is worse because more insulin is required than at age 6 or 7 years. This needs interpretation to them.

The nurse should give the insulin in a syringe that is specially made to facilitate the accurate dosage of insulin. If lente or NPH insulin is ordered, it can be placed in the same syringe as modified insulin.

The nurse should make a plan of locations at which the insulin should be injected. Others caring for the child on different tours of duty should know this plan and adhere to it so that insulin is not injected in the same place each time. Alternate thighs and arms can be used.

Health instruction. A definite plan for health instruction should be made so that the nurse is aware of the part she is to play. She must know what the doctor and nutritionist tell the child and his family and what the doctor wishes her to teach. Also, the nurse has a responsibility to see if the parents and the child have understood what the doctor has explained. Written directions in addition to verbal ones are helpful if the child and his family can read.

Usually, the nurse is the one who teaches the child how to test his urine, what the significance of the test is, and how to give his insulin. Even a 6-year-old child can be taught to test his urine and give insulin under supervision. The nurse can indicate how far back to pull the plunger of the syringe. The child should have a chance to practice this many times before leaving the hospital. The child's mother should be shown how to test urine and give insulin also. The child has to be familiar with figures before he can draw up the dose of insulin. A child 9 or 10 years old who is in the fourth or fifth grade should be able to do this; sometimes an 8-year-old child can. It depends on the child. A 10-year-old child requires less supervision in testing urine and in giving insulin, but a parent needs to see that the child takes time from his play to do it. The child should be given increasing responsibility as he gets older. By adolescence he should be able to regulate his diet and insulin with a minimum of supervision.

If the nutritionist could teach the child about his diet and also teach the mother how to adapt the child's diet to the family menu, it would be ideal, but sometimes this is not possible and the hospital nurse has to do this teaching. Sometimes the school health nurse has to do such teaching if it has not been done previously. If the child is of school age, taking his lunch to school may be better than eating lunch at home; however, if there is a school cafeteria, the child can be taught to select foods suitable for his diet.

Activities of the child need discussion. The child should be allowed freedom and outdoor exercise, but there should be an understanding that with additional exercise such as a long hike with scouts and then swimming, the school-age child will need either more food or less insulin.

It is reasonable to suppose that additional activity will increase his appetite.

Untoward symptoms suggestive of insulin shock or acidosis should be specifically taught to the child and his parents. The child should carry sugar in his pocket. Candy in his pocket is tempting for the child to eat, so that sugar is preferable. At home sweetened orange juice could be given if there are signs of insulin shock. At the same time the child and his family need to be taught the promotion of health in order to try to avoid illnesses with resultant changes in insulin needs. (For a discussion of health promotion refer to Chapter 9; for discussion of psychological aspects of a child with prolonged illness refer to p. 465.)

Discharge. When the child is ready for discharge, referral should be made to the public health nurse. For continuity of care the hospital nurse should be sure that the referral contains information about what has been taught to the child and his parents. If the child's home is in a city and there is a school health nurse, it is assured that the county health nurse will contact the school nurse to avoid duplication of work and to best serve the child. The school nurse can, as stated previously, interpret the child's needs to the school personnel and give guidance as necessary.

The mother may need continuing help in planning family meals so that the child will not feel different from the rest of the family. The family of the child may wish to join the American Diabetes Association through a local chapter. It may be comforting for them to know that there are many other parents whose children have diabetes.

If the family is receiving aid for dependent children from the welfare department, then that department should be notified of the condition of the child, since it may be able to give financial help with the insulin that the child requires.

Since emotional stress has a particularly negative effect on the child's physical status, the emotional climate in the home is important as well as the child's social and emotional health. If the parents have domestic conflicts, the nurse should make every effort to get them to talk with their minister or go to a particular community resource agency that gives family or marital counseling.

NEPHROTIC SYNDROME (NEPHROSIS)
Nature of the condition

The nephrotic syndrome is not a disease entity but a group of clinical and laboratory manifestations caused by a loss of protein in the urine. Proteinuria is the sine qua non of the nephrotic syndrome. Hypoalbuminemia, hypercholesterolemia, and generalized edema are usually present. The severity of these findings depends upon the duration and extent of the proteinuria. Most children with nephrosis are markedly pale, almost waxy. The blood pressure is normal, as is often the child's temperature, unless the child has an infection. Although there is generalized edema, the ascites is very prominent. During periods of severe edema, there is marked proteinemia and albuminuria. The urine volume is low, and the urine has a high specific gravity. Results of renal function tests such as urea clearance are normal.

The average age of onset is about 2½ years; it is uncommon in the first year. It occurs in about 8 children per 100,000 population under the age of 10 years. Etiology is unknown. In most instances it is not possible to relate the onset of nephrosis to another disease. There is reason to believe that there is an abnormal immune response to chemical substances, tissue antigens, or both in the child affected with this disorder. Nephrosis may be associated with such diseases as disseminated lupus erythematosus, amyloid disease, diabetes mellitus, or chronic glomerulonephritis. It may also follow a bee sting or poison oak dermatitis or ingestion of nephrotoxic agents such as penicillamine, gold salts, and mercury.

The most important clinical feature is proteinuria, although edema is the symptom that commonly suggests the diagnosis. The onset of edema is usually insidious and is first noted by the parents rather than the physician. As the swelling advances, it may involve the legs, arms, back, and abdomen. Accumulation of fluid in the scrotum and pleural cavity is common. The children appear to be very pale, more so than would be the case in anemia. Susceptibility to infections is increased during the periods of edema and hypoproteinemia. Pneumococcal peritonitis and pneumonia are the two most common infections diagnosed in these patients. Malnutrition may result because of a severe loss of protein in the urine and a lack of protein intake as a result of a poor appetite. The child's behavior and attitude may range from being irritable and depressed to being in remarkably good spirits even in the presence of massive edema.

The laboratory examinations play an important role in establishing the diagnosis as well as being used as guides to treatment and predicting prognosis. Urine analysis reveals a large amount of protein and on some occasions a few red blood cells. The daily urinary output of protein varies from 50 mg. 10 15 gm. per day. The blood protein and albumin levels are decreased, while the blood cholesterol is markedly elevated. The blood cholesterol level varies from 300 to 1,800 mg. per 100 ml. as compared to a normal level of 200 mg. per 100 ml. or less. The sedimentation rate is markedly elevated, but the serum complement is low.

It is not possible early in the disease to predict which children will recover and which will not. The average length of time of the active clinical disease with and without remissions is 12 to 18 months. Recent follow-up studies of children treated with steroids and antibiotic therapy reveal that 70% to 75% of the children could expect a favorable outcome.

The treatment is a long-term problem because of the chronicity of the disease. The parents must receive more than the usual amount of psychological support from the physician and nurse since these children will experience many exacerbations and remissions with an uncertain outcome. The diet of the nephrotic child is that suitable for the normal child. Salt intake is restricted only when severe edema is present. Antibiotics should be administered after exposure to bacterial infections promptly and more liberally to patients with possible bacterial infections. The continuous prophylactic use of antibiotics is not recommended. Adrenocorticosteroids (prednisone) are given to most children with nephrotic syndrome. In approximately 95% of children given steroids in large doses, there is a clinical and biochemical remission in 6 to 8 weeks. Diuresis usually occurs within 14 days after the beginning of steroid therapy. After the remission occurs, the steroid dosage is tapered rapidly and replaced by intermittent therapy, either every other day or 3 days in the week. Whenever the child has been free of proteinuria for several months, slow reduction in dosage is attempted until the steroids can be discontinued completely. Diuretics may provide important symptomatic relief in refractory patients or before diuresis has occurred in very edematous patients who are being treated with steroids. Immunosuppressant drugs (chlorambucil, cyclophosphamide) are reserved for the child with nephrosis who is nonresponsive to steroids or one who does respond to steroids but relapses frequently. Since these immunosuppressive agents are considered experimental they should be used by investigators actively engaged in studying the effects of these drugs in patients with the nephrotic syndrome.

Role of the nurse

Observations. Observations that help to indicate the condition or progress of the child's condition include the presence and location of edema and the color and general behavior of the child. If the child is irritable or lethargic, he is not feeling well. Sometimes these children become depressed. Behavior is symptomatic. Although there is generalized edema, any increase in the amount of abdominal distention is of particular interest since it may interfere with respirations; thus the child has respiratory distress. If this happens, an abdominal paracentesis may be done. As these children are susceptible to respiratory infections, the presence of a cough or nasal discharge should be noted and reported.

Skin care. During an acute episode, when the child is severely edematous, skin care, next to administration of medications, is probably the most important single aspect of the child's care. The child's eyes should be bathed gently with cotton balls, going from the inner canthus to the outer canthus. There may be dried secretions on the eyelids. Eye care should be given several times a day. Bathing the entire body of the child helps to promote circulation. Special skin care should be given to the child's back, buttocks, and bony prominences several times a day to prevent the skin from breaking down. The scrotum can be elevated or supported with a T binder. When the child lies on his side, a pillow should be placed under the knee and leg that are uppermost to support them and keep the child comfortable. A pad of foam rubber might be used under the child's hips. The child's position should be changed at least every 2 to 3 hours and every 4 hours at night when he is awake for comfort and to prevent bedsores.

Nutrition. Since the child is losing protein in his urine, the protein intake should be increased. Salt added to food is withheld because of the generalized edema. Also, fluid intake is restricted during the period when the child is edematous.

In the acute phase of nephrosis the child's appetite is poor. Because of the edema of the peritoneal wall, the child's digestion is disturbed. He may have a feeling of fullness. Getting the child to eat frequently provides a real challenge to the nurse. Whether the child is more comfortable sitting on the nurse's lap while he eats or sitting up in the bed with a tray in front of him depends on the child. Ingenious methods of making mealtime pleasant are important if the nurse is going to encourage the child's intake Pieces of ice or hard rock candy are good items to offer a child who is on limited fluids. The candy will add needed calories.

An accurate record should be kept of the child's fluid intake and his urinary output on each tour of duty. This is a means of determining fluid retention and in ascertaining the functions of the kidney. In addition, an accurate record of the fluid intake indicates whether the child is getting the right amount of fluid.

Administering medication. As stated previously, steroids are usually given and sometimes diuretics. Since children are susceptible to respiratory infections, especially pneumococcal infections, antibiotics may be prescribed prophylactically. A spontaneous pneumococcal peritonitis may simulate acute appendicitis, so that blood cultures, blood counts, and probably a peritoneal tap may be done in such instances. Large doses of penicillin are administered when a pneumococcal infection is present.

Weighing. The child should be weighed on admission and thereafter each day at the same time with the same amount of clothing. This is usually done daily before breakfast. The scales should be carefully adjusted before the child gets on them. Accuracy of weight is very important. A gain or loss of weight is one way of knowing whether edema is worse or better. A gain of 500 mg. (0.5 kg.) is equivalent to 500 ml. of fluid. In addition, weight is a helpful guide in judging the child's nutritional status and general health.

Blood pressure. Blood pressure is usually routinely taken twice a day. Hypertension is not associated with nephrosis; however, steroids cause an elevation of the blood pressure.

Assisting with tests. The nurse needs to explain to the child what the test is and what it involves. Some of the frequent tests ordered are blood urea nitrogen, cholesterol, and urea clearance tests; 24-hour urine collection for total protein excreted; intravenous pylogram; and renal biopsy. Abdominal paracentesis is commonly performed in a child with nephrosis. The nurse should explain the procedure to the child so that he will be prepared to cooperate. Voiding is recommended before the procedure to help prevent the puncture of the bladder. The nurse should sit the child at the edge of the table, hold his hands, turn his head away from the site of the puncture and talk to him during the procedure. The ascites fluid is removed slowly and sent to the laboratory for culture and chemistries. When the procedure is over, the abdomen is wrapped with a binder and careful observation of the amount of drainage is recorded by the nurse.

Also, the nurse assists the physician when kidney biopsies are done. It is only by kidney biopsy that the lesion can be put into a pathological classification and therefore into a prognostic group. The child is well medicated before he is taken into the treatment room. During the biopsy, the nurse holds the child in the desired position. He is usually left flat on his back for a few hours after the biopsy. Blood pressure and pulse are taken at frequent intervals for several hours after the biopsy is done. Hemorrhaging into or around the renal capsule could occur.

Activity and recreation. During an acute phase of generalized edema, the child lies in bed or may wish to be held by his parents. Even when the child is feeling ill, he may wish to hold some favorite toy or have it near him. During a remission, the child is active. Recreational diversion is in accordance with the child's condition. Having another similar-aged child in the room is helpful.

Emotional support. The child's parents may be discouraged because of the child's frequent admissions to the hospital. These feelings can be easily communicated to the child, so empathy and emotional support of the parents are part of the nurse's care of the child.

The nurse should share the child's care with the mother. Helping to bathe the child or hold him while his crib is being made helps the mother to feel useful. In addition, the nurse should try to see that the mother leaves the child for her own meals. Also, there should be some provision for the mother's rest. When the child has his nap, the mother may wish to lie down also. For her own welfare she should be encouraged to go outside the hospital for a short time daily.

The child is fussy and irritable in the acute phase of the disease, and the nurse needs to be patient. Irritability itself indicates that the child is not well. (For other psychological aspects of the care of the child with a long-term illness see p. 465.)

Preparation for discharge

The physician describes the future treatment and course of the disease to the parents; actually often he reviews what he has already told them. The nurse should be present at the conference. She can teach the parents the exact dose of any medication that the physician wishes the child to take at home. Depending on the plan of the physician, the parents may be taught to test the child's urine for protein content and keep a record of this. This record can be shown to the physician in return visits to his office or to a clinic.

The nurse may further discuss the diet, prevention of infection, and significant factors in promotion of his health (Chapter 9). The importance of the mother getting adequate rest should be pointed out, also that she have some time to herself without the child being present. It is difficult (and undesirable) to be with the child 24 hours a day, 7 days a week.

CYSTIC FIBROSIS

The hospital nurse may meet the child with cystic fibrosis in the newborn nursery since a small percentage of neonates develop a condition known as meconium ileus—intestinal obstruction due to abnormally viscous secretions.

The public health nurse in a health conference may see a child who has failed to thrive and grow even though his diet is adequate. The child seems fretful and malnourished. On the other hand, the public health nurse, the office nurse, and the out-patient clinic nurse may see this child with repeated respiratory infections. Depending on his state of illness, he may or may not be admitted to the hospital for diagnostic purposes.

Cystic fibrosis is such an important cause of chronic pulmonary disease in children that there are many clinics just for cystic fibrosis in connection with medical centers. Research projects are supported by the National Cystic Fibrosis Foundation. About one half of the children who have this condition die by 10 years of age and over three fourths of them by 20 years. Before 2 or 3 years of age the majority of patients have symptoms relating to indigestion, malnutrition, and persistent respiratory symptoms. The chief cause of death is related to the degree of lung involvement. Right-sided heart failure can occur.

When the child is admitted to the hospital, what are the nursing responsibilities? This depends a good deal on the severity of his illness and the particular symptoms he has. There is considerable variability among patients.

Nature of the condition

Cystic fibrosis is a disease of the exocrine glands in which there is generalized dysfunction. It is transmitted as a recessive trait and is seen in both sexes, but rarely develops in blacks. The exact cause is unknown.

The disease was differentiated from celiac disease in 1936. At first the disease was thought to be due to a deficiency of the pancreas; later the disorder was called mucoviscidosis because investigators thought it was a mucus-secreting gland defect. The inaccuracy of this was shown when other investigators later pointed out that the disease was generalized and affected many (perhaps all) exocrine glands, some of which were mucus producing and some of which were not. The mucus-producing glands have abnormally viscous secretions, and the nonmucus-producing glands, like the sweat glands, have abnormal chemical composition of their secretions. Chloride and sodium levels in sweat are two to five times above the normal.

Symptoms relating to the digestive and/or respiratory systems develop early. Symptoms relating to the digestive system are failure to gain weight, undernourished appearance, protuberant abdomen, wasted buttocks, a haggard appearance, and either watery stools or foul-smelling bulky stools. The lack or deficiency of pancreatic enzymes (trypsin, lipase, amylase) impairs digestion. Vitamin A and D deficiencies often occur from failure to absorb fat-soluble vitamins.

In the newborn period, as already stated, intestinal obstruction (meconium ileus) may result from abnormally viscous secretions. Obstruction often occurs near the ileocecal valve. Viscid meconium is found on operation. The same infant may develop respiratory distress from bronchial obstruction by viscous secretions. Atelectasis, pneumonia, or emphysema could result. However, as previously stated, only a few infants develop meconium ileus and have difficulties in the newborn period.

The child may have no digestive disturbances but have repeated respiratory infections and signs of bronchial obstruction. There is increased viscosity of pulmonary mucus, which causes partial obstruction and prevents full aeration of the lung. There is stagnation of the secretions, which in turn is conducive to growth

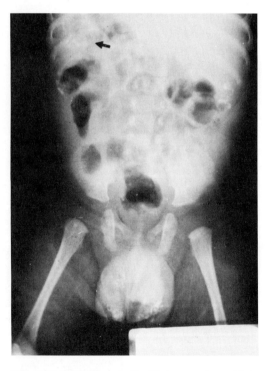

Fig. 16-1. Meconium peritonitis in a newborn. Note presence of calcified meconium particles in peritoneal cavity (end of arrow) and scrotum. Intestinal perforation occured earlier and sealed spontaneously. Meconium that escaped through perforation became calcified.

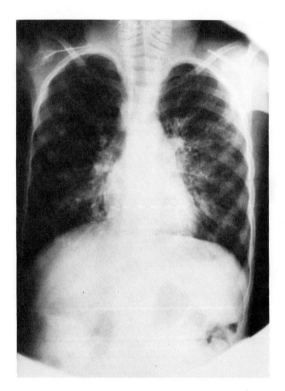

Fig. 16-2. Cystic fibrosis in a 9-year-old child. There is a diffuse infiltrate with thickening of the walls of the bronchi and dilatation of bronchi. Note evidence of hyperaeration.

of microorganisms; an infection results. After the infection is treated there is usually some fibrosis left. The child continues to have a dry, unproductive cough and later develops increasing dyspnea and then clubbing of fingers and toes.

Because of loss of chloride and sodium in sweat, the child with cystic fibrosis may have heat prostration in hot weather or if exposed to a very hot environment. The mother of an infant with cystic fibrosis may say the infant has a salty taste when she kisses him. This is due to the excessive sodium in his perspiration.

In general, the treatment is directed toward controlling pulmonary infection, maintaining good nutrition, and preventing abnormal loss of salt.

Complications of cystic fibrosis include pulmonary fibrosis, lobular atelectasis, bronchiectasis, and pulmonary insufficiency. Cirrhosis of the liver, rectal prolapse, pansinusitis, and nasal polyposis may occur. Diabetes is sometimes encountered in patients with cystic fibrosis.

Role of the nurse

The nurse should be aware that the nursing care plan for a child with cystic fibrosis must be individual. Some children are sicker than others; some have problems relating mostly to the respiratory system; some have problems relating to the digestive system; and some have problems relating to both.

Observations. At the time of admission of the child the nurse should observe and record a description of the child, as for any child newly admitted. Particular signs for which she should look include color, signs of dehydration, muscle tone, protuberant abdomen, wasted buttocks, cough and nature of cough, sputum, dyspnea, clubbing of fingers and toes, and behavior (listless, vigorous, irritable, cheerful). In her daily observations on each 8 hour tour of duty the nurse should observe and record on the nurses' notes any changes manifested, so those caring for the child will be aided in formulating a nursing care plan. The child's reaction to treatments and tests is also important to know.

Description of stools. All stools need to be described according to their amount, color, consistency, and anything unusual. The stool may be hard and small. Fecal impactions can occur, but also the stools may be bulky and foul smelling. With diet therapy (including pancreatic extract) the stool may change.

Weighing. The child's weight should be taken accurately at the same time and with the same amount of clothing each day. It is necessary to see whether he is gaining weight, remaining stationary, or losing weight.

Assisting with diagnostic tests. When a test is done, an explanation should be given to the child in accord with his age and understanding. The presence of a familiar nurse is especially helpful to the younger child. No explanation can be given the infant, but after the unpleasant experience he should be lifted and cuddled.

The nurse assists with venipuncture for blood chemistries and sends sputum specimen for culture and urine specimen for evaluation. A sweat test is done to see if there are abnormal elevations of sodium and chloride. Up to 20 years of age a level of more than 60 mEq. per liter of sweat chloride is diagnostic. This is considered one of the most reliable tests.

Duodenal contents may be aspirated by passing a small Levin tube to see if there are any pancreatic enzymes present. Trypsin is the most important of these. This test is done only for research purposes.

X-ray films are taken of the chest, and stool specimen is examined for steatorrhea. The latter test is not a specific diagnostic test, since there are other conditions in which fat is not absorbed.

Nutrition. Once the diagnosis is established, nutrition is part of the therapy for cystic fibrosis. The child should have a high-caloric, high-protein diet with vitamin supplementation and pancreatic enzyme replacement. Since absorption of food is incomplete, the caloric intake must be larger than normal. Total fat in the diet is decreased but not severely limited.

The nurse's role is especially important in trying by various methods to get the child to eat. (Refer to p. 283 for a discussion of mealtime.) Pancreatic extract (powder, capsule, or granular form) is given with a small amount of food such as applesauce or something else that he accepts. This should be given before other foods because the child is hungry when he begins his meal. There is always a possibility that an infant will not take all of his formula so the pancreatic extract should not just be added to his regular formula bottle but given to the infant either mixed with a little formula in a separate bottle or in a cup or even by teaspoon. The pancreatic extract aids the digestion, and as stated previously, there is an absence of normal pancreatic enzymes. An older child may take tablets or capsules with each meal.

Vitamins A and D in twice the usual dosage are given. A multiple vitamin solution is given in regular amounts twice daily.

Administering medication. Aerosol therapy should come before postural drainage. This is done three to four times daily for 10 or 15 minutes. It can be given with a nebulizer or

tent. This further hydrates the secretions and facilitates expectoration.

Antibiotic therapy usually consists of broad-spectrum antibiotics. The antibiotics used are selected in accord with sensitivity tests from throat swabs or sputum. These may be given intramuscularly, orally, and/or by inhalation (aerosol therapy).

Expectorants are often used to thin the bronchial mucous secretions. Saturated solution of potassium iodide (SSKI) is frequently prescribed; also, syrup of hydriodic acid may be used. Robitussin is sometimes used instead of iodides. The nurse should be aware that prolonged use of iodides is conducive to hypothyroidism. Bronchodilators are often used.

Mist tent. Depending on the severity of pul-

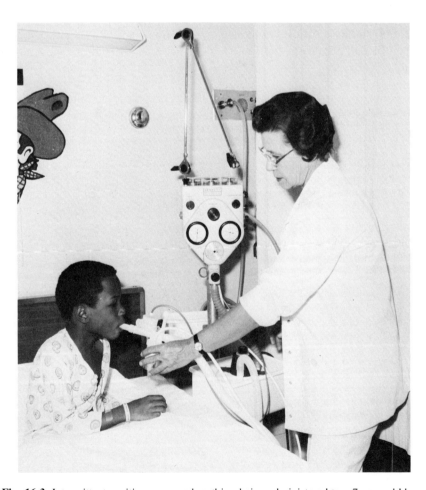

Fig. 16-3. Intermittent positive pressure breathing being administered to a 7-year-old boy.

monary involvement, a mist tent may be placed over the child at night and during nap time. Two neubulizers are commonly used to make a water-saturated atmosphere. The mist tent facilitates loosening of secretions and thus expectoration.

If the child requires a mist tent at home, it is well for the nurse to know that a list of available equipment can be obtained from the National Cystic Fibrosis Research Foundation.

Physiotherapy. Postural drainage and breathing exercises are done by the physiotherapist. The timing of these procedures is important. At least 1 hour should have elapsed since mealtime; in addition, the procedures should follow nebulization.

In postural drainage the child's position must be one that facilitates gravity in the expectoration of mucus. If the child is small, he may be placed on a board, tilted crib mattress, or the adult's lap. With his head lowered the child might look at interesting pictures or play games with his fingers or have some form or diversion that would help him to relax. If the child holds himself tense, he does not cough or expectorate. Sometimes he is afraid of vomiting. He needs to be reassured that it is all right if he does. Many times if he vomits, considerable mucus is seen in the vomitus.

Clapping with cupped hands over the areas that are to be drained helps dislodge secretions. The physician, of course, has to designate which areas are the affected ones. Clapping and vibrating are two techniques that are used to loosen secretions. Postural drainage must be done regularly several times a day according to the physician's orders.

Breathing exercises are given to increase the duration of exhalation. The child is taught to exhale very slowly. Sometimes other exercises are given, such as trunk bending and twisting, all of which are intended to improve ventilation by mobilizing the thorax. Physical fitness exercises are used as the patient can tolerate them.

Preparation for discharge. When the child is ready to go home, it is important that the parents receive explicit explanations regarding diet, medications, postural drainage, and exercises, according to the child's tolerance. Parents should give the child the exercises under supervision of the physiotherapist before taking the child home.

A referral should be made to the public health nurse just as in the case of any children with long-term or chronic illness. The referral form should include specific directions regarding diet, postural drainage, exercise, and medications. If indicated, the public health nurse should come to the hospital to watch a demonstration by the physiotherapist.

The public health nurse and the parents should be aware of the following general health measures. This child should receive immunizations and booster shots for communicable diseases the same as any other child. Measles vaccine should be given early in infancy (6 months) since there is often pulmonary deterioration after a child has measles. Gamma globulin should be given to those who have not had vaccine and are exposed to measles. Susceptibility to heat prostration should be guarded against in hot weather. Increased salt should be given at that time.

The play and school activities of the child depend on the severity of his illness. Each child has to be considered individually.

For general measures to maintain and promote health refer to Chapter 9.

Prevention. Cystic fibrosis cannot be prevented, but it can be kept under control, complications can be lessened, and the child may be aided to a longer life. The earlier the diagnosis, the better is the general prognosis for the child.

The nurse must be particularly careful to look for infants who do not have a steady gain in height and weight or who, although they consistently gain some, are far below the expected standard. In her home visits and in child health conferences the public health nurse needs to be alert to children who look undernourished and/or have foul-smelling bulky stools. If a mother says her infant "tastes salty" when she kisses him, the infant should be referred for a medical examination. Also, if one child in the family has this disease, the nurse needs to be aware that another sibling may develop it. The school nurse needs to be on the alert for children with absence due to repeated respiratory infections.

GLUTEN-INDUCED ENTEROPATHY (CELIAC DISEASE)

Gluten-induced enteropathy is one of a group of conditions in which there is malabsorption. Gee, in 1889, first named this condition celiac disease. It is characterized by malnutrition, abnormal stools, and a distended abdomen. In the late 1930's cystic fibrosis was shown to be a separate disease entity, not part of celiac disease. Later, in the 1960's, gluten-induced enteropathy was identified as one of the most important causes of malabsorption.

Nature of the condition

In gluten-induced enteropathy there is a defect in enzymatic metabolism, which is precipitated mainly by the ingestion of wheat and rye gluten, although oats and barley could also be the cause. An allergic reaction may be a factor in the etiology.

There are two fractions of gluten: glutenin (relatively unharmful) and gliadin, which causes malabsorption. Glutamine is an amino acid that is responsible for much of the weight of wheat gliadin; however, when susceptible patients have ingested this amino acid itself, it has not made their condition worse. To have an adverse effect it must be in a bound state in the form of gliadin.

This condition is seen in both sexes, but is uncommon in blacks and in the Mongolian race. The disease does show an increased familial incidence.

The public health nurse may see this child at home or in the child health conferences before a physician has diagnosed the condition. Although this condition is seen in infants especially between 6 and 18 months of age, symptoms may be present in the first few weeks. If the infant fails to gain steadily in height and weight, the physician's attention should be called to this child. Bulky, greasy stools that have a foul odor are characteristic. The malabsorbed fat in stools causes the greasy appearance. The infant may be fretful, and often has a poor appetite.

As the child gets older, further symptoms are apparent as the result of impaired digestion and, of course, in accordance with the severity of the condition. Malnutrition manifests itself in the thinness of the body, poor musculature, skin hanging in folds, pallor, and distended abdomen, as well as retardation of growth and development. Anemia is often present. With increased severity of symptoms the emotional behavior pattern is more than that of a fretful child. There may be moodiness, fits of temper, and even hysterical behavior. At times there may be periods of unusual timidity.

The hospital nurse may see this child if a physician refers him to the hospital for diagnostic purposes, or she may meet him if a "celiac crisis" occurs. Sometimes, after or during an acute infection (often a respiratory one), the child develops watery diarrhea and vomiting. This usually occurs when the child is under 2 years of age and his electrolyte balance is less stable. The child is prostrate and dehydrated and shows manifestations of acidosis. He is gravely ill. Oral fluids are withheld, and he is given intravenous therapy. When the child is able to retain oral fluids, a fat-free formula made of special protein milk or skimmed milk may be given. Banana powder can be added to the formula as a treatment for the diarrhea. Depending on the age of the child, simple carbohydrate foods such as fruit juice, ripe mashed banana, or cooked pureed fruits may be given to meet the child's caloric requirement. All starches and cereals are usually avoided until the diagnosis of gluten-induced enteropathy has been established. This regimen may continue for 1 to 6 months, according to the severity of the condition and the child's individual response.

Once the child shows a steady gain in weight and an absence of symptoms, the diet can be liberalized to include pureed cooked vegetables, pureed meats, and hard-cooked eggs. All wheat and rye products must be avoided. Since gluten also occurs in barley and oats, these grains are also restricted. Corn and rice will serve as the major cereals in the child's diet.

Since diet is the major therapy in celiac disease, it is imperative that the parents receive specific instructions concerning which foods the child may or may not eat from each of the basic four food groups. Parents must also be aware that, whereas the offending grains are easy to recognize in typical cereal foods, they may also be present as thickeners and fillers in noncereal products. Parents should be told to read the package labels. A dietitian can be helpful in supplying recipes for preparing low-gluten dishes, which can be included in the family's menu pattern.

The prognosis for gluten-induced enteropathy is excellent; however, the child will have to remain under close medical supervision. As he grows older, foods appropriate for his age will be added to the diet to meet nutritional requirements for normal growth. Foods containing wheat may be cautiously included if there are no symptoms; however, each child has to be considered individually. Some children may never be able to tolerate the reintroduction of wheat. During the adolescent period, weight should be frequently checked if wheat has been reintroduced, since retardation of growth may be the only observable adverse effect. An acute infection may cause a recurrence of the symptoms.

Role of the nurse

Child's behavior. In approaching the fretful infant or young child with temper outbursts, the nurse should exercise patience. It is trying to care for a child who is often resistant, but she should remember that this unhappy behavior is part of the disease process. When his condition improves, his disposition will improve also. In the meantime it is especially important to socialize routines of bathing, dressing, and preparation for rest hour or the night's sleep. Commands should be avoided. Tact is necessary. The behavior of the child should be charted daily on the nursing notes, since irritability and management problems are a manifestation of gluten-induced enteropathy.

Weighing. Even if the child is not admitted in celiac crisis, the child should be weighed daily and care taken to ensure an accurate weight. With dietary treatment, gain in weight signifies that there is physical improvement and that food is being assimilated.

Feeding. For technique in formula feeding see p. 68, and for mealtime in the hospital see p. 283. The child often has anorexia, and every effort should be exerted to make mealtime pleasant. Small portions should be given. It is easier to give more food later than to get the child to eat a large amount if he is not hungry.

As the diet is the main method by which gluten-induced enteropathy can be controlled, it is impossible to overemphasize the importance of the nurses' role at mealtime and in encouraging the child to improve his dietary habits.

Recreation. Recreational diversion should be in accord with the severity of the child's illness and his age. If the child feels like playing with a toy, play materials should be provided. Perhaps he would just like to be held in an adult's lap or sit in a stroller and be pushed down the hall into the playroom. How he reacts when recreation is offered will often cue the nurse as to his need for diversion.

Avoiding infection. As any child with this condition is very susceptible to respiratory infections, personnel with colds should keep away from him or wear a double mask if they are going to be in the room for only a brief time. The child should not be placed in a room with a child who has any infection. Also, when it becomes colder at night, it is essential that the child be covered adequately. Often young children kick off their bedclothing before they fall asleep. If the child is not covered, he could easily develop a respiratory illness.

Administering medication. Water-soluble multivitamins (especially vitamins A and D) are given in two to four times the usual dosage. If there is a hypothrombinemia, vitamin K is given. If the child has been on broad-spectrum antibiotic therapy for an infection, vitamin B complex may be given. Calcium lactate may be given orally if milk is excluded from the diet. Iron and liver extract are prescribed if there is anemia.

Assisting with tests. A sweat test may be done to rule out cystic fibrosis. There is no increased chloride or sodium in the sweat of a child with gluten-induced enteropathy. Stools are sent to the laboratory to see if there is fat in them; however, if excess fat is present, this only shows malabsorption of fat and is not diagnostic of the cause of the condition in this patient.

Blood chemistries are done. The nurse should know that the amount of total serum protein helps to indicate the severity of the disease. The child whose total serum protein is less than 5 gm. per 100 ml. in a sick child. An intercurrent infection could be very serious. The red blood count often shows anemia, and the microscopic examination reveals hypochromic red blood cells.

A microscopic examination of the mucosa of the small intestine is usually done. There are significant changes in it if the child has gluten-induced celiac disease. An oral glucose tolerance test is low with severe malabsorption. The xylose tolerance test may be performed. This shows absorption in the upper part of the small intestine. An oral dose of xylose is administered. The child's urine is collected for 5 hours. Normally 20% of the xylose is recovered; a low percentage indicates less functioning of the small intestine.

Preparation for discharge. A referral should be made to the public health nurse. A specific list of foods that the child can have should be given to her as well as to the parents. The hospital nurse should ascertain whether the parents understand directions about the diet and vitamin therapy before they leave the hospital. The parents should also understand that, even if the child seems well, eats well, and has normal stools, there should still be strict adherence to the prescribed diet. In addition, the nurse should make sure that the parents appreciate the fact that the child will need to be seen at regular intervals by a private physician (or in a pediatric clinic) for a long time. Even though he seems well, the appointment with a clinic or private physician should be kept. If the child develops a respiratory illness, prompt medical attention should be sought in order to avoid the possibility of a celiac crisis.

The emotional climate of the home is important to a child with this condition. Parents need to have patience with the child and to avoid conflicts with each other or emotional upsets in front of the child. The services of a medical social worker are useful if there is domestic discord.

RHEUMATIC FEVER

Rheumatic fever represents one of the common illnesses that require prolonged medical supervision. Rheumatic carditis (one manifestation of rheumatic fever) is among the first five leading causes of death in children from 5 to 14 years of age. Rheumatic fever can be prevented by adequate control of streptococcal infections.

Since rheumatic fever is most prevalent in children 5 to 15 years of age, the school health nurse (or the public health nurse in a rural area) often has contact with this child prior to hospitalization as well as after hospitalization. The hospital nurse sees the child during an acute attack of illness, whereas the public health nurse in a large city is most likely to see a child who has been hospitalized and is referred for follow-up care.

Nature of the condition

Rheumatic fever may follow an infection caused by streptococci, such as pharyngitis or scarlet fever. Rheumatic fever is associated with an urban rather than a rural community and with the lower socioeconomic level. There is a high familial incidence of the disease. Another etiological factor is climate. Rheumatic fever is prevalent in temperate zones. The season varies according to the locality. In the United States it is especially seen in March and April on the eastern seaboard and in January and February on the western seaboard.

Rheumatic fever is a nonsuppurative inflammation. The four major manifestations of rheumatic fever are carditis, polyarthritis, chorea, and erythema marginatum. The child might exhibit just one manifestation or a combination of two, but chorea and polyarthritis are not usually seen together.

In polyarthritis the large joints at the elbow, knee, ankle, or wrist are usually swollen, warm to touch, and painful. The pain may or may not travel from one joint to another. Several joints may be affected or only one joint. The child usually has an elevated temperature, complains of pain when he moves around, and prevents anyone from touching or rubbing the joints that are involved.

In chorea (Saint Vitus' dance) muscular weakness, emotional instability, and uncoordinated muscle movements are seen. (Refer to p. 490 for nursing care of chorea.)

Carditis occurs in approximately 50% of all cases of rheumatic fever, and it is found in every fatal case. The presence of a pansystolic murmur at the apex that was not present before the acute onset of rheumatic fever is pathognomonic of rheumatic carditis. The mitral valve is most commonly affected and the aortic valve is second. Tachycardia or bradycardia may be observed. The child appears to be fatigued with a tired pale facial expression. Epistaxis is frequent. Roentgenograms of the chest reveal cardiomegaly, with the left ventricle and atrium being the chambers most enlarged.

Erythema marginatum is present in cases of severe rheumatic fever. It is characterized by a circinate macular and erythematous rash appearing on the trunk or extremities.

Subcutaneous nodules are a specific manifestation of rheumatic fever and occur almost exclusively in the severest types of rheumatic fever with carditis. They remain present from several weeks to months. They are loosely attached to joint capsules or tendon sheaths. Most commonly they are found over the joints, scalp, and vertebrae and are not painful or tender.

The general signs of inflammation consist of (1) fever in the range of 101° to 103° F., (2) moderately elevated white blood cell count, (3) elevated erythrocyte sedimentation rate, (4) increased antistreptolysin O titer, and (5) mild anemia secondary to depressed erythropoiesis and decreased red blood cell survival. The onset of the inflammation process usually begins 10 to 14 days after an antecedent streptococcal infection that was inadequately treated or not treated at all.

Treatment

There is no specific treatment for acute rheumatic fever in an attempt to prevent cardiac damage. However, the acute manifestations can be suppressed by the use of hormones, salicylates, anticongestive measures, and general supportive care. The child is kept for about 2 weeks at strict bed rest during the acute attack. Gradual ambulation is started as the acute symptoms subside and the discomfort passes. The child will usually become very rebellious about being restricted to bed when he begins to feel better. This is a good observation for which to look when determining when to begin ambulation.

Restriction of salt intake is recommended for children with congestive heart failure who are receiving steroids. Caloric intake restrictions may have to be instituted in some of the patients on steroids because of their enormous appetites. They should be given a diet high in protein, carbohydrates, and vitamin C.

Adequate doses of penicillin should be administered for 10 days, or long-acting benzathine penicillin should be administered immediately to eradicate the *Streptococcus* organism. After the eradication of *Streptococcus,* penicillin prophylaxis should be started immediately.

Steroids are given to the child with evidence of severe rheumatic heart disease. Severe rheumatic heart disease is diagnosed by the presence of myocarditis, endocarditis, and pericarditis. The child with only minimal evidence of heart involvement may or may not be placed on steroids, depending upon the preference of the individual physician. The steroids do not prevent residual valvular damage but suppress the inflammatory signs more quickly and certainly than salicylates do.

Patients with rheumatic fever without clinical evidence of heart involvement should not be given steroids. If steroids are used, they should be given early in the disease and high dosages ordered. Examples of large dosages are hydrocortisone, 300 mg. daily, and prednisone, 150 mg. daily. Most authorities begin tapering the dosage after 2 weeks of therapy and hope to have the child off steroids completely by 4 to 6 weeks after the initial dose. During steroid therapy, potassium chloride is added to the diet to compensate for the urinary losses of potassium. Some of the more common complications of steroid therapy are Cushing's syndrome (weight gain, striae, hirsutism), peptic ulcer, diabetes mellitus, psychosis, and infections.

Salicylates have been used for many years to achieve symptomatic relief in acute rheumatic fever. Salicylates are the drugs of choice today for children having acute rheumatic fever without heart disease. When the salicylates have been administered for 24 to 48 hours a serum salicylate level should be obtained to determine if proper absorption is occurring. The dosage should be continued for 2 to 4 weeks, when gradual "tapering off" may be introduced. The salicylates are usually continued as long as there are signs of rheumatic activity present.

Rheumatic fever patients in congestive heart failure should receive anticongestive drugs in essentially the same fashion as do other patients with congestive heart failure. (See p. 489 for management of heart failure.)

Course and prognosis

Gross cardiomegaly and congestive heart failure secondary to rheumatic fever have the worst prognostic implications. If the heart remains large, the murmur remains loud, and there is extensive residual valvular damage after treatment of the acute condition, it is more likely that evidences of heart disease will persist for many years or for life. Mitral stenosis is the most common valvular lesion developing as a consequence of rheumatic endocarditis. It is rare in children and it takes 5 to 10 years after the acute episode for its development. The majority of patients who are given rigid penicillin prophylaxis will become free of heart disease 5 to 10 years after the acute episode.

Complication

Subacute bacterial endocarditis is an infection of the heart that usually develops at the site of the damaged cardiac valve secondary to the rheumatic carditis. The most common causative organism is alpha-hemolytic *Streptococcus,* which is normally found in the nose and throat. The infection usually destroys the endocardial lining of the valves and the surrounding muscle. This may lead to perforation of the valves or septa.

The most frequent symptoms are fever, chills, malaise, weight loss, anemia, and systemic embolization in various parts of the body, which may include the spleen, liver, kidneys, and lungs. The embolic phenomenon is characterized by petechiae in the conjunctiva and oral mucous membranes and by splinter hemorrhages under the toenails and fingernails. The diagnosis is established by identification of the causative organism by blood culture. Penicillin and streptomycin are the drugs of choice and are given intravenously for 2 to 4 weeks. Bac-

teriological studies are used to confirm that the correct antibiotics are being used.

Most children recover completely when early and adequate treatment is provided. Inadequate treatment usually means a high rate of recurrences.

Prevention of recurrence

To prevent a recurrence of rheumatic fever, prophylactic antibiotics (penicillin or sulfadiazine) are given to the child for an indefinite number of years, certainly throughout childhood. Also, when an attack of pharyngitis or respiratory infection occurs, parents need to secure prompt medical attention for their child.

Case finding

The physician may discover the child has rheumatic fever in the course of a routine medical examination. Also, Chahen (1975) writes of a streptococcus screening program. On the other hand, the child's teacher may refer the child to the school nurse because of listlessness, loss of weight, pallor, or joint pain. Sometimes the school child is referred to the nurse because of fumbling, awkwardness, dropping of objects, or general nervousness. (These last symptoms are characteristic of the child with chorea.)

Role of the nurse

For nursing care of a child with chorea refer to p. 490.

If the child has polyarthritis, the nurse should see and feel which joints are warm to touch, swollen, and painful. Care should be taken in turning or handling this child because of his pain. Salicylates usually relieve joint symptoms. Sometimes heat is applied to painful joints. Polyarthritis tends to occur alone more than with carditis. The child with polyarthritis who does not have cardiac involvement has a comparatively brief hospital stay (2 weeks).

In caring for a child with rheumatic carditis, the following are important considerations.

Selection of a room. The child should preferably be placed with children of his age and sex; however, the child with rheumatic fever should never be in the same room with a child who has a draining wound or an infection of any kind. Since he will probably be in the hospital for more than a few days, he should be placed next to windows so that he can have some pleasant diversion.

Observation. On each 8-hour tour of duty the nurse needs to know the quality of the pulse (weak, strong, irregular, thready) and respiration. She should look for any signs of dyspnea. If the child does not wish to lie down at any time and persistently sits up, this is a point to note on the bedside chart. Other observations include color, behavior (apathetic, irritable, listless, playing with toys), weakness, appetite, precordial pain, edema, skin rash, and abdominal pain. Cyanosis, dyspnea, orthopnea, and tachycardia are symptoms suggestive of congestive heart failure.

Assisting with diagnostic measures. The nurse often assists the doctor in venipunctures for blood count, erythrocyte sedimentation rate, antistreptolysin titer, and C-reactive protein determination. Even if the nurse does not assist the physician, she can explain to the child that he will feel a prick from the needle but, if he holds still, it will be over quickly. Blood is going to be drawn many times during the child's stay, and this is something he needs help in accepting. How the child reacts to the second and third time blood is drawn depends a good deal on how skillfully the procedure was managed the first time. The presence of the nurse and her acceptance of his behavior, even if he cries, aids the child.

An electrocardiogram is done soon after the child's admission and frequently thereafter. This shows heart abnormalities. Interpreting this diagnostic measure to the child in accordance with his age is necessary. It is well to tell him how his heart works: It is a big muscle that is like a pump; it makes the blood go around the body.

An x-ray film of the chest is taken also. Not only will this show heart enlargement but it also will show evidence of any infection such as pneumonia, which the child may have in his lower respiratory tract.

Administering medications. When the child is first admitted, the physician may prescribe penicillin for him. This is not to combat rheumatic fever but to combat the presence of streptococci that may be present. Drugs such as salicylates and corticosteroids are given to suppress and control the acute phase of the disease. It is believed that children with carditis may improve more rapidly with steroids than with salicylates.

When steroid therapy is given, the nurse needs to take the child's blood pressure at least daily. If the diastolic pressure rises to 100 mm. Hg or above, she should notify the physician at once. Other possible reactions from steroid therapy are a moonface, acne, hirsutism, increased pigmentation, striae, and abnormal deposits of fat. These symptoms are called Cushing's syndrome. When the drug is withdrawn, the nurse needs to watch to see if the symptoms of discomfort return again to the child.

If salicylates are given, toxic reactions for which to watch include nausea, vomiting, headache, and tinnitus.

Phenobarbital is sometimes ordered for a restless child and morphine for the child with precordial pain. If heart failure occurs, digitalis or digoxin and diuretics are usually ordered. The nurse needs to be particularly careful to watch for signs of nausea, vomiting, gastric distress, or a sudden slowing of the pulse when digitalis preparations are given.

Position. The child should be in the position that is most comfortable to him. If he feels like playing with toys or if he is having dyspnea, the head should be elevated. At night children with severe heart disease have a headrest somewhat lowered but not flat.

Rest. In general, the child remains in bed (no bathroom privileges) until improvement is shown by laboratory data and examination (negative C-reactive protein, normal pulse rate, and decreased sedimentation rate). A comfortable night's sleep helps, as well as an hour's rest period after lunch in a darkened, quiet room. Reading and letter writing should not be permitted in rest hour. (For making rest hour conducive to sleep see p. 286.)

If the child has severe carditis, the nurse should make every effort to conserve his strength and energy. Care should be individualized. The nurse may or may not need to let the child rest after breakfast before making his bed. She may or may not need to feed him.

When the child feels better, he will want to do this himself. The nurse should so organize her work that she does not need to continually disturb the child. She should also note if visitors disturb or tire the child. The environment should be so arranged that it is conducive to relaxation.

Nutrition. The child with rheumatic carditis should have an adequate diet high in vitamins, proteins, and carbohydrates. The child's appetite tends to be poor unless steroids are being administered. It is up to the nurse to use ingenuity in encouraging the child to eat. Mealtime should always be made as pleasant as possible (p. 283). Fluids should be urged unless the child is in congestive heart failure.

If the child has severe carditis, a low-sodium diet is usually prescribed.

The child with rheumatic fever has an elevation of temperature during the acute phase of the disease. When fever is present, metabolism is more rapid; there is also tissue destruction.

The child's appetite, as well as what food he ate, should be recorded on the bedside notes.

Fluid intake and output. The nurse needs to record carefully all fluids and food given to the child since this helps to indicate how the child is feeling and his progress. A child in heart failure is on restricted fluids, whereas other children with rheumatic fever are urged to take fluids in view of the presence of an infection and elevated temperature.

General hygiene. Attention to oral hygiene prior to meals sometimes aids the child to eat better. A daily bath improves circulation, refreshes the child, and helps to keep the skin in good condition. The child's back, buttocks, and bony prominences need to be rubbed several times a day to increase comfort and to prevent skin irritation. Position should be changed periodically both for comfort and to avoid pressure areas. If the child has severe carditis and sits up in bed most of the time, he may need to have a foam rubber mattress. A rubber air ring could be used on which the child could sit. Attention should be given to bowel elimination. Straining from constipation should be avoided.

Mental hygiene. It is hard for the child to be away from his family for a period of time. The child who is in the hospital may become de-

pressed. Letters from various members of the family help, or even postcards. The nurse should be sure to make the most of every contact she has with the child to let him see that she likes and is interested in him. During the acute phase of the disease, physical comfort and skilled care may be the best emotional support she can give. When the child feels better, he may become bored. An unhappy child does not eat well, and, if a child is not eating well, he makes slower progress toward recovery. Diversional therapy plays an important part in the child's care. The amount and kind of recreation he is allowed should be discussed with the physician. An occupational therapist may come to his bedside, or the child might be taken to the playroom, according to the severity of his illness. During convalescence, a schoolteacher should come to the bedside if the patient cannot go to a schoolroom.

Ambulation. When the child is permitted to be out of bed and ambulate, the nurse must be sure to take his pulse first and then again when the child gets back into bed. The rate of the pulse helps to indicate how well the child is able to tolerate ambulation.

Preparation for discharge. The nurse should make sure that the child and his parents understand (1) when the child is to return to the pediatric outpatient clinic or private physician's office, (2) exactly what activities the child can do, and (3) the importance and necessity of taking daily whatever medication the physician has prescribed.

The nurse can be helpful to both the child and his physician by ascertaining what particular activities the child enjoys—bicycle riding, horseback riding, swimming, or projects in a 4-H club or a scout group. Then she can be sure that his pet activities are discussed with the doctor.

Either penicillin or sulfadiazine is recommended to be taken daily in order to prevent a recurrence of rheumatic fever. It is sometimes difficult for an adolescent patient to understand why he should take medicine when he feels no pain. This may be an opportune time to explain to the child that when he has any dental work done, he will also need additional medicine. The parents or the adolescent himself must be sure to let the dentist know he has had rheumatic fever.

If the child has had severe carditis, it is especially important that a referral should be made to the public health nurse. Sometimes problems in care at home arise that medical personnel in the hospital did not anticipate. Also, the public health nurse can be helpful in seeing that the health instructions are understood and are being followed.

For other psychological aspects of care of a child with a chronic health problem refer to p. 465.

CONGESTIVE HEART FAILURE

Congestive heart failure is a clinical syndrome associated with heart disease in which the heart is unable to supply the body with the cardiac output it demands or is unable to dispose adequately of the venous return or, most likely, shows a combination of the two. This may be seen in infants with congenital heart disease or in children with rheumatic heart disease. The heart may fail for many reasons: poor coronary artery blood flow resulting in myocardial ischemia, increased systemic vascular resistance as in hypertension, obstruction of a valve causing undue strain on the ventricle, or direct infection of the heart muscle as in myocarditis.

Right-sided failure is identified by increasing systemic venous pressure, enlargement of the liver, dependent edema, ascites, and oliguria. Left-sided failure is characterized by weakness, fatigue, dyspnea on exertion, pulmonary edema, pulmonary rales, and cardiac asthma. Cardiac enlargement is present in both; cyanosis may or may not be present in either.

The treatment of cardiac failure is an emergency. Digitalis should be administered intravenously or intramuscularly. The function of digitalis is to improve the contraction and function of the heart as well as to slow the heart rate by prolonging diastole. The dose of digitalis is calculated according to the child's age and size and is given every 6 to 8 hours until the child is fully digitalized. The two most frequently used preparations are digoxin and digitoxin. Digoxin reaches its peak action in 4 hours and is fully excreted in 48 to 72 hours,

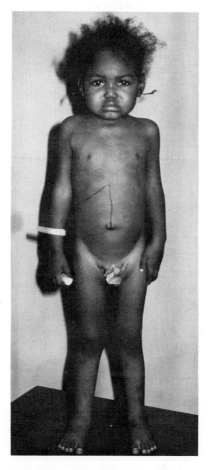

Fig. 16-4. Congestive heart failure due to severe anemia and parasitosis in an 8-year-old child. Note edema of the face, outline of enlarged liver, and apathetic look.

whereas digitoxin levels peak in 8 hours and it is excreted more slowly, taking 10 to 14 days for it to disappear from the body. Accurate records of time and dose should be maintained during digitalis administration.

Oxygen is indicated to improve the oxygenation of the blood and cardiac muscle. Diuretics are used to decrease the increased blood and interstitial fluid volume. The most commonly used diuretics are furosemide (Lasix), mercurial diuretics (meralluride [Mercuhydrine]), and enzyme inhibitors (acetazolamide [Diamox], chlorothiazide [Diuril]). The limitation of intake of fluids and sodium may be helpful in controlling the increased fluid retention. Bed rest for older children is advisable. Elevation of the head of the bed for older children or the use of a cardiac chair (infant seat) for infants may relieve the dyspnea. Morphine sulfate (0.1 mg. per kilogram) is indicated every 8 hours if the child appears anxious or agitated.

The nursing care is directed towards relieving dyspnea, conserving energy, skin care, attention to nutrition (oral or intravenous), and general emotional support of the child and his parents. Special attention should be given to the accurate administration of drugs, especially digitalis or its derivatives. Careful frequent assessment of the child's condition is essential to adjustment of the nursing care plan and thus to meeting the child's nursing needs. For details in care turn to p. 486 for a discussion of care of the child with rheumatic carditis.

CHOREA (SYDENHAM'S CHOREA)
Nature of the condition

Chorea is one of the major manifestations of rheumatic fever, as stated on p. 484. It is characterized by emotional instability, muscular weakness, and uncoordinated muscular movements. During sleep, no involuntary twitching or motion is seen. When chorea is not accompanied by carditis, the prognosis is excellent. It seldom recurs after adolescence unless there is cardiac involvement. Girls seem to be affected more than boys.

Treatment

The usual antirheumatic agents are not effective in the control of the signs and symptoms of chorea. Complete mental and physical rest is essential. The room should be kept quiet. The child should be protected by padding the bed to prevent injury to himself. The drugs most frequently used to help in control of the exaggerated emotional instability are phenobarbital and the phenothiazines (Thorazine). Chorea is a self-limited disease that is usually not followed by significant neurological sequelae after the child recovers from the disease.

To prevent a recurrence of rheumatic fever, prophylactic penicillin is given to the child, either by monthly injection of benzathine penicillin (Bicillin) or daily oral penicillin G.

School health nurse

The school nurse or public health nurse may see this child before the hospital nurse does. The child's teacher might have drawn the nurse's attention to this child because of awkwardness, trembling, and garbled speech. The child might even have been punished for making faces or grimaces at his parents or teacher. The child may be irritable and restless. That the child is ill might not occur to either parents or teacher. Untreated, the child becomes progressively weaker until he is unable to stand up and walk.

Hospital nurse

When the nurse is notified that a child with chorea is going to be admitted, she should get side rails for his bed and pad them. (As the child is usually over 5 years of age, he is too large for a crib.)

If possible, these children should not be in a room with more than one other child. Opinions vary as to whether the room should be darkened. The fewer children there are in the same room, the more restful it is. The child with chorea is fully aware he cannot control his speech or his movements, which embarrasses him. He may not be able to control sphincter muscles if a urinal or bedpan is not offered frequently. Considering the age of the child, this can be very upsetting to him.

Daily nursing care

Approach to the child, prevention of injury, skin care, supervision of mealtime and rest periods, and administration of prescribed medications are the main problems for the nurse.

Deliberate, unhurried movements in caring for the child are helpful in preventing further tenseness. Quick motions and speech of the nurse may result in even more aimless uncoordinated movements.

Since the child may have difficulty in expressing himself verbally, the nurse should try to anticipate his needs. He will have to be fed and bathed since he cannot do these things for himself; moreoever, the nurse can expect the child to be moody—to laugh easily or to cry easily. This behavior is part of his physical condition. As he gets better, his behavior changes and there is increased coordination of movements.

Padding the side rails, using a spoon to feed the child rather than a fork, and using a plastic cup rather than a glass help to prevent possible injury; so does avoiding play materials with which the child could hurt himself, such as scissors or Tinker Toys.

A daily bath plus special care several times a day to the child's back, buttocks, and bony prominences are important since his skin may become irritated by so much friction against the sheet. Attention to dietary needs is particularly important. Nourishing fluids like eggnog should be offered between meals.

Seeing that the child is comfortable and that environmental conditions are conducive to rest or sleep during rest hour and at night is also important in his care.

Medications ordered by the physician may vary in different medical centers and hospitals. In general, some form of sedative is used; tranquilizers are used also. Whatever is ordered, the nurse should know the expected results, as well as possible toxic reactions.

As soon as movements are better controlled, the child is allowed to help with his physical hygiene, to have school lessons at the bedside, and to receive diversional therapy.

If the child with chorea has carditis also, the nurse can refer to p. 486 for a discussion of the appropriate nursing care.

CONVULSIVE DISORDERS

A convulsive seizure is a *symptom* of an abnormal process in the brain. It is not a diagnosis in itself. Mental retardation is sometimes associated with convulsive disorders.

There are certain differences between adult seizures and childhood seizures. In the first place, more seizures occur during the first 3 years of life than at any other time. The causes of seizures are more easily recognized in childhood, convulsions are more localized, convulsions can be more readily controlled, and electroencephalograms are more abnormal.

For convenience, nursing care of a child with convulsive seizures will be discussed from a developmental viewpoint. Although the etiology of some seizures in children is known, most seizures in children fall into a group called "idiopathic epilepsy," for which no organic cause can be found. It is a condition to which the child and his parents have to learn to adjust and must live with. This is one of the reasons that the subject of convulsive disorders is placed in this chapter with other conditions that need prolonged medical supervision.

Causes of seizures
Early infancy

The nurse in the newborn nursery and the public health nurse in the home may see infants who have convulsions as a result of developmental disorders—infants with malformed brains or biochemical defects such as galactosemia and phenylketonuria. (Refer to pp. 548 and 549 for discussion of these conditions.)

Neonatal tetany and hypoglycemia are other causes of seizures. In neonatal tetany there is a low serum calcium and a raised phosphate level. Administration of calcium to infants with this condition will relieve their symptoms. Glucose is given to an infant with hypoglycemia. Infants of diabetic mothers are likely to have hypoglycemia, likewise, infants of mothers with toxemia. An infant with hypoglycemia might also have seizures. The character of seizures in infants is different from that in older children.

Later infancy

In later infancy, convulsions might be due to a high elevation of temperature during a respiratory or systemic acute infection. These are called *febrile convulsions*. In caring for infants and young children with acute infections, the nurse needs to be on the alert for a rise in temperature and apply appropriate temperature-reducing measures.

Certain specific *infectious cerebral diseases* are associated with convulsions: meningitis, encephalitis, and tetanus. In caring for children with these conditions, the nurse should be alert to symptoms of possible sequelae that might signify the development of a brain abscess or subdural hematoma. Convulsions, along with other signs such as persistent drowsiness, bulging fontanel, and projectile vomiting, are signs of increased intracranial pressure.

Toddler and preschool period

Acute poisonings are associated with twitchings or convulsions, as in poisoning from salicylates, lead, or insecticides. Another cause of seizures might be a cerebral neoplasm or renal insufficiency.

School years

During the school years, the nurse may see a child either at home or in the hospital who has a *degenerative disease* of the central nervous system (such as tuberous sclerosis), which is associated with convulsions. As the child gets older, there is an increase in the amount of damage to the brain in these children. However, during the school years, a nurse is most likely to come in contact with a child who has *idiopathic epilepsy*. This disorder may be manifested at 3 or 4 years of age but is seen with increasing frequency as the child becomes older. The majority of seizures in children do not have an organic cause and are classified as idiopathic epilepsy. This type of epilepsy, as has previously been stated, is most frequent during childhood.

Types of seizures

Infantile spasms are often associated with developmental defects and birth injuries. The character of seizures in infants younger than 12 months may vary from mild twitchings to spasms of all voluntary muscles of the body or to a sudden flexing forward of the head and trunk; or possibly the spasm is such that the child assumes an opisthotonic position. After a tonic phase in which there is rigidity of the body, the infant may relax or he may have a few convulsive clonic jerks. Sometimes infantile spasms of the whole body follow each other in quick succession. After the spasms he may be pale, red, or even cyanotic. He may or may not show increased saliva. Sometimes the infant may cry weakly and whimper after a spasm. Whatever the infant does, the nurse should be accurate in her description.

After the seizure the nurse should turn the infant on his side to lessen the possibility of aspiration from increased salivation. She should stroke the infant and speak softly to him. Although infants cannot be verbally interviewed, it is possible that having a seizure was an uncomfortable experience that both frightened and startled him. The infant needs comforting. If he falls asleep after the seizure, this too should be recorded.

Minor seizures include petit mal, myoclonic, and akinetic seizures. Petit mal means "small sickness." The child may stare into space for a few moments and then resume what he was doing. A myoclonic attack may consist of several or only one jerking movement of an extremity. The child does not lose consciousness. An akinetic seizure is of brief duration and is associated with a loss of postural tone and a short period of unconsciousness. The child may fall to the floor if he is standing. After the seizure he is perfectly alert.

Grand mal seizures are major seizures. After the infant is 17 or 18 months old the grand mal attacks are more like adult seizures. The older child may have an aura or warning. He utters a sharp cry or falls unconscious to the floor; then there is a tonic phase of rigidity of the body. Apnea and cyanosis occur. This is followed by a clonic stage in which there are contractions of the musculature of the trunk and jerking movements of the extremities. There may be urinary or fecal incontinence. Sometimes there is frothing at the mouth because of increased salivation. The child may be alert or, more often, drowsy after the seizure.

Older children may be able to describe an aura. The child may have an epigastric aura in which he feels nausea, sudden hunger, or a queer sensation in the epigastric region; a peculiar sensation in his head or a feeling of fright, in which he tries to run away; or an auditory aura wherein he sees flashes of light or hears various sounds.

Focal seizures are common in children. They are seizures that repeatedly begin with the same characteristic behavior or manifestations. Electroencephalograms show repeatedly the same localized abnormality. In motor seizures there may be tonic or clonic movements. These may only involve one side of the child or occur on alternate sides at different times.

A jacksonian convulsion is a type of focal motor seizure that is not common in children. There is a definite sequence of the part of the body involved. The seizure may begin in a thumb and gradually spread to the hand, the arm, and over one side or all of the body. Sometimes the term *jacksonian march* is used.

In the sensory type of seizure there may be a sensation of numbness that begins in one area and spreads to the entire side of the body; other sensory attacks may relate to the special senses and auditory, visual, and gustatory phenomena may appear.

Psychomotor seizures are uncommon in early childhood but increase with age. The manifestations are complex. There may be semipurposeful or stereotyped movements like lip sucking. Speech may be irrelevant. There may be disturbances in thinking, feeling, or motor activity. An aura or anxiety often precedes the attack. There may be auditory, olfactory, gustatory, or psychic experiences or phenomena. Some authorities believe that temporal seizures and psychomotor seizures are the same.

Status epilepticus is a condition in which the child goes from one grand mal seizure into another.

Idiopathic epilepsy
Role of the nurse

Because the nurse is most likely to come in contact with a child who has idiopathic epilepsy, a discussion of her role is given here in some detail.

Importance of medical evaluation. In a home visit, a child health conference, or a school visit, a nurse's attention may be called to the child who has "fits," "blackouts," "attacks," or convulsions known by whatever name lay persons give them. The nurse should try to have the child taken to a physician for evaluation. A convulsion is a symptom and not a disease in itself. The child needs to be examined and his illness evaluated to be certain that there is no organic cause for his seizures. If the child has idiopathic epilepsy, the sooner treatment is started, the better it is for the child and his family.

Because social stigma is so often attached to epilepsy, the nuse may encounter difficulties in getting the parents to take the child to a doctor or even acknowledge that something is wrong. The nurse might point out to the parents that

every child should have a yearly physical examination, not because he is ill but to make sure he is well and to obtain guidance to help him maintain health. The nurse's presence when the parents take the child to the doctor may, in some instances, be helpful to the parents, giving them emotional support. She has accepted both them and their child.

If the nurse can win the confidence of the parents, she should try to find out something about the child's convulsions prior to the medical examination. How old was the child when he first began to have these attacks? How many months or weeks has he had them? Had the child injured himself in any way previous to these attacks? How often do the attacks occur? Do they occur at any particular time of day or night? What does the child do during a convulsion? Does he become stiff and rigid, then have rapid jerking movements? Does he just have a period of rigidity? Does any part of his body begin to jerk before the rest? Is his whole body affected or just part? Does the child urinate during the convulsion? Does the child fall to the floor and remain relaxed? Does the mother (or teacher) ever notice the child just staring into space for a few minutes? Any details regarding the nature of the convulsion should be reported to the physician. Hospitalization is usually needed in order to evaluate the child thoroughly and prescribe treatment.

Hospital admission. If the nurse knows in advance that a child is being admitted with convulsions, she should select a room for him which has both a suction and oxygen outlet. Oxygen mask and connecting tubes should be available in the room as well as a catheter for suctioning. Padded side rails should be placed on his bed. (When the child is in bed, these should be fastened in place securely.) A tracheotomy set and an endotracheal catheter also should be available.

The nurse's approach to the child should be the same as to any other child, unless by her observations it is obvious he is either subnormal or superior in intelligence. In either of these instances she would have to adjust her approach accordingly. Recreation should be provided for the child according to his age and ability. Other means of helping the child to feel at ease in a new situation have been discussed on p. 277. An older child should be asked if he knows or can tell when he is going to be sick (have an attack). If he has an aura or any kind of warning, the nurse should tell him to lie down at that time and so prevent possible self-injury. The child may or may not have ambulatory privileges. If he has, he may wish a tub bath, but because the child could have a seizure in the tub and drown a nurse has to remain with him while he bathes.

Care during a seizure. If the child has a convulsion while he is ambulating and falls to the floor, the nurse should not try to move him. Any objects on which he might injure himself during a convulsion need to be moved away. If the child is in bed when he has a convulsion, the nurse should first use a bell cord or light to summon help.

No matter where the child is when he has the convulsion, the nurse should note the duration and nature of the convulsion. She should be able to describe afterward in what part of the body the seizure began, to where it traveled, what the child did during the convulsion, and his behavior after it. Usually the child sleeps.

During the convulsion, the nurse should loosen tight clothing, especially around the neck, and turn the child on his side, if possible, to prevent pooling of secretions he might aspirate.

She can place the tongue depressor between his teeth, not in a tonic stage but later, as a means of obtaining a better passageway for oxygen. The main danger in a convulsion is respiratory obstruction, either from a spasm of the respiratory muscles or from mucus and secretions. If the child's color is very poor, she can give him oxygen by mask until the doctor arrives.

In summary, the nurse's responsibility during a convulsion of a child is to prevent injury to the child, prevent aspiration of secretions, maintain an open airway, and observe the convulsion as accurately as possible.

Diagnostic tests. The child should receive explanations in advance about the diagnostic tests that are given to him. These include venipunctures for blood examinations, urine examination, skull x-ray films, brain scan, and an electroencephalogram. A spinal tap may be done. A brain scan, a pneumoencephalogram, or an arteriogram may be done if an organic cause is suspected.

Administering medication. The medication ordered by the physician varies somewhat with the type of seizure the child has.

Drugs. In drug therapy for epilepsy the child is usually begun on a small dose of the selected drug, and then the dose is increased until the seizure is controlled or toxic symptoms appear. The child may remain on medication for a lifetime or, if seizures do not recur for several years, the drug may be slowly withdrawn.

The medications most frequently used for *grand mal* and *focal* seizures are phenobarbital, diphenylhydantoin sodium (Dilantin), and primidone (Mysoline). A combination of phenobarbital and Dilantin may be given. Other drugs are available if these do not control the seizures, but the ones named are the most frequently used.

In *psychomotor seizures* Dilantin, phenobarbital, benzedrine, and Mysoline are often used, although there are other medications available. For *petit mal,* ethosuximide (Zarontin) is sometimes called the drug of choice because of effectiveness and low toxicity. Benzedrine, dextroamphetamine (Dexedrine), and methsuximide (Celontin) have been recommended. Trimethadione (Tridione) and paramethadione (Paradine) are effective but very toxic. In *status epilepticus,* sodium phenobarbital, Dilantin, paraldehyde, or ether may be used. In *minor seizures* such as akinetic and myoclonic types, phenobarbital, Nebard, meprobamate, and acetazolamide (Diamox) are often prescribed. New drugs for the treatment of seizures are being developed and are rapidly becoming available.

Nursing responsibilities. In order to judge the effectiveness of the medication the nurse needs to chart the frequency, duration, and severity of the seizures so that an accurate comparison to earlier seizures can be made. Also, the nurse should be on the alert for toxic reactions and report them promptly to the physician. Possibly important toxic manifestations of the drug she is giving should be listed on the back of the medicine card for that drug.

Particular attention is called to the appearance of skin rash or skin reactions, since the drug may be withdrawn on their appearance. If abnormal symptoms such as drowsiness or ataxia are seen, the nurse should consult the physician before administering the medication, since these reactions are usually regulated by the size of the dose. With adjustment of the dose the drug is still given. Hyperactivity in relation to phenobarbital may denote idiosyncrasy to that drug. Hyperplasia of the gums and hypertrichosis may be side effects of Dilantin. Certain anticonvulsive drugs such as Tridione and Paradione cause depression of the bone marrow. For that reason periodic examinations are done of the blood of children receiving any of these drugs. In addition, the urine examination and kidney function tests are done on children receiving Tridione and Paradione, as the genitourinary system may be affected.

Surgical treatment

Surgery is sometimes performed in certain situations when the convulsions are not controlled by medications. A hemispherectomy is performed when a child has hemiplegia from a developmental defect or birth injury. Sometimes a temporal lobectomy is performed if the seizure originated with atrophy of the temporal lobe. Sometimes surgery is also done when there is believed to be scarring of the brain due to previous head injuries. This scarred tissue may act as an epileptogenic focus, and the tissue around the scar is removed. Anticonvulsant medications are used after surgical treatment.

Preparation for discharge

When the child leaves the hospital, what guidance do the parents need? What should the child understand? The doctor and nurse need to discuss teaching and home guidance of the child before he is discharged so there is an understanding and classification of the teaching to be done and who will do it.

Medications. Depending on the age and the depth of understanding of the child, he should be told about the importance of taking his medication and how much to take. His dosage should be written out for him (and his parents)

on paper so there will be no mistake about it. If he is taking Tridione capsules, it is essential that they be stored in a cool place, since the drug evaporates when exposed to excessive temperatures.

The parents and the child together might keep a diary of each attack and bring it to the physician's office or pediatric outpatient clinic on their return visit. Parents should understand that with medication the seizures should lessen in frequency until none appears but that sometimes it takes time to find the drug most suited to that particular child. If the drug that he is taking does not have desired results, another drug or a combination of drugs could be used. Parents sometimes need assurance that the medications are not narcotics and the child will not be a drug addict as a result of taking them.

Parental attitudes and adjustment. As with any child who has a handicap, the manner in which the parents accept the situation is going to influence the child. Much social stigma is attached to epilepsy, which causes parents to have deep emotions about it, ambivalent ones. They may love the child but feel anxious, frightened, and inadequate in their care of the child. They often feel guilt, as well as bitterness, that they produced such a child. Ambivalence may cause them discomfort in his presence. Before the child is discharged the services of a social worker or even those of a psychiatrist may be necessary in order for the child to have the family emotional climate so essential to him. Sometimes a foster home placement may be beneficial.

In regard to neighbors it is better to let them know the child has "attacks" than to hide the child. Neighbors can be told frankly that the child is receiving medicine to lessen and to prevent his having more attacks.

Health guidance in child's adjustment

Activities. The child with epilepsy needs companionship of other children, just as any child does.

Prior to discussing the home care of the child the nurse can find out what particular activities he usually enjoys so the doctor can set any necessary limits. In general, children with epilepsy should receive the same supervision that any child should and enjoy the same activities; however, the parents should be warned that climbing trees, swimming, and horseback riding are not without danger. If the child swims, someone should be with him. (This is a safe rule also for any well child or adult.) Whether he should enter a competitive sport when he is a teenager may be questioned. It needs discussion. How well the medication controls the seizures is really the important factor. Older children like to talk or ask questions of the doctor directly; especially is this true of the teenager who is interested in driving a car, marriage, and gainful employment. Each child is an individual so no one set of rules can be applied. There is often more danger in forbidding activities in which other children indulge than in permitting these activities because it makes the child feel "different" and lessens his self-confidence. There are no statistics to prove that epileptic children have more accidents than other children. Learning to roller-skate, swim, or ride a bicycle develops courage. Some camps accept epileptic children. A change of environment and wholesome outdoor living may prove very beneficial to the child.

Although all children need outlets for their emotions and activities in which they take pleasure, this is particularly important for the child who has a handicap; and epilepsy is a handicap. Swimming, driving, playing musical instruments, playing tennis, or gardening may give the child the emotional outlet he needs.

Discipline. The child should have the same discipline as other siblings. Discipline means teaching the child acceptable ways of behavior. (Refer to a discussion of this on pp. 210 and 225.) Overprotection and special privileges may injure the child. He needs the companionship of other children and needs to learn to share, take turns, and participate in play with them.

School attendance. Children can attend school as others do unless they are mentally retarded. In that case they may be placed in a special class or special school. The school should be informed of the child's condition and care. Further knowledge by the schoolteacher and school authorities about a particular child and his particular condition may change a negative attitude to a positive one. The school nurse often can be very helpful in interpreting the child's care to the school. If the teacher knows what to do specifically if the child does have a seizure, she will likely be better prepared for such an emergency.

Organizations for epilepsy. The nurse should know whether there are local organizations for epilepsy. The parents may be interested in joining because knowing other parents who have a child with a similar condition is often helpful.

In some cities clubs are formed by those interested in children with epilepsy, to which parents, professional personnel, and others belong. Some of these clubs have joined the National Epilepsy League at 130 North Wiles Street, Chicago, Ill. The National League helps to keep others informed about epilepsy and any new developments and facts.

Of general interest to the parents might be the knowledge that state departments of education have specialists for education of handicapped children, of whom the child with epilepsy is one.

Prognosis

When children with epilepsy do not receive treatment, the seizures may become worse. Approximately one half of the children with epilepsy gain complete suppression of seizures with adequate therapy. If the medication is discontinued, most of the children will have a recurrence of seizures.

Children with petit mal attacks may cease to have them by adolescence, but these attacks may be replaced by grand mal attacks.

The outcome of convulsions other than idiopathic epilepsy depends on the organic cause. A small percentage of all children with febrile convulsions develop seizures later in life.

Summary

A convulsion is a symptom of an abnormal process in the brain. Although there are numerous organic causes, no specific cause is known for most seizures in children. The name *idiopathic epilepsy* is given to this group.

The role of the nurse is in case finding, accurate observation and reporting of convulsive seizures, proper care of the child during a seizure, and (together with other members of a health team) education of both the parents and the affected child in how to live with this handicapping condition.

RHEUMATOID ARTHRITIS (STILL'S DISEASE)

In other readings that the student does she may find rheumatoid arthritis classified under *collagen diseases,* likewise rheumatic fever. They both have one common feature, which is destruction and deterioration of connective tissue. In addition, certain manifestations of the disease may be the same, but each one has separate characteristics. As the child with rheumatoid arthritis has to have medical supervision over a period of years, a discussion of rheumatoid arthritis appears in this chapter.

Nature of the condition

The exact etiology of rheumatoid arthritis is unknown. Some authorities believe it is a hypersensitivity response and others, a direct infection from unknown infectious agents. Rheumatoid arthritis is rare in infants under 1 year of age. The median age of onset is 5 years and it is more common in girls than boys. There appears to be a genetic factor, since rheumatoid arthritis has a high familial incidence. Psychological stress may be related to both the onset of the disease and acute exacerbations. Climate has some influence; the disease is seen more often in the spring months and in temperate zones.

The onset of the disease can be insidious or it can be sudden with fever, an arthralgia (articular neuralgia), adenopathy, splenomegaly, and anemia. There may be stiffness, swelling, and gradual limitation of motion of a single joint or of more than one joint. The joint may be warm to the touch. Joints in the lower part of the body may be affected fiirst, but eventually all joints may be involved. In young children there may be just pain and stiffness of joints without any other manifestations of the disease.

Flexion contractures may occur due to limitation of motion rather than to the process of the disease itself. The affected child may have a salmon pink, macular rash. The rash may appear blotchy if some of the spots coalesce. Subcutaneous nodules may be present on the occiput, spine, and ulna. The hands and feet of the child may be cold. Sedimentation rate is elevated in the acute phase, and there is leukocytosis, albuminuria, and anemia; C-reactive protein is present in the serum. Carditis is sometimes a complication of the disease.

Treatment

There is no curative agent for rheumatoid arthritis. Palliation of the signs and symptoms necessitates the use of anti-inflammatory drugs. Acetylsalicylic acid (ASA) in large doses is the most commonly used drug. If the child does not respond to aspirin therapy, then corticosteroid therapy is started. The corticosteroids are used with caution and in the lowest dosage possible because of their side effects of growth disturbances, osteoporosis, gastric ulceration, endocrine imbalance, and decreased resistance to infections. The amount of drugs and the length of therapy should be determined by the amount and time it takes to permit the child to engage in a normal amount of physical activity. Attendance at school is encouraged, and the parents should actively participate in the overall care of the child. Physical therapy should be used to prevent contractures and severe deformities.

To prevent deformity, to maintain motion in the affected joints, and to help the child toward normal mental and emotional growth are all aims in therapy of the child with rheumatoid arthritis. As stated earlier, the disease may continue for years, although there are periods of remission.

Role of the nurse

Hospital admission. When a child is admitted with a tentative diagnosis of rheumatoid arthritis, he should be placed, if possible, in a room with a child of similar age. As the child will be in the hospital for several weeks, it is good for him to have a like-age companion. The room should be away from the nurse's station so there is less chance of the child's rest at night or during rest hour being disturbed by noise and commotion. A room away from the elevator is also advantageous.

Observations. On admission and daily the nurse needs to note whether there is redness, swelling, and pain in the joints, the general behavior of the child (irritable, relaxed, quiet), the child's facial expression, and the way he uses his body functionally.

When the parents are present, the nurse should be observant of the parent-child relationship. She should be careful not to chart such a phrase as "domineering mother," but rather, note the action of the mother and the interaction between the mother and the child. Nurses' notes are a means of communication with the physician and, since psychological stress so often plays a part in the disease, some understanding of the parent-child relationship is important.

Emotional support. It is the physician's responsibility to tell the parents about the nature of the disease. A school-age child also needs an understanding of his physical condition.

If the child is in the hospital for a period of time and many people come and go from the room, the thoughtful charge nurse on each shift should visit the child daily, even if the visit is brief. This provides a continuity of care and helps the child to know that there are certain people on each tour of duty who are present to look after him. Staff nurses and nursing aids change assignments so there is only the charge nurse on each shift who really sees the child with some consistency. School should be provided in the hospital for this child, the same as for any child during a long-term illness. Also, there should be recreational activity for afternoon and early evening. (See p. 465 for further discussion of psychological aspects of any long-term illness.) It is sufficient to call attention here to the fact that every effort should be made not to have the child unduly dependent on others.

General nursing measures. Some physicians suggest that a board be used under a child's mattress and as few pillows be used as possible; certainly none should be under the child's knees. A small pillow under his head should be adequate.

Since the stiffness in joints is usually worse in the mornings, the nurse should have the child wash his hands before breakfast in fairly hot water. Just to lay hands in the water and to exercise fingers in it may serve to alleviate some of the discomfort, and the child will eat breakfast better. A warm tub bath is helpful after breakfast.

Nutrition and daily weight records are important. Any weight gain indicates improved health. The child is usually anemic, so watching food intake or whether there is continued loss or gain of weight is part of nursing care. Eating with others in the recreation room and having pleasant surroundings is more conducive to the child's eating than if he remains alone in his room. If the child is not ambulatory, his bed might be pushed into the recreation room at mealtime.

Exercise. Whether the child remains in bed or is ambulatory depends on how acute the disease process is. After the acute phase of the disease the child is encouraged to ambulate, if only for a limited time. Ambulation and participation in normal activity in which the child is interested are part of physiotherapy.

In addition, the child usually has specific exercises to take, either in his own room or in a physiotherapy department. Communication between the physiotherapist and the nurse is necessary so that the nurse will be aware of the aims and treatments given by the therapist; this will enable her to be consistent with the therapist in caring for the child on the unit.

Rest. In the acute phase when the child is on bed rest, and even after he is ambulatory, a night's restful sleep is very helpful emotionally and physically; likewise, he should have at least 1 hour of bed rest in the middle of the day.

Administering medication. Salicylates are usually prescribed for inflammation and pain. They are ordered in sufficient amounts to maintain a blood level around 20 mg. per 100 ml.

Steroids (especially prednisone) may be given when the child is acutely ill, but they are not continued over a period of time because of the side effects.

Whatever drugs are given, the nurse's responsibility is not only in the actual administration of the drug and in watching for side effects but also in seeing if there is improvement of the symptoms.

Psychiatric guidance. Sometimes the services of the psychiatrist are sought by the child's physician to aid both the child and the parents in the long-term illness. If so, free communication between the psychiatrist and the nurse is essential so that the child and his parents can be guided with consistency. Sometimes the services of a social worker are utilized. The nurse should be cognizant that a team approach for the care of the child is necessary. The nurse can contribute best if she understands the total medical care plan for the child.

Preparation for discharge. Before the child is discharged the nurse needs to discuss with the physician whether the services of a public health nurse might be helpful. A medication and special exercises are continued over a period of time. If the child is of school age, he will be attending school either in a regular class or in a special class, depending on the severity of the handicap.

Parents should receive guidance or general factors relative to promotion of health, the same as for any other child. (Refer to Chapter 9.)

SCOLIOSIS
Nature of the condition

Scoliosis is a lateral curvature of the spine. Although it could be caused by congenital lesions such as hemivertebra or infections like poliomyelitis, most of scoliosis is idiopathic. Scoliosis may be mild, with the spine a C shape, or it can be so severe that the spine may assume an S shape. The condition is more frequently seen in girls and is associated with the adolescent.

Early recognition of scoliosis is important in order to prevent an increase in it. If the child has a severe scoliosis, one shoulder appears higher than the other, one hip is more prominent, and shoulder blades project. In addition, there may be shortness of breath because of the diminished respiratory capacity as well as gastrointestinal upsets from crowding of the abdominal organs.

In treatment of scoliosis, corrective exercises are often first prescribed in order to mobilize the spine, and a Risser jacket or Milwaukee brace may be applied to prevent further increase in scoliosis and to correct the curve. A spinal fusion is done to stabilize the spine and prevent further curving. Following surgery a cast is still worn, and then a brace for many months. Some orthopedic surgeons correct the curve by performing a rib resection, then straightening the spine. A cast is worn for a period of time afterward.

Role of the nurse

Nursing care of a child with a cast is described on p. 341. If the child has a Risser jacket, particular attention needs to be given to possible irritation of the skin around the neck of the child. The cast may need further trimming or further padding.

See p. 415 for psychological aspects of operations and pp. 296 and 297, respectively, for general preoperative and postoperative care.

The child can continue in school with either a brace or a cast. Postoperatively either a cast or a brace is worn for a long time to maintain the corrected position. Insofar as possible, the adolescent girl or boy should continue his usual activities and interests.

OSTEOCHONDROSIS (LEGG-CALVÉ-PERTHES DISEASE)

In osteochondrosis there is an aseptic necrosis of the head of the femur. It occurs most frequently in boys of age 3 to 12 years. The first sign noticeable is usually a limp; also, the child may complain of pain. There is some limitation of motion and muscle spasm. Changes in the hip bones are seen on roentgenograms. It is a self-limiting disease.

The aim of treatment is to prevent flattening of the femoral head. To accomplish this the child may first be placed in traction, which helps to overcome any muscle spasm. Then he is allowed up, but no weight is to be placed on the affected hip. Often a Thomas walking caliper splint is used with crutches. The lower part of the affected leg is placed in a sling that goes to the shoulder of the opposite side. Sometimes a nonweight-bearing splint with a patten bottom is used. The shoe on the affected leg is built up several inches.

The child is examined at regular intervals by the doctor. This may be continued for 2 to 4 years before the child is permitted to bear weight on his leg. During this time, the child may attend school and enter general family activities.

CEREBRAL PALSY
The problem

Care of children with cerebral palsy constitutes a social and economic problem as well as a medical problem. Cerebral palsy is among the leading causes of crippling. Frequently the child has more than one handicap. For this reason a team approach to the care of the child is essential. There is no cure for the condition, but sufficient help may be given to some of these children to make them better able to live with this problem and contribute to society.

Nature of the condition

Cerebral palsy is a term that is used rather loosely to designate the disorder of those children whose motor centers of the brain do not function normally. Cerebral palsy is characterized by paralysis, weakness, and incoordination of voluntary movements. There are often other manifestations of brain damage such as seizures, visual and hearing handicaps, speech problems, and mental retardation.

Anoxia in the perinatal period and trauma in the natal and postnatal period are two of the most important etiological factors, although cerebral palsy could follow an infection such as meningitis and encephalitis or be due to kernicterus.

Manifestations

The commonest manifestations of cerebral palsy are *athetosis* and *spastic paralysis.*

In athetosis, constant, irregular, and involuntary slow movements are seen.

There are several different types of spastic paralysis. If one extremity is affected, it is called monoplegia; both lower extremities, paraplegia; one side of the body, hemiplegia; three extremities, triplegia; or all four extremities, quadriplegia.

The child with spastic paralysis has hyperirritability to all stimuli. Reflexes are exaggerated. His movements are jerky and uncertain. There is spastic rigidity of the parts of body involved. Possibly the child is in opisthotonos position. Spasms of the muscles and tendons may cause a position of scissoring of the legs or be such that the child cannot straighten his legs or arms as he stands. The child is unable to relax even in his sleep. Spasticity of facial muscles produces difficulties in chewing food. Drooling is common. Eye defects are very common. The child shows delayed motor development.

It is difficult to judge the intelligence of the child with spastic paralysis, especially one who is severely handicapped. Both the child's verbal and nonverbal means of communication are highly limited. Speech of the child may be too indistinct to understand, and he cannot control voluntary motions and actions. He makes grimaces when he tries to talk or even smile because he is unable to control facial muscles. Expression of the child's eyes may help the nurse to understand what he is feeling or whether he is understanding what she is saying.

The ultimate aim in treatment of the child with cerebral palsy is to help develop his potentials to the fullest extent so in adulthood he can be a contributing citizen. To this end treatment is directed toward aiding the child in physical independence, providing schooling in accordance with his mental capacity, providing vocational training, and guiding the child and his family to adjust both emotionally and socially to his condition.

To achieve these goals requires the combined efforts of several types of medical specialists, plus the use of educational and social resources in the community. The attitude of the child's family and the community toward this child influences very much whether the child will put forth his best efforts to cooperate and try to help himself.

Some of the children with cerebral palsy are so handicapped physically and mentally that custodial care in an institution or in the home is required, whereas other children may be of normal intelligence and can be aided with treatment.

Parent teaching

In her guidance of the child with spastic paralysis, the public health nurse should instruct the mother how to encourage self-help activities such as eating and dressing. The child may be 5 or 6 years of age before he is toilet trained. The nurse needs to interpret the child's health needs to the mother. The social and emotional needs of this child are the same as for any healthy child, except that this handicapped child has an even greater need of being accepted and liked. This child, like any other, needs companionship and play. (For ways to promote his general health see Chapter 9.)

The nurse should know if there are special classes for the handicapped in the community. Such information is available from the board of education. Sometimes there are camps for handicapped children, to which a child with this condition could go in the summer. The nurse should also be familiar with community resources for speech therapy and know whether there is a local organization of the United Cerebral Palsy National Association. Parents may derive benefit and comfort from a discussion of their problems with other parents who have a child with a similar condition and similar problems.

HYPERTHYROIDISM (THYROTOXICOSIS)
Nature of the condition

Hyperthyroidism in childhood occurs as a result of diffuse hyperplasia of the thyroid gland. This results in an increased amount of thyroid hormone secretion. It occurs approximately five times more commonly in girls than in boys, and the majority of the cases occur between 10 and 15 years of age. The onset of the disease is gradual and occurs most often near the time of puberty. There is a high incidence of a family history of thyrotoxicosis, suggesting a genetic basis as a possible etiological factor. Another causative factor entertained is that of an intrinsic abnormality within the thyroid gland itself, causing a disturbance in the iodine metabolic pathway of the gland.

Manifestations

The clinical symptoms of hyperthyroidism develop because of the excessive thyroid hormone secretion. These include increasing appetite, sweating, and increased heart rate. Even with the increased appetite the child may continue to lose weight. The child may become overtly anxious and frightened with minimal excitation. Fine tremor of the fingers and tongue is present. The thyroid gland becomes

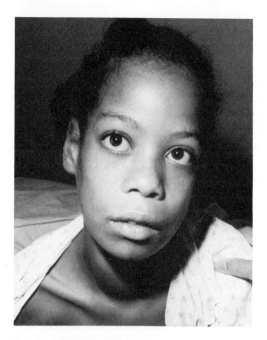

Fig. 16-5. Hyperthyroidism in a 10-year-old child. Note presence of exophthalmos and enlarged thyroid gland.

gradually enlarged and may be felt by palpation of the neck. The eyeballs may become very prominent (exophthalmos) as the disease progresses.

Laboratory determinations ordered to assist in the diagnosis are (1) protein-bound iodine (P.B.I.) determination, (2) butanol-extractable iodine (B.E.I.) determination of blood, (3) uptake of radioactive iodine, and (4) T_3 suppression test. The levels measured by these tests are characteristically elevated in hyperthyroidism.

The prognosis of thyrotoxicosis in childhood is good with early and adequate treatment. The course of the disease varies, but the illness is more benign in children than in adults.

Treatment

The treatment of hyperthyroidism must be directed toward the reduction of excessive thyroid hormone secretion. The two principal methods used to reduce these secretions are: (1) drugs such as propylthiouracil and methemazole (Tapazole) to suppress the formation of thyroid hormone and (2) subtotal thyroidectomy. Most authorities are presently using the conservative medical management. The treatment must be carefully monitored by clinical evaluation and laboratory studies to determine the amount of effects of the drugs being used. The treatment may have to be continued for 2 to 5 years before the child is symptom free and the thyroid gland is normal in size and function.

If the medical treatment fails, surgical removal of part or all of the thyroid gland is performed. Surgical removal of all of the thyroid gland requires the administration of exogenous thyroid preparations for an indefinite period of time.

REFERENCES

Bain, H. W., and Chote, A.: Diabetes in school children, Pediatr. Clin. North Am. **12:**919, November, 1965.

Baird, H.: The child with convulsions, New York, 1972, Grune & Stratton, Inc.

Bakwin, H., and Bakwin, R.: Behavior disorders of children, ed. 4, Philadelphia, 1972, W. B. Saunders Co.

Bray, P. F.: Neurology in pediatrics, Chicago, 1969, Year Book Medical Publishers, Inc.

Brewer, E.: Rheumatoid arthritis in childhood, Am. J. Nurs. **65:**66, June, 1965.

Burgess, L.: Morale boosting in cystic fibrosis, Am. J. Nurs. **69:**332, 1969.

Chahen, N.: Strep screening: from project to ongoing program, Am. J. Nurs. **75:**1489, September, 1975.

Crate, M.: Nursing function in adaptation to chronic illness, Am. J. Nurs. **65:**72, October, 1965.

Dekaban, A.: Epilepsy. In Neurology of early childhood, Baltimore, 1970, The Williams & Wilkins Co.

DiMaggio, G.: The child with asthma, Nurs. Clin. North Am. September, 1968.

Ellis, R., and Mitchell, R. G.: Disease in infancy and childhood, ed. 7, Baltimore, 1973, The Williams & Wilkins Co.

Farmer, T., editor: Pediatric neurology, ed. 2, New York, 1975, Harper & Row Publishers.

Feeney, R.: Preventing rheumatic fever in school children, Am. J. Nurs. **73:**265, February, 1973.

Fielding, W. J., and Waugh, T.: Postoperative correction of scoliosis, J.A.M.A. **182:**541, 1962.

Foley, M. F.: Pulmonary function testing, Am. J. Nurs. **71:**1134, January, 1971.

Ford, F.: The epileptics and paroxysmal disorders of the nervous system. In Diseases of the nervous system in infancy, childhood, and adolescence, ed. 6, Springfield, Ill., 1973, Charles C Thomas, Publisher.

Gellis, S., and Kagan, B., editors: Current pediatric therapy, ed. 6, Philadelphia, 1973, W. B. Saunders, Co.

Goldman, L.: Prevention and treatment of eczema, Am. J. Nurs. **64:**112, March, 1964.

Gordis, L., et al.: Studies in the epidemiology and preventability of rheumatic fever, Pediatrics **43:**173, 1969.

Johnson, M. I., and Fassett, B. A.: Bronchopulmonary hygiene in cystic fibrosis, Am. J. Nurs. **69:**320, 1969.

Keith, J. M.: Heart disease in infancy and childhood, New York, 1967, The Macmillan Co.

Kurihara, M.: Postural drainage, clapping and vibrating, Am. J. Nurs. **65:**76, November, 1965.

Lerner, M.: The juvenile diabetic and the visiting nurse, Am. J. Nurs. **68:**106, 1968.

McCollum, A. T., and Gibson, L. E.: Family adaptation to the child with cystic fibrosis, J. Pediatr. **77:**571, 1970.

McLean, R. H., and Roger, H.: Childhood nephrosis; the influence of infection in therapy, J. Pediatr. **65:**558, 1964.

National Cystic Fibrosis Research Foundation: Guide to drug therapy in patients with cystic fibrosis, New York, 1972, The Foundation.

Raney, R. B., and Brashear, H. R.: Shand's handbook of orthopedic surgery, ed. 8, St. Louis, 1971, The C. V. Mosby Co.

Roberts, F. B.: The child with heart disease, Am. J. Nurs. **2:**1080, June, 1972.

Sather, M.: Environmental care of the asthmatic child, Am. J. Nurs. **68:**816, 1968.

Saxena, K. M., Crawford, J. D., and Talbot, N. B.: Childhood thyrotoxicosis: A long term perspective, Br. Med. J. **2:**1153, 1964.

Sheldon, J., Lovell, R., and Mathews, K.: A manual of clinical allergy, ed. 2, Philadelphia, 1967, W. B. Saunders Co.

Shirkey, H. C., editor: Pediatric therapy, ed. 5, St. Louis, 1975, The C. V. Mosby Co.

Stadnyk, S.: A camp for children with cystic fibrosis, Am. J. Nurs. **70:**691, August, 1970.

Steele, S.: The preschooler with nephrosis, Nurs. Outlook **12:**50, October, 1964.

Sultz, H., et al.: Longterm childhood illness, Pittsburgh, 1972, University of Pittsburgh Press.

Turk, J.: Impact of cystic fibrosis on family functioning, Pediatrics **34:**67, 1964.

Vaughan, V. C., III, and McKay, R. J.: Nelson's textbook of pediatrics, ed. 10, Philadelphia, 1975, W. B. Saunders Co.

17

Nursing care of
THE CHILD WITH A GRAVE PROGNOSIS

The fact that only a small percentage of those who die of cancer are children is actually misleading. When the pediatric nurse refers to mortality statistics of children, she can better evaluate the importance of malignancy in children. Among children from ages 1 to 4 years, malignancies are the fourth leading cause of death. In children 5 to 14 years of age, they are the second leading cause; the first is accidents.

Of interest is the fact that leukemia accounts for the largest proportion of the malignancies in children. Other common types of malignancy seen in children include tumor of the brain, neuroblastoma, nephroblastoma (Wilms' tumor of the kidney), retinoblastoma, and bone sarcoma. Hodgkin's disease is not as common in children as in adults.

In general, nursing care is directed toward making the child physically comfortable, giving emotional support to the parents, and aiding the physician in diagnostic and therapeutic measures. Because of medications, surgical measures, and radiation therapy, many of these afflicted children have remissions in which they feel well. During those periods of time the child's activities should continue in as normal a manner as possible. (Refer to paragraphs under common psychological factors for a fuller discussion of other psychological factors.) Here let us emphasize that the way the nurse feels about illness that has a grave prognosis is important since her feelings can so easily be transferred to the child in nonverbal communication. Also, because the child is likely to be readmitted several times before the terminal stage of illness, his adjustment to the hospital and hospital personnel is a matter of even more concern than that of children admitted for an acute episode of illness and then discharged.

Since the hospital nurse most frequently meets a child with leukemia, more attention is given to the nursing care of this condition than to nursing care of children with other types of malignancy. The school nurse may see the child with leukemia or other malignancy in school both prior to his illness and later, at the time of remissions of the disease, when the child feels well enough to carry on his usual interests and activities.

COMMON PSYCHOLOGICAL FACTORS

Children whose ultimate prognosis is poor present a challenge to parents, nurses, and all personnel who participate in their care—namely, their philosophy toward life and death. What the nurse, the mother, or others believe influences each in her behavior toward the child. This is true whether the child has leukemia, a malignant tumor, or any other condition with a poor prognosis.

Nurse's attitude. What the nurse does for the child in relation to meeting his spiritual needs depends on her own attitudes. Should the county public health nurse see that a pastor of the family's faith is informed of the child's condition or should she leave this to the family of the child? Should the hospital nurse request the chaplain to come to visit a toddler and to pray for the child? Should the nurse herself talk to the child about the meaning of life and death? Are the spiritual needs of a child met if a chaplain visits him daily? Are the spiritual needs of like-age children met in the same way? What is the attitude of the nurse toward death?

503

Between the time of the child's diagnosis and the terminal stage of the disease, there may be an interval of months or years. A child with Cooley's anemia or progressive muscular dystrophy may live until early adulthood and die of an intercurrent infection. A child with leukemia who is under medical supervision has periods of remission when he feels fine. In the interval between the diagnosis and the terminal stage of the disease, should the child learn something more of religion in general? Should the child be told the prognosis for leukemia? Should the child and his parents talk together concerning their beliefs about the hereafter? Would the truth help to relieve tension between parents and child? The answers of each nurse to these questions vary in accord with her own beliefs.

Reactions of parents. What the news of the child's prognosis may mean to the parents depends on their relationship to the child. If the parent-child relationship is a close one, the news may be overwhelming. The parents may refuse to believe it and may take the child to several different private physicians or hospital clinics before they can accept the diagnosis and prognosis for the child. In this crisis religion may be more meaningful to the parents than it was formerly. A pastor may be able to bring comfort to such a family. In caring for the child the nurse needs to take into consideration the parents' reactions to the child's illness. She should express sympathy but not pity. The mother who feels hostility toward the child may cover this up by an oversolicitous and protective attitude. She may be the mother who showers attention on the child.

The stages of grief may be considered as (1) shock, denial, and disbelief, (2) sadness, anger, and anxiety, and (3) adaptation and acceptance.

Going to one doctor after another is part of denial of the diagnosis and the prognosis. It takes some people a longer time to pass through the stage of denial than it does others. Sometimes a family friend may help, sometimes a social workers, a doctor, or a minister. From denial the parent moves to the stage of anger or sadness. A parent may say, "Why does this have to happen to *my* child?" In this stage of awareness, which may sometimes last for

months, there needs to be an adaptation to the situation on the part of the child and the parents. Parents may go through another stage of grief called "bargaining." "If my child will only live, I will . . ." The parents are ready to promise something in return for the child's health or perhaps a longer period of remission. Parents may move into the stage of adaptation or acceptance by themselves or they may need help.

Care in remissions. In the period when the child is at home during a remission of symptoms, it is generally conceded that the family's usual routine and pattern of living should be followed. Extra privileges or changes may confuse the child and make him anxious. The child may attend school and participate in activities he enjoys. One 11-year-old child wrote an article entitled Is It So Awful? (Timmons, 1975). Between her remissions, this child led a full life with various school activities and apparently gave pleasure to herself and others. Apparently she had worked through the stages of grief, including adaptation or acceptance.

To act the same as usual may be difficult for parents. Their knowledge of the child's prognosis is hard on them. Each time the child with leukemia returns to have his blood count checked, there is a period of painful suspense. Is the child going to be readmitted or can he remain at home still? If he is readmitted, the question is "Is this admission terminal?" In order to give their best to the child, both parents, especially the mother, need to get away from the child for their own recreational and emotional needs. Irritability, fatigue, and even rebellious hostile feelings are possible results if the mother devotes her entire time to the child.

Terminal stage. When the terminal stage of the disease approaches, should the child be told he is going to die? Death to a small child means absence. Children often have seen the death of a pet. Sometimes an elderly relative has died. Parents may have said the relative "has gone up to God."

Children sometimes have an awareness that they are seriously ill without anyone saying anything. Sometimes there is a nonverbal communication through facial expression, gestures, method of touching, etc. An older child may wish to express himself but does not know how to begin. Sometimes an older child has been afraid to let his parents know that he understands his condition for fear it would worry them more. Talking things over together is usually considered supportive to both the child and the parent. Tension may be relieved.

During the terminal illness the presence of the nurse is comforting to the parents. She cannot stay with the child constantly unless she is his own private duty nurse, but she should visit the child frequently and keep him as comfortable as possible. Often parents like to participate in the child's care since to help him in any way gives them a feeling of usefulness. A small child likes to be held.

Sometimes after the child has died, parents, especially the mother, may like to come into the hospital to speak with some of the nurses and doctors who knew him. This may aid the stage of resolution. The funeral has aided the parent toward the reality of the fact that the child has gone to another life, but the parent still needs time before they can reorganize their own life without the presence of the child who died. Talking to the nurse about the child's last illness may help the mother. One mother brought to the hospital various toys for other children to use that had belonged to her child. A thoughtful public health nurse may call on the parents (if she has known them previously) and allow the parents to express their feelings. Parents cannot immediately resolve their feelings and their life without the child. They need to know of people's interest and sympathy, that their child is not forgotten even though he has gone.

If the child has had to receive considerable physical care before his death, the mother may be very tired. Her health also should be the concern of the nurse. The mother might like to discuss the reactions of the siblings to the child's death. On questions about the explanation of death, the nurse should refer the family to their pastor. This is in his area of training and concern; however, if the mother does say to the nurse, "But what do you really believe?" it is hoped that the nurse will have found a philosophy that enables her to give an answer that can comfort the parents.

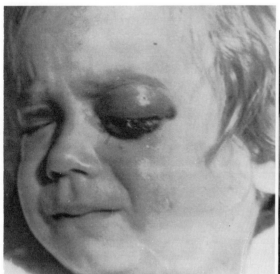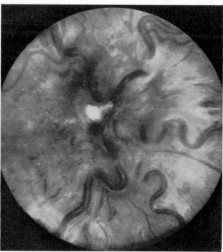

Fig. 17-1. A, Intraocular and orbital hemorrhage in monocytic leukemia. The globe later ruptured. **B,** The fundus in acute myelocytic leukemia, showing papilledema, enormous engorgement, tortuosity of retinal veins, and hemorrhage on disk. (From Donaldson, D. D.: Trans. Am. Ophthalmol. Soc. **62:**429, 1964.)

MALIGNANCIES
Leukemia
Nature of the condition

In leukemia there is uncontrolled proliferation of leukocytes and their precursors. The disorder is characterized by bone marrow dysfunction, increased metabolism, and infiltration of various tissues and organs by the leukemic process. These characteristics account for the signs the nurse sees and the symptoms the child feels when he is admitted to the hospital. His blood count may show leukopenia. Sometimes there are infections of the mouth and pharynx due to a deficiency of normal granulocytes.

The incidence of leukemia is high in the first 5 years of life, and again at 8 or 9 years of age. It occurs more in boys than girls. In contrast to leukemia in adulthood, the disease in childhood is usually very acute.

Leukemia may be classified, according to the predominating cell seen, as lymphocytic, myelocytic, and monocytic. Often in children the predominating cell is lymphocytic, although it is sometimes undifferentiated and is called a stem cell. Acute lymphoblastic leukemia is regarded as the most common form of leukemia in childhood.

The etiology of leukemia is unknown. The disease usually has a fatal outcome. Some children have prolonged remissions with drug therapy, thus making the prognosis undeterminable.

Clinical manifestations

The onset of the disease may be gradual, and a frequent history is that of weight loss, fever, pallor, and easy bruising in a previously normal child. Bleeding from the gums, epistaxis, or persistent hemorrhage after a minor operation may be the first evidence of acute leukemia. The disease may be ushered in by an upper respiratory infection from which the child does not recover as expected with routine treatment.

The most common abnormal physical findings are usually enlargement of the lymph nodes, especially of the cervical region, hepatomegaly, splenomegaly, petechiae, purpura, and ecchymoses. Almost all body organs may become infiltrated with leukemic cells, thereby becoming abnormal in size and function.

Treatment

The aim of therapy in children with leukemia is the destruction of the leukemic process in the blood and tissues and the return of hematopoiesis to normal. There is no curative method or agent that permanently controls the disease process. The three principal therapeutic agents used in childhood leukemia are (1) the antileukemic chemotherapeutic agents such as methotrexate, mercaptopurine (Purinethol), and cytarabine (Cytosar), (2) the cytotoxic agents such as radiation, busulfan (Myleran), cyclophosphamide (Cytoxan), and vincristine (Oncovin), and (3) immunotherapeutic agents such as ACTH and corticosteroids. Appropriate management depends upon the selection of these agents for administration alone or in combination. Most of the chemotherapeutic agents are used because they inhibit one or more of the steps in nucleic acid biosynthesis. Methotrexate is a folic acid antagonist and is effective because leukemia cells requre more folic acid than do normal cells. Cyclophosphamide is a polyfunctional akylating agent. The corticosteroids are beneficial because of their effects on blood vessel integrity and suppression of the leukemic process in the bone marrow. The use of steroids is the treatment of choice when serious bleeding occurs and the patient's condition is critical. Rapid and dramatic remissions have resulted by the use of these hormones in critically ill patients with acute leukemia within several weeks of treatment. A remission is defined as eradication of morphological evidence of leukemia from the blood and bone marrow with the return of normal health. At least three remissions are possible before the child becomes refractory to all therapy.

One or two of the chemotherapeutic drugs are usually continued in the form of maintenance therapy to prolong the remission period. When the leukemic process recurs, a new attempt at eradication of the abnormal cells is initiated with a different drug. Cyclic drug therapy has been used by some authorities to prevent the development of resistance to the chemotherapeutic drugs.

Blood transfusions are administered frequently to combat anemia and to control hemorrhage. Also, fresh whole blood has been reported to have caused an occasional remission. Infusions of platelet concentrates may be needed if severe bleeding is secondary to thrombocytopenia. Leukocyte transfusions are ordered when the child develops severe leukopenia due to the drug therapy or the disease process.

The disease and the therapy tend to lower the body's defense mechanism to infections. Antibiotics are used to treat and control infections. The most frequently used antibiotics are methicillin, ampicillin, gentamicin, and carbinicillin. Fungal infections such as moniliasis are treated with antifungal antibiotics such as nystatin (Mycostatin).

In some special leukemia care units, facilities for a strict sterile environment may be available. It is provided by a plastic "life island" over the whole bed with portholes through which the needs of the child may be met.

Prognosis

Of children with leukemia, 10% to 15% respond poorly to all therapeutic attempts. An appreciable number of children now survive from 2 to 3 years after diagnosis, while a few children are alive 5 years or longer after the initial diagnosis.

Role of the nurse

Observations. As the nurse assists with the admission of the child to the hospital and cares for him daily, she should carefully evaluate the new patient's condition so she can formulate a nursing care plan to meet his particular needs. The condition of the child on admission is so variable that he may be very weak and in pain or he may be pale but in no distress.

Both on admission of the child and in her daily observations the nurse needs to be aware of various possible manifestations of the disease and record them. Because of bone marrow dysfunction there may be manifestations of pallor, listlessness, weakness, and hemorrhage. The nurse should note the skin for signs of bruising or petechiae; also, she should note whether there is any sign of bleeding from the gums and nose. The color of the urine may be dark red, as hematuria is sometimes present. Because of leukemic infiltration there may be bone and abdominal pain. If the central nervous system is involved, there may be such symptoms as headache, cerebral palsies, and (in an infant) separation of the cranial sutures.

As the posture and activity of a child may indicate the location of pain, the nurse should see whether the child moves all extremities freely, flexes his legs on his abdomen, lies predominantly in one position, or cries when he is moved.

When medications that suppress leukemia are administered, the nurse needs not only to watch for toxic symptoms but also to see if the child seems in any way worse, the same, or better. Some drugs have a more rapid effect than others. In general, after medications are begun the nurse should observe whether the child seems to eat better, act more sprightly, have less pain, and be less lethargic. Also, urine output should be recorded, since the urinary tract could be obstructed by precipitations of urate crystals. The urinary excretion of uric acid is considerable, especially after antileukemic drugs are begun.

Assisting with diagnostic measures and treatments. Because diagnostic procedures are so often repeated (such as venipunctures or bone aspirations) it is especially important to explain in simple terms to the child what is going to be done. Explanations may vary with the age and understanding of the child. After the procedure is completed the nurse should try to see that the child has some pleasant experience—possibly giving him a glass of fruit juice and a cookie, rocking the young child, or taking the older child into the playroom. As the presence of a familiar person lends support, it is helpful to the child if the same nurse who is assigned to his care is present when blood is drawn or when bone marrow aspiration, intravenous pyelogram, or x-ray examinations are done.

Reading the report of diagnostic treatments helps the nurse to understand the degree of illness of the child. The total number of leukocytes may be reduced at the beginning of the disease; however, the number is not as important as the characteristics of the cell. Immature cells, often lymphoblasts, are present.

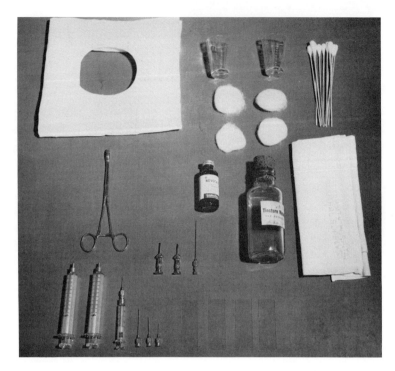

Fig. 17-2. Equipment for bone marrow puncture. (From Varga, C.: Handbook of pediatric medical emergencies, ed. 4, St. Louis, 1968, The C. V. Mosby Co.)

There is a decrease in the number of erythrocytes, and sometimes a severe anemia is seen. The x-ray film may reveal characteristic changes in bones as well as mediastinal lymph nodes, and an enlargement of liver, spleen, and kidney. After treatment with medication is begun these changes may disappear. The report of the intravenous pyelogram may show an enlarged kidney and other changes. Renal failure could occur as a result of leukemic infiltration. The report of the bone marrow biopsy, if the child has leukemia, shows immature or abnormal white cell precursors, as well as an overgrowth of abnormal leukopoietic tissue.

Blood transfusions are given as indicated. X-ray therapy may be done over the entire skull if the meninges are involved.

Administering medications. Once the diagnosis of leukemia is established, medications are ordered that will help the child to have a remission of the disease. Most of the medications are given orally because of easy bruising and bleeding from injections. Since the medica-

tion is so vital to the child, it is important to know how the child prefers to take the medicine. Does he pick up the tablet or capsule in his fingers, or does he tip up the cup to let the tablet drop in his mouth? What fluid does he like with his medications? This should be on the Kardex or other form that is used for the nursing care plan.

The nurse should watch for toxic symptoms of each of the drugs ordered and observe the child's appearance and behavior after the drug is started to see if there is a change. The nurse should also be aware that reexaminations of the blood and bone marrow are done to learn the effectiveness of the drugs on leukemia.

The deficiency of normal granulocytes predisposes toward the development of an infection. Analgesics and sedatives may be ordered for pain and antibiotics for any infection.

Nutrition. A nutritious diet high in calories, proteins, vitamins, and liver is helpful to the child. When acutely ill, the child may not be

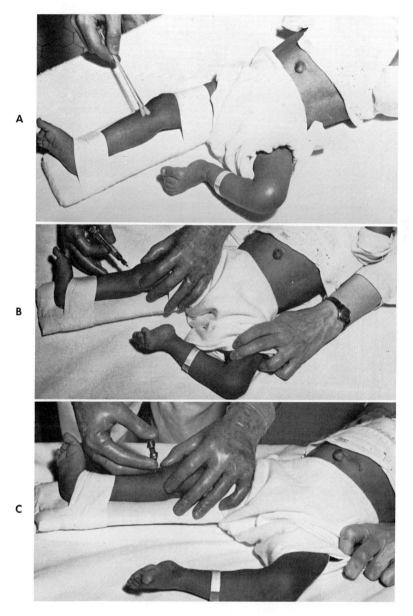

Fig. 17-3. Tibia bone marrow puncture. **A,** Painting skin with 2% iodine followed by 70% alcohol. **B,** Local anesthesia with 1% procaine. **C,** Insertion of trocar. (From DeSanctis, A. G., and Varga, C.: Handbook of pediatric medical emergencies, ed. 3, St. Louis, 1963, The C. V. Mosby Co.)

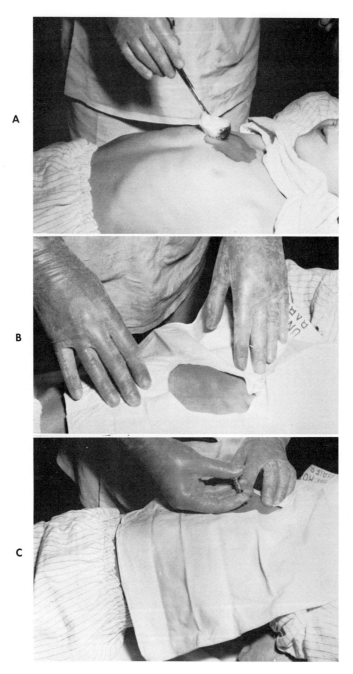

Fig. 17-4. Sternal bone marrow puncture. **A,** Skin antisepsis. **B,** Sterile draping prior to local anesthesia. **C,** Insertion of cannula. (From DeSanctis, A. G., and Varga, C.: Handbook of pediatric medical emergencies, ed. 3, St. Louis, 1963, The C. V. Mosby Co.)

hungry or feel like eating, so the nurse needs to be resourceful. (Refer to p. 283 for discussion of mealtime.) As the child begins to feel better, his appetite improves.

Physical comfort. Physical comfort measures are the best supportive care when the child is acutely ill. Oral hygiene is especially important if there is bleeding from the gums or if there are ulcerative areas in the child's mouth. Applicators, well-padded with cotton, can be substituted for a toothbrush and used to cleanse the child's teeth and gums. Afterward the child can rinse out his mouth with a solution. These oral hygiene measures should be done before and after eating. Although the child may wish to sit up for oral hygiene, he probably would be most comfortable with the headrest lowered afterward.

Turning the patient and propping him on alternate sides should be done gently and carefully because of the possibility of fracture. A bottom and drawsheet pulled tight is more comfortable than one full of wrinkles. Because of anemia the child's feet and legs may be cold. Possibly a small blanket tucked around the feet may warm the child and help him to relax. Suitable, attractive clothing helps the child to feel at ease. A warm bath every morning is refreshing, likewise having back and buttocks bathed and rubbed before nap time and bedtime.

If the central nervous system is involved and the child's head aches, the nurse might darken the room and try to reduce the noise outside the room as well as reduce stimuli within the room. Analgesics for pain should be given freely.

The afternoon nap and night's sleep are important to the child. Every effort should be made to see that he is comfortable and the environment conducive to rest.

Several times during every tour of duty, the nurse needs to return to the child's bedside so the child will know that "his" nurse is looking after him.

Recreation. The child should have diversion and occupational therapy in accordance with his condition, his age, and his interests. When he feels like playing, he should be provided with play materials. A small child who feels acutely ill may wish to be held and rocked or want to keep some favorite toy next to him. If the child is well enough to take an interest in his surroundings, he may like to have his bed pushed beside a window or want to go into the playroom with other children.

Interim care. When the blood and bone marrow show a remission of the disease and the child is again feeling well, he is discharged with instructions to return at periodic intervals to the clinic or doctor's office. This period of remission may last several months before he again returns to the hospital.

In this interim the child should be allowed to continue his usual interests. The same factors are conducive to good health as those outlined in Chapter 9. In the care of a particular child the nurse should refer to the section appropriate for his age. Activities should be geared to the child's condition. As long as he feels well, he can play outdoors, attend school, belong to scout or other organizations, etc.

Visits by a public health nurse are valuable, both to give the mother emotional support and to help judge whether the child needs to return to the clinic or private doctor before the scheduled date of a periodic examination. (For further discussion of psychological factors in his care refer to p. 503.)

Terminal stage. The child may be readmitted to the hospital several times before he returns in the terminal stage of the disease. Intracranial hemorrhage may cause the death of the leukemic child. He may be in a coma prior to his death, and medications should be administered freely to relieve the child of pain. He should be handled gently and carefully. All possible physical measures to make him comfortable should be employed. Care needs to be exercised in talking in front of the child because he understands more than is realized, even when he appears to be sleeping.

Each child should be judged as an individual and *his* particular needs evaluated. If he is used to seeing grandparents and parents at home, then the presence of four people is not disturbing to him; however, a steady stream of visitors is tiring. If any particular visitor seems upsetting to the child, the nurse or doctor can discuss the advisability of that person's visiting again.

If visitors come to see the parents, they should be received in the visitors' room, not the child's. Those people who are important to the child should see him, but not necessarily to talk to him. The effort of talking is sometimes tiring.

The child knows he is sick because he feels bad and hurts. At this point the question arises as to whether he should be prepared for the fact he is leaving this world. It is the prerogative of the parents, not the nurse, to make the decision. The nurse can inquire if the family wishes a pastor of their faith to be called, and she can ask the parents if the child knows what is happening. However, the child belongs to the parents, and it is their privilege to explain or not explain death to the child. The presence of a minister may be helpful to the parents.

The nurse can be helpful in making the child as comfortable as possible, in talking with parents and seeing that the mother and/or father have their meals and have the opportunity to rest at night. Returning often to the child's room lets the parents know that the nurse cares about both the child and them.

After the child does die the parents may wish to be alone with him for a few moments before they leave the hospital. The nurse should see that they have this opportunity if they wish it.

Brain tumor
Nature of the condition

Next to leukemia in childhood, malignancies of the central nervous system are the most common (Murphy, 1972). This group includes tumors of the brain and eye. With the exception of the cystic cerebellar astrocytoma tumor, the prognosis is grave for children with brain tumors. The location of the tumor often makes removal difficult or impossible since they tend to be below the tentorium in the *posterior fossa* of the skull. The medulloblastoma is the most common type of brain tumor. It is seen more often in boys than girls around the age of 5 years. It metastasizes rapidly to the meninges of the brain and cord.

Early case finding

By noting unusual symptoms in a child and referring him to a doctor or pediatric clinic,

the nurse may save the child undue suffering. There is a possibility that the brain tumor may not be malignant. In that case the tumor can be treated. During home visits the public health nurse should watch vigilantly for unusual symptoms that may denote increased intracranial pressure—morning nausea and vomiting, unsteadiness in walking, irritability, drowsiness, and any sign that may indicate the child's head hurts. The small child does not readily complain and cannot express himself well, so it is hard to tell if he has a headache. In small children the size of the head increases when there is separation of cranial sutures. This again points to the importance of measuring the circumference of the skull in a child health conference. Nystagmus is often seen. Papilledema, nuchal rigidity, and seizures are seen more often as late signs after other behavior changes have occurred.

If the child has a tumor of the brain stem, instead of signs of intracranial pressure, he may show a change in disposition and behavior. Motor weakness or spasticity might be seen in some cases. The school nurse, who sees the child both prior to his operation and afterward, should be aware of unusual behavior or manifestations of illness.

Role of the nurse

When the child is admitted to the hospital, the nurse needs to be observant of unusual symptoms. Even if the child vomits in the morning, he can be served his breakfast; nausea after vomiting does not continue. Vomiting, to a certain extent, relieves intracranial pressure. Various procedures such as lumbar puncture, ventriculogram, pneumoencephalogram, and angiogram are used to make the definitive diagnosis of a brain tumor.

The child usually has a craniotomy, followed by intensive radiotherapy. A biopsy of the tumor is done at the time of the craniotomy. (Refer to p. 296 for explanation of general preoperative and postoperative care.) During the immediate recovery period after the operation, the nurse should not turn the patient onto the side operated on, as that causes more pressure. In addition, she should watch his temperature carefully; sometimes it rises rapidly.

(See p. 292 for a discussion of temperature-reducing measures.) Attention is also called to the importance of giving the first fluids postoperatively slowly, as the swallowing reflex may not be functioning well. After the operation the nurse should note whether both eyes close when the child is sleeping and whether the child has any limitation of motion of any extremity.

During the postoperative period, the child and his parents may be embarrassed by the sight of his head, which is covered with bandages. This may make the child feel self-conscious and different from others. A doctor's scrub cap might be obtained for him and put over the head dressings. The child could be told he is "a little doctor," dressed like the doctors in the operating room. A small child may be pleased by this. As other children are going to look at him anyway, this is a positive method of handling the situation.

Radiotherapy is often employed after surgery. Medications that may be given include actinomycin D. The life-span of a child with a malignant tumor of the brain is limited. During the period of remission of his symptoms, he should pursue his usual activities and interests. His physical condition and energy govern the extent to which he wishes to play. In the terminal stage, general comfort measures are employed. Medications to alleviate pain should be freely given. If a medication appears ineffective in relieving pain, the nurse should report this to the physician. (For general psychological factors in his care at home and in the hospital refer to p. 503.)

Retinoblastoma

Retinoblastoma is a rare malignant tumor of the eye, most commonly seen in infants and young children. Although the tumor is present at birth, it may not be observed until later in infancy. The tumor often occurs bilaterally.

A strong hereditary tendency has been observed. The diagnosis is established by careful ophthalmoscopic examination. Strabismus because of impairment of vision may often be the presenting symptom.

The only acceptable treatment is enucleation of the affected eye and removal of a portion of the optic nerve. Radiotherapy or drug therapy may be used following enucleation. If the tumor is not removed, the eyes become grossly deformed and large tumor masses may protrude from the orbits before death occurs.

Psychological factors and care during periods of remission in the acute stage do not differ from those applicable to children with other malignancies. (For general comfort measures see p. 511; for general preoperative and postoperative care see p. 290.)

Neuroblastoma
Nature of the condition

Neuroblastoma is seen most often in young children and infants. It may occur anywhere that there is sympathetic nervous tissue. The condition may first draw attention by exophthalmos and proptosis or by a swelling of the abdomen due to an adrenal tumor. Pain in an extremity, extreme hepatomegaly, and cervical and axillary lymphadenopathy may be present. The child may look pale, feel ill, and lose weight. The diagnosis is made by measurement of the urinary excretion of catecholamines and their metabolites. If the tumor arises in the adrenal area, intravenous pyelogram shows displacement of the kidney. Calcification may be visible within the substance of the tumor. Roentgenograms of the body skeleton may reveal bone destruction by the tumor. Biopsy of the tumor or bone marrow aspiration will confirm the presence of tumor cells. Surgery is done even if the tumor cannot be completely excised. Irradiation and drugs such as vincristine, actinomycin D, or cyclophosphamide are given. The prognosis is more favorable for young children than for older ones. Metastases to bone, demonstrable by either x-ray films or bone marrow aspiration, are with rare exceptions indicative of a fatal outcome within a few months. The child who has no evidence of disease 2 years after treatment can be regarded as cured.

Role of the nurse

The role of the public health nurse is largely that of early case finding and referral. An eye or eyes that are different from usual should at once draw the nurse's attention, and she should try to see that medical evaluation and advice is sought. Pain anywhere in the body is something that calls for investigation. The role of the nurse in the hospital is one of helping with diagnostic tests, giving preoperative and postoperative nursing care, and being supportive to the parents.

Nephroblastoma (Wilms' tumor)
Nature of the condition

Nephroblastoma is a fairly common type of malignancy in children, affecting the kidney. The child whom the nurse sees with this condition is usually under 3 years of age. Often the mother has noted a very large abdominal mass; sometimes there is pain and fever. The tumor, in contrast to neuroblastoma of the adrenal, does not cross the midline.

Role of the nurse

When the child is admitted to the hospital, the nurse should be on the lookout for hematuria, although this is not common, and hypertension. X-ray films are taken, and an intravenous pyelogram is done. Although abnormalities of the renal pelvis on the affected side are usually seen, the real importance of the x-ray examination is to see whether there is one normal kidney before any surgical procedures are done.

It is not unusual for the nurse to be asked to hang a sign on the child's crib, saying "Do *not* palpate my abdomen." This is because handling and palpation of the tumor accelerate the spread of malignant cells into the bloodstream. The nurse can omit bathing the affected side if she is giving a bed bath.

Sometimes preoperative radiotherapy is done, but often the child is taken to surgery for a nephrectomy as soon as the diagnosis is made. (See p. 296 for general preoperative and postoperative care and p. 415 for a discussion of psychological factors in surgical nursing.) After the operation, radiotherapy is done, and actinomycin D is often prescribed. Nitrogen mustard, cyclophosphamide, and vincristine are also sometimes given. The prognosis is grave, but with prompt surgery, use of drugs, and irradiation the prognosis is better than formerly. Children under 1 year of age who are treated have the best possibility of a cure. In other children if there is no recurrence or metastasis 2 years after the tumor is removed, the prognosis is good. The commonest site of metastasis is the lungs.

When the child returns home after surgery, he should be allowed to participate in his usual activities. (See p. 503 for a discussion of psychological factors in care of the child.)

Osteogenic sarcoma
Nature of the condition

The two most common types of bone tumors are osteogenic sarcoma and Ewing's tumor. Of these, the former is the more common. Osteogenic sarcoma is seen more often in preadolescent children than in younger ones. It is characterized by pain, swelling, rapid growth, and metastasis. The end of the diaphysis of a long bone is usually affected. The condition most often occurs in the upper tibia, the lower femur, and the upper humerus. Roentgenograms show bone destruction and new bone formation. This malignancy commonly metastasizes to the lungs.

Role of the nurse

Since the child first complains of pain in an extremity and believes he has injured himself on the playground, the school nurse may see him; otherwise, perhaps it is the office nurse or nurse in an outpatient clinic of a hospital. When he is referred to the hospital for study and diagnosis, the nurse in the hospital unit meets the child.

Particular observations the nurse should make (when she knows there is a question of sarcoma) include the following: pain, swelling, and limitation of motion of the affected extremity. The child may not wish to bear weight on the limb involved. In moving around in his bed he may be very careful of it. The nurse should aid the child in his adjustment to the hospital, as she does any child (Chapter 11), and assist in diagnostic measures.

When the physician has made the diagnosis, it may come as a surprise and shock to the parents. The term *malignancy* does not usually mean much to a child, but if the plan is to amputate the extremity, certainly the child should be told the reason, in accordance with his ability to understand. The explanation of the proposed medical plan is the prerogative of the physician; however, the nurse should know what the physician has said to the child. An explanation that in time he will have an artificial leg should also be given to the child.

Prior to an amputation, radiation therapy is usually given. If there is metastasis, amputation may or may not be done. Some physicians believe it best to remove the original site of the tumor. In addition, radiation therapy, nitrogen mustard, or actinomycin D may be tried.

For general preoperative and postoperative care see p. 296; for psychological factors in the care of children who have surgery see p. 415. Specific factors in the nursing care of a child with an amputation include *not* placing the stump on a pillow in order to avoid a contracture. Also, medications for pain should be given freely. The child may complain of pain in the foot or leg that was amputated. Since the attitude of adults is easily communicated to a child, it is important for the nurse to be objective although accepting and sympathetic. The child must not feel that the nurse pities him. The nurse should be aware that, if treatment is given early, there could be a remission of symptoms for several years, although the ultimate prognosis is poor.

After the child is fitted for a prosthesis the nurse should note whether there are any signs of redness, irritation, or swelling of the stump. The child learns to use the prosthesis under the direction of a physiotherapist.

THALASSEMIA, SICKLE CELL ANEMIA, AND APLASTIC ANEMIA
General nursing measures

The nursing care of children with these blood disorders is discussed together because the role of the nurse is essentially the same in all of them. The public health nurse may see a child with such a condition in her home visits. If he exhibits untoward symptoms, she should encourage the parents to have him examined by a doctor; if she sees the child in a child health conference, she should draw the attending physician's attention to what the mother has said about behavior such as anorexia, listlessness, or fatigability.

The role of the hospital nurse is somewhat similar to that described for care of the child with leukemia. As she assists with diagnostic tests and in supportive therapy, she should make the child as comfortable as possible. The prognosis in each disease is grave; the life-span of the patient varies with the severity of the disease. The child with sickle cell anemia may live to early adulthood.

A brief discussion is given on the following pages about the nature of thalassemia, sickle cell anemia, and aplastic anemia.

Thalassemia (Cooley's anemia, erythroblastic anemia, Mediterranean anemia)

Thalassemia is a chronic hypochromic type of anemia that is seen most frequently in children of Mediterranean ancestry, although it is also seen in other children. It is hereditary. There are two forms: the major and the minor. In thalassemia minor the patient may have either no symptoms or such minor ones that no treatment is necessary unless particular stress occurs, such as an infection. In thalassemia major the child may have manifestations of varying degrees of severity. The child may require transfusions frequently or only occasionally. These transfusions are usually done before the hemoglobin value drops lower than 6.5 to 7.5 gm. per 100 ml. in order to avoid the possibility of heart failure (Smith, 1972). Particular features noted in children with thalassemia include pallor, lethargy, diarrhea, fever, anorexia, skeletal changes, stunted growth after 8 to 10 years of age, enlarged abdomen, and poor musculature. Laboratory findings—besides markedly lowered hemoglobin and reduction in the number of erythrocytes—may show leukopenia, thrombocytopenia, and increased serum iron level. (There is a rapid destruction of immature and defective blood cells.) Repeated transfusions and sometimes a splenectomy are done. Congestive heart failure may occur. The outlook for children with thalassemia major is very grave, but those with thalassemia minor may live normal lives. If cardiac failure develops, it is treated with digitalis and diuretics and the physical activity of the child has to be limited. (Refer to p. 489 for discussion of congestive heart failure.)

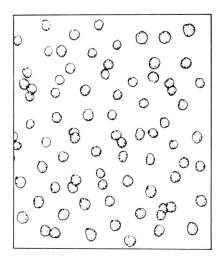
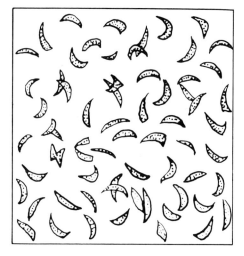

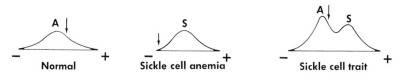

Fig. 17-5. Diagram of normal red blood cells and hemoglobin A electrophoretic pattern compared to sickled red blood cells and hemoglobin S pattern. Note electrophoretic pattern of SA hemoglobin.

Sickle cell anemia

Sickle cell anemia derives its name from the abnormal structure of erythrocytes seen in children with this type of chronic hemolytic anemia. Sickle cell anemia is an inherited disease that is seen most often in blacks.

If the disease is inherited from both parents, the child has sickle cell disease, or the homozygous form. On the other hand, if the disease is inherited from only one parent, the child has sickle cell trait, or the heterozygous form. In both forms the hemoglobin is abnormal hemoglobin S rather than normal hemoglobin A. The greatest percentage of hemoglobin S is produced in the homozygous form of sickle cell anemia, therefore making it the most severe of the two. The hemoglobin S is responsible for forming the red blood cells into a sickle shape, which causes the malformed cells to clump together and obstruct capillaries. This results in pain in an area (pain crisis) because of the obstruction of blood vessels and infarction result-ing in hypoxia of different parts of the body such as the spleen, kidneys, lungs, heart, and bone.

In children with sickle cell trait there are no clinical symptoms. In sickle cell disease the child may not have difficulties until late childhood, or there may be clinical manifestations by the preschool period. An elevated temperature, anorexia, easy fatigability, vomiting, and pain in the back, joints, and abdomen may be the main manifestations seen. The pain may be acute. The small child under 5 years may have symmetrically swollen hands and feet (hand-foot syndrome). Bone changes are seen on x-ray films. Besides anemia, laboratory findings might include (in a crisis) leukocytosis, hematuria, proteinuria, and urine of low specific gravity. Crises are less frequent as the child gets older. Between crises the child enjoys normal health.

At the time of a crisis the child needs adequate hydration, antibiotics for any infection

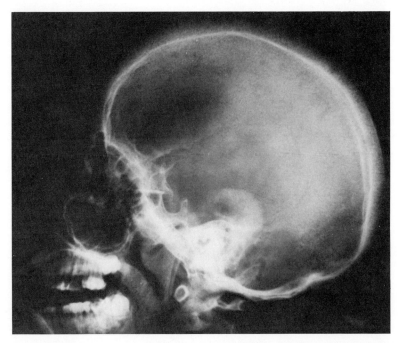

Fig. 17-6. X-ray film of skull in 4-year-old child with sickle cell anemia showing "hair-on-end" appearance.

present, and analgesics for pain. Blood transfusions are avoided whenever possible, for they add to the content of iron in the body and in time may lead to abnormal deposition of iron in the tissues of the body (hemosiderosis). High concentrations of oxygen administered by mask may help decrease tissue hypoxia and help relieve the pain. Other drugs frequently used, which have not proved very effective, are tolazoline (Priscoline) as a vasodilator, sodium bicarbonate to alter the pH of the blood, and dextran or plasma to increase plasma volume.

Because of treatment the life of the child may be prolonged so that he reaches early adulthood, or he may succumb to cardiac failure, renal failure, or cerebral infarction. With the use of antibiotics, chemotherapy, transfusions, and oxygen therapy, life expectancy can be prolonged. Many of the crises can be prevented by the early management of acute illnesses in these patients by their physician or clinic.

Many patients with homozygous sickle cell anemia survive the fourth decade. Women with sickle cell anemia who become pregnant develop more complications than normal women.

They should be given early and adequate prenatal care to permit them to go to term and deliver a healthy infant.

Aplastic anemia

According to Smith, aplastic anemia can be classified as either idiopathic or as secondary—caused by a drug, chemical, or ionizing radiation. Idiopathic aplastic anemia refers to anemia in which the cause is unknown. One type of this is associated with multiple congenital anomalies (Fanconi's syndrome), and another occurs without congenital anomalies.

Aplastic anemia is characterized by failure in granulocyte, platelet, and erythrocyte formation. In consequence of this, infections and bleeding are likely to occur.

Drugs that can produce bone marrow depression include nitrogen mustard, folic acid antagonists such as aminopterin, 6-mercaptopurine, and busulfan. The hospital nurse often has occasion to administer these drugs to children suffering from leukemia or certain malignancies. Another group of drugs that could cause bone marrow depression are those sometimes used in treatment of seizures such as trimethadione (Tridione) and mephenytoin (Mesantoin). The prolonged use of chloramphenicol, tetracyclines, or sulfonamides can also induce bone marrow depression. Chemical agents such as DDT, gasoline, cleaning solutions, and insecticides can be dangerous if used in areas where there is little or no ventilation. If the anemia is caused by a drug or chemical, the offending agent should be removed.

In home visits the public health nurse needs to note any child who seems unduly pale or listless, bruises easily, or may have dyspnea after playing, since these are early symptoms of aplastic anemia. Such a child needs referral to a doctor or pediatric clinic for diagnostic evaluation.

Later in the course of the disease other signs may be observed, such as recurrent epistaxis, bleeding from the gums, hematuria, retinal hemorrhage, a considerable amount of ecchymosis, and menorrhagia. Ulcerations of the mouth and pharynx may be present.

The diagnosis is established by performing a bone marrow aspiration, which discloses aplasia or hypoplasia of the blood-forming elements. The other abnormal laboratory findings are (1) the red blood cell count is low, fluctuating between 1.5 and 3.0 million per cubic millimeter, (2) the hemoglobin value is low, (3) the white blood count is low, ranging from 1,500 to 4,000 per cubic millimeter, and (4) the platelet count falls below 50,000 per cubic millimeter.

The first step of treatment is the removal of the causative agent (such as a drug, chemical, or insecticide). Small repeated blood transfusions are given to combat the anemia and provide platelets. Adrenocorticoids and testosterone are administered to stimulate bone marrow regeneration. Platelet-rich plasma transfusions may be needed if the platelet count remains very low and the patient suffers from persistent severe bleeding. This procedure may be lifesaving. Splenectomy is performed if all other available measures fail. Every effort is made to prevent and/or control infection, since infections depress bone marrow function and aggravate hemorrhagic manifestations. Bone marrow transplantation has been used on occasions with fair results.

In general, if the cause of the aplastic anemia is known, the prognosis is better. The results of the use of androgen-corticosteroid therapy are favorable, whereas prior to their use the disease was almost uniformly fatal. Death may occur from intracranial hemorrhage and/or septicemia.

HODGKIN'S DISEASE (MALIGNANT LYMPHOMA)

Hodgkin's disease is characterized by progressive painless enlargement of the regional lymph nodes. As the disease progresses, involvement of other parts of the body such as the spleen, liver, bone marrow, central nervous system, and lungs occurs. Etiology of the disease is unknown.

The signs and symptoms depend on the site of involvement. The presence of painless large lymph nodes in the neck is the most common initial manifestation. In some patients the first evidence of Hodgkin's disease may be a mediastinal mass in the chest observed on a roentgenogram ordered for some other reason. Other symptoms include weight loss, nausea, fever, and weakness. Cough and dyspnea may occur if the glands in the mediastinum press on the trachea and bronchi.

Laboratory findings early in the disease are not characteristic, especially if the disease is localized. When the disease becomes more extensive, hypoplastic anemia develops. Leukopenia and lymphopenia often occur in the advanced cases. Bone marrow and/or lymph node biopsy are used to confirm the presence of Reed-Sternberg cells, which are characteristically found in patients with Hodgkin's disease.

The treatment plan consists of the use of radiotherapy and chemotherapy. Radiotherapy is used when localized disease is present. If there is systemic spread of the disease, chemotherapy and radiotherapy are used in combination. Some of the frequently used chemotherapy drugs are the nitrogen mustards and antileukemic drugs. General supportive therapy for infections and hemorrhagic complications are employed.

The prognosis is generally poor. The average survival time following diagnosis is 2 to 3 years. Some patients have survived more than 20 years after diagnosis. Possible and probable cures may be anticipated with modern treatment.

HEMOPHILIA
Hemophilia A (classic hemophilia)

Hemophilia A is due to an inherited defect of factor VIII production. It is inherited as a sex-linked recessive character transmitted directly by unaffected females to male offspring. There is usually a family history of hemophilia. The clinical severity of the disease is dependent upon the level of factor VIII in the plasma. In severe cases the factor VIII levels may fall to 3% of the normal level.

The clinical signs and symptoms become evident in infancy because of either spontaneous bleeding or bleeding from slight trauma or minor surgery. Subcutaneous and intramuscular hemorrhages are frequent and extensive. Bleeding from the mucous membranes is frequent and, like that from other significant wounds, difficult to control. Repeated hemorrhage into the joints is especially characteristic and eventually produces a form of arthritis with deformity and limitation of motion. Low abdominal pains may be caused by bleeding into the colonic wall, mesentery, or retroperitoneal tissues. Bleeding may take place into the urinary tract and may be very difficult to stop. Fortunately, hemorrhage into the central nervous system is rare. If a large amount of blood is lost, pallor, weakness, and tachycardia may become apparent.

The hematological findings in hemophilia A reveal that the peripheral blood elements are normal. The bleeding time is usually normal, whereas the clotting time is extremely long. Normal blood clots in 3 to 6 minutes; hemophiliac blood may require an hour or more for clotting. A test to measure the specific level of factor VIII in the plasma is available. The partial thromboplastin time (P.T.T.) is the simplest and most sensitive test to detect milder deficiencies of factor VIII.

Treatment begins with the avoidance of injury and requires psychological adjustment to the restrictions of the disease. The use of cold compresses will frequently limit the extent of hemorrhage into the tissues. Hemarthroses of the elbows, knees, and ankles are best treated by conservative orthopedic and physiotherapeutic measures. Pain requires relief by sedatives, analgesics, immobilization of the joints, and applications of cold to the part. External bleeding can be controlled by gentle cleansing and approximation of the edges of the wound without sutures. Careful handling of the part involved is necessary to prevent further bleeding. The open wound may be powdered with thrombin, and local packing with absorbable packs such as a fibrin foam or oxidized cellulose (Oxycel, Surgicel) may be applied. Transfusion of fresh whole blood or packed red cells should be administered if the patient has suffered extensive blood loss. The use of fresh frozen and lyophilized plasma (cryoprecipitate) is the treatment of choice to raise the level of factor VIII in the plasma. Antihemophilic plasma, which contains factor VIII in high levels, may also be used. These plasma preparations may be given in preparation for surgical operations or to prevent or abort early bleeding episodes. The factor VIII level should be maintained above 25%. Venipunctures should only be performed from superficial veins since severe uncontrollable bleeding may result if femoral or internal jugular punctures are done.

Hemophilia B (Christmas disease)

Hemophilia B is an inherited defect of the production of factor IX (PTC). It accounts for 15% of the cases of hemophilia. The disease is transmitted as an X-linked recessive trait. The disease cannot be distinguished clinically from classic hemophilia but can be readily diagnosed by laboratory tests. Treatment of choice for this disease is by the use of fresh frozen plasma since there is no factor IX concentrate available commercially. The other supportive measures used in the management of classic hemophilia are also used in these patients.

Hemophilia C (PTA deficiency)

Hemophilia C produces mild bleeding episodes due to a deficiency in factor XI. It is inherited as an autosomal dominant trait. The disease may be seen in both sexes. The usual clinical manifestations are easy bruising and nosebleeds. Severe hemorrhagic episodes and hemarthroses are very rare. The laboratory tests for evaluation of clotting and coagulation are used to confirm the decreased level of factor

XI. The use of plasma therapy corrects the deficiency of factor XI and controls the hemorrhage.

Nursing care

The child will be admitted to the hospital on many occasions for treatment of his disease. The nurse should help the parents and child develop a healthy attitude toward the disease and treatment. The child should be handled with extreme care to prevent further bleeding. Toys with smooth and soft edges should be made available to these children. Older children should be permitted to ambulate with supervision and play, but their environment should be free of potentially dangerous obstacles. The nurse should be aware of any new or recurrent sites of bleeding and, if they occur, be capable of handling these until the physician is notified.

When the child is admitted with hemarthrosis he will be in severe pain. The method of moving or turning this child with the least pain should be determined and used. If the child can talk he will be able to tell the nurse which method is the best, thereby lessening the pain and sense of uncertainty. Injections are given slowly and pressure applied to the site for at least 4 to 5 minutes. If possible, oral medications should be used. Venipunctures are performed in the superficial veins with pressure being applied for a long time afterwards.

The child and parents should be aware of the daily dangers of trauma at home and school. Persons at home and school coming in contact with the child should be aware of his disease and the problems it creates.

The child should be allowed activity within the limits of safety and not be overprotected by his parents and teachers.

The child will have to visit the physician or clinic many times a year. When the child is free of symptoms, medical care does not seem necessary and is often neglected by the parents. The nurse should provide encouragement and emotional support of the parents so that they recognize the importance of preventive medical care. Good dental care is essential to avoid extraction of teeth.

A child with a chronic disease such as hemophilia may use it to control his parents or teachers. He may demand a favor by threatening to hurt himself if it is not complied with. The child and parent may need professional counseling if it persists. The child should be allowed to develop initiative and independence as normal children do.

The parents will probably need financial assistance since the disease is long term. The child will need repeated hospitalizations, blood or plasma transfusions, and care for repeated episodes of hemarthrosis. These services are very costly, and very few families have the financial resources to pay for them. The physician and the nurse should refer the family to agencies interested in helping hemophiliac patients. These agencies could provide financial assistance, crippled children's services for care of the orthopedic deformities, and other special services that the child might be in need of but the parents could not afford.

PSEUDOHYPERTROPHIC PROGRESSIVE MUSCULAR DYSTROPHY

A brief discussion of muscular dystrophy is placed in this section of the book not because the disease itself is fatal but because the dystrophy grows progressively worse until the child is severely crippled. The child usually dies of an intercurrent disease before he reaches adulthood, or he may die of heart failure. The condition is seen more often in boys than girls, but it is transmitted as a recessive characteristic by females. There is weakness and atrophy of skeletal muscles. Disability and deformity increase as the child grows.

In a home visit the public health nurse may notice that the child pushes on one knee and then the other as he mounts steps. Weakness in the legs is usually seen first. The child may fall frequently, have a mildly waddling gait, and show lumbar lordosis. As the disease progresses, weakness extends to the trunk of the body, and the child has difficulty getting up when he falls down. Muscular atrophy continues with progression of the disease and extends to the legs, spine, pelvis, and shoulders. There is no specific treatment for this condition.

If the public health nurse sees the child in his home, she should encourage him to be as active as possible and to exercise his muscles, since inactivity increases the weaknesses. As long as the patient is able, he should continue in school and follow his usual interests. In the later stages of the condition the services of a visiting teacher may be needed. The child's mentality remains unhampered, and he needs diversion and opportunity to join in the family activities. A pet such as a dog may be a source of pleasure to the child, even when he becomes severely crippled. Watching a potted plant or flower grow may relieve monotony. Visits from family friends are helpful. Orthopedic appliances, perhaps a back brace or a leg brace, may be used to correct contractures. Sometimes lengthening of the tendon of Achilles is done if it is contracted sufficiently to interfere with walking. The public health nurse may teach the child and his mother exercises that the physician advises for the child. Her visits should prove to be an emotional support for both the mother and the child.

REFERENCES
Common psychological factors

Beigh, R.: Let's talk about death, Am. J. Nurs. **66:**71, 1966.

Chodoff, P., et al.: Stress, defenses and coping behavior; observations in parents of children with malignant disease, Am. J. Orthopsychiatr. **120:**743, 1964.

Easson, W.: The dying child, the management of the child or adolescent who is dying, Springfield, Ill., 1970, Charles C Thomas, Publisher.

Engel, G. L.: Grief and grieving, Am. J. Nurs. **64:**93, September, 1964.

Goldfogel, L.: Working with the parent of a dying child, Am. J. Nurs. **70:**1674, August, 1970.

Green, M., and Solnit, A.: Reactions to the threatened loss of a child; a vulnerable child syndrome, Pediatrics **34:**58, 1964.

Gyulay, J.-E.: The forgotten grievers, Am. J. Nurs. **75:**1476, September, 1975.

Maxwell, M. B.: A terminally ill adolescent and her family, Am. J. Nurs. **72:**925, May, 1972.

Prattes, O. R.: Helping the family face an impending death, Nurs. '73 **3:**40, February, 1973.

Telling the truth to the leukemic child, Nurs. Clin. North Am. **1:**167, March, 1966.

Timmons, A.: Is it so awful? Am. J. Nurs. **75:**988, June, 1975.

Specific conditions

Auscombe, A. R.: Surgery in hemophilia, Nurs. Mirror **132:**3, April 23, 1971.

Boggs, D. R., et al.: The acute leukemias, Medicine **41:**163, 1962.

Brinkhouse, K. M.: Changing prospects for children with hemophilia, Children **17:**222, 1970.

Brubaker, C. A., et al.: Cyclic chemotherapy for acute leukemia in children, Blood **22:**820, 1963.

Control of hemophiliac bleeding, Nurs. Mirror **130:**43, March, 1970.

Craver, L. F.: Some aspects of the treatment of Hodgkin's disease, Cancer **7:**927, 1954.

Creative nursing care for acute leukemia, Nurs. '73 **3:**19, June, 1973.

Dameshek, W., et al.: Therapy of acute leukemia, 1965 (editorial), Blood **26:**220, 1965.

Diggs, L. W.: The crisis of sickle cell anemia: hematologic studies, Am. J. Clin. Pathol. **26:**1109, 1956.

Diggs, L. W., et al.: Pathology of sickle cell anemia, South. Med. J. **27:**839, 1934.

Dorfman, R., and Reinhard, E.: Hodgkin's disease, J.A.M.A. **208:**325, 1969.

Green, P.: Acute leukemia in children, Am. J. Nurs., **75:**1709, October, 1975.

Kenney, G. M., Staubitz, W. J., and Murphy, G. P.: Wilm's tumor, Cancer Bull. **23:**6, January-February, 1971.

Murphy, M. L.: Chemotherapy of neoplastic diseases. In Shirkey, H. C., editor: Pediatric therapy, ed. 4, St. Louis, 1972, The C. V. Mosby Co.

Pochedly, C.: Sickle cell anemia, Am. J. Nurs. **71:**1948, October, 1971.

Sergis, E.: Hemophilia, Am. J. Nurs. **72:**2011, November, 1972.

Shirkey, H. C., editor: Pediatric therapy, ed. 5, St. Louis, 1975, The C. V. Mosby Co.

Smith, C. H.: Blood diseases of infancy and childhood, ed. 3, St. Louis, 1972, The C. V. Mosby Co.

Staudt, A.: Femur replacement, Am. J. Nursing **75:**1346, August, 1975.

Sutow, W. W., Gehan, E. A., Heyn, R. M., et al.: Comparison of survival curves, 1956 versus 1962, in children with Wilms' tumor and neuroblastoma, Pediatrics **45:**800, 1970.

Thomas, T. W.: Hemophilia—a teacher's view, Nurs. Times July 9, 1970.

Vaughan, V. C., III, and McKay, R. J., editors: Nelson's textbook of pediatrics, ed. 10, Philadelphia, 1975, W. B. Saunders Co.

Venick, J., and Lunceford, J.: Milieu design for adolescents with leukemia, Am. J. Nurs. **67:**559, 1967.

Whitmore, W. F.: Wilms' tumor and neuroblastoma, Am. J. Nurs. **68:**527, 1968.

18

Nursing care of
THE CHILD WITH A
COMMUNICABLE DISEASE

Prevention

The nurse's most important role relative to communicable diseases is to teach the parents to have their children protected against diseases for which there are specific preventive measures (Table 9-3). The public health nurse, the school nurse, the office nurse, and the hospital nurse all have opportunities to do this. Not included in the table are preventive measures that can be taken by those in a family exposed to meningitis. Sulfadiazine administered to them will limit the spread of the disease. For those allergic to sulfadiazine, penicillin may be given.

Also, antirabies serum and a vaccine are available to prevent rabies (hydrophobia) if a child is bitten by a rabid animal. The wound should be thoroughly cleansed. The animal should be apprehended and observed for 10 days. The decision to administer serum and vaccine immediately or during the observation period depends somewhat on the behavior of the animal, the presence of rabies in the area, and the circumstances of the bite (Berenson, 1975). No treatment is given unless the skin is broken or a mucosal surface has been contaminated by the animal's saliva. (Berenson describes the management of an animal bite adapted from the Sixth Report of the WHO Expert Committee on Rabies by the USPHS Advisory Committee on Immunization Practices.)

Public education is essential to all pet owners. Preventive vaccination can be given to all dogs and cats. Dogs should be registered and licensed. They should be kept on a leash unless confined to the owner's premises.

Bites on the face and neck are even more serious than those on the legs because they are closer to the brain. The virus from a rabid animal is on the saliva, so a bite can be the portal of entry if the skin is broken. The rabies virus goes from the portal of entry to the spinal cord and brain.

If no protection is given, an acute encephalitis, possibly fatal, may occur.

COMMON VIRAL
AND BACTERIAL DISEASES

The discussion of nursing care here will be limited to care of children who are ill with the communicable diseases that are more commonly seen in childhood.

The public health nurse may see children at home with infectious parotitis (mumps), rubeola (red measles), rubella (German measles), or varicella (chickenpox). A few pertinent comments about the care at home of these childhood communicable diseases are included, but a more detailed discussion of the care of a child with meningitis is given since an infant or child with this condition is frequently seen in the pediatric unit of a large general hospital during the winter or spring months. The hospital nurse may see a child with pertussis or diphtheria, but this is fortunately becoming rare because of immunizations.

Measles
Rubella (German measles)

Rubella is a mild disease usually, and the child is often up and around the house with it. Symptoms include an elevation of temperature, catarrhal symptoms, and maculopapular red rash. Lymph glands are swollen, especially the occipital, postauricular, and postcervical glands. If there is a temperature elevation to over 100° F. or if the child seems to feel ill, he should remain in bed. Nutritious foods should be urged. Reading and watching television should be avoided, since the eyes are sometimes inflamed.

Rubella is now preventable. Immunizations can be given to children prior to school entrance; if not then, at least before puberty.

Congenital rubella syndrome. Rubella acquired during the first trimester of pregnancy is associated with an increased number of congenital malformations, stillbirths, and abortions. Central nervous system involvement is striking, with the fontanel being very large and tense. Microcephaly and mental retardation are usually the end result if the child survives the first year of life. Muscular hypotonia is common. Other clinical manifestations that these infants may exhibit are (1) low birth weight, (2) congenital lesions of the eyes such as cataracts, glaucoma, retinitis, and coloboma, (3) deafness, (4) congenital heart disease, particularly patent ductus arteriosus and peripheral pulmonary stenosis, (5) thrombocytopenia purpura, (6) hepatomegaly, (7) splenomegaly, (8) jaundice (hepatitis), and (9) bone lesions. Infants with congenital rubella infection may continue to excrete virus from the pharynx and urine for several months after birth. Rubella of these infants is contagious, and they should be isolated from presumably susceptible women early in their pregnancy. The disease should be considered contagious for 3 to 4 months after birth. The treatment of such infants will depend upon the severity and type of the abnor-

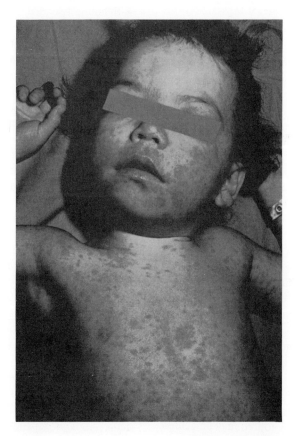

Fig. 18-1. Infant with typical rash of measles. Note confluent maculopapular lesions on face. (From Krugman, S., Ward, R., and Katz, S. L.: Infectious diseases of children, ed. 6, St. Louis, 1977, The C. V. Mosby Co.)

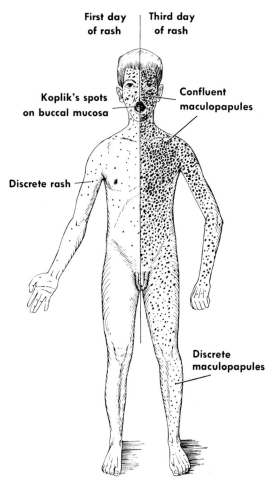

First day of rash | Third day of rash

Koplik's spots on buccal mucosa

Confluent maculopapules

Discrete rash

Discrete maculopapules

Fig. 18-2. Schematic drawing illustrating the development and distribution of measles rash. (From Krugman, S., Ward, R., and Katz, S. L.: Infectious diseases of children, ed. 6, St. Louis, 1977, The C. V. Mosby Co.)

malities identified. Many of these infants are institutionalized. If the child remains at home, the physician and public health nurse should be aware of the many crippled childrens' programs that attempt to help the child with congenital rubella syndrome obtain his full potential.

Rubeola (red measles)

In contrast to rubella, children may be acutely ill with rubeola. Complications that can occur include otitis media, mastoiditis, pneumonia, and encephalitis.

Characteristics of rubeola are, initially, signs of coryza, inflamed conjunctiva, photophobia, hard brassy cough, Koplik's spots, elevated temperature, and a fine macular pink rash of tiny spots. The rash may first appear on the neck or face around the hairline, then progress downward. The spots become brighter and bigger, and several may coalesce. Koplik's spots are usually seen in the buccal area prior to a rash but at the same time as signs of coryza and coughing.

On a pediatric ward, especially during the spring, the nurse should be sure to note any child with a metallic-sounding cough. The child may be developing measles. The nurse should look for any further signs of measles such as coryza, rash, or sudden elevation of temperature and call the physician's attention to any such findings.

At home a room that is warm (even at night), with humidity added by means of a pan of water or a steam inhalator, may relieve the cough somewhat. If the cough keeps the child awake or is so hard that it causes him to vomit, the physician should be so informed. Sometimes cough syrup containing codeine is necessary. If the temperature goes above 100.6° F. (as frequently happens), aspirin may be ordered. Temperature-reducing measures such as a sponge bath should not be given if there is any danger of chilling the child. After the rash appears the temperature often decreases. Nonirritating fluids can be urged. A light diet of gelatin, cream soups, eggnogs, and the like can be given. Rest in bed during the acute phase of the disease may help to prevent complications; certainly as long as there is any elevation of temperature the child should stay in bed. On the other hand, a small child may find considerable comfort in being held and rocked; however, every effort should be made not to let him get chilled. The room should be kept at an *even* temperature.

Since the child often has photophobia, his bed or crib should be turned away from the light. The room does not necessarily have to be darkened. This depends on the child; however, the use of a strong or direct light should be avoided for all children with measles. Coloring pictures, looking at television, reading, and

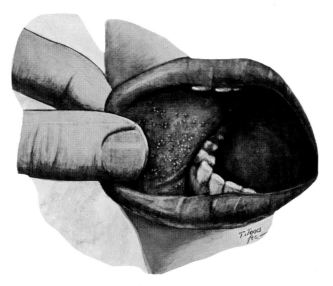

Plate 1. Koplik's spots. (From Zahorsky, J., and Zahorsky, T. S.: Synopsis of pediatrics, ed. 6, St. Louis, 1953, The C. V. Mosby Co.)

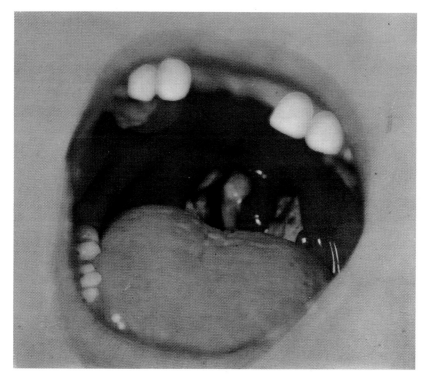

Plate 2. Tonsillar diphtheria. (Courtesy Franklin H. Top, M.D., Professor and Head of the Department of Hygiene and Preventive Medicine, State University of Iowa, College of Medicine, Iowa City, Iowa, and Parke, Davis & Company's Therapeutic Notes.)

similar activities should be discouraged, even if the child feels fairly well. Secretions in the eyes should be gently washed and wiped away. Eyes may need bathing several times daily. Soap should not be used in bathing the child because this may irritate his skin.

Since the source of the infection is secretions from the nose and throat of infected people, tissues used by the child should be placed in a paper bag rather than dropped on the floor, rug, or bed.

If a young child appears unusually drowsy, pulls at his ear, or seems to have pain in the mastoid area, this should be reported to the physician because an ear or mastoid infection could be occurring. A sudden rise in temperature after the temperature has started to decrease may also be a danger signal. Complications include pneumonia and encephalitis.

States vary in their regulations about isolation, but many require 7 to 10 days of isolation after the rash disappears. When the child is well again, there should be a thorough cleansing of his room and washing of any articles contaminated by secretions from the nose and throat.

Varicella (chickenpox)

The mother may discover the rash on a small child's body when bathing him. It appears first on the trunk of the body and then spreads to other areas. Since the onset of the chicken pox is often abrupt, there may have been nothing unusual before the appearance of the rash to suggest illness. The child is often not ill enough to need to stay in bed. If infection is severe, encephalitis, pneumonia, and septic complications can occur in children. Some elevation of temperature, general malaise, and headache are more often seen in older children and adults than in young children.

Young children are often out of bed and playing during an episode of chickenpox. The child's greatest complaint, as a rule, is the severe itching of the rash. At first the rash is macular and very small. The tiny red spots change to papules and then to a vesicular stage; some may then change to blisters. Crusting occurs after the blisters break. Sometimes the spots increase in size. The rash comes in crops, so the eruption is in varying stages on different parts of the body. The lesions are most numerous over the trunk of the body but are present in the mouth and upper respiratory tract as well.

Scratching of the lesions could cause a secondary skin infection, so the child's fingernails need to be cut short. Cotton gloves may be worn if the child will keep them on his hands. Gentle application of calamine lotion with cotton helps to allay itching. Some physicians order an antihistamine such as Chlor-Trimeton. Soap is not used in bathing because it is likely to irritate the skin. A starch or soda bicarbonate

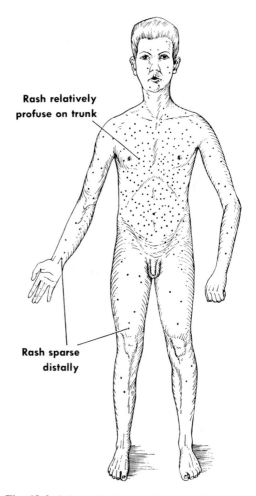

Rash relatively profuse on trunk

Rash sparse distally

Fig. 18-3. Schematic drawing illustrating the typical distribution of the rash of chickenpox. (From Krugman, S., Ward, R., and Katz, S. L.: Infectious diseases of children, ed. 6, St. Louis, 1977, The C. V. Mosby Co.)

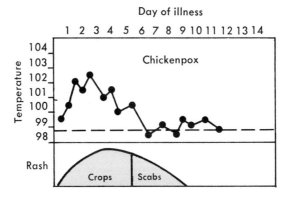

Fig. 18-4. Schematic diagram illustrating clinical course of typical case of chickenpox. (From Krugman, S., Ward, R., and Katz, S. L.: Infectious diseases of children, ed. 6, St. Louis, 1977, The C. V. Mosby Co.)

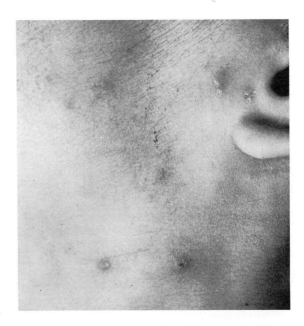

Fig. 18-5. Chickenpox lesions in various stages. (From Krugman, S., Ward, R., and Katz, S. L.: Infectious diseases of children, ed. 6, St. Louis, 1977, The C. V. Mosby Co.)

bath may help the child to relax before nap time or bedtime. A light nourishing diet can be offered. Because of the rash in his mouth, liquids and soups are taken better than solid food.

When the child is well again, his room should be thoroughly cleansed, as mentioned also in relation to measles.

Infectious parotitis (mumps)

Mumps is another viral disease. There is a vaccine available that can prevent mumps, but it does not provide protection for more than 2 years and, in contrast, one attack of mumps gives lasting immunity to the disease. Some physicians believe that it is preferable to let the child have the disease if he has not yet reached puberty, since adults are often sicker than children. After puberty more serious complications such as meningitis, encephalitis, and deafness can occur; also the testicles and ovaries may be affected.

Mumps is characterized by swelling on one

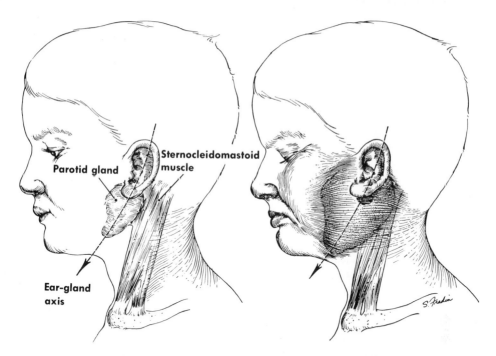

Fig. 18-6. Schematic drawing of parotid gland infected with mumps compared with normal gland. An imaginary line bisecting the long axis of the ear divides the parotid gland into two equal parts. These anatomical relationships are not altered in the enlarged gland. An enlarged cervical lymph node is usually posterior to the imaginary line. (From Krugman, S., Ward, R., and Katz, S. L.: Infectious diseases of children, ed. 6, St. Louis, 1977, The C. V. Mosby Co.)

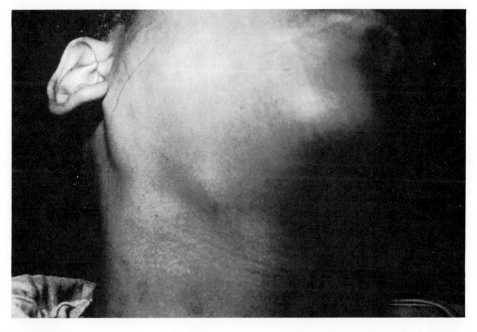

Fig. 18-7. Patient with mumps showing right parotid and submaxillary swelling. Note displacement of ear and characteristic location of both glands. (From Krugman, S., Ward, R., and Katz, S. L.: Infectious diseases of children, ed. 6, St. Louis, 1977, The C. V. Mosby Co.)

side or both sides of the neck. It involves the parotid gland especially, but often salivary glands are tender and enlarged also. In respiratory infections in children the cervical glands are sometimes swollen. In order to tell whether the child has a cervical adenitis or has mumps, a pencil should be held against the line of the lower jaw. If there is swelling above the pencil (on the cheek), the child has mumps.

If his neck is painful, the child prefers to lie quietly in bed. Hot-water bottles, partially filled and placed on each side of his neck, may make him more comfortable. Usually warm fluids such as cream soups are easier for the child to take than cold fluids. A soft diet may be offered, but because chewing is painful nourishing foods such as cream soups, custards, and eggnogs are taken better. Aspirin may be ordered for the comfort of the child. The patient should remain in bed until the swelling has subsided or until the physician believes that it is safe for him to ambulate.

Disinfection after illness is the same as after measles.

Pertussis (whooping cough)

Unless the child with pertussis has a complication, it is not likely that he will be admitted to the hospital with this ailment. The public health nurse may see a child with this condition in the home, but since pertussis is preventable, it is hoped that she will encounter no one with this disease.

Pertussis is caused by the pertussis bacillus. It affects the respiratory tract and is characterized by spasmodic attacks of coughing. At the end of the cough there is an inspiratory, high-pitched whoop in which the child has difficulty in getting his breath. Clear, tenacious mucus is usually expelled with a violent cough. Not all infants and very young children have this characteristic whoop.

In children who are under 3 years of age, pneumonia is a common complication. (Refer to Chapter 14 for a discussion of pneumonia in children.) Atelectasis can result from a plug of mucus in a bronchiole. Other complications are related to the increased intracranial, intrathoracic, and intra-abdominal pressure during these spasmodic attacks of coughing. Included

in these complications are umbilical hernia, emphysema, bronchiectasis, hemorrhage, encephalitis, and encephalopathy associated with anoxia.

The prognosis is serious for children less than 4 years old and especially so for infants under 6 months. There is no specific drug for this disease, but tetracycline is used prophylactically against secondary infection. In an effort to lessen the paroxysms of coughing, paregoric, phenobarbital, and codeine are sometimes used; however, coughing helps to remove mucus and in this respect is desirable.

In general, there are three stages of pertussis: the catarrhal, the paroxysmal, and the convalescent. In the first stage the child has a persistent cough, which is worse at night. A mother, because of signs of coryza, may believe that he has a cold. After the child's illness is diagnosed he should be kept in isolation. His room should be well ventilated and kept at an even temperature. In warm weather he may be placed on a porch that is screened. The head of the crib or bed should be elevated. When the child coughs, his abdomen should be supported. Since the infant or child may vomit when coughing, his nutrition may suffer. An infant very sick with pertussis often begins to cough when his position is changed. It may be well for the nurse (or mother) to pick the infant up for his feeding, place him over her lap with his face downward, let him cough and bring up mucus, and then feed him. Aspiration pneumonia may be avoided this way. Feedings are best given to infants every 3 hours rather than every 4 hours. Careful charting of the amount of fluid and food taken by the infant is essential, as this may need to be supplemented by infusions. If the infant is sick enough to be in the hospital, the nurse should organize her work with care so that the infant does not have to be constantly disturbed. Rest is very essential. After the infant is discharged the room used should be thoroughly cleansed and aired. All articles with any discharges on them need to be carefully washed.

Diphtheria

Diphtheria is caused by the Klebs-Loeffler bacillus. It is an infectious disease affecting the upper respiratory system. A dirty grayish membrane is seen in the throat. It is surrounded by an area of redness. When the membrane is scraped with a tongue depressor, it bleeds. The severity of the disease is due to absorption of toxin from the gray membrane, which may extend into the trachea. This is referred to as tonsillopharyngeal diphtheria. The child usually has an elevation of temperature, general malaise, and hoarseness. An increasing stridor denotes increased respiratory distress. This is particularly evident in children under 5 years of age, since the lumen of the respiratory passages is small and swelling obstructs breathing more than in adults. Suffocation can occur.

Between 2 and 5 years of age, laryngeal diphtheria is commonly found. Nasal diphtheria is diagnosed by the presence of a white membrane on the nasal septum. The toxin is absorbed poorly from this site, which accounts for the mildness of the disease.

It particularly important that the nurse be able to recognize symptoms of this disease and see that the child have immediate medical attention because of the severity of the disease. There is real danger in asphyxiation of the child in laryngeal diphtheria due to development of edema of the trachea and respiratory passages.

If the child is admitted to the hospital, equipment that the nurse should get immediately is a tracheotomy set.

Isolation of the patient is necessary. Sources of infection are nasal discharges and discharges from skin lesions or other lesions of infected patients.

Children who are exposed to diphtheria may be given, prophylactically, diphtheria antitoxin and a series of diphtheria toxoid inoculations.

In treatment of diphtheria, large doses of antitoxin are given either intramuscularly or intravenously. Penicillin and erythromycin are administered in association with the antitoxin. A Croupette may be used to facilitate breathing of the child. Constant nursing care is required. Rest is especially important, since heart damage (myocarditis) can occur. Nourishing fluids and a soft diet are given. Swallowing may be painful because the throat is sore.

Meningitis

It is not unusual for the nurse to see infants and children admitted to the hospital with meningitis, especially during the winter and spring. Meningitis is seen most commonly in children and young adults. Boys seem to be affected more often than girls.

Nature of the condition

Meningitis is an inflammation of the meninges. It can be caused by several different organisms. In the very young infant the *Escherichia coli* and the *Staphylococcus* are common causes; in older infants and children the commonest organism causing meningitis is the *Haemophilus influenzae*. Meningitis due to the pneumococcic or meningococcic organism is also frequently seen. The organisms mentioned have a purulent exudate.

Aseptic meningitis is caused by a virus. No organisms are found on a direct smear from throat culture or spinal fluid.

Sometimes a chronic meningitis may be seen, which extends over a long period of months. The child appears very emaciated and may be in an opisthotonos position. Hydrocephalus and cranial nerve palsies may be present.

Characteristics of the various types of purulent meningitis that the infant may exhibit are more or less the same, except that in meningococcal meningitis a purpuric eruption over the child's body is often seen. Frequent manifestations in meningitis include abrupt onset (except in tuberculous meningitis, where the onset is insidious), irritability, elevated temperature, projectile vomiting, headache, convulsions, prostration, and general muscular rigidity. If the patient is an infant, his anterior fontanel may be tense or bulging. Chills at the onset of the disease and delirium may be seen in older children. Urinary retention and constipation may be present. The child may be in an opisthotonos position. Brudzinski and Kernig signs are both positive, as is the Babinski reflex. When the doctor raises the child's head and tries to flex it on his chest, the patient bends his knees and hips. Finding it painful, the child utters a high-pitched, shrill cry. His back is rigid. This response is called the Brudzinski sign. A Kernig sign is elicited when the child's leg is brought to a 90-degree or right angle to his body and an attempt is made to straighten the leg. The attempt causes the child to cry in pain.

The diagnosis is established by culture of the organism in the spinal fluid. The spinal fluid in bacterial meningitis shows an increased number of white cells, which are predominantly polymorphonuclear cells. A lymphocytic response is the usual in viral meningitis. The sugar (glucose) concentration of the spinal fluid is decreased in bacterial meningitis. Gram stain of the spinal fluid frequently reveals the organisms on microscopic examination. The peripheral blood count shows a leukocytosis.

The type of treatment of meningitis is determined by the causative organism identified. *Escherichia coli* meningitis is treated with kanamycin and penicillin. The antibiotic of choice for meninginococcal meningitis is penicillin, whereas chloramphenicol is most effective in patients with *Haemophilus influenzae* meningitis. Children with pneumococcal meningitis respond well to aqueous penicillin. Ampicillin has been used for some forms of bacterial meningitis. The antibiotics are administered intravenously for the first 48 to 72 hours of therapy and then given intramuscularly or orally. Careful administration of fluid and electrolytes is also necessary.

If meningitis is treated early and adequately, the prognosis for life is good, but there may be complications and sequelae such as hydrocephalus, impaired intellectual ability, subdural collections of fluid, otitis media, optic atrophy, and other eye conditions.

Role of the nurse

Isolation. When a child is admitted with either a tentative or a positive diagnosis of meningitis, he should be placed in isolation. Isolation is usually discontinued after 24 hours of treatment with chemotherapeutic agents and antibiotics. In isolation technique particular attention is given to the care of nasal and mouth secretions or discharges from the ears, since they are sources of infection. Also special care must be taken of the spinal fluid after a spinal puncture. The offending organism is in this fluid.

Rest. Every effort should be made to reduce stimuli and noise. The room should be quiet. Shades should be pulled down. Sudden movements should be avoided, and quietness should prevail. Paraldehyde or another sedative may be ordered for restlessness.

Care in convulsive seizures. See p. 494 for discussion of nursing care for convulsive seizures.

Assisting with a spinal puncture. See p. 301 for general discussion of assisting with a spinal puncture. It should be emphasized that the nurse is responsible for seeing that specimens (usually three) of spinal fluid are sent to appropriate laboratories: one specimen for direct smear and cell counting, one for bacterial culture, and one for determinations of protein, chloride, and sugar. The nurse should record on the nurses' notes the character of the spinal fluid (cloudy or clear) and the amount of pressure of the spinal fluid if that is measured.

Care of intravenous infusion. See p. 301 for nursing care with intravenous therapy.

Fluid intake and output. An accurate record should be maintained of oral fluids, intravenous fluids, and urine output. Often these patients suffer from retention of urine. At the height of the illness the child may be incontinent, or he may void in small amounts frequently.

Diet. When the infant or child can take an oral diet, fluids high in calories should be urged such as fruit juices, eggnogs, milk, and creamed soups. After the acute stage of the condition a diet as tolerated is given. In view of possible retention of urine it is especially important to urge fluids. In feeding the infant with meningitis it may cause him less pain to be left in bed than to be lifted and held in the nurse's arms. In that case the head of the bed could be temporarily elevated. The infant's back and spine pain him, especially when moved.

General hygiene. Bathing the child, turning him gently and slowly, and rendering special attention to the bony prominences are important if problems with pressure areas are to be avoided. Because movement causes pain, the nurse needs to handle the child carefully and avoid any sudden, abrupt motions. In changing diapers of an infant or taking his temperature, she should lift and move his legs as little as possible. If the patient is unable to close his eyes because of paralysis, the eyes need to be irrigated with sterile water or saline twice a day and covered. Yellow oxide of mercury may be ordered for use in the eyes.

Administering medication. Chemotherapeutic agents to be administered are selected in accordance with the particular organism causing the disease. Drugs in large doses are administered intravenously and/or intramuscularly. After the laboratory report of the organism found in the spinal fluid is available, the antibiotics may be changed.

Paraldehyde may be ordered for restlessness or convulsions, as may chloral hydrate, diazepam (Valium), or other sedative and/or anticonvulsive drugs.

Avoiding aspiration. The patient needs to be turned from one side to the other and not left on his back if aspiration of vomitus is to be avoided during the acute stage of the disease. Suction should be used as indicated.

Watching for complications. With adequate treatment the number of complications formerly associated with meningitis should be greatly reduced; however, subdural effusions may still be seen in the child who has either *Haemophilus influenzae* or pneumococcal meningitis. The nurse should be alert to symptoms of increased intracranial pressure such as tense or bulging fontanel, vomiting, lethargy or undue drowsiness, convulsions, and weakness or paralysis in any part of the body. Redness is sometimes seen over the fontanel.

As the older child begins to convalesce, special notation should be made of any motor weakness in an arm or leg, indistinct speech, retarded behavior, or anything unusual. Recording intake and output of fluids should be continued throughout his convalescence because these children often have retention, and if insufficient fluids are given, the urine becomes very concentrated.

Guillain-Barré syndrome (infectious polyneuritis)

The etiology of infectious polyneuritis is unknown, although a viral cause has been suspected by many researchers. The polyneuropathy is frequently preceded by an infection and is considered by many to be a toxic effect of the first infection. The cause of the infection can be found in some cases if a diligent search is made. Some of the diseases that have been associated with polyneuritis are diphtheria, mumps, influenza, measles, upper respiratory infections, infectious mononucleosis, and some enterovirus infections.

The disease involves the nervous system and manifests itself by causing varying degrees of motor and sensory disturbances. The clinical picture of this syndrome is variable but is usually characterized by acute ascending motor paralysis and cranial nerve involvement. Weak-

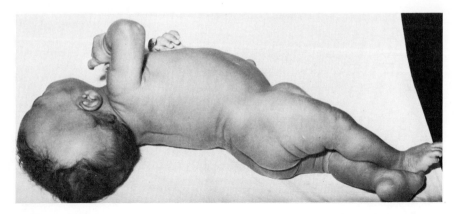

Fig. 18-8. Opisthotonus resulting from *Haemophilus influenzae* meningitis in a 5-month-old child.

ness in the lower extremities may be the first symptom. Paresthesia in the hands and feet is a common initial symptom. The paresis is usually ascending and frequently involves the intercostal nerves, thus causing varying degrees of respiratory paralysis. The paralysis is symmetrical. The third to the twelfth cranial nerves may be involved, with resultant facial weakness and impaired gag, swallow, and cough reflexes. Impaired sensation and loss of position sense are common sensory abnormalities found during neurological examination. Urinary retention and constipation may result due to weakness of the abdominal muscles.

Physiotherapy should be dealyed during the acute stage, except for proper positioning and passive full range-of-motion exercises. Cortico-

steroid therapy has been used early in the course of the disease with doubtful results.

Complete recovery without residua is the most common end result. The most common complication is pneumonia. Respiratory paralysis is the most dreaded hazard, which frequently requires constant artificial respiratory ventilation for weeks. The time necessary for complete recovery varies from 2 to 18 months.

The spinal fluid usually contains a markedly increased level of protein with a normal amount of white blood cells. The protein is slightly elevated during the first week, with a peak concentration in about 4 weeks.

Treatment is supportive. Good nutrition, adequate hydration, skillful nursing care, and prevention of contractures and deformities

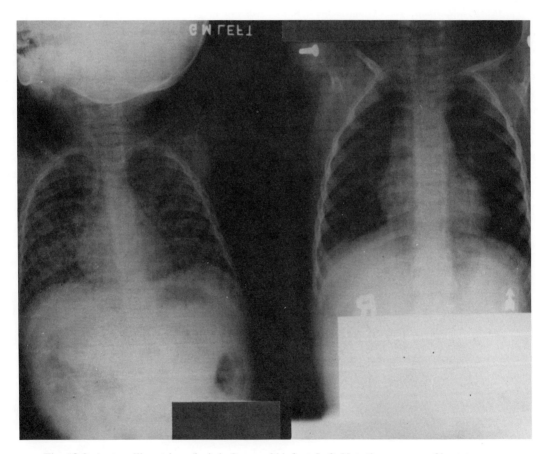

Fig. 18-9. Acute miliary tuberculosis in 2-year-old infant. Left: Note the presence of hematogenous dissemination in the lungs. Right: Same child after 1 year of therapy with streptomycin, isoniazid, and PAS.

are elements of a good supportive program. Tracheostomy and/or assisted ventilation may be lifesaving in the presence of respiratory embarrassment.

Tuberculosis

The mortality rate from tuberculosis is highest in infancy and adolescence, although tuberculosis is not among the first five leading causes of death in the age periods just mentioned. Its prevention is possible through measures that include avoiding contact with tubercle bacilli, drinking pasteurized milk, early identification of tuberculosis contacts, and development of artificial immunity by means of BCG or isoniazid given prophylactically to children exposed to tuberculosis contact. (For a discussion of BCG and the use of tuberculin tests refer to p. 186.)

Tuberculosis is caused by the bacillus *Mycobacterium tuberculosis*. Chronic illness, chronic fatigue, and malnutrition may be disposing causes. Although the disease can affect almost any tissue or organ of the body, the majority of these children have some form of intrathoracic tuberculosis. The incidence of tuberculosis of the central nervous system, genitourinary tract, or bones and joints is much lower.

When there is any indication that the child may have tuberculosis, a careful and complete medical examination is done because he may have tuberculosis of the lung or other parts of the body. As a preventive measure, isoniazid is given for 1 year to those who have converted to a positive skin test and to all young people who have positive tuberculin tests. Children under 3 years of age are especially susceptible, as are adolescents and young adults (Berenson, 1975).

The positive diagnosis of tuberculosis is made by (1) isolating the tubercle bacillus in sputum, cerebrospinal fluid, and discharges from other sources; (2) inoculating a guinea pig with the suspected material; and (3) culturing the lavaged contents of a fasting stomach. (Young children often swallow sputum.) X-ray studies of the lungs are helpful, although often difficult to interpret in childhood because tuberculosis lesions may be similar to lesions seen in other conditions such as histoplasmosis. Sedimentation rates, blood cell counts, general malaise, and an elevated temperature help to indicate if the tuberculosis infection is active.

Drugs used in the treatment of tuberculosis include isoniazid (INH), streptomycin, and para-aminosalicylic acid (PAS), ethambutol, kanamycin, and rifampin. INH and PAS are frequently given together.

The child should remain in bed during the active stage of the disease. It is specifically essential that the child receive adequate amounts of proteins, minerals, and vitamins. Large doses of vitamin C and vitamin B complex also are considered beneficial. Since the treatment of tuberculosis takes a long time, the psychological factors applicable in any illness requiring prolonged medical supervision play an important part in the child's recovery. (Refer to p. 465.)

Streptococcal infections

Streptococcal infections in children are due to beta-hemolytic streptococci. The beta-hemolytic streptococci produce many different clinical syndromes in children, such as acute pharyngitis, acute tonsillitis, scarlet fever, erysipelas, and impetigo. The streptococci pathogenic for humans are for the most part members of group A, of which there are approximately 50 serological types. Group A streptococci produce a number of substances that have a bearing on the type of illness that results. Two of the most common substances produced are erythrogenic toxin, which is responsible for the rash of scarlet fever, and streptolysin O and S hemolysins, which produce antistreptolysin O and S antibodies. The antistreptolysin O antibody laboratory test is widely used as an indicator of a recent streptococcal infection.

The clinical manifestations of streptococcal disease vary according to the portal of entry, the patient's age, and the immunological response. Streptococcal infection (streptococcosis) in infants under 6 months of age is characterized by a nasopharyngitis with a thin mucopurulent discharge and excoriations around the nose. The infant may have slight elevation in temperature at the onset. The nasal discharge and irritability may last 6 weeks. The illness may clinically resemble a common cold.

Streptococcal infection in a child 6 months to 3 years of age will usually have an insidious onset of low-grade fever and mild nasopharyngitis. The anterior cervical lymph nodes become enlarged and tender. The nasal discharge becomes purulent, and the complications of sinusitis and otitis media are common. Culture of the nasopharynx will establish the presence of *Streptococcus.*

Children 3 to 12 years of age with a streptococcal infection will usually present with acute follicular tonsillitis or pharyngitis or scarlet fever. Streptococcal tonsillitis is scarlet fever without a rash. The diagnosis is established by nasopharyngeal culture.

Scarlet fever in a child is streptococcal tonsillitis with an erythematous rash. The rash results from an erythrogenic toxin–producing *Streptococcus.* The rash blanches on pressure, is pinhead in size, and gives the skin a rough, sandpaper-like texture. The rash of scarlet fever resembles a ''sunburn with goose pimples.'' The other clinical symptoms are high fever, vomiting, headache, chills, and malaise. The diagnosis is established by nasopharyngeal culture.

Treatment

Penicillin is the drug of choice for all types of streptococcal infections. Adequate penicillin dosage should be administered to maintain an adequate blood level for a minimum of 10 days to eradicate all of the streptococci from the site of infection, prevent septic complications, and reduce the incidence of rheumatic fever and acute glomerulonephretis. Bed rest, adequate fluid intake, and regular diet as tolerated are general supportive measures that are recommended. Aspirin and analgesics are given for fever and pain. Patients allergic to penicillin may be given erythromycin, the second drug of choice.

Prevention

Streptococcal infections can be prevented by the administration of penicillin *prior to exposure.* On only a rare occasion is the prophylactic use of penicillin indicated for the prevention of streptococcal disease. Prophylactic therapy may be indicated for (1) an obvious epidemic in a school or institution, (2) a previous history of rheumatic fever in any member of a family, (3) an intimate household exposure, and (4) an intercurrent illness in the exposed person. Patients allergic to penicillin may be treated with erythromycin.

Impetigo

The nurse may see a child with impetigo in the home or even in the school. It is associated with poor hygienic conditions, and it is more common in children under 10 years of age than in older ones. It is hoped that the nurse will not see impetigo in a newborn nursery.

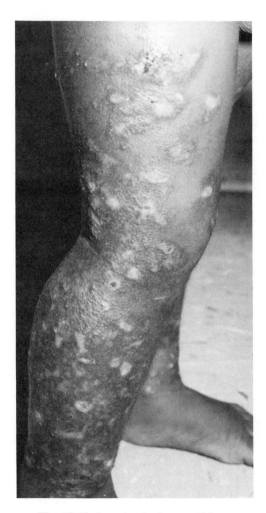

Fig. 18-10. Impetigo in 3-year-old boy.

Impetigo affects the superficial layers of the skin. Presence of vesicles and crusts with an area of redness around them is typical. The vesicles become seropurulent, and pustules form. Various strains of *Staphylococcus* and *Streptococcus* are the responsible organisms. A child can get impetigo from contact with a person who is an asymptomatic carrier of staphylococci and streptococci from a person who has lesions. Skin abrasions serve as a portal of entry. The anterior nares is the major location where a large colonization can be found.

Preventive measures are essential. The importance of personal hygiene and cleanliness in general should be part of school health instruction. That each member of the family should have his own towel and washcloth may need to be stressed. Personnel responsible for caring for infants and young children in a hospital or in any institution should be free from infections of any kind. In some hospitals nasal cultures are made of personnel caring for newborn infants. Infants have less resistance than others, even young children.

In infants, impetigo may be called pemphigus neonatorum or bullous impetigo. Lesions are most commonly first seen in diaper areas of the infants. If the nurse sees any lesions, she should be on the lookout for other signs of infection such as diarrhea or an elevated temperature. Septicemia could follow. It is easy for the lesions to become secondarily infected if not treated quickly and adequately.

The infant in the hospital or institution with this skin condition should be isolated at once. At home this is not practical, but if an infant at home has this condition, other children should be told not to handle him; adults should carefully wash their hands after caring for him. A young child or older child with this disease should sleep by himself and, of course, have his own towel and washcloth.

Intramuscular administration of penicillin (long-acting benzathine penicillin G [Bicillin]) is the drug of choice for the treatment of impetigo. The skin of infected infants should be washed thoroughly with hexachlorophene solution several times daily. Because of the danger of inducing sensitivity by applying an antibiotic drug topically, the drug used in topical ointments should be one that is rarely used systemically, such as neomycin or bacitracin. Topical ointments mentioned are not dependable in the treatment of impetigo.

Infectious hepatitis (epidemic hepatitis, viral hepatitis)

Infectious hepatitis is caused by a virus that has been very difficult to isolate in tissue cultures and animals. This disease is the most common cause of jaundice in children after infancy. Recent findings demonstrate that jaundice occurs in the minority of cases.

It appears that man is the only susceptible host to this virus. Humans acquire the disease by ingesting food and water contaminated with feces containing the infectious hepatitis virus. Serum hepatitis virus is passed from one individual to another by way of parenteral injections. Serum hepatitis and infectious hepatitis produce a similar disease.

The clinical manifestations vary greatly. It is a milder disease in children than in adults. Jaundice, the major manifestation, may be very mild to completely inapparent. In the more severe cases anorexia, fever, nausea, vomiting, and abdominal pain may be present. The liver frequently becomes enlarged and tender. In rare cases of hepatitis, it may be fulminating and result in cirrhosis or death in 1 to 2 weeks.

There is no specific laboratory test to establish the diagnosis of hepatitis. The peripheral blood count reveals a leukopenia during the preicteric phase. Bile may be detected in the urine, and the bowel movements become clay colored. The direct serum bilirubin and serum transaminase (S.G.O.T.) levels become markedly elevated.

Treatment

There is no specific treatment. Adequate diet and bed rest are recommended for a period of a few weeks. The diet should be nutritious, well balanced, and palatable and should contain supplemental vitamins. The length of restricted activity should be determined by the clinical response and liver function test results.

Prognosis

Complete recovery without residua is the most common result. The majority of the children who develop the fulminant type of hepatitis will die during the first 10 days of the disease or develop chronic hepatitis or cirrhosis.

Infectious mononucleosis (glandular fever)

Infectious mononucleosis is an acute, mildly contagious disease presumably caused by a virus. The disease occurs most frequently in adolescents and adults but is not uncommon in children between the ages of 3 and 10 years. Experience has shown that patients with mononucleosis can be treated on an open ward without fear of cross-infection. Direct oral contact such as kissing is the most commonly accepted hypothesis to explain how the disease is transmitted.

The disease may begin abruptly or gradually with headache, chills, anorexia, fever, lymphadenopathy, and sore throat. The symptoms are usually mild in children as compared to adults. Hepatomegaly and splenomegaly are fairly common. Jaundice and abnormal liver function tests are signs of hepatic involvement. An erythematous maculopapular rash may occur during the course of the illness. Some of the children will have a prolonged fatiguing illness that may last for months. Rupture of the spleen, thrombocytopenia purpura, pericarditis, and myocarditis are some of the dreaded complications.

The diagnosis is usually made by the presence of an elevated heterophil antibody titer. The titers are lower in children than in adults. Atypical lymphocytes (Downey cells) in the peripheral blood are a characteristic finding during some stage of the disease.

Treatment is largely supportive. Bed rest is recommended initially, with gradual return to normal activity depending upon the patient's temperature and evidence of fatigue. Prolonged periods of decreased physical and social activity may be necessary before a state of normalcy returns. Patients with liver involvement may be given corticosteroids to improve liver function, but they should not be given in uncomplicated cases.

The prognosis is generally excellent. Severe cases of mononucleosis may have to be followed for months because of asthenia. Rarely does the disease produce neurological residua or rupture of the spleen.

PARASITIC INFESTATION

Although the hospital nurse does not see a child admitted primarily for treatment of a parasitic infection, she sees children admitted for another reason who are found to have such infections after admission. The public health nurse in home visits, the school nurse, and the hospital nurse in the pediatric and/or dermatology outpatient clinic are most likely to see children with parasitic infestations.

Oxyuriasis (pinworm)

Oxyuriasis (pinworm infestation) is very common, especially in children of preschool or school age. A child may exhibit a variety of symptoms such as picking the nose and other nervous habits, irritability, and itching of the anus. There may be inflammation of the vagina and perineum of little girls. The itching is worse at night. Eggs hatch in the intestinal tract and migrate to the anus. The diagnosis of pinworm is made by placing a bit of Scotch tape (sticky side down) against the anus before the child rises in the morning. The tape is then placed (sticky side down) on a glass slide. The slide is examined under a microscope by the physician.

Specific treatment for the condition includes the administration of piperazine citrate (Antepar) or pyrvinium pamoate (Povan) (Berenson, 1975).

The bed linen and clothing of the infected child should be boiled or put in the usual washing machine. Attention should be given to washing hands before eating and after defecating and to the use of clean underclothing and bed linen. In schools, toilet seats should be washed daily with a disinfectant. There should be adequate handwashing facilities. If one child in the family has pinworm infestation, other members of the family may be infected also. If there are any suggestive symptoms, others should also be examined for the presence of pinworms.

Ascaris lumbricoides (roundworm)

Sometimes roundworms cause no symptoms until the child vomits one or passes one in a stool; however, if the child is very infested, he may have abdominal pain, vomiting, restlessness, and disturbed sleep. The condition is most commonly seen in southern United States in preschool and elementary school children.

The eggs hatch in the intestinal canal, migrate by way of the lymphatic and circulatory system to the liver and lungs, ascend the bronchi, are swallowed, and go to the small intestine. Eggs from the female worm are passed from the body in feces; therefore, when there is inadequate sanitary disposal of feces, the soil is a source of infection. Proper sewage disposal and adequately constructed privies are important in preventing the condition. Children and adults should be taught to wash hands before eating and cooking and after defecation. Raw fruits and vegetables should be washed

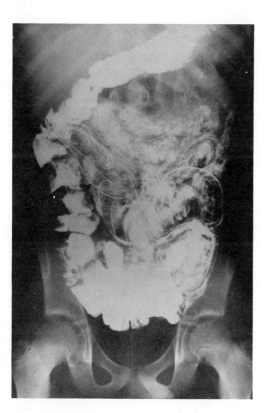

Fig. 18-11. Ascariasis in 5-year-old child. Note barium-filled adult ascaris in intestinal lumen.

before they are eaten. In treatment of ascariasis a piperazine derivative is used.

The public health nurse has a responsibility to try to determine the source of the infection. She can request the help of the sanitation department in the local board of health if necessary. Education of the child's family is her responsibility and must be given attention, or the child who is under treatment will continue to be reinfected. The hospital nurse has a responsibility in the education of parents and child in hygienic habits. In addition, she should refer the child and his family to the public health nurse for continued search for the source of infection. Also, the teaching done in the hospital needs to be reinforced.

Trichuris trichiura (whipworm)

Trichuriasis is an infection of the human intestinal tract caused by the nematode *Trichuris trichiura*. Whipworm is a cosmopolitan parasite, being most abundant in the warm, moist regions of the world. The parasites are whiplike in shape. The adult worms live in the cecum with their anterior portions buried in the mucosa. The female lays barrel-shaped eggs, which are passed in the stool every day. The eggs develop in moist warm soil over a 10-day period. After ingestion the infective eggs hatch in the upper duodenum and the larvae become attached to the villi of the intestines, where they continue to grow. At maturity the adult parasites leave the duodenum and pass down to their final habitat in the cecum. The site where the parasite is attached becomes inflamed and may become secondarily infected. This may lead to colitis, mucosal erosion, and rectal prolapse. Severe infections produce hypochromic microcytic anemia and moderate eosinophilia.

Many children have mild trichuriasis without clinical symptoms. Young children tend to acquire heavier infections and some of them experience nausea, irritability, sleeplessness, abdominal pain, protuberant abdomen, and edema of the legs. Diarrhea with bloody mucus may occur in severe infections. If the diarrhea is associated with tenesmus, rectal prolapse occurs eventually.

The diagnosis depends upon the recovery

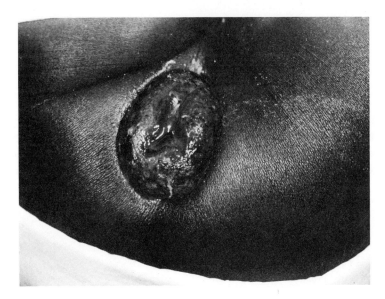

Fig. 18-12. Rectal prolapse due to severe trichuiriasis in 18-month-old child.

from the feces of characteristic double-shelled, bile-stained eggs.

Treatment is unsatisfactory. The drug of choice is Mebendazole. There are a few mild side effects of the drug. Complete eradication of the parasites is very difficult.

Prevention depends upon sanitary disposal of human feces, washing of the hands before eating, and sanitary toilet facilities. The maintenance of a safe water supply is also important.

Necator americanus (hookworm, uncinariasis)

A public health nurse's attention may be drawn to a child with hookworm disease, since he may look malnourished and anemic. This is due to the blood-sucking activity of the worm. A heavily infected child may develop a hypochromic microcytic anemia.

The diagnosis of hookworm disease is made by examination of the feces of the suspected person. If the child is infested, the eggs of the worms will be present in the feces.

Hookworm is particularly prevalent when there are sandy soil, warm weather, and inadequate disposal of human excreta. The eggs in the feces hatch and are on the ground. If children go barefooted in contaminated areas, they get the infection through penetration of the skin by the larvae. The larvae go to the

lungs and up to the throat, are swallowed, and descend to the small intestine. They attach themselves to the intestinal wall and produce eggs after several weeks.

A child who has this infection is treated with tetrachloroethylene or hexylresorcinol. The hospital nurse, whether on the unit or in the outpatient department, should refer the child and his family to a public health nurse.

Again, the source of infection should be found, and all members of the child's family should be examined; probably they too have the disease. Better personal hygiene, including wearing shoes, and education about soil contamination and sanitary privies are necessary if the child is not going to be reinfected.

Pediculosis

Pediculosis is infestation of people by lice (pediculi). The eggs are called nits. Pediculosis of the head is caused by *Pediculus capitis;* that of the body by *Pediculus corporis;* and that of the pubis, by *Pediculus pubis.*

The nurse may see a child with this condition in school, in the hospital, or in a summer camp. Contact with an infected person or his belongings is a source of infection. If one person in the family has it, the chances are that all of them do. A common symptom of pediculosus capitis is a repeated scratching of the head.

The scalp can become very irritated. When the hair is inspected for pediculi, it should be parted and examined, then again parted about an inch from the first part, etc., until the head has been thoroughly examined. The nit, or egg, adheres close to the hair, whereas the pediculi move. The condition is embarrassing to children.

Treatment with gamma benzene hexachloride (lindane), 1% dusting powder or 1% shampoo (Kwell), is effective. After a shampoo, an adult should inspect the hair of the affected child. The shampoo may need to be repeated several times before the hair is free of all nits and live pediculi. If the eyelids are infected, the use of an ophthalmological ointment containing 0.25% physostigmine (eserine ointment) is curative.

When the nurse visits a home to give treatment to an infected child, she should observe other members of the household for pediculosis and treat them also or the child will become reinfected. School children should be kept out of school until they are free of lice. The nurse has the opportunity of teaching personal hygiene and the need of changing personal clothing and bedclothes often.

FUNGUS INFECTIONS
Histoplasmosis

Histoplasmosis is a disease caused by a fungus, the *Histoplasma capsulatum,* which grows as a mold in soil and as a yeast in animal and human hosts. The source of infection is in soils with a high organic content (as in old chicken houses).

There are several forms of histoplasmosis: (1) the asymptomatic benign infection, (2) the acute progressive disseminated form, and (3) the symptomatic benign infection. The diagnosis is made by laboratory tests and finding the fungus in sputum, exudates of ulcers, blood, or bone marrow. The disease is uncommon in the Rocky Mountains and most common in central United States. Adults and children are both affected.

The nurse may first become aware of this condition if it is hospital routine to have children on admission tested for histoplasmosis as well as for tuberculosis. The test can indicate that the child has had contact with the organism producing the disease. Just as when a child exhibits a positive tuberculin test he is carefully examined for evidence of disease, so he is if the test for histoplasmosis is positive.

Case finding, as in tuberculosis, is essential. Other members of the household should be examined if a child has a positive histoplasmin test because they are likely to have been infected by virtue of being in the same environment.

Symptoms of this disease are variable: fever, anemia, failure to gain weight, hepatosplenomegaly, ulceration of skin or mucous membranes, purpuric manifestations, and atypical pneumonitis.

Medications used in treating the condition include amphotericin B and triple sulfonamide suspension.

The child is not isolated, but care should be taken of discharges from skin lesions and sputum. Because the primary lesion of histoplasmosis is in the lung, it is essential to differentiate whether the child has tuberculosis or histoplasmosis if there is evidence of a disease process.

Ringworm

Ringworm is a mycotic infection. It may affect the scalp (tinea capitis), the body (tinea corporis), or the nails (tinea unguium).

Tinea capitis (ringworm of the scalp)

Ringworm of the scalp can come from infected animals such as dogs, cats, and cattle, or the reservoir of infection can be man. The condition is more prevalent in children than adults. The affected area on the head may begin as a pimple but spread and cause hair to become brittle, lose its lustre, and break off. Baldness (alopecia) may occur. As long as there are lesions present, the disease is communicable.

The diagnosis of ringworm is made by microscopic examination of the hair or skin scrapings. To identify the species, culture is necessary. In addition to this, Wood's light is often used for diagnostic purposes. Under the light the affected hair will fluoresce if the infection is due to a species of *Microsporum;* however, the hair will not fluoresce if the infection is due to *Trichophyton mentagrophytes* or less common species.

The head of the child should not be shaved. The hair should be clipped, and the head should be washed daily. Ointments containing salicylanilide, copper undecylenate, or similar compounds are used in treatment. Griseofulvin given orally is recommended. Topical antifungal medications such as Whitfield's ointment may be used concurrently (Berenson, 1975).

Culture and microscopic examination are done to ascertain if the child is cured. The use of Wood's light is not always reliable.

In trying to find the source of infection, animal pets should be examined. Parents should be told that the child can get ringworm from contact with an infected person. Caps, hats, and scarfs should not be used interchangeably between children.

Tinea corporis
(ringworm of the body)

Ringworm of the body usually causes flat, round-shaped lesions. All age groups are susceptible. The source of the infection is the skin lesions of infected people or animals. Contaminated articles (for example, towels) are also a source of infection.

The child with ringworm should have the lesions washed thoroughly before using ointments prescribed by the physician. Whitfield's ointment or any ointment containing salicylic acid may be ordered. Vioform ointment is sometimes used. Griseofulvin may be given orally in addition to an effective topical fungicide (Berenson, 1975).

In prevention of this condition the school nurse who is active in the school health program may inquire about general housekeeping measures utilized in showers and dressing rooms. Also, there should be an investigation of household pets. In addition, this child should be excluded from the swimming pool and gymnasium. This is true of children having any type of ringworm because the condition is communicable.

Tinea pedis (ringworm of the foot, athlete's foot)

Tinea pedis is seen more frequently in the adolescent than in the small child. There are several infectious agents of mycotic origin. Children can get it from contaminated floors (as in a bathroom, shower, or area around a swimming pool), from direct contact with skin lesions of affected persons, or through indirect contact with personal belongings of the latter.

Characteristics of tinea pedis are scaling or peeling of the skin of the foot, especially between the toes, or the appearance of blisters containing thin watery fluid.

In treating this condition, topical fungicides are used. Griseofulvin is given orally in a severe or resistant case (Berenson, 1975). In summer the affected persons should be encouraged to wear sandals so the foot is exposed to the air. Daily bathing and careful drying between the toes are necessary in general personal hygiene. Socks and stockings should be changed daily.

In prevention of an outbreak in school the school nurse could see whether housecleaning measures used for showers, dressing rooms, and the like are adequate. No one with any skin infection should use the swimming pool or take gymnasium classes if he has to use the same school shower and dressing room as other children.

VENEREAL DISEASES
Gonorrhea

Gonorrhea is not frequently seen in young children, although it can cause a *vulvovaginitis*. Vulvovaginitis in children is more likely to be nonspecific in origin. Gonorrhea is seen in increasing frequency in the late-adolescent group of children. The newborn may get *ophthalmia neonatorum* from the birth canal of an infected mother in the process of birth. To prevent its development a 1% silver nitrate solution should be placed in the infant's eyes immediately after birth (Chapter 4).

The public health nurse should be alert to notice any edema, redness, or discharge from a young infant's eyes. Ophthalmia neonatorum occurs 24 to 72 hours after birth. The discharge may be serous or serosanguineous at first, later becoming purulent, thick, and profuse. Diagnosis is made by examination of a smear from the exudate. The condition is treated with penicillin.

The role of the nurse in reference to gonorrhea is more one of education and early case finding than the actual care of patients. The disease is treated with penicillin. If he is admitted to a hospital, the adolescent is on isolation for 24 hours after administration of the antibiotic. The patient admitted to the hospital is more likely to be one with salpingitis (inflammation of a uterine tube). Untreated gonorrhea can cause sterility.

The fact that gonorrhea is increasing among teenagers draws attention to the fact that every community needs to provide adequate supervised recreational activities for young people. Also, thought should be given to the question of whether the topic of gonorrhea and its prevention should not be included in school health instruction, along with other communicable diseases, preferably in junior high school.

When an adolescent is found with this condition, there should be an investigation of contacts of the patient if gonorrhea is going to be controlled, since it is spread by sexual intercourse. The infectious agent is the gonococcus. The incubation period is only 3 or 4 days.

Congenital syphilis

The nurse's role is not so much in giving care to infants with congenital syphilis, since it is now less prevalent than formerly, but rather in making sure that pregnant mothers are under medical supervision so they will have a blood test done. The fetus in utero can be affected through placental transfer by a mother who has syphilis. If syphilis in the mother is adequately treated before the fifth month of pregnancy, it is not very likely that the infant will have syphilis. The mother's blood often is tested both early and late in pregnancy, since the mother may have contracted syphilis after the first test was done. The presence of active syphilis in the mother can cause premature birth of the infant or cause the infant to be stillborn. If the blood test of the mother is positive, she is given penicillin.

Testing of the cord blood at birth is not a reliable diagnostic tool for ascertaining whether the infant has syphilis. Examinations of the placenta and x-ray films of the long bones will indicate something about the condition of the infant, but his blood can be tested by 6 months of age for a positive diagnosis.

If the infant does have congenital syphilis, there may be nothing unusual in his appearance during the first couple of weeks of his life. Characteristic manifestations for which to watch are constant snuffles, a maculopapular skin eruption, and fissures and cracking of the lips. Healing of fissures causes a scarring that is called rhagades—mucous patches on the hands and soles of the feet. Osteochondritis and periostitis sometimes occur. There may be a pseudoparalysis due to pain in the long bones.

Late manifestations of congenital syphilis are Hutchinson's teeth (notched teeth), saber shins (outward curving of the tibias), interstitial keratitis, eighth nerve deafness, and osteomyelitis. Neurosyphilis is the same as in an adult and can lead to mental deficiency.

A seropositive, asymptomatic newborn of a mother who did not receive treatment for syphilis during her pregnancy should be treated with penicillin G for 10 days. If the mother received adequate penicillin therapy during her pregnancy, the newborn usually is seropositive but does not require antibiotic therapy. The seropositive state will become negative during the first 6 months of life.

The school health nurse may have occasion to see the child with interstitial keratitis at the time that eye examinations are made. He should be referred for medical evaluation if there is any redness or inflammation of the eye. Sometimes the child complains of photophobia.

If the nurse cares for an infant with syphilitic infection, she should place the infant on isolation. It is best for her to wear gloves. The diapers of the infant should not be fastened with pins. Feeding is usually the greatest problem because of the infant's snuffles. A rubber bulk syringe may be used to suction out the mucus from the infant's nose before he is fed.

REFERENCES

Ahern, C.: I think I have V.D., Nurs. Clin. North Am. **8:**77, March, 1973.

Benenson, A., editor: Control of communicable diseases in man, ed. 11, New York, 1975, American Public Health Association.

Brooksaler, F. S., et al.: Cat scratch disease, Postgrad. Med. **36:**336, 1964.

Brown, W. J.: Acquired syphilis—drugs and blood test, Am. J. Nurs. **71:**713, April, 1971.

Dubay, E. C., and Grubb, R. D.: Infection: prevention and control, St. Louis, 1973, The C. V. Mosby Co.

Ellis, R., and Mitchell, R.: Disease in infancy and childhood, ed. 7, Baltimore, 1973, The Williams & Wilkins Co.

Krugman, S., Ward, R., and Katz, S. L.: Infectious diseases of children, ed. 6, St. Louis, 1977, The C. V. Mosby Co.

Larsen, G. I.: What every nurse should know about congenital syphilis, Nurs. Outlook **13:**52, March, 1965.

Lenz, P. E.: Women, the unwitting carriers of gonorrhea, Am. J. Nurs. **71:**716, April, 1971.

Monif, G.: Infectous diseases in obstetrics and gynecology, New York, 1974, Harper & Row, Publishers.

Mushlen, I., and Ambuson, J.: Tracking down tuberculosis, Am. J. Nurs. **65:**91, December, 1965.

O'Grady, R., and Dolan, T.: Whooping cough in infancy, Am. J. Nurs. **76:**114, January, 1976.

Top, F. H., and Wehrle, P. F., editors: Communicable and infectious diseases, ed. 8, St. Louis, 1976, The C. V. Mosby Co.

Woody, N., et al.: Congenital syphilis; a laid ghost walks, J. Pediatr. **64:**63, 1964.

19

Nursing care of
THE CHILD WITH MENTAL
RETARDATION

DEFINITION

Who is the mentally retarded child? He is the child who has subaverage intellectual functioning that has originated during the developmental period. He has difficulty in adjusting to everyday living needs. The retarded child's intelligence quotient (I.Q.), as measured by tests, is below 70. Children who have I.Q.'s between 70 and 85 are considered borderline.

The degree of retardation of a child may vary from mild to profound or very severe (Table 19-1). The majority of the retarded children fall into the classification of mild retardation. These are children whose development is slow but who are usually able to achieve academic learning to approximately the sixth grade. Also, they can attain, with guidance, both social and vocational skills that may enable them to be self-supporting. The *moderately retarded* child can learn to care for himself and can work in a sheltered environment. The *severely retarded* child may have poor motor development, is quite retarded in speech and language,

but can learn to communicate. He profits from habit training. Physical handicaps often accompany severe retardation. The *profoundly retarded* child needs constant care and supervision throughout the 24 hours. His physical coordination and sensory development are very impaired.

The terms *trainable* and *educable* are often used: trainable to denote a child capable of habit training, and educable to denote the child who has ability for some academic learning.

THE PROBLEM

Mental retardation is now recognized as both a major social problem and a major health problem. Six million people are affected in the United States, or approximately 3% of the general population; however, the figure of 3% of the population needs some analysis. The percentage of those affected varies with socioeconomic level of the population and the chronological age of the child. The number of children identified as mental retardates increases at 6 years of age, or the time of entry into school, and decreases after 16 years of age. In a segment of the population where the socioeconomic level is high, there may be less than 1% of mental retardates, yet in another segment of population where the socioeconomic standards are very low, there may be more than 7% of mental retardates.

The extent of the problem may be further seen when it is realized that only about 5% of the mentally retarded are institutionalized; others are living with relatives or with their own family. As stated previously, the greatest number of mental retardates (85%) fall into the

Table 19-1. Distribution of I.Q. ranges in mentally retarded individuals*

Description	I.Q.	
Mild retardation	55 to 70	85%
Moderate retardation	40 to 55	10%
Severe retardation	25 to 40	3%
Very severe retardation (profound)	0 to 25	2%

*From Report of Pediatric Subcommittee on Prevention and Etiology of Mental Retardation, Atlanta, 1965, Georgia Department of Public Health.

classification of mild retardation. To provide adequate habit training and academic and vocational guidance for these people places a heavy responsibility on every community within each state, on every state, and on the nation as a whole.

Further insight into the problem is gained when one understands that the cause of retardation of approximately three fourths of the mild and moderately retarded children is due to cultural and familial factors. The reproductive capacity of this group of mental retardates is usually normal, so that many of the offsprings from matings of this group will have subnormal intelligence. As a result of this, there may be many retarded children in a single family unless measures are taken to prevent conception. Furthermore, a child born into a deprived family environment has less chance of attaining his potential capacity. His health needs may not be met; later, a young woman is less likely to have proper prenatal care, and her child will be affected by her health. In turn, her child may not receive adequate care.

A final factor in the problem of the retardates is the economic burden to the tax payer. In one tax-supported institution for the mentally retarded, it cost $13.96 per child per day for

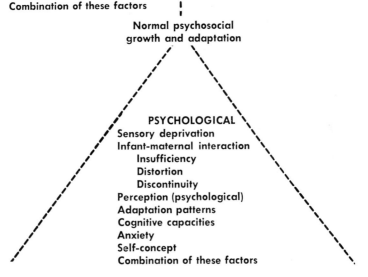

Fig. 19-1. Factors relative to the etiology of mental retardation. (Courtesy Georgia Department of Public Health; from Richmond, J. B., and Lastman, S. L.: J. Med. Educ. **29:**23, 1954.)

the fiscal year of 1969. In 1976 the cost had risen to $35.00 per day (in a multipurpose residential facility in the South). Multiply that figure by 1,000 children in one institution, and the economic problem may be better understood. Actually, in some institutions the cost per child per day is higher than this; in some it may be lower. Outside of institutions the government has put millions of dollars into various programs to aid the mentally retarded.

ETIOLOGICAL FACTORS

Biological, sociocultural, and psychological factors may affect the normal intellect (Fig. 19-1). They may operate singly or together, both in children without demonstrable brain damage and those with brain damage.

The exact cause of retardation of children in the group *without* demonstrable brain damage is unknown. Subnormal intellectual functioning may be the only manifestation, or the retardation could be associated with environmental deprivation or with emotional disturbance. The emotional disturbance may vary from a mild to a major personality disorder, such as childhood schizophrenia. The cultural-familial retardate is included in the classification of children without brain damage. In this instance, besides subnormal intellectual functioning, there is intellectual retardation of at least one parent and of one or more of the siblings. In addition, there is some cultural deprivation.

Table 19-2. Etiological factors in severe retardation*

A.	Autosomal chromosome aberrations (mainly mongolism)	20%
B.	Sex chromosome aberrations	2%
C.	Genetic disorders (phenylketonuria, galactosemia) cretins, amaurotics, some hydrocephalics, some microcephalics	10%
D.	Nongenetic microcephalics, cretins, hydrocephalics	10%
E.	Prenatal upsets in prematures, birth injuries, infectious disease, accidents, etc.	40%
F.	Other	18%

*From Report of Pediatric Subcommittee on Prevention and Etiology of Mental Retardation, Atlanta, 1965, Georgia Department of Public Health.

The mental retardation of the group of children *with* brain damage is due to causes that can be identified. It is worthwhile to note in Table 19-2, which depicts causes of severe retardation, that prenatal upsets in prematurity, birth injuries, infectious diseases, accidents, etc. rank highest; genetic factors such as Down's syndrome (mongolism) are second.

Identifiable causes of retardation
Genetic considerations

Possibly the commonest *chromosomal abnormality* that influences mental retardation is found in *Down's syndrome,* or *mongolism.* Children with this condition account for 10% of the inmates of an institution for the mentally retarded. Down's syndrome occurs in 1.5 per 1,000 births. There are three patterns of chromosome abnormality; the commonest is trisomy of chromosome 21, in which there are 47 chromosomes instead of the normal 46. This type is rarely familial and is more likely to occur in children born to older women. The translocation type of Down's syndrome is rare. It is characterized by an exchange of material between a number 21 chromosome and some other chromosome. The most frequent type of translocation in Down's syndrome patients is a condition in which one of the chromosomal pair 15 is joined to one of the pair 21. The translocation type is familial, and the affected child generally is of younger parents. Mosaicism in Down's syndrome is very rare. It is the result of an error in division of an early embryonic cell, leading to the coexistence in one individual of cells with different chromosome counts.

The cell most commonly used for study of the mitotic chromosomes is the small lymphocyte of peripheral blood. The lymphocytes are grown in a nutrient medium for 72 to 96 hours. Bone marrow and fibroblast tissue cultures may also be used.

Down's syndrome is a disorder of growth that affects many systems and organs of the body. The signs of the syndrome may be recognized at birth. A chromosomal analysis is used to confirm the clinical diagnosis. The face of the child with Down's syndrome simulates one of the Oriental race; hence the name *mongolism*

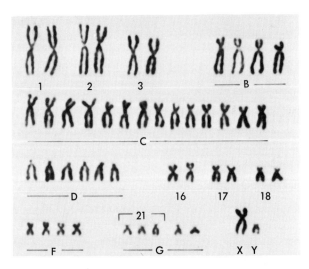

Fig. 19-2. Chromosomes of patient with Down's syndrome, trisomy 21. Note total count of 47 chromosomes due to the presence of an extra 21 chromosome. (Courtesy G. Rogers Byrd, Ph.D., Medical College of Georgia.)

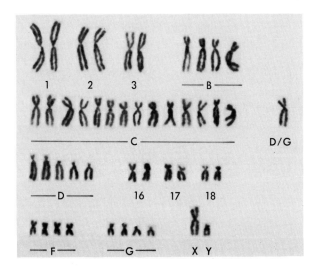

Fig. 19-3. Chromosomes of patient with the translocation type of Down's syndrome. Note the presence of compound 15/21 (D/G) chromosome. (Courtesy G. Rogers Byrd, Ph.D., Medical College of Georgia.)

was formerly given to this condition. The term *Down's syndrome* is more commonly used at present.

There is an oblique slanting of the eyes, with an epicanthic fold at the inner canthus. The iris may show white or light-colored spots (Brushfield spots) just within the margin of the iris. The bony orbits of the eye may be smaller than usual. The skull is flattened anteriorly and posteriorly. (The term *brachycephalic* is often used to describe the head of the child afflicted with Down's syndrome.) The tongue often protrudes and appears too large for the mouth. There may be deformities of the ears, especially the lobules. Since both the metacarpal bones and phalanges tend to be short, the hands and feet of the child are usually short and also broad. The fifth finger is frequently incurved.

There is a wide space between the first and second toes. In place of the usual creases in the palm there may be one prominent transverse line. There are skeletal abnormalities in pelvic bones as seen by x-ray examination. There are hypotonia and relaxation of muscles of the child. In general, the child's physical and motor development are delayed. His mental retardation may vary from mild to severe; occasionally there may be only borderline retardation.

The child with Down's syndrome usually functions at a much higher level in his home environment. The prognosis for good health and longevity is below normal because these children suffer more severely from the common childhood diseases.

Other abnormal conditions associated with Down's syndrome are congenital heart diseases and abnormality of the white blood cells. Leukemia occurs in this group with greater frequency than in the general population. Also, respiratory and fungal conditions are frequent.

Other conditions that may be due to genetic factors are *microcephalus* (a condition in which the brain is abnormally small) *craniosynostosis* (a condition in which there is premature closing of the cranial sutures), and *hydrocephalus* (a condition in which there is an excess amount of cerebrospinal fluid within the subarachnoid and ventricular spaces of the brain). Microcephalus, hydrocephalus, and craniosynostosis also may be acquired.

There is no treatment for microcephalus, but if hydrocephalus and craniosynostosis are diagnosed and treated early, brain damage may be avoided in some children. In both untreated hydrocephalus and craniosynostosis the brain lacks space to expand. These conditions are discussed elsewhere.

The final genetic factor to be considered here is the *metabolism* of the individual. Normal metabolic functioning is important for optimum growth and development. Hypothyroidism (cretinism) and inborn errors of metabolism are disorders that represent faulty metabolism and thus affect mental development of the individual. Congenital hypothyroidism may be due to iodine deficiency in the mother during pregnancy or due to impaired or absent function of the thyroid gland. If recognized and treated in early infancy, further retardation may be prevented. In general, the older the child is before the condition is identified, the greater the damage will be. The damage is not reversible.

Early signs of hypothyroidism include lethargy, drowsiness, constipation, and feeding

Table 19-3. Identifiable biochemical disorders often associated with mental retardation, characterized by elevated blood amino acids*

Disease	Amino acid accumulated in blood	Chief clinical features in patients with biochemical defect
Phenylketonuria	Phenylalanine	Mental retardation; convulsions; eczema; fair hair and skin
Maple-syrup urine disease	Valine; leucine; isoleucine	Mental retardation; spasticity; myoclonic seizures
Tyrosinosis	Tyrosine	Myasthenia gravis
Hyperprolinemia	Proline	Congenital genitourinary tract anomalies; renal disease; photogenic epilepsy; mental retardation
Hydroxyprolinemia	Hydroxyproline	Mental retardation; microscopic hematuria
Histidinemia	Histidine	Delayed speech development; mental retardation
Citrullinuria	Citrulline	Mental retardation; convulsions; vomiting
Hyperglycinemia	Glycine	Mental retardation ketosis after leucine ingestion; neutropenia, thrombocytopenia; hypogammaglobulinemia
Homocystinuria	Methionine (homocystine in urine)	Mental retardation; seizures; dislocated lenses; thromboembolic phenomena
Oasthouse urine disease	Valine; leucine; isoleucine; methionine; phenylalaine; tyrosine	Mental retardation; white hair; edema; unpleasant odor of urine

*From Report of Pediatric Subcommittee on Prevention and Etiology of Mental Retardation, Atlanta, 1965, Georgia Department of Public Health.

Table 19-4. Identifiable biochemical disorders often associated with mental retardation, characterized by increased urinary amino acid but little or no increase in blood concentration*

Disease	Chief clinical features	Amino acids in excess in urine
Hartnup disease	Mental retardation; ataxia; pellagra-like rash	"Neutral" amino acids, many
Joseph's syndrome	Infantile convulsions; increased cerebrospinal fluid protein	Proline; hydroxyproline; glycine
Argininosuccinicaciduria	Mental retardation; convulsions; friable hair; ataxia	Argininosuccinic acid
Cystathioninuria	Mental retardation; congenital anomalies; psychosis; pituitary disease	Cystathionine
Hypophosphatasia	Bone disease; low alkaline phosphatase	Phosphorylethanolamine
Glycinuria, with nephrolithiasis	Nephrolithiasis	Glycine
Galactosemia	Mental retardation; jaundice; cataracts	Many
Hepatolenticular degeneration	Cirrhosis; tremor	Many, especially cystine and threonine
Cystinosis	Vitamin D–resistant rickets; acidosis; dehydration; early death	All plasma amino acids

*From Report of Pediatric Subcommittee on Prevention and Etiology of Mental Retardation, Atlanta, 1965, Georgia Department of Public Health.

problems. The baby sucks or nurses poorly and may show a lack of interest in eating. Sometimes respiratory distress and choking are associated with his feedings. The tongue may be so large that it interferes with his swallowing. A weak, hoarse, and rather slow cry is frequently present, as well as an umbilical hernia and usually dry skin. The extremities are often cool to touch. There is a tendency toward prolonged jaundice in the neonatal period. Although heavy at birth, the infant fails to meet the expected growth in length at recurrent examinations. Manifestations seen later include continued delayed physical growth and development, absence of sweating, profound apathy, and sometimes a goiter. There is considerable apparent adipose tissue.

Laboratory studies on the infant immediately after birth are not valid since there may be maternal thyroid hormone still circulating in the infant's blood; however, by 2 to 6 weeks of age, blood thyroid studies as the serum concentration of protein-bound iodine (P.B.I.) and butanol-extractable iodine (B.E.I.) should reflect the infant's problem. Also, x-ray films of the foot and knee of the infant show retarded bone growth, even at birth. Desiccated thyroid U.S.P. is given throughout life.

Certain inborn errors of metabolism that can result in mental retardation are described in the following paragraphs: phenylketonuria, galactosemia, and cerebral lipoidosis.

Phenylkentonuria (PKU). Phenylpyruvic oligophrenia is an inborn error of metabolism manifested by an inability of the body to convert phenylalanine (an amino acid) to tryosine. High levels of phenylalanine can be detected in blood serum after an infant has received milk feedings for 24 hours. The clinical symptoms are mental retardation, seizures, and poor hair pigmentation. Early diagnosis and treatment appears to prevent some of the mental deficiency that would otherwise be expected if treatment is delayed. Routine testing of infants for elevated blood levels of phenyllalamine is carried out by most hospitals before discharge from the nursery. The test must be performed after the infant has had milk feedings for 2 or more days.

Treatment of the disorder is directed toward the restriction of the dietary intake of phenylalanine. A commercially available protein hydralysate (Lofenalac) from which phenylalanine has been removed is utilized. The child must be carefully monitored clinically and by phenylalanine blood levels to determine if child has a serum amino acid level between 4 and 10 mg. per 100 ml. Milk and other proteins may have to be used to supplement the Lofenalac formula if signs of amino acid deficiency develop while the child is on the restricted diet. With the patient maintained on a low-phenylalanine diet, seizures disappear and the electroencephalogram returns to normal. The effect of therapy on mental ability is not as clearcut. The hair color regains its natural color. The duration of treatment is controverisal; various centers are advocating terminating dietary restrictions between 4 and 15 years of age.

If the child is not treated, most infants will show signs of mental retardation before the age of 2 years. Unless the abnormality is suspected before 6 months, irreversible central nervous system damage may have occurred. Dietary control is in all probability useless after the age of 2 years.

Galactosemia. In galactosemia, which is an inborn error of carbohydrate metabolism, there is an inability to convert galactose to glucose, so there is an accumulation of galactose in the bloodstream. In addition to mental retardation, jaundice and cataracts frequently occur if dietary treatment is not begun early in infancy. Milk and milk products are omitted from the diet. The infant is placed on a specially prepared milk-free formula made from either casein hydrolysate or soybeans. Since galactose is derived from lactose (the principal carbohydrate of milk), milk and milk products are omitted from the diet.

Cerebral lipoidosis. The commonest disorder of lipid metabolism is cerebral lipoidosis (formerly called amaurotic familial idiocy).

There are several different kinds of cerebral lipoidosis, the best known being the infantile form, also called Tay-Sachs disease. Cerebral lipoidosis is characterized by different times of onset of the degenerative process. There is a lipid disturbance of the cells of the nervous system. It is seen especially in Jewish children and in children of parental consanguinity. The child may appear normal during the first months of life; then there is progressive deterioration. Motor skills are lost, and neurological disorders are seen. Spasticity, blindness, convulsions, and paralysis may occur. This represents another condition for which there is no treatment at present. Genetic counseling is of value to parents who know that this condition exists in a relative.

Perinatal factors

Health of mother. The health of the mother at the time of conception and throughout pregnancy has a bearing on the fetus (Table 2-1). Infections such as rubella and chronic diseases such as diabetes, hypertension, cardiovascular conditions, and chronic nephritis may affect the fetus adversely. Toxemia of the mother may cause anoxia of the fetus. Blood incompatibility of the mother and the fetus (Rh and ABO disease) may cause a high level of bilirubin, which in turn can produce brain damage (kernicterus). The infant may be born prematurely if laboratory results indicate that interruption of the pregnancy is necessary for survival of the fetus. The ingestion of certain drugs such as methotrexate may have a harmful effect on the fetus (p. 50). Excessive radiation is not without potential damage to the fetus. A final consideration is the nutritional status of the mother. Several studies have indicated that there may be a relationship between maternal malnutrition and mental retardation in the infant.

Mechanism of labor. In the mechanism of labor there are several possible causes of anoxia of the infant that could result in brain damage. Hemorrhage of the mother due to abnormal uterine implantation may result in anoxia to the fetus. Also, anoxia could be caused by several other factors such as premature separation of the placenta, prolapse of the umbilical cord prior to delivery, prolonged labor, cord knots and entanglements, breech deliveries, and abnormal presentation and other complications of the birth process. In addition, there may be brain trauma as a result of cephalopelvic disproportion.

Birth weight. If the mother is well and the infant is of average birth weight, the infant tends to grow and develop normally. On the other hand, the infants of low birth weight, especially those weighing less than 1,500 gm. (3 pounds 5 ounces) at birth, have a greater number of developmental defects and disorders. The premature infant has many handicaps. He develops at a slower rate. He is more difficult to feed and more susceptible to infections. All of his body organs and tissues are immature and do not function as those of an infant weighing over 2,500 gm. (5½ pounds). He also has a tendency toward hypoglycemia and hemorrhage. There is even a greater need for careful delivery of the premature infant than the full-term infant, especially in view of his tendency to hemorrhage.

Postnatal causes

Severe maternal, nutritional, cultural, or socioeconomic deprivation may keep a child from attaining his potential. Head injuries, tumors, the ingestion of poisons, and infectious diseases like meningitis or encephalitis may also cause varying degrees of retardation. A rare encephalitic reaction to pertussis immunization could cause mental retardation and brain damage. An emotional disorder may prevent a child from functioning at the level of which he is really capable. By a similar process a child suffering from handicaps such as hearing, speech, neurological, or orthopedic defects cannot function at his optimum potential.

BROAD APPROACHES TO PROBLEM OF MENTAL RETARDATION

There is need of considerable education for parenthood, since in tax-supported hospitals many mothers come to be delivered without ever seeing a physician during pregnancy. In school the principles of nutrition and healthy living should be part of the curriculum. Some high schools have a class in family life education, but this may be too late. In the elementary school the preteenager and early teenager can be taught that a mother should go to a physician prior to marriage and all through pregnancy. In addition, means of family planning should be available to those parents who want it. Some parents may be desirous of genetic counseling.

The provision of increased facilities for prenatal and infant care is another approach. There should be careful evaluation and supervision of the high-risk mother (Table 2-1). Good obstetrical care aids in the prevention of prematurity and in the control of certain other conditions of the mother that may be potentially harmful to the infant. Increased availability of facilities should include provision for careful medical supervision of the infant, especially during the first year of life. Any deviations from normal growth and development can be noted. Neurological, orthopedic, and sensory difficulties might then be identified early. Guidance in nutrition and general care of infants

should be given as well as education in prevention of accidents. The need of the infant for mothering, for sensory stimulation, and for prompt relief from tensions in part of this teaching. Immunization (Table 9-3) is a necessary component of medical supervision of the infant for elimination of some communicable diseases that may have a sequela of brain damage. In some locations, before the newborn infant is discharged from hospital, tests are done for identifiable metabolic diseases, especially phenylketonuria. Early treatment of both galactosemia and phenylketonuria is mandatory to prevent brain damage.

A high quality of medical and nursing care of infants in all newborn nurseries gives the infant a better start toward good health. In addition, the premature infant in the nursery has need of careful medical and nursing care.

Head Start programs for preschool children may help to offset cultural disadvantages. In the school-age child an increased number of special classes are needed, especially for those who cannot achieve as the average child yet are capable of a certain amount of academic learning. Classes for retardates who are trainable but not educable help to enable them to realize their optimum potential. Vocational training and sheltered workshops at a later age may help some of the children toward gainful employment.

Antipoverty programs that better the housing and living conditions help to offset cultural-social disadvantages. Regional evaluation centers are needed for the retarded child and his family. These centers not only evaluate retarded children but help to give positive guidance to those families with retarded children.

Further research into the etiology of mental retardation, including inborn errors of metabolism and chromosomal and sex abnormalities, is a necessary requisite for a solution for one of today's most active health problems.

ROLE OF THE NURSE

The nurse contributes to the field of mental retardation through preventive health teaching, recognition and reporting of unusual signs and behaviors, counseling parents, guiding the retardate toward self-help and socialization, and caring for the child with a poor prognosis for life (as the child with cerebral lipoidosis or classical Hurler's syndrome).

Preventive health teaching

Medical supervision in pregnancy. Since factors in the prenatal period affect the mental development of the fetus, prevention of mental deficiency includes careful prenatal supervision. Factors influencing the growth and development of the fetus were discussed in Chapter 2. Specific to mental retardation are the effects of toxic substances such as certain drugs taken in pregnancy, excessive radiation during pregnancy, maternal infections, maternal malnutrition, any conditions interfering with the supply of oxygen to the fetus such as maternal hemorrhage, compression of the umbilical cord, excessive use of depressant drugs in labor and delivery, and trauma of the infant during the birth process.

Because the health of the expectant mother is so important to the health of the unborn child, junior as well as senior high school students should be taught the importance of medical supervision of the expectant mother throughout pregnancy and the perinatal period. The school nurse, in her role as a consultant to the health curriculum in school, is in a position to influence this teaching.

In her home visits the public health nurse should be alert to note the expectant mother and ascertain whether she is seeing a private physician or is attending a prenatal clinic. Of course, the expectant mother may attend clinic once, but her decision whether or not to return is influenced by the manner in which those at the clinic speak to her and take care of her. The nurse has the opportunity to guide the expectant mother in her general hygiene and nutritional habits. Of interest to the mother also is how the fetus grows and develops in utero, and then finally what he is like at birth. In addition, the nurse can teach the mother danger signals in pregnancy, such as abdominal pain, bleeding, or visual disturbances, and to seek medical help immediately if any of these occur.

Prevention of accidents. All possible opportunities should be utilized by the nurse for teaching parents about the prevention of accidents that could lead to mental impairment, whether she be in institutional public health, private duty, or office nursing. Posters and/or drawings are helpful, in a hospital waiting room, doctor's office, school clinic, or pediatric clinic. Possibly a 15-minute talk on prevention of accidents in the infant and toddler period could be one of several planned educational ventures with a group of mothers in a child health conference. Such a talk might be given prior to the doctor's examination of the infants. Care needs to be taken that too much is not included in one session. Prevention of neurological damage by accidental ingestion of toxic substances could be one subject alone.

Ingestion of lead and insecticides can cause neurological damage as well as severe mental retardation. Ingestion of toxic substances is a danger at the time when the infant begins to crawl and when the toddler and young preschool child is busy investigating his environment. The chief source of lead poisoning is from old paint flaking off walls of houses. This is seen more commonly in blacks than whites and in families of low socioeconomic status. (See p. 445 for a discussion of the child with this condition.)

The chief offending insecticides and weed killers are those that contain arsenic plus those insecticides and rodenticides that contain thallium. The containers of these substances should be carefully tightened also in order to prevent easy access or loosening by little fingers. Parents need to read the labels of insecticides and rodenticides before buying them. There are many available that do not contain substances potentially dangerous to children. As children grow out of the toddler period, they should be taught the right use of any objects around the house.

Another topic of importance is the prevention of head injuries. In accidents the head is the most frequently injured part of the body. Although not every head injury is accompanied by brain damage, neurological impairment is always a serious threat, particularly at a time when the brain is developing.

Maintenance of a healthful environment should be a part of school health programs, as discussed earlier in the book. Safety education should be taught as part of health instruction.

Protection against specific diseases. Since pertussis and measles are sometimes followed by encephalopathy, preventive measures include protection against these dissases. Before parents leave the hospital with their new infant they should have information about protecting the infant from communicable diseases. Also, the nurse can utilize opportunities for teaching about immunizations in her home visits, in clinics, and anywhere she has contacts with parents.

At the time an infant is immunized, his mother should be told that, if the infant seems ill and has a prolonged temperature elevation, this should be reported to the family doctor or the child should be taken to a pediatric outpatient clinic in the emergency unit of a hospital. Encephalopathy, although rare, can occur as a result of immunizations, particularly that for pertussis.

Assessing development

It is important to assess the physical growth and development of the infant to see if there is significant deviation from the normal. As stated earlier, delayed growth and development often are associated with mental retardation. On the other hand, there may be abnormalities such as a head that is enlarging too rapidly, early closure of the anterior fontanel, or premature fusion of the cranial bones. Also, the nurse should bear in mind that impairment of any of the sensory organs influences the responsiveness of the infant.

Physical growth. In weighing the infant the nurse should note whether he has gained, lost, or remained stationary in weight. Has he grown in length since his last examination? Have teeth started to erupt? If so, how many are there?

Has the circumference of his head increased more than 1 cm. during each month? If it has increased as much as 2 cm., hydrocephalus may be developing. At 6 months the circumference of the chest and the head should be the same. Is the head of an infant who is 6 months old or older obviously larger than the chest? If the child has hydrocephalus, early surgical treatment is imperative if brain damage is to be avoided (p. 419).

On the other hand, is the head unusually small? The child with microcephalus has a small skull and brain. The nurse should notice, too, the shape of the infant's head. An odd-shaped head may be a clue to craniosynostosis (p. 383).

Responsiveness. Next, after measuring the height and the head circumference, inspecting the head, and weighing the child, the nurse should note as she handles the infant whether his body seems rigid, limp (hypotonia), or of normal tonus. At the same time the nurse can observe the alertness of the infant and how he responds to the stimuli of being weighed, measured, and handled. Does he seem either apathetic or unduly irritable, or does he seem to adapt himself to the ministrations and overtures of the nurse? (Of course, the nurse must remember that infants respond more favorably to a smiling face, gentleness, and a soft tone of voice than they do to sudden abrupt movements and a harsh commanding voice.) If an infant cries, is the sound weak or has it a good full quality? Does the older infant appear interested in his surroundings? Does he vocalize in any way except by crying? Can the toddler say single words, short sentences, or only expressive jargon? Does he understand a simple suggestion?

Motor development. The healthy infant is active when he is awake. Is this infant apathetic and quiet, does he move both arms and legs, or does one arm remain more less motionless? Are twitchings of any muscles noted?

The nurse should be thoroughly familiar with the milestones of motor development so that she can call the physician's attention to delayed development.

Sensory organs. The sensory organs are often involved in children with neurological impairment. The nurse can use a single article to see if the infant can focus on it and follow it with his eyes. She can shake a rattle behind the infant's back and see if he turns toward the sound of the noise. If the infant makes no kind of response, perhaps he does not hear it. This must be brought to the doctor's attention.

Mental ability. The nurse must remember that the infant's mental ability is judged largely on the basis of skills that are part of his motor, social, language, and physical development. Sensory impairment may influence the infant's development and keep him from obtaining abilities he might otherwise have shown.

In assessing the health of children over 1 year of age, in addition to observing the height, weight, and general development, the nurse should especially note the child's language development, his means of communication, and his ability to follow simple suggestions. The way in which he walks and handles objects gives a clue to his motor coordination. It is of value to know the child's grade placement in school. Most children begin school at 6 years of age so it is not hard to calculate what grade he should be in. The way in which the child is progressing in school is pertinent information.

Early recognition of untoward or unusual manifestations

The nurse, whatever the type of health service to children in which she is engaged, has a responsibility for calling the physician's attention to signs, symptoms, and behavior of infants and young children. Even though prevention of mental retardation is not possible in all instances, abnormalities cited early can either be verified or disapproved with careful medical attention and supervision. Some disorders such as hypothyroidism and phenylketonuria can be aided with treatment, but others such as Down's syndrome (mongolism) cannot. Referral of children with such conditions for expert evaluation followed by counseling of the parents should be done as early as possible in the best interest of the child and his future.

Observations of infants and young children can be made in newborn nurseries, home visits, pediatric clinics, or anywhere that health service is rendered to children.

There are certain manifestations to which a nurse caring for a *newborn* infant should be particularly alert, whether the infant is in the hospital or in the home. If the skin of the infant is even slightly yellow, this should be reported to a physician, or if at home, the infant should be referred to a physician. The nurse should not wait until deep jaundice is seen. Although jaundice could be due to several possible causes, it may be the first indication that the level of the infant's bilirubin is high. *Kernicterus,* a condition in which there is extreme neurological damage, may develop if the level of the total serum bilirubin rises above 20 mg. per milliliter. Kernicterus is a condition that is caused by blood incompatibility between the mother and the fetus (an Rh factor or an ABO incompatibility). Brain damage may include motor and mental retardation, disturbed hearing and speech, and involuntary movements. Exchange transfusions of whole blood are given, possibly several successive ones. In addition to showing jaundice the infant may be drowsy, apathetic, and little interested in nursing. Twitching or convulsions may be seen, and rigidity of the body may be felt as the nurse handles the infant. Head retraction, hypotonia, and weakness may be observed by the nursery nurse, or they could appear later. It is important for the nurse to know that jaundice develops prior to neurological damage.

Signs of *hypoglycemia* (an abnormally low level of blood glucose) may be present in infants born of diabetic mothers or toxemic mothers. Indications for which the nurse needs to watch include twitching, listlessness, drowsiness, limpness or hypotonicity, irritability, pallor, sweating, or convulsions.

The nurse may be called upon to collect urine specimens or assist the physician as he takes blood from the infant or young child to rule out certain identifiable inborn errors of metabolism (Tables 19-3 and 19-4). *Galactosemia* and *phenylketonuria* represent two metabolic conditions for which the newborn infant is tested in many hospitals before being discharged to go home; indeed, testing for phenylketonuria is mandatory in some states. These two conditions have been discussed earlier in this chapter, but emphasis is placed again on the fact that the earlier the treatment (dietary) is begun, the less will be the brain damage. The nurse has a responsibility for teaching the mother how to make the formula and later to help her with meal planning as the child grows older.

Hypothyroidism (cretinism) has been discussed earlier in this chapter, but emphasis here is placed on the need for recognition of early

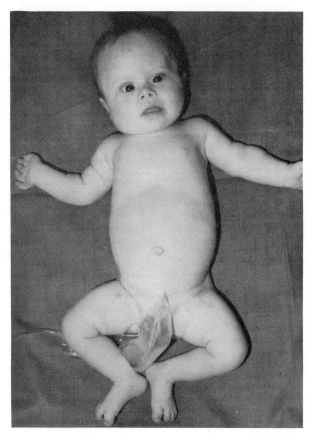

Fig. 19-4. Down's syndrome in 4-month-old girl. Note characteristic facies, protruding tongue, and protuberant abdomen.

symptoms that appear during the very early months of the infant's life, such as lethargy, feeding difficulties, a large tongue, constipation, a weak, rather slow cry, lack of linear growth, and cool, possibly mottled extremities. By the time typical symptoms of cretinism appear, such as adipose tissue, etc., brain damage has already taken place.

Other manifestations during infancy that may denote abnormal neurological pathology include weak sucking movements, lack of responsiveness, feeding difficulties, hyperirritability, seizures, peculiar odor of urine or body, spasticity, and failure to thrive and grow as evidenced by height and weight charts. Such infants should be referred to a physician for further evaluation.

Down's syndrome (mongolism). The nurse in the newborn nursery who sees an infant with Down's syndrome will not have any difficulty in recognizing that he is different from other infants because both his appearance and his behavior are suggestive of this condition. As was discussed earlier in the chapter, there is an oblique slanting of the eyes as in the Oriental population. The head is small, is brachycephalic, and has a flat occiput. An elongated tongue occasionally protrudes from the mouth. The face is broad with a nasal bridge that is flat. The ears often show absence of lobule or other deformities. In the eye the iris may show white or light-colored spots (Brushfield spots) just within the margin of the iris. The hands of the infant are short and broad with short or tapering fingers. The little or fifth finger of the hand is short and incurved. In place of the usual creases in the palm there may be one prominent transverse line. There may be a large space between the first and second toe. When holding him, the nurse may notice that the infant is usually relaxed and limp (hypotonic). Later, delayed physical and motor development is seen.

Counseling parents

The parents of the mentally retarded child may have the same feelings about their child as the parents of the child who has a congenital defect. Their child is "different" from others. They mourn the well infant who did not come, and it is difficult to accept this defective infant. Indeed, parents may deny the existence of mental impairment and visit many different doctors before finally acknowledging to themselves that their child is not the same as others. They may have feelings of guilt and shame. Everything that was said about parents' attitudes toward children with congenital defects is true about parents of retardates p. 338).

The nurse needs to be on the lookout for clues as to the parents' relationship to the child. What are their feelings toward him? Do they accept and love him in spite of his handicap, or do they reject him? If parents are rejecting the child, he usually knows it by the way that he is handled. He learns this through his sensitivity to touch and sometimes from facial expressions and tone of voice. It takes real fortitude for parents to see that the child is different from others and yet acknowledge that the child is part of them and belongs to them.

If the parents seek help from the nurse, she should first urge them to take their child to a private physician, a pediatric clinic, or a community mental health center for a thorough examination of his condition. The physician may refer the child to an evaluation center for children who are mentally retarded. There the child has psychological tests and a physical examination that includes hearing and vision. A social service worker interviews the parents and the child and usually visits the home. A plan for the child's care is the outcome of several experts' evaluation of the child. If institutionalization is recommended, parents must be told that there is a long waiting list of children to be admitted and that preference will be given in accordance with the needs of the child. Many times this requires interpretation to the parents.

It may be hard for the parents to decide whether or not they wish institutionalization for their child, and they may approach many people about it, including the public health nurse. The nurse can be of help to parents by discussing with them the advantages and disadvantages of institutional placement. If the young child is placed in an institution, he may suffer from environmental deprivation and so be judged more subnormal than he really is, since some of the best institutions are overcrowded and understaffed. A young child needs individual protection and mothering. He needs companionship, play materials, experiences, and stimulation to help him develop his potential. The subnormal child has the same psychological needs as the well child: warmth of affection, a feeling of belongingness, and a chance for achievement and recognition. The nurse can interpret to the parents the use of facilities within a community if the child remains at home—special classes, day care center, etc. The nurse can discuss, too, whether the mother can care for the child or whether he will need more specialized attention, such as the child with seizures and spasticity. If the child has a degenerative condition, like cerebral lipoidosis, in which he gradually regresses and loses achievement abilities, it is possible the parents may wish to keep him at home until he becomes so handicapped that they cannot give him the physical care he needs. If the child is hyperactive and unpredictable in his behavior, the parents need to consider whether they can give him enough supervision to avoid having the child hurt himself or others.

The effect of the subnormal child on siblings needs discussion. Is the care of the subnormal child so great that other children will be deprived of mothering and supervision? On the other hand, other siblings may have the opportunity of learning attitudes of protection, sympathy, and helpfulness toward the subnormal child. If the child is institutionalized, the parents and the siblings still know that there is one member of the family different from them, whether he is with or away from the others. Visiting the child in an institution may be very trying for the whole family.

The parents need to be given time to make up

their minds about what they wish to do for the child. If the nurse pressures them for a decision, they may withdraw from her and/or the doctor. Rapport between the nurse and the parents should be such that the latter feel free to express feelings of hostility, warmth, or ambivalence toward team members at the evaluation center. The nurse should not be critical or pass judgment on the parents but, instead, try to gently guide them toward acceptance of the experts' decision for the child's care. Perhaps the family wish to care for the child while he is small and later consider institutionalization.

At all times the nurse must remember that it is the parents' responsibility and prerogative to decide whether to follow the physician's recommendation or not. The nurse must not inject her own feelings about the child and about placement into the situation.

Guiding the retardate toward self-help and socialization

Whether the nurse is in contact with the child at home, in a general hospital, in an institution for mentally subnormal children, or in a community health center, she needs to understand the goals toward which guidance of the subnormal child is directed. Primarily these involve helping each child to his optimum potential, whether that be in activities of daily living, attendance at an appropriate school, or in a sheltered workshop. In an institution the nurse either teaches the child directly or shows aides how to teach the child in activities of daily living. In the home and the community health center she works with the mother and sometimes with school personnel. Often the nurse is the liaison between the home and the school. The nurse, in whatever situation she may be, needs to know the results of any testing of the child, as well as any recommendations made by a private physician or by the experts in an evaluation center.

For practical purposes the nurse working with these children needs to know the mental age of the child in order to assess his abilities more easily and know what to expect from him. For example, a child may be 10 years old but actually function at the level of a 4-year-old.

Also, the nurse needs to know what to expect of the well or normal 4-year-old child in order to handle such a subnormal child's needs successfully.

The nurse also needs to interpret to the parent the capabilities of the child in a realistic manner. If adults have too low or too high an expectation of his behavior, the child can be emotionally distressed and frustrated.

The child who is trainable or educable is taught activities of daily living: dressing, washing, eating, control of elimination, combing hair, using play material, etc. If the child at home is taught these things, his care is less burdensome to his mother and to his family. The child himself feels a certain joy of accomplishment rather than a growing sense of unworthiness. The same principles of learning (repetition, satisfaction, readiness) influence the subnormal child as a normal child; likewise, other factors in learning are relative to the physical state of the child (health, fatigue, illness, mental capacity, past experiences, amount of practice, motivation, and state of maturation). Curiosity and hope of social approval provide the strongest motives for learning. The methods of learning of the subnormal child are much the same as those of the normal child, only the subnormal child takes longer to learn. Further research in methods of learning of subnormal children is needed. Association and example, particularly example, are common methods of learning; names of objects are learned by association. Developing a sense of trust in people is essential. The washing of hands is learned partly by seeing the example of siblings and parents, partly by doing it, and partly by positive adaptation ("Johnny, rub your soapy hands together"). Whether the child repeats the performance and finally takes care of it himself depends on the satisfaction he has obtained from doing it. Was the water warm and pleasant? Was it fun to let his fingers pat the water and have them play with each other? Was he praised for his efforts? Did others smile at him afterward?

In guiding the child's learning experience the adult finds that certain principles must be remembered. The child's attention must be gained before he is given directions. The directions should be given by one adult at a time and with simplicity, explicitness, and care. There must be consistency in the way the task is performed each time. The child must be given time enough to do the particular task, and then he must be kept up to a standard of accomplishment.

The adult teaching the child must be patient and calm. A tearful or domineering mother has a negative effect in a learning situation. The same can be said for the domineering nurse or teacher. Important considerations for the adult in teaching the child problem solving are when to enter the situation and what type of help to give. Since success stimulates further efforts and failure means dissatisfaction and unwillingness to attempt to solve the problem, the adult should give some help if necessary rather than allow complete failure. If the child is having difficulty with buttoning a coat, the nurse might give encouragement by saying, "You have almost gotten it." If the child still has trouble, she could give explicit directions like, "Push the button into the hole." If still unable to do it, she could do part of the task for him, such as holding the buttonhole widely so the button can easily go through it.

Progress in learning must be from the simple to the complex. The child with a mental age of 3 years but a chronological age of 6 to 7 years can pull on his own shoes, but the adult needs to place the right shoe on the right side and the left on the left side. In eating, this same child can drink from a cup himself if the cup is straight sided and has no handle. Until smooth motor coordination has been achieved, it may be easier for the child to have finger foods so he can pick up food with his hands. Also, a spoon is easier for the child to use than a fork in order to get food into his mouth. Serving food in a bowl rather than on a plate makes it easier for the child to get food on the spoon.

As the child matures, motor coordination improves, but the nurse must remember that the rate of development is slow. When the retarded child seems to understand what a toilet is for and is able to walk by himself, then plans for toilet training should proceed just as for a normal child. (See p. 207 for a discussion of toilet

habits.) The nurse should remember that a normal child throughout his second year is kept dry only by an adult's taking him to the toilet and that he is 3 years old before he himself begins to voice his needs and take responsibility for dryness. By 4 years of age the child should be able to keep a dry bed at night. Again, the nurse needs to know the mental age of the child, since that is her guide of what she can expect.

The emotional and social growth of the subnormal child are equally as important as learning specific skills and the activities of daily living. The child's social adjustment is going to be important to him in terms of being accepted in a special class for the retarded in school, and ultimately his social adjustment will influence his ability to hold a job. When a child is happy, there is less likelihood of his hitting and hurting other people.

When a child is still an infant, he needs to associate warmth, food, and physical comfort with adults; by association he will then learn friendliness toward them. It is more by nonverbal communication than by verbal communication that the infant or young child learns when others have real affection for him.

Discipline (teaching a child acceptable ways of behavior) is just as important to the subnormal child as to the well child. (Refer to p. 210 for a discussion of discipline.) The same principles apply here. First and foremost, let the child know that he is accepted and loved. Second, and of almost equal importance, have reasonable expectations of behavior. The young child is noisy and active and needs space in which to run and play. Unless he has suitable play materials, he may well get into mischief. Again, in selection of play materials, be sure to remember the child's mental age. He might be 4 years old chronologically but enjoy large wooden beads, since his mental age is possibly 1½ years.

Being reasonable includes understanding. The behavior of a child is not as good in the evening as it was in the morning because he is now tired. Have only a few things the children cannot do. Even a normal child cannot remember many rules. When it is necessary to say "Don't," also tell what he can do. "Don't throw blocks—build with blocks.'' Be consistent. What is wrong one day is wrong another, and what is right one day is right another. Minimize commands. Change a command into a statement when possible: ''It's time to have dinner now,'' rather than ''Come to dinner now''; and not ''Wash your hands,'' but ''It's time to wash your hands.'' Associate satisfaction with the right way of acting. A word of praise, a lollipop, or an ice cream cone as a reward helps sometimes. Adequate rest both at night and in rest hour is important since rest contributes to emotional stability. If a child gets up irritable and cross in the morning, perhaps he should be put to bed earlier at night. Routines such as going to bed and washing hands need to be socialized; make them a pleasant game. If a behavior problem occurs, try to motivate the child more by associating greater satisfaction with desired behavior.

When the child with mental retardation is playing with siblings or other children, the play needs supervision so that he will learn to share and take turns with others. Also, supervision is needed to see that the children do not hurt each other. For the adult supervising play, again, the mental age of the subnormal child needs to be understood. The child who is only 2 years old mentally is not ready to share. He is aware of what another child is doing, but he is not ready to play with another child. The 2-year-old does not have the ability to understand what sharing is. Subnormal children with a mental age of 2 years should have duplicate toys and not be expected to share them with each other.

In planning a play period in any institution the nurse should remember that normal children under 6 years of age are not ready for group games. The normal preschool and kindergarten child still has more individual than group play, although the nature of the play material (blocks, dolls, and doll equipment) may be conducive to more than one child playing with it at the time. This is desirable in encouraging social behavior.

Music, singing, short stories, or picture books may be used together when the children are in a group. Clapping hands to music or using some single instrument, such as bells to keep time with, is enjoyable and helpful to the children.

It is through play together that learning to share, take turns, and participate takes place. Recreation is a valuable tool to use in teaching social development. Also, the way that adults act toward each other and toward the child is meaningful in terms of his learning the right way to behave.

Behavioral modification program. Bijou (1968) has discussed behavior modification programs used by teacher, nurse, parents, social workers, and psychologists in some detail in a volume of the *Pediatric Clinics of North America* devoted to mental retardation. Through a carefully considered plan it is hoped that a retarded child's behavior will be more acceptable. Particular problem areas of behavior include toilet training, self-destructive behavior, feeding behavior, and speech development. A behavior modification program is the application of behavior principles in teaching the child.

There are three main characteristics of such a program: (1) a behavioral objective, (2) contingencies to be used (events or objects that the child likes), and (3) specification of the starting point and steps that will help the child to attain the desired behavior (objective). The contingencies are for desired behavior and are withheld when undesirable responses are shown. The contingencies used have to be selected for a particular child. What is pleasing to one child may not be to another.

In general, the goal in guidance is to help the child in social adjustment, to teach him to care for himself, and to give him academic learning in accordance with his capability. Of course, the profoundly retarded child needs 24-hour care. Again, how much the child can do is dependent upon the extent of his mental capacity plus any physical handicap. Communication is considered a part of social adjustment. The child whom the nurse sees in the public school system is usually the mild or moderately retarded child. Even so, if his social adjustment is poor, he may be excluded from school.

Caring for the child with a poor prognosis

When working with retarded children, the nurse has contact with some who have conditions that are characterized by degenerative processes. The problems that these children present are unique. As newborn infants they may appear normal, but gradually they lose skills and abilities possessed at an early age. Their condition grows worse until they become bed patients, and from that status they deteriorate until death occurs.

The nurse has the responsibility for seeing that the parents have really understood what the doctor has told them about the child. The parents may reject what has been said by one doctor in the clinic and wish the child to be seen by another doctor. That is their privilege. The nurse's role is one of emotional support to the parents who have been told that their child cannot be helped and that his life-span is limited.

Because of the poor prognosis, parents may wish to have such a child remain with them while they are able to care for him. In some instances the child may appear normal and should be cared for as would a normal child until evidence of degenerative processes appears. The age varies with the disease. For example, in Hurler's syndrome evidence of deterioration appears within the first 3 to 4 years of life.

In order to make a valid plan of care for these patients, either in the home or in the hospital, the nurse has to note the abilities and problems of each individual child with such a disease and the ability of the mother to care for the child. The plan for care cannot indefinitely remain the same since the child's physical condition worsens, as well as his mental state. In a terminal stage of degenerative diseases, hospitalization or institutionalization is usually necessary since the care of the child at that point becomes too much for the parents. The child not only is bedridden but also has to be tube-fed and possibly suctioned. Careful skin care and frequent turning are essential. Prevention of respiratory infection is necessary. If convulsive seizures develop, anticonvulsive medications are prescribed. Anticonvulsive medications are continued daily. (Refer to p. 494 for care of a child in a convulsion.)

In the following paragraphs is a brief description of a few conditions in which the child grows progressively worse. It takes a nurse with unusual qualities to care for these children day after day: someone with patience, compassion, love of children, and a mature philosophy.

Niemann-Pick disease. Niemann-Pick disease is characterized by lipid degeneration of bodily organs, including the brain. It occurs chiefly among Jews, especially girls. It begins gradually in the first 6 months of life. The mother may first notice that the infant eats poorly. The infant loses weight and may become emaciated. Acquired motor achievements are lost. There is mental deterioration, and anemia, hepatomegaly, and splenomegaly develop. Sometimes there is brown discoloration of the skin. Blindness occurs late. The infant usually dies in the second year of life.

Tuberous sclerosis. Tuberous sclerosis is an inherited disorder in which there is mental retardation, convulsions, and cutaneous lesions. There are usually tumors of other organs as well as cardiac tumors. Motor defects are unusual, unless mental deficiency is severe. Around 4 years of age lesions of pink or yellow color appear over the bridge of the nose and part of the face. There is retarded physical development. Mental ability may vary from borderline to severe retardation.

In the mild form the child might live for a long time, but in the severe form the infant or young child may die of cardiac tumors or in later childhood die of a pulmonary infection.

The mucopolysaccharidoses. The mucopolysaccharidoses are autosomal recessive inherited disorders of mucopolysaccharide metabolism. Included in this category are six different disorders: (1) classical Hurler's syndrome, (2) Hunter's syndrome, (3) Sanfilippo syndrome, (4) Morquio's disease, (5) Scheie's syndrome, and (6) Maroteaux-Lamy syndrome. Former names to describe this group are gargoylism, lipochondrodystrophy, dysostosis multiplex, and Hurler's syndrome.

The intellectual ability is normal or only mildly impaired in Morquio's disease and in Scheie and Maroteaux-Lamy syndromes. It is the child with classical Hurler's syndrome (MPS-I), Hunter's syndrome (MPS-II), and the Sanfilippo syndrome (MS-III) whom the nurse is most likely to see in an institution for the mentally retarded. Eventually there is physical as well as mental deterioration, and the child becomes a bed patient.

The child with Hurler's syndrome may develop normally for a few months, then he begins to regress both mentally and physically. The head of the child is large, the bridge of the nose flat, the face somewhat coarse and ugly, and the expression apathetic. There is retinal degeneration. The neck is short and the thorax deformed. The child is short in stature. There is limitation of extensibility of joints. Orthopedic deformities such as talipes equinovarus occur often. The abdomen is prominent. Because of deposits of mucopolysaccharides, both the liver and spleen are enlarged. The fundamental defect of the child is due to an increased urinary excretion of chondroitin sulfate B and heparitin sulfate.

The urinary excretion in Hunter's syndrome (MPS-II) is the same as in classical Hurler's syndrome; however, mental deterioration progresses at a slower rate. The child has stiff joints, is dwarfed in appearance, and has hepatosplenomegaly. His facial appearance is suggestive of gargoylism. Hunter's syndrome does not occur as frequently as Hurler's syndrome, which is about 1 in 40,000 births.

The Sanfilippo syndrome is characterized as excretion of excessive amounts of heparitin sulfate in the urine. The intellect of the child may not deteriorate until school age. Eventually there is severe mental retardation. Dwarfing and stiffness in joints are less severe than in other types described.

The child with classical Hurler's syndrome has the shortest life; possibly he will not survive the first decade of life due to respiratory infection or cardiac failure.

Cerebral lipoidosis. Cerebral lipoidosis is discussed on p. 549.

SUMMARY

Mental retardation constitutes one of the major social and health problems today. Over three fourths of the children thus affected are mildly or moderately retarded. This places a responsibility on every community to provide appropriate services for them, such as special classes, day care centers, sheltered workshops, etc. Some of the retardation is due to demonstrable brain damage; some is not.

As more is learned about the needs of these children, the role of the nurse may change. In her present status, suggestions have been discussed that the nurse can contribute through health teaching (medical supervision in pregnancy and perinatal period, prevention of accidents, and protection against communicable diseases), careful assessment of a child's health status, referring to a physician infants or children with unusual manifestations, counseling parents, guiding the retardate toward self-help and socialization, and caring for the child with a poor prognosis.

REFERENCES

Anderson, M. L.: Care of the retarded child in the home, Nurs. Forum **6:**403, 1967.

Bernstein, N., editor: Diminished people: problems and care of the mentally retarded, Boston, 1970, Little, Brown & Co.

Bijou, S.: Behavior modification in the mentally retarded, Pediatr. Clin. North Am. **15:**969, 1968.

Buck, P.: The child who never grew, New York, 1950, The John Day Co.

Burr, A.: Learning to care for the mentally retarded children, Am. J. Nurs. **62:**1000, 1962.

Dingham, H.: Mental retardation: a demographic view, Pediatr. Clin. North Am. **15:**825, 1968.

Fackler, E.: The crisis of institutionalizing a retarded child, Am. J. Nurs. **68:**1508, 1968.

Grossman, H. J., editor: Symposium on mental retardation, Pediatr. Clin. North Am. **15:**819, 1968.

Hallas, C. H.: The care and training of the mentally subnormal, ed. 4, Baltimore, 1970, The Williams & Wilkins Co.

Kanner, L.: Parents' feelings about retarded children, Am. J. Ment. Defic. **57:**375, 1953.

Keogh, B., and Legeay, C.: Recoil from the diagnosis of mental retardation, Am. J. Nurs. **66:**778, 1966.

Logan, H.: Me and my shadow, Nurs. Outlook **14:**54, 1966.

Menkes, J.: In Textbook of childhood neurology, Philadelphia, 1974, Lea & Febiger, Chap. 1.

Milligan, G. E.: History of the American Association on Mental Deficiency, Am. J. Ment. Defic. **66:**375, November, 1961.

Milumsky, A.: The prevention of genetic disease and mental retardation, Philadelphia, 1975, W. B. Saunders Co.

O'Neal, J.: Siblings of the retarded, Children **12:**226, 1965.

Patterson, E. G., and Rowland, G. T.: Toward a theory of mental retardation nursing; an educational model, Am. J. Nurs. **70:**731, 1950.

Pounds, V. A.: The severely distressed subnormal child—admission and observation, Nurs. Times **64:**226, 1968.

Santostefano, S., and Stayton, S.: Training the preschool retarded child in focusing attention; a program for parents, Am. J. Orthopsychiatr. **37:**732, 1967.

Segal, A.: Some observations about mentally retarded adolescents, Children **14:**223, 1967.

Sloane, H. N., Jr., and MacAulay, B. D., editors: Operant procedures in remedial speech and language training, Boston, 1968, Houghton Mifflin Co.

Smith, D. W., et al.: The mental prognosis in hypothyroidism of infancy and childhood, Pediatrics **19:**1011, 1957.

Stone, N. D.: Family factors in willingness to place the mongoloid child, Am. J. Ment. Defic. **72:**16, 1967.

Thompson, T., and Grabonski, J., editors: Behavior modification of the mentally retarded, New York, 1972, Oxford University Press, Inc.

Van Nyk, J., and Arnold, M.: Early recognition of cretinism, Pediatrics **26:**732, 1960.

Watson, L.: Child behavior modifications: a manual for teacher, nurse, and parents, New York, 1973, Pergamon Press, Inc.

White, H.: Metabolic diseases. In Merritt, H. H., editor: Textbook of neurology, ed. 5, Philadelphia, 1973, Lea & Febiger.

Whitney, L. R.: Behavioral approaches to the nursing of the mentally retarded, Nurs. Clin. North Am. **1:**641, 1966.

Whitney, L. R., and Barnard, K. B.: Implications of operant learning theory for nursing care of the retarded child, Ment. Retard. **4:**26, 1966.

Appendix A: CHILD DEVELOPMENT

Behavior characteristics	Health problems*	Health needs
Neonatal period: birth to 28 days		
Active when awake; has random, uncoordinated movements	Postnatal asphyxia and atelectasis	Help in adjusting to extrauterine living
Vigorous cry	Immaturity	1. Warmth
Sucks well	Congenital malformations	2. Food
Lifts head momentarily when placed on abdomen	Birth injuries	3. Cleanliness (tub bath given after cord is off)
Can urinate and defecate	Ill-defined diseases peculiar to early infancy, including nutritional maladjustment	4. Relief from tension (Prolonged periods of crying are stressful.)
Sleeps in naps of 3 to 4 hours; wakes to be fed and/or have needs met, then returns to sleep		Careful and frequent observation
Lies in crib with thighs flexed on abdomen and arms bent upward at elbows with hands clenched in a fist		Protection against ophthalmia neonatorum
		Clean environment and free from infection
		Frequent change of position
		Sensory stimulation: movement, sound (as voice or music) and touch (being held closely, stroked, bathed, clothed, carried, etc.)
Infancy: 28 days to 11 months		
2 months	Influenza and pneumonia	Continued need of nurturing, relief from tension, warmth, food, sensory stimulation
Can focus eyes on object	Congenital malformations	Guidance of parents about nutrition of infant and introduction of only one new food at a time
Will return an adult's smile	Accidents	
3 months		Medical supervision to see if growing and developing normally
Eyes follow moving object		
Spontaneous smile		Protection against communicable diseases (may begin immunizations 4 to 6 weeks of age)
4 months		
Holds head erect and steady		
Plays with fingers; reaches with both hands for object with wavering approach; vocalizes, laughs; makes anticipatory adjustment to being lifted		Prompt attention to respiratory infections, any handicap or malformations, and any illness
5 months		Keeping infant away from crowds and people with infections
Cries at scolding voice		
Can turn over		Protection from inhalation or ingestion of objects that could cause obstruction or suffocation (infant mouths objects through 2 years.)
6 months		
Recognizes difference between strange and familiar people so may withdraw from strangers		Protection from other accidents: burns, drowning, falls, etc.
Active vocalization		Enlarging circle of acquaintances, but needs to have feeling of belonging to family
Reaches directly with one hand to grasp object		Learning to depend on other people than mother to meet needs
7 months		
Sits alone unsupported		Teething ring or equivalent to bite on when teeth are erupting

Adapted from Ilg, F. L., and Ames, L. B.: Child Behavior, New York, 1955, Harper & Brothers, Publishers, and Gesell, A., Ilg, F. L., and Ames, L. B.: Youth; the years ten to sixteen, New York, 1955, Harper & Brothers, Publishers.
*Health problems are based on mortality rates. Only the leading causes of mortality are listed.

Behavior characteristics	Health problems	Health needs
Infancy: 28 days to 11 months—cont'd		Encouragement of vocalization
9 months		Needs to be with others (children and adults)
Crawls or some form of locomotion; can pull self to feet		for socialization after 4 months
Plays peak-a-boo and waves hand		
10 months		
Uses thumb and finger in picking up objects		
May imitate simple syllables as "da-da"		
Toddler: 1 to 3 years	Accidents	Continued need of nurturing, affection, feeling
Says two or more words	Influenza and pneumonia	of belonging, sensory stimulation, relief
Walks with help	Congenital malformations	from tension, and guidance of parents about
Cooperates in dressing	Malignant neoplasms	nutrition
Follows suggestion as "Give it to me"		Chance for achievement and recognition
Friendly; loves an audience		Learning to be comfortable with adults other
Repeats performances laughed at		than immediate family for short periods of
15 months		time
Walks alone with feet wide apart		Continued protection against communicable
Wants to be very independent		diseases
Ceaselessly active; little or no inhibition; gets into everything; pokes fingers into holes, explores environment		Medical supervision; dental supervision and care by 3 years
May point to what he wants		Protection from being burned, drowned, or hit
18 months		by cars; protection from accidents resulting
Walks but balance unsteady; climbs		from child's lack of inhibition or judgment
Can build tower of two or three cubes		as swallowing poisonous substance or objects
Expressive jargon; small vocabulary; "No" chief word; understands much more than he can say		Opportunity for physical activity because of boundless energy of toddler
Seldom obeys verbal command, but attention can be easily diverted		Safe place to play—indoors and outdoors; play materials and supervision
Has quick temper and wants to have everything done immediately		Opportunities for independence
2 years		Learning self-care: eating, dressing, toileting, washing, and enjoyment of these activities
Parallel play; cannot share		Afternoon nap (Mother needs sleep when child
Imitates circular scribble		does, since child care is very fatiguing at
Puts two or more words together in a sentence; nouns predominate in vocabulary		this age.)
Knows 200 or more words; can name familiar objects in picture		Regular time for certain activities during day (dressing, bathing, eating, nap time, playing)
Can use language effectively to express needs		May begin toilet training at 18 months to 2 years in accord with child's development,
Can be warmly responsive; frustrated less easily		interest, and understanding
Climbs and runs more smoothly		Needs to hear good speech pattern from adults
2½ years		—not baby talk
Vigorous, energetic; ritualistic, rigid, inflexible: everything needs to be in its proper place and done in a certain way		
Preschool child: 3 to 4 years	Accidents	Continued need for:
3 years	Influenza and pneumonia	Affection, feeling of belonging, achievement, recognition
More mature; less need of being ritualistic	Congenital malformations	Medical, dental, and nutritional supervision
Increased ability to use language, vocabulary near 600 words	Malignant neoplasms	Protection against communicable diseases

Continued.

Behavior characteristics	Health problems	Health needs

Preschool child: 3 to 4 years—cont'd

3 years—cont'd

Beginning to share, but play is largely individualistic; enjoys housekeeping toys, doll equipment, blocks, etc.

Can stand on one foot momentarily, ride tricycle, draw a cross (+), walk with alternate feet up and down steps

Wishes to please adults

Feeds self well

Usually keeps dry in daytime (begins to take responsibility for this)

4 years

Aggressive (hits, kicks), defies authority; boastful, uses profane language, may tell tall tales

Can draw a man with head and legs; can skip

Keeps dry at night

Engages in play rather than playing games; preeminently a toy period with much imagination and imitation; enjoys activity for activity's sake

Plays in shifting loose group but more by self than with others

Asks questions for information

Childhood: 5 to 11 years

5 years

A time of equilibrium: friendly, calm, stable

Likes to be instructed and to get permission

Enjoys being near mother; proud of father

Skips, names colors, and can count ten objects correctly

Little or no infantile articulation

Uses all types of sentences; defines words in terms of use

Prefers companionship to solitary play

6 years

Emotions fluctuate to opposite extremes; cannot accept criticism, blame, or punishment well; demanding of others; aggressive

Enjoys activities which involve running and jumping; games of chase as tag

Tension seen by constant body activity

7 years

Somewhat withdrawn; may at times be moody, complaining and unhappy; tends to feel adults do not like him

Wants adult approval as well as peers

May shift blame to others

Employs speech to express thinking

Enjoyment still of games of chase, simple table games, and outdoor materials as jungle gym, slide, wheel toys as bicycle

---

Health problems (Childhood: 5 to 11 years):

Accidents: motor vehicles, drowning, fire

Malignant neoplasms (including leukemia)

Congenital malformations

Influenza and pneumonia

Health needs (Preschool child):

Protection against accidents

Play materials, play space, supervision in play

Learning about self-care (eating, dressing, toileting, washing)

Companionship of other children

Learning to express emotions in socially acceptable ways (should be given means and opportunity for self-expression)

Learning to accept authority even though it is in conflict with desires

Direct, simple, and truthful answers to questions (including origin of babies) in relation to their curiosity and ability to understand

Differentiation between fact and fiction (children often tell tall tales at this age)

Simple responsibilities

Health needs (Childhood: 5 to 11 years):

5 years

To facilitate adjustment in the first grade, 5-year-old should learn to:

Manage his own clothing

Play cooperatively with other children

Be able to express his ideas

Follow simple directions

Be happy with adults other than parent for short period of time

Know name, address, and telephone number

Know how to cross street with traffic light; know to ask help from policeman if necessary

Take full responsibility for toilet needs (including flushing toilet and washing hands)

5 to 11 years

Need of a few home rules for comfort and safety of entire family

Opportunity to talk about school experiences

Opportunity for role playing of school authority figures

Patience and sympathetic understanding for the aggressive 6-year-old child and moody, withdrawn 7-year-old child

Need of wholesome outlet for energy

Education in nutrition; safety (motor vehicle, water, fire)

Continued need for:

Behavior characteristics	Health problems	Health needs

Childhood: 5 to 11 years—cont'd

8 years

Exuberant and expansive; ready for anything

Interested in playmates and school activities

Interest in collecting objects as shells, rocks, etc.

Play interests about same as for 7-year-old

9 years

Tends to defy adult authority if it conflicts with his desires

Growing independence from parents; more interested in friends than family

Competitive in school; may fear failure; tends to worry

May complain of physical illness if dislikes particular task or school

Play interests about same as for 7-year-old

Enjoys reading

10 years

Usually straightforward; boundless energy; "the gang" or particular play group becoming increasingly inportant; more rules in games and sports; socially able to accept them

Girls tend to play with girls and boys with boys

Interested in perfecting skills such as bicycle riding, roller skating, swimming

"Smutty jokes" popular

Early adolescence: 11 to 14 years

11 years

Self-assertive; rebellious against parents; resists imposed tasks; critical of parents; may be rude to them; begins to see them as individual people; adjustment to school may be smoother than at home; best behavior away from home

Restless, intense, variable moods; likes to argue and talk

Height of interest in "gang," 10 to 15 years

Increased facility in mental and social activity

Boys interested in electricity and construction

Girls interested more in domestic science and housekeeping

Slumber parties popular

Health problems (8–10 years column): *(none listed)*

Health needs (8–10 years):

Affection, feeling of belonging, achievement, and recognition

Medical and dental supervision and care (permanent teeth start to erupt by 6 years)

Protection against communicable diseases

Protection against accidents (building code for schools should be enforced, environmental safety)

Play materials and play space; supervision of play up to 10 years to make sure children do not hurt themselves or each other

Peer age companionship

Learning to express emotions in acceptable way

Health problems (11 years):

Accidents: motor vehicles, drowning, fire

Malignant neoplasms (including leukemia)

Congenital malformations

Influenza and pneumonia

Health needs (11 years):

Opportunity for independence and responsibility as arranging room, spending allowance, participation in family plans

Information about body changes in both sexes during adolescence, reproduction, smoking, alcohol, venereal diseases

Motor activity for tensional outlets

Adequate sleep and some quiet activities that would be restful

Additional food for growth (especially protein and calories)

Role model of both father and mother

Continued need for:

Affection, feeling of belonging, achievement, and recognition

Medical and dental supervision and care

Protection against communicable diseases

Education for safety, nutrition, and general health

Continued.

Behavior characteristics	Health problems	Health needs

Early adolescence: 11 to 14 years—cont'd

12 years

More stable than 11-year-child; cheerful, sociable, more responsible, more companionable; more capable of organizing his energy than 11-year-old

Interest in sex, newspapers, magazines (wide range of variations in physical growth of boys and girls)

Still enjoyment of peer group of same sex; wishes to conform to values of peers as in dress

Interests broader than those of 11-year-old; desires adventure, excitement; interest in various forms of speech as reading, ghost stories, symbols, songs, codes, foreign language, "pig Latin," charades, guessing games

13 years

Self-absorption; has periods of musing and reverie

Tendency to worry; critical of self and others—sensitive to moods of others; may withdraw from family to room for further privacy; before going to sleep, often thinks about self

Interest in body image and changes; hence interest in personal appearance, clothing, hair, and general hygiene

Interest in schoolwork and school activities

Desires more independence and freedom

14 years

Feels more secure; new self-assurance; expresses self well in language; more congenial and outgoing

Relations with younger siblings better

Interested in people; increasingly aware of personality differences; gregarious; tireless communication with friends; very active on telephone

Interested in team games and group activities; may overplan activities

Still enjoys particular peer group of same sex but beginning to show interest in opposite sex

Concerned about body image and appearance

Hypercritical of parents but less tense relationship with them than at 13 years

Provisions for group experience with peer group of same sex, particularly from 10 to 15 years (camp, scout organization, Y.W.C.A., etc.)

13 years

Same needs as above

Sympathetic understanding and patience

Instruction in personal hygiene

14 years

Same needs as above

More specific information about boy-girl behavior, dating, etc.

Appendix B: NORMAL LABORATORY VALUES

HEMATOLOGICAL VALUES FOR INFANTS AND CHILDREN (FORMED ELEMENTS)

	Birth	12 weeks	6 months to 5 years	6 to 12 years
Hemoglobin (gm./100 ml.)	14.0-20.0	9.5-15.0	10.5-14.0	11.5-16.0
Hematocrit (vol. packed cells/100 ml.)	43-63	30-40	30-42	35-40
Reticulocytes (per 100 red blood cells)	4.5-5.0	1.0-2.0	1.0	1.0
Platelet count (per mm.^{3})	100,000-350,000	100,000-350,000	250,000-350,000	250,000-350,000
White blood cells (per mm.^{3})	9,000-28,000	6,000-18,000	6,000-14,000	4,500-13,000
Neutrophils (%)	40-80	30-40	45-50	55-60
Lymphocytes (%)	30-35	60-70	40-50	40-45
Eosinophils (%)	2	2	2	2
Monocytes (%)	6	5	5	5

HEMATOLOGICAL VALUES FOR INFANTS AND CHILDREN (BLOOD CHEMISTRY)

	Newborn	Child
Albumin (serum)	3.5-4.5 gm./100 ml.	3.5-4.5 gm./100 ml.
Alkaline phosphatase (serum or plasma)	10-15 Bodansky units	5-10 Bodansky units
Amylase (serum or plasma)	40-160 Somogyi units	40-160 Somogyi units
Bicarbonate (serum)	18-22 mEq./L.	22-26 mEq./L.
Bilirubin, direct (serum)	1-2 mg /100 ml.	Up to 0.4 mg./100 ml.
Bilirubin, total (serum)	1-10 mg./100 ml.	Up to 1 mg./100 ml.
Blood gases		
CO_2 content	24-28 mEq./L.	24-28 mEq./L.
pCO_2	36-44 mm. Hg	36-44 mm. Hg
O_2 content (arterial blood)	15-23 vol. %	15-23 vol. %
O_2 saturation (arterial blood)	96%-98%	96%-98%
pO_2	90-100 mm. Hg	90-100 mm. Hg
Calcium (serum)	4.5-5.5 mEq./L. or 9-11 mg./100 ml.	4.5-5.5 mEq./L. or 9-11 mg./100 ml.
Chloride (serum)	98-109 mEq./L.	98-109 Eq./L.
Cholesterol, total (serum or plasma)	17-59 mg./100 ml.	39-69 mg./100 ml.
Creatinine (serum)	0.5-1.2 mg./100 ml.	0.5-1.2 mg./100 ml.
Fibrinogen, (plasma)	0.2-0.4 gm./100 ml.	0.2-0.4 gm./100 ml.
Globulin (serum)	1.5-2.2 gm./100 ml.	1.9-2.2 gm./100 ml.
Glucose (serum)	20-80 mg./100 ml.	70-100 mg./100 ml.
17-Hydroxycorticosteroids (plasma)	10-15 μg./100 ml.	10-15 μg./100 ml.
Iodine, protein-bound (serum)	3.0-7.0 μg./100 ml.	4.0-8.0 μg./100 ml.

Continued.

HEMATOLOGICAL VALUES FOR INFANTS AND CHILDREN (BLOOD CHEMISTRY)—cont'd

	Newborn	Child
Iron, total (serum)	65-150 µg./100 ml.	65-175 µg./100 ml.
Iron-binding capacity (serum)	225-262 µg./100 ml.	215-475 µg./100 ml.
17-Ketosteroids, total (plasma)	25-125 µg./100 ml.	25-125 µg./100 ml.
Lactic acid (blood)	5-20 mg./100 ml.	5-20 mg./100 ml.
Lead (serum)	<0.06 mg./100 ml.	<0.06 mg./100 ml.
Lipids, total (serum)	550-700 mg./100 ml.	450-1,000 mg./100 ml.
Magnesium (serum)	1-2 mEq./L.	1-2 mEq./L.
pH (serum)	7-30-7.44	7.35-7.44
Phenylalanine (serum)	Up. to 2 mg./100 ml.	Up to 2 mg./100 ml.
Phospholipids (serum)	100-175 mg./100 ml.	150-250 mg./100 ml.
Phosphorus (serum)	1.45-2.8 mEq./L. or 2.5-4.8 mg./100 ml.	1.45-2.8 mEq./L. or 2.5-4.8 mg./100 ml.
Potassium (serum)	14.0-21.5 mg./100 ml. or 3.6-5.5 mEq./L.	16-20 mg./100 ml. or 4-5 mEq./L.
Protein total (serum)	5.5-7.0 gm./100 ml.	6.2-8.5 gm./100 ml.
SGOT (serum glutamic-oxaloacetic transaminase)	13-105 units	<40 units
Sodium (serum)	135-145 mEq./L.	135-145 mEq./L.
Triglycerides (serum)	30-135 mg./100 ml.	30-135 mg./100 ml.
Urea nitrogen (serum)	5-25 mg./100 ml.	9-15 mg./100 ml.
Uric acid (serum)	3.0-4.5 mg./100 ml.	3.0-4.5 mg./100 ml.

URINANALYSIS VALUES FOR INFANTS AND CHILDREN

	Newborn	Child
Specific gravity	1.007-1.020 units	1.007-1.030 units
pH	4.5-6.0	4.5-8.0
Protein	Trace	None
Glucose	None	None
Ketones	None	None
Microscopic examination (unspun)		
Red blood cells	0-2/hpf	0/hpf
White blood cells	0-3/hpf	2-4/hpf
Hyaline casts	2-3/hpf	1-2/hpf
Addis count		
Protein	<5 mg./12 hours	<10 mg./12 hours
Red blood cells	<250,000	<250,000
White blood cells	<500,000	<1,000,000

CEREBROSPINAL FLUID VALUES FOR CHILDREN

Total protein	15-45 mg./100 ml.
Sugar (glucose)	40-80 mg./100 ml.
Chlorides	120-132 mEq./L.
Cell count (lymphocytes only)	0-10/mm.^{3}
GOT (glutamic-oxaloacetic transaminase)	7-49 units
VDRL test	Nonreactive
Lactic dehydrogenase	15-71 units
Sodium	140-166 mEq./L.
Potassium	0.27-0.53 mEq./L.
Nonprotein nitrogen	8-20 mg./100 ml.

Appendix C: COMPOSITION OF FLUIDS USED FOR PARENTERAL THERAPY IN CHILDREN

	Calories/L.	Na (mEq./L.)	K (mEq./L.)	Cl (mEq./L.)	NCO_3 (mEq./L.)	Ca (mEq./L.)	P (mEq./L.)
Isotonic saline solution	0-200	154		154			
1/2 isotonic saline solution	100-200	77		77			
3% saline solution		500		500			
M/6 sodium lactate		167			167		
7.5% sodium bicarbonate solution		892			892		
Ringer's lactate	0-400	130	4	109	28	3	
Darrow's KNL solution		122	35	104	53		
Ordway's solution	140-400	26	27	53			
Amigen protein solution	345-515	30	15	22		5	30
50% glucose solution	2,000						
5% glucose solution	200						
Plasma (with acid citrate dextrose solution)		146	5	75	60		
Blood		95	4	50	40		2

Appendix D: HEALTH HISTORY AND IDENTIFICATION FORMS

```
                           Earl K. Long Hospital
                             Pediatric Clinic
   Name_____    EKL #:_____

   Date_____    WB #:_____
                              NURSE INTERVIEW
```

Age: Mos.	**SUMMARY OF FEEDING AND DEVELOPMENT**
Weight lbs. oz.; %tile	<u>Milk:</u> (Type of formula, dilution, amt. / 24 hrs.)
Height in. cm.; %tile	<u>Solid foods:</u> (Circle kind & amt. / 24 hrs.)
Head Circ. in. cm.; %tile	Cereals ( ) Fruits ( )
Hemoglobin gms. %	Vegetables ( ) Eggs ( ) Meats ( )
DDST Pass Fail (Circle)	Dinners ( ) Juices ( )
	Iron ( ) Vitamins ( )

DEVELOPMENT:

First tooth at	Sat alone at	Walked alone at
mos.	mos.	mos.
Talked at	Bowel control	Bladder control
mos.	mos.	mos.

Problems with baby:

_____

NURSE'S SIGNATURE

Description of abnormal physical examination findings:

CIRCLE IMMUNIZATION GIVEN:	
DPT #1	Trivalent #1
DPT #2	Trivalent #2
DPT #3	Trivalent #3
DPT B	Trivalent B
Measles Vaccine	Tine / TB-I
Smallpox Vaccine	

IMPRESSION:

RECOMMENDATIONS:

_____ M.D.

PHYSICIAN'S SIGNATURE

Admitted to the: EARL K. LONG HOSPITAL	□ Male □ Female	□ White □ Non-White	Birth / /	Time □ A.M. □ P.M.
Weight	Length	Chest Circ.	Head Circ.	Gestational Age
gms. lbs. ozs.	cm. in.	cm. in.	cm. in.	wks.

* Code Each Item as Follows: O—No Abnormalities X—Abnormality (Describe Abnormal Findings Objectively)	Code*	EXAMINATION DESCRIPTION OF ABNORMAL FINDINGS
1. GENERAL APPEARANCE (Maturity, Activity, Tone, Cry, Color, Nutrition, Edema)		
2. SKIN (Icterus, Rashes, Hematoma)		
3. HEAD, NECK (Molding, Caput, Craniotabes Cephalohematoma)		
4. EYES (Abnormalities, Conjunctiva, Red Reflex)		
5. EARS, NOSE & THROAT (Lips, Gums, Palate)		
6. THORAX (Including breast hypertrophy)		
7. LUNGS		
8. HEART (Including Femoral Pulse)		
9. ABDOMEN (Including Umbilicus)		
10. GENITALIA (Testes, Circumcision, Meatus, Discharge)		
11. ANUS		
12. TRUNK AND SPINE		
13. EXTREMITIES (Including Clavicles and Abduction of Hip Joints)		
14. REFLEXES (Moro, Grasp, Sucking, Swallowing)		

IMPRESSION:

Date:_____   _____ M.D.
                              Signature

EKLH 305 (R 10/69)
PHYSICIAN'S RECORD OF NEWBORN INFANT

EARL K. LONG MEMORIAL HOSPITAL
Baton Rouge, Louisiana

NEWBORN IDENTIFICATION

MOTHER—Name	Hospital No.	INFANT—Name		Hospital No.

I D E N T - A - B A N D		Infant's Birth Date	Time	Sex
Printed Number	Signature, Person Applying			

PRINTS		Color or Race	Weight	Length
Signature, Person Taking				

MOTHER'S RIGHT INDEX FINGERPRINT	INFANT'S LEFT FOOTPRINT (or palmprint)	INFANT'S RIGHT FOOTPRINT (or palmprint)

TO BE COMPLETED IN DELIVERY ROOM

Signatures, Persons Confirming Sex and Identification	Physician	Delivery Room Nurse	Nursery Nurse

UPON DISCHARGE - Affix Infant's Ident-A-Band below and have statement signed and witnessed.

Date _____

I CERTIFY that during the discharge procedure I received my baby, examined it and determined that it was mine. I checked the Ident-A-Band parts sealed on the baby and on me and found that they were identically numbered _____ and contained correct identifying information.

Signed _____

Witness   Mother

_____
Hospital Representative

Appendix E: SCHEDULE FOR WELL CHILD CONFERENCES*

	Physical examination	Immuni-zations	Developmental landmarks	Measurements	Discussion and guidance
First 3-5 days	Complete (at birth)		Can lift head momentarily when prone Flexes thighs on abdomen; lower arms bent upward at elbow Likes knee-chest position	Weight Height Head circumference PKU test	Concern for mother's and father's welfare† Diapering, cleaning of body, care of cord Crying: a sign of distress Need of affection: touching, rocking, holding Signs of hunger, feeding technique
6 weeks	Complete	DTP No. 1 Trivalent oral-polio	Lifts head off table when prone Eyes follow object to midline Smiles in response to adult smile	Hemoglobin Weight Height Head circumference	Explanation of immunization† Nutrition and feeding techniques Bathing, dressing Need for T.L.C. and relief from tension (crying)‡ Protecting from falls (crib sides up, etc.) Own bed Exploration of mother's feelings and her action when baby cries†
3 months		DTP No. 2 Trivalent oral polio	Lifts head off table 45 degrees Eyes following moving object Spontaneous smile	Hemoglobin Weight Height Head circumference	Review of nutrition and feeding technique Schedule to fit family Need of sensory stimulation Safe toys
6 months	Complete	DPT No. 3 Trivalent oral polio	Sits briefly leaning forward No head lag when pulled to sitting position Reaches for objects with either hand Transfers cube from one hand to other Active vocalization	Hemoglobin Weight Height Head circumference	Nutrition and clothing (review) Safety of toys, prevention of aspiration and/or small objects, protection from falls, in auto, bed, high chair Use of teething ring or rattle Play and exercise

*Earl K. Long Hospital Pediatric Department.

†This is explored each time baby is brought to well child conference or clinic.

‡Interpretation of and reminder of need of immunizations done at each visit.

Continued.

	Physical examination	Immuni-zations	Developmental landmarks	Measurements	Discussion and guidance
6 months—cont'd			Rolls from supine to prone position and vice versa		
9 months			Sits without support Has some form of locomotion Turns to voice Feeds self cracker Plays peek-a-boo Works for toy out of reach.	Hemoglobin Weight Height Head circum-ference	Nutrition and eating: sitting at table as family member; encouraging use of cup in daytime; eating with fingers Continued need for affection, sensory stimulation, relief from tension Play and exercise Safety: preventing aspiration or swallowing of small objects or poisons, preventing drowning and burns, care in auto
12 months		Time test Measles Smallpox	Says two or more words Responds to "Give it to me" Stands alone briefly Walks with one hand held or holding onto furniture Tries tower of two cubes Plays pat-a-cake.	Hemoglobin Weight Height Head circum-ference	Nutrition: use of table food and whole milk, encouraging use of cup as much as possible, use of spoon Toys and materials: safety and appropriateness Exercise: outdoors and indoors Setting limits to behavior Having own equipment and place for it: toys, crib, drawer, etc. Learning words through association Giving good speech pattern (not baby talk) Nap and sleep Avoiding temper tantrums, allowing child to be as independent as possible Review of characteristics, good clothing
15 months	Complete	DTP Trivalent oral polio	Stands alone, walks alone, toddles Points and vocalizes wants Six cubes into cup, takes tower of two cubes Four to six words	Hemoglobin Weight Height Head circum-ference	Nutrition: off bottle completely, decreased appetite Review prevention of accidents: safe place to play, poisons, falls, burns, drowning, aspirating or swallowing tiny objects Play and play toys Reemphasis of right speech pattern, learning words through association Encouraging increasing independence: eating,, dressing, playing Continuing to set limitations in behavior Toilet training

	Physical examination	Immuni- zations	Developmental landmarks	Measurements	Discussion and guidance

30 months	Complete	Rubella	Imitates circular scribble
			Feeds self fairly well
			Jumps, runs
			Helps undress self
			Names body parts
			Likes to be independent
			Helps with simple house-
			  hold tasks
			Joins two to three words
			  in short sentences
				Hemoglobin
				Stool (ova,
				  cysts,
				  parasites)
				Weight
				Height
				Head circum-
				  ference
					Dental referral
					Review prevention of acci-
					  dents: burns, drowning,
					  poisons, falls
					Encouraging independence
					Continuing to set limits
					  in behavior
					Toilet training
					Safe place to run and
					  play (danger of street)

INDEX

A

Abdomen
  of infant, examination of, 173
  of neonate, 61
Abdominal paracentesis, 476
Abduction test for unilateral dysplasia of hip, 343
ABO incompatibility, hemolytic disease caused by, 328
Abruptio placentae, 25
Abuse, child, 457-462
Abusive parents, 459-460
Accident victim, child as, 434-462
Accidents, prevention of
  to infant, 182
  to prevent mental retardation, 551-552
  of school-age child, 230
  to toddler and preschool child, 212-213
Acetaminophen
  after immunization, 186
  for nasopharyngitis and tonsillitis, 397
  to reduce temperature, 293
Acetazolamide
  for congestive heart failure, 489
  for minor seizures, 494
Acetylsalicylic acid for rheumatoid arthritis, 497
Achievement and recognition, 279
Achievement tests, 247-248
Acidosis, diabetic, 472
Acoustic blink reflex, 62
Acquired dyslexia, 259
Acrocephalosyndactyly, 386
Acrocyanosis, 55, 57-58
ACTH for leukemia, 506
Actinomycin D
  for brain tumor, 513
  for nephroblastoma, 514
  for neuroblastoma, 513
  for osteogenic sarcoma, 515
Active immunization and tuberculin testing of infants and
    children, 184
Acyanotic cardiac defects, 350-352
Addiction
  drug, 156
  to heroin, 156
  neonatal narcotic, 335
Addis count test, 312
Adenoidectomy, tonsillectomy and, 418-419
Adenoids, 96
Administration of pediatric unit, 279-280
Adolescence, 130-158; *see also* Adolescents
  accelerated growth during, 132-136
  calcification of cartilage in, 134-135
  changes in body conformation during, 132, 134

Adolescence—cont'd
  defining, 130-132
  early, summary of development in, 565-566
  identity realization in, 130
  muscular development in, 135-136
  physical development and leadership in, 137
  physical growth in, 132-137
  promotion of health in, 231-240
  psychological and social behavioral change in, 137-148
  skeletal development in, 134-135
  social interaction in, 141-144
  rejection in, 142-143
  reproductive organs in, 136
Adolescent girl, iron for, 223
Adolescent value systems, 144-145
Adolescents; *see also* Adolescence
  alienation of, 149-150
  behavior characteristics of, 234
  calcium absorption of, 235
  characteristics of, 149
  community resources for, 240
  conflict of, with society, 149-151
  deaths and death rates for, 231
  desirable characteristics of, 143
  eating and, 234-236
  education for family living of, 240
  emotional, social, and intellectual needs of, 236-238
  and father, relationship between, 148
  general hygiene of, 234-236
  group psychotherapy with, 156
  health of
    assessment of, 232-234
    guidance toward, 234-240
  help for, 156-157
  height and weight tables for, 133-134
  idealism of, 149
  intelligence tests for, 249
  modern, 149-157
  and mother, relationship between, 148
  nonprescription drugs used by, 153
  nurse and, 231
  nutrition instruction for, 239
  nutritional needs of, 234-235
  nutritional problems of, 235-236
  obesity in, 235-236
  parents and, 131
    problems of, 148-149
  personal hygiene of, 240
  physical examinations for, 238
  pregnant, 236, 238-239
  psychological assessment of, 271
  rebellion among, 150-151